Sobotta
Atlas of Human Anatomy

Volume 2 Trunk, Viscera, Lower Limb

Sobotta
Atlas of Human Anatomy

Edited by: R. Putz and R. Pabst
with assistance of Renate Putz

Volume 2 Trunk, Viscera, Lower Limb

13th English Edition
Nomenclature in English
21st German edition

755 colored figure tables
40 tables

Translated and edited by:

Andreas H. Weiglein, M.D.
Associate Professor
Institute of Anatomy
Medical School
Karl-Franzens-University Graz
Graz, Austria, Europe

LIPPINCOTT WILLIAMS & WILKINS
A **Wolters Kluwer** Company
Philadelphia • Baltimore • New York • London
Buenos Aires • Hong Kong • Sydney • Tokyo

Correspondence and criticism to:
Urban & Fischer, lecturer for medical students, Dr. D. Hennesseen, Karlstrasse 45, 80333 Munich

Editors:

Professor R. Putz, M.D., Chairman
Institute of Anatomy
Ludwig-Maximillian-University
Pettenkofferstrasse 11, 80336 Munich

Professor R. Pabst, M.D., Chairman
Department of Functional and Applied Anatomy
Medical School
Carl-Neuberg-Strasse 8, 30625 Hannover

The atlas consists of two separate volumes:

Vol. 1: Head, Neck, Upper Limb

Vol. 2: Trunk, Viscera, Lower Limb

Program Director:	Dorothea Hennessen, M.D.
Lecturer:	Alexander Gattnarzik
Production:	Renate Hausdorf
Graphics Design:	Carsten Tschirner, Munich
Cover Design:	prepress, Ulm
Cover Illustration:	Michael Budowick

German Library Cataloging-in-Publication Data

Sobotta, Johannes:
Atlas der Anatomie des Menschen/ Sobotta [Hrsg. Von R. Putz und R. Pabst unter Mitarb. Von Renate Putz]. - München: Jena: Urban und Fischer
  Further editions in non-European languages.- until 20th edition by Urban und Schwarzenberg, Munich, Vienna, Baltimore
  Engl. Edition titled: Sobotta, Johannes: Atlas of human anatomy. -
  French edition titled: Sobotta, Johannes: Atlas d'anatomie humaine. -
  Turkish edition titled: Insan anatomisi atlasi

Vol. 2 Trunk, Viscera, Lower Limb: 40 tables. - 21st revised edition - 2000
ISBN 3-437-41950-1

All rights reserved
21st edition January 2000
©2000 Urban & Fischer – Munich – Jena

ISBN 0-7817-3174-7
for the 13th English/English edition
© 2001 Lippincott Williams & Wilkins

00 01 02 03   5 4 3 2 1

This book including all its parts is protected by copyright. Every utilization outside the tight borders of the copyright law without permission from the copyright owner is illegal and liable to punishment. This is particularly true for reproduction, translation, microphotography and storage in electronic systems.

Setting: Typodata, Munich
(Set in type in 9 Point Corporate in Quark Xpress in Apple Macintosh)
Reproduction: Typodata, Munich
Printing and Binding: Appl, Wemding
(Printed on Nopacoat 115 g)
Printed in Germany

The founder of this atlas, Johannes Sobotta; M.D. †, was the former Professor of Anatomy and Director of the Anatomical Institute of the University of Bonn.

German Editions and year of publication:
1st Edition: 1904-1907 J.F. Lehmanns Verlag, Munich
2nd - 11th Editions: 1913-1944 J.F. Lehmanns Verlag, Munich
12th Edition: 1948 and following editions Urban & Schwarzenberg, Munich
13th Edition: 1953
14th Edition: 1956
15th Edition: 1957
16th Edition: 1967 (ISBN 3-541-02826-2)
17th Edition: 1972 (ISBN 3-541-02827-0)
18th Edition: 1982 (ISBN 3-541-02828-9)
19th Edition: 1988 (ISBN 3-541-02829-7)
20th Edition: 1993 (ISBN 3-541-17370-X)
21st Edition: 2000 (ISBN 3-437-41950-1)

Licensed Editions:
Arabic Edition
Modern Technical Center, Damascus

Chinese Edition
Ho-Chi Book Publishing, Taiwan

Croatian Edition
Naklada Slap, Jastrebarsko

Dutch Edition
Bohn Stafleu van Loghum, Houten

English Edition (English Nomenclature)
Atlas of Human Anatomy
Lippincott Williams & Wilkins

English Edition (English Nomenclature)
Atlas of Human Anatomy
Urban & Fischer

French Edition
Atlas d'Anatomie Humaine
Tec & Doc Lavoisier, Paris

Greek Edition (Greek Nomenclature)
Maria G. Parissianos, Athens

Greek Edition (Latin Nomenclature)
Maria G. Parissianos, Athens

Hungarian Edition
az ember anatómiájának atlasza
Semmelweis Kiadó

Indonesian Edition
Atlas Anatomi Manusia
Penerbit Buku Kedokteran EGC, Jakarta

Italian Edition
Atlante di Anatomia Umana
UTET, Torino

Japanese Edition
Igaku Shoin Ltd., Tokyo

Korean Edition
Panmun Book Company, Seoul

Polish Edition
Atlas anatomia cztowieka
Urban & Partner

Portuguese Edition (Portuguese Nomenclature)
Atlas de Anatomia Humana
Editora Guanbara Koogan, Rio de Janeiro

Portuguese Edition (Latin Nomenclature)
Atlas de Anatomia Humana
Editora Guanbara Koogan, Rio de Janeiro

Spanish Edition
Atlas de Anatomia Humana
Editrial Medica Panamericana, Buenos Aires/ Madrid

Turkish Edition
Insan Anatomisi Atlasi
Bera Basim Yayim Dagitim, Istanbul

Contents

Preface	VI
General Terms	VII
Instructions for colored figures	VII
Acknowledgements	VIII

Back — 1-47

Surface anatomy	1
Vertebral column	2-26
Muscles of back, suboccipital muscles, muscles of neck	27-40
Sections through vertebral column	41
Blood vessels and nerves of back and occiput	42-45
Blood vessels and nerves of vertebral canal	46-47

Thoracic and abdominal walls — 48-75

Surface anatomy	48
Ribs	49-50
Sternum	51-52
Thoracic cage	53
Breast, mammary gland	54-55
Blood vessels and nerves of thoracic and abdominal walls	56
Segmental sensory innervation	57
Muscles of thorax and abdomen	58-66
Inguinal ring	67
Diaphragm	68-70
Lumbosacral plexus	71
Anterior abdominal wall	72-73
Section through abdominal wall	74-75

Thorax — 76-131

Heart	76-91
Trachea	92-93
Lungs	94-102
Silhouette of heart	103
Projection of trachea, borders of lung and pleura	104-105
Esophagus	106-110
Thymus	111-113
Pleural cavity and mediastinum	114-115
Aorta	116-117
Posterior mediastinum	118-119
Autonomic division of nervous system	120-121
Sections through thorax	122-123

Abdominal and pelvic viscera — 132-261

Stomach	132-136
Small intestine	137-139
Colon	140-141
Liver, gallbladder, and biliary duct system	142-149
Pancreas	150-152
Spleen	153
Abdominal cavity, development	154-155
Position of abdominal viscera	156-167
Celiac trunk, superior and inferior mesenteric arteries and veins	168-177
Hepatic portal vein	178-179
Kidney	180-186
Suprarenal [adrenal] gland	187
Urinary bladder	187-188
Male urogenital system	189-193
Female urogenital system	194-204
Rectum	205-207
Renal artery	208
Blood vessels and nerves of retroperitoneal space	209-221
Pelvic diaphragm [floor]; male and female external genitalia	222-239
Sections through pelvis	240-261

Lower Limb — 262-388

Surface anatomy	262
Bones, joints, ligaments	263-307
Muscles of lower limb	308-347
Blood vessels and nerves	348-378
Sections through lower limb	379-386
Distribution of lumbosacral plexus	387-388

Supplement — 389-405

Index	389-405

Preface

After the excellent acceptance of the 20th edition of the Atlas, that was founded in 1903 by J. Sobotta, the editors and the publishers considered what could be improved in a standard book like this. From many letters and from many discussions with both students and colleagues it became obvious that the concept still fits into the "study landscape," due to the fact that gross anatomy—besides the other basic sciences—unquestionably is one of the pillars of medicine, particularly with a practical point of view. Although this atlas primarily focuses on the pre-clinical student, it—as a "book for a life as a physician"—nevertheless meets all requirements to accompany the student throughout the clinical years and also as a reference book for the later professional activity. Following the most important wishes of the users, the 21st edition presents a number of innovations:
In the new edition we have
- drawn 133 new figures based on original prosections, e.g. the serial sections of the brain and the thorax,
- replaced the black and white figures,
- updated the figures according to technical development, e.g. endoscopic views or X-rays,
- introduced diagrams on joint load,
- completely redone the diagrams on the muscles.

As a second important goal we improved the readability by:
- the introduction of signal colors for the chapters,
- a color code of the labels of topographical figures,
- consistent introduction of orientation sketches for slice direction and visual angle,
- revision and renewal of the well accepted tables,
- the introduction of small "wind roses" referring to adjacent figures in different directions and sections.

Of course, the new nomenclature (Terminologia Anatomica) valid since October 1998 has been used consistently. The glossary builds a bridge of understanding for those interested in the background of our terminology.

With the exception of discussion about general concepts and mutual correction, the editors have maintained the division for the revision of the chapters as follows:

R. Putz: general anatomy, upper limb, brain, eye, ear, back, lower limb;

R. Pabst: head, neck, thoracic and abdominal walls, thorax, abdomen, pelvis

For the large number of new figures the following medical illustrators deserve our acknowledgment: Mrs. Ulrike Brugger, Mr. Ruediger Himmelhan, Mrs. Sonja Klebe, and Mr. Horst Russ. It is owing to them that the familiar and successful "Sobotta style" has essentially been maintained. The electronic processing of photographs and the production of graphs have been accomplished by Mr. Michael Budowick. We also owe a debt of gratitude to our clinical colleagues, who again made several figures available for this edition (see acknowledgements). We also would like to thank the involved members of the institutes and departments for their insight and their suggestions. Mr. Dr. N. Sokolov and Mr. A. Buchhorn have done the delicate dissections to serve as the basis for many new illustrations; Mrs. S. Fryk and Mrs. G. Hoppmann supported us in text processing. The glossary was critically reviewed by Mr. cand. phil. T. Lederer.

The editors would also like to express their gratitude to the lecturers, particularly to Mrs. Dr. D. Hennessen and Mr. A. Gattnarzik, who despite some external turbulence helped us to consistently pursue the accomplishment of this new edition. In the beginning the production was assisted in the proved way by Mr. P. Mazzetti and later on by Mrs. R. Hausdorf with great effort. Mrs. Renate Putz was responsible for both the realization of the Nomina Anatomica and for the standardization of references and text. We would like to express our special thanks to all ladies and gentlemen who devoted themselves to the nerve-wracking job of the correction and the assembly of the index. It is only possible that the "SOBOTTA" now is published with lots of new contents and in new brilliance with the constructive collaboration of all people involved. We also wish to thank our families for their understanding for this time-consuming project.

Many innovations of this atlas are based upon the critiques and the suggestions of both students and colleagues. This is highly appreciated by the editors, and we would like to ask the users of this edition not to hesitate to send us their comments.

Munich and Hannover, September 1999
R. Putz and R. Pabst

General Terms

The following terms indicate opposite positions of organs and parts of the body, partially regardless of the position of the body, as well as the position and direction in the extremities. These terms are not only used in human anatomy, but also in practical medicine and comparative anatomy.

General terms

anterior-posterior = in front of-in back of (e.g. anterior and posterior tibial arteries)
ventral-dorsal = closer to the belly-closer to the back
superior-inferior = higher-lower (e.g. superior and inferior nasal conchae)
cranial-caudal = closer to the cranium-closer to the tail
internal-external = inward-outward
superficial-deep = close to the surface-in the depth
middle, intermediate = between two other structures (e.g. the middle nasal concha lies between the superior and inferior nasal conchae)
median = in the median plane (anterior median fissure of the spinal cord). A "median section" divides the body into two symmetrical parts.
medial-lateral = closer to the middle of the body, closer to the side of the body (e.g. medial and lateral inguinal fossae)

Terms for directions and positions in the extremities

proximal-distal = closer to the root of the extremity-closer to the end of the extremity (e.g. proximal and distal radio-ulnar joints)

for the upper limb:
radial-ulnar = on the side of the radius-on the side of the ulna (e.g. radial and ulnar arteries)

for the hand:
palmar [volar]-dorsal = on the palm of the hand-on the back of the hand (e.g. palmar aponeurosis, dorsal interossei)

for the lower limb:
tibial-fibular [peroneal] = on the side of the tibia-on the side of the fibula (e.g. anterior tibial artery)

for the foot:
plantar-dorsal = on the sole-on the dorsum of foot (e.g. lateral and medial plantar arteries, dorsalis pedis artery [dorsal artery of foot])

Instructions for colored figures

The multicolored figures of this book are based on didactic considerations: contrasts should be enhanced, structures that are difficult to distinguish should be more obvious. The colors used for different tissues (such as tendons, cartilage, bone, muscles) and pathways (such as arteries, veins, lymph vessels, nerves) differ from those in the living or dead body or the embalmed cadaver. Arteries are colored in red, veins in blue, nerves in yellow, lymph vessels and nodes generally in green.

In addition to the artists (K. Hajek, Professor E. Lepier, F. Bathe, H. von Eickstedt, K. Endtresser, J. Kosanke, J. von Marchtaler, J. Dimes, U. Brugger, N. Lechenbauer, I. Schnellbaecher, and K. Schuhmacher) that produced the base for the entire figure set together with Professor Sobotta and the later editors Professor Becher, Professor Ferner, and Professor Staubesand, the following artists worked for this present issue: Mrs. Ulrike Brugger, Mr. Ruediger Himmelhan, Mrs. Sonja Klebe, and Mr. Horst Russ. A series of original photographs were processed electronically by Mr. Michael Budowick. Some CT-scan diagrams were produced by Mrs. Henriette Rintelen.

The following figure numbers indicate both newly developed figures and new drawings due to main corrections:
U. Brugger
707, 923, 924, 927-932, 934, 936, 937, 1266, 1378
R. Himmelhan
1367, 1368, 1370, 1372, 1374, 1375
S. Klebe
1162, 1174, 1175, 1218, 1222, 1223, 1250, 1349
H. Russ
788, 798, 1281-1284, 1302-1304

Acknowledgements

The authors are greatly obliged to the following clinical colleagues for their contribution of ultrasound, computer-tomographic, and magnetic resonance images as well as endoscopic photographs and color photographs of surgical procedures:

Prof. Altaras, Center of Radiology, University of Giessen (Figs. 964, 979, 980)
Dr. Baumeister, Department of Radiology, University of Freiburg (Fig. 1095)
Prof. Daniel, Department of Cardiology, Hannover Medical School (Figs. 862–864, 935)
Prof. Galanski, Dr. Kirchhoff, Department of Diagnostic Radiology I, Hannover Medical School (Figs 924, 1144 a, b, 1154, 1155)
Prof. Galanski, Dr. Schäfer, Department of Diagnostic Radiology I, Hannover Medical School (Figs. 838 a, b, 888, 933, 958, 1139, 1147, 1150, 1152)
Prof. Gebel, Department of Gastro-enterology and Hepatology, Hannover Medical School (Figs. 253 a, b, 966, 975, 976, 981, 990, 991, 1026, 1043)
Dr. Goel, Radiology, Heerlen, Netherlands (Figs. 1010, 1011) (with permission: Radiology 173: 137–141, 1989)
Dr. Greeven, St. Elisabeth Hospital, Neuwied (Figs. 166, 1182)
Prof. Von der Hardt, Clinic of Pediatrics, Hannover Medical School (Fig. 893)
Dr. Hennig, Department of Radiology, University of Freiburg (Fig. 529)
Prof. Jonas, Urology, Hannover Medical School (Figs. 1050 a, b, 1051)
Prof. Kremers, Policlinic of Preservative Dentistry and Parodontology, Munich University (Fig. 182)
Prof. Kunze, Clinic of Pediatrics, Munich University (Figs. 15–18)
Dr. Meyer, Department of Gastro-enterology and Hepatology, Hannover Medical School (Figs. 906, 949 a, b, 959, 1086)
Prof. Pfeifer, Division of Radiology, Clinic of Surgery, Munich University (Figs. 306, 319, 321, 748–751, 789–792, 1199, 1230, 1231, 1260, 1261)
Priv.-Doz. Rau, Department of Radiology, University of Freiburg (Figs. 875, 886, 887)
Prof. Ravelli, Institute of Anatomy, Innsbruck University (Fig. 746)
Prof. Reich, Clinic of Orofacial Surgery, Bonn University (Figs. 133, 134)
Prof. Reiser, Dr. Glaser, Institute of Clinical Radiology, Munich University (Figs. 307, 578–582, 705 a, b, 771, 1369, 1371, 1373, 1377)
Prof. Rudzki-Janson, Policlinic of Pediatric Orthopedics, Munich University (Figs 80, 81)
Dr. Scheibe, Department of Surgery, Rosman Hospital, Breisach (Figs. 1233 a–c)
Prof. Schillinger, Women's Clinic, Freiburg University (Figs. 1072–1074)
Dr. Dr. Schliephake, Orofacial Surgery, Hannover Medical School (Figs. 167, 212, 213)
Prof. Schloesser, Center of Gynecology, Hannover Medical School (Figs. 1071 a, b, 1080, 1082, 1083, 1130)
Prof. Schumacher, Neuroradiology, Department of Radiology, Freiburg University – (Figs. 448 a, b)
Dr. Sommer and Priv.-Doz. Bauer, Radiologists, Munich (Figs. 650, 1234–1236)
Prof. Stotz, Policlinic of Orthopedics, Munich University (Fig. 1193)
Prof. Vogl, Policlinic of Radiology, Munich University (Figs. 440, 442, 631, 632)
Prof. Vollrath, Clinic of ENT Surgery, Moenchengladbach (Figs. 246–248)
Prof. Wagner †, Department of Diagnostic Radiology II, Hannover Medical School (Figs. 914, 1014, 1017, 1020, 1023, 1090)
Prof. Wenz, Department of Radiology, Freiburg University (Fig. 747)
Dr. Willfuehr, Abdominal and Transplant Surgery, Hannover Medical School (Fig. 1001)
Priv.-Doz. Wimmer, Department of Radiology, Freiburg University (Fig. 778)

Additional illustrations were taken from the following books:

Birkner, R.: Das typische Roentgenbild des Skeletts. (The Typical Radiograph of the Skeleton.) Urban & Schwarzenberg, Munich-Vienna-Baltimore, 1990 (Fig. 1200)
Welsch, U. (ed.): Sobotta-Histologie (Sobotta-Histology), 5th edition, Urban & Schwarzenberg, Munich-Vienna-Baltimore, 1997 (Figs. 635, 646)
Wicke, L.: Atlas der Roentgenanatomie (Atlas of Radiological Anatomy), 3rd edition, Urban & Schwarzenberg, Munich-Vienna-Baltimore, 1985 (Figs. 905 a, b, 1076)
Wilhelm, K.R., R. Putz, R. Hierner, R.E. Giunta: Lappenplastiken in der Handchirurgie (Flaps in Handsurgery). Urban & Schwarzenberg, Munich-Vienna-Baltimore, 1997 (Fig. 58)

Back, surface anatomy 1

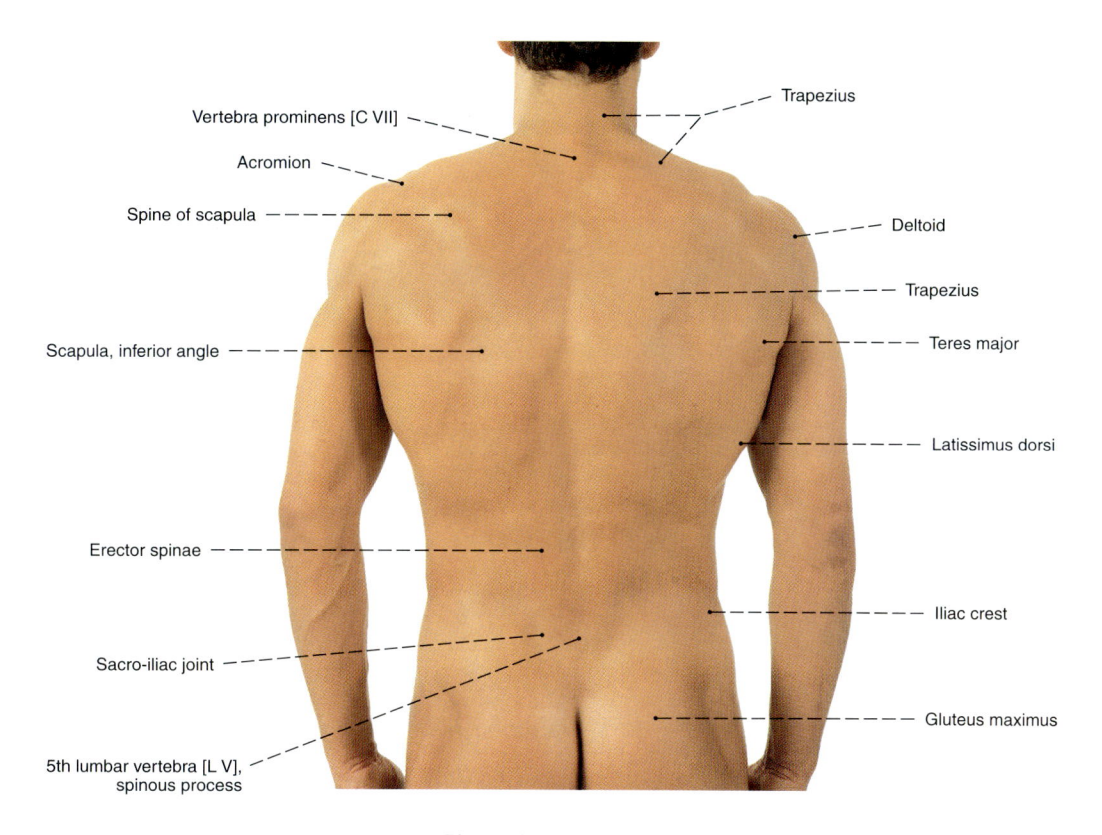

Fig. 706 Back, surface anatomy.

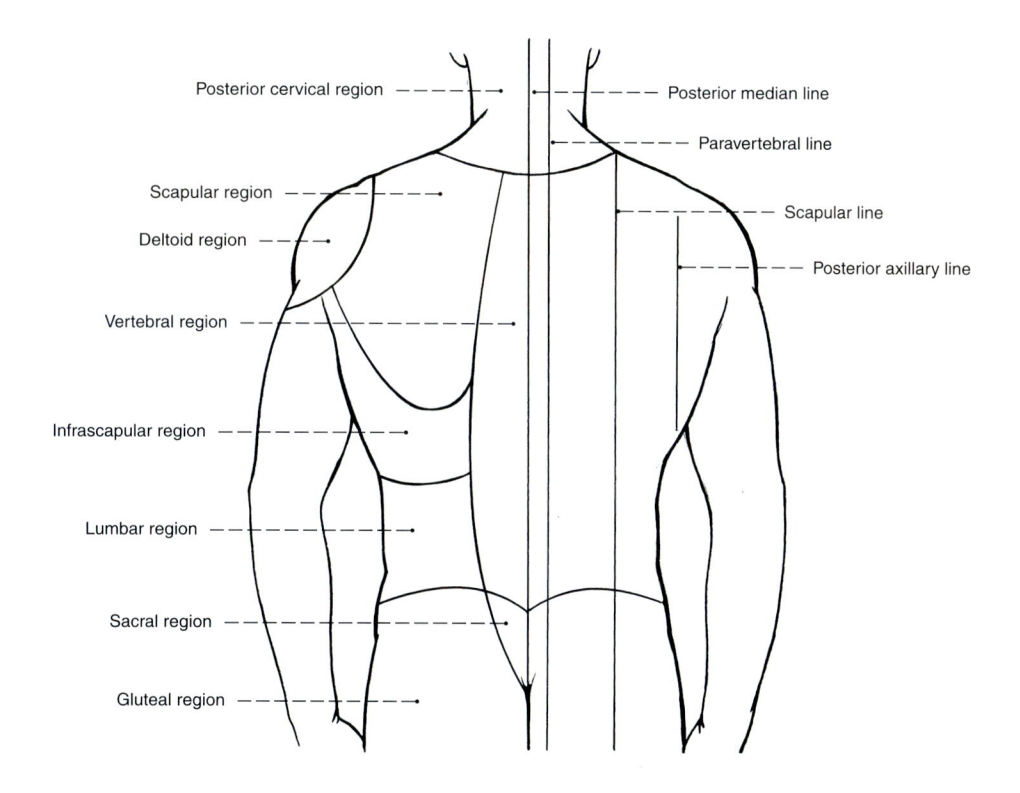

Fig. 707 Posterior planes and axes of the human body.

2 Back

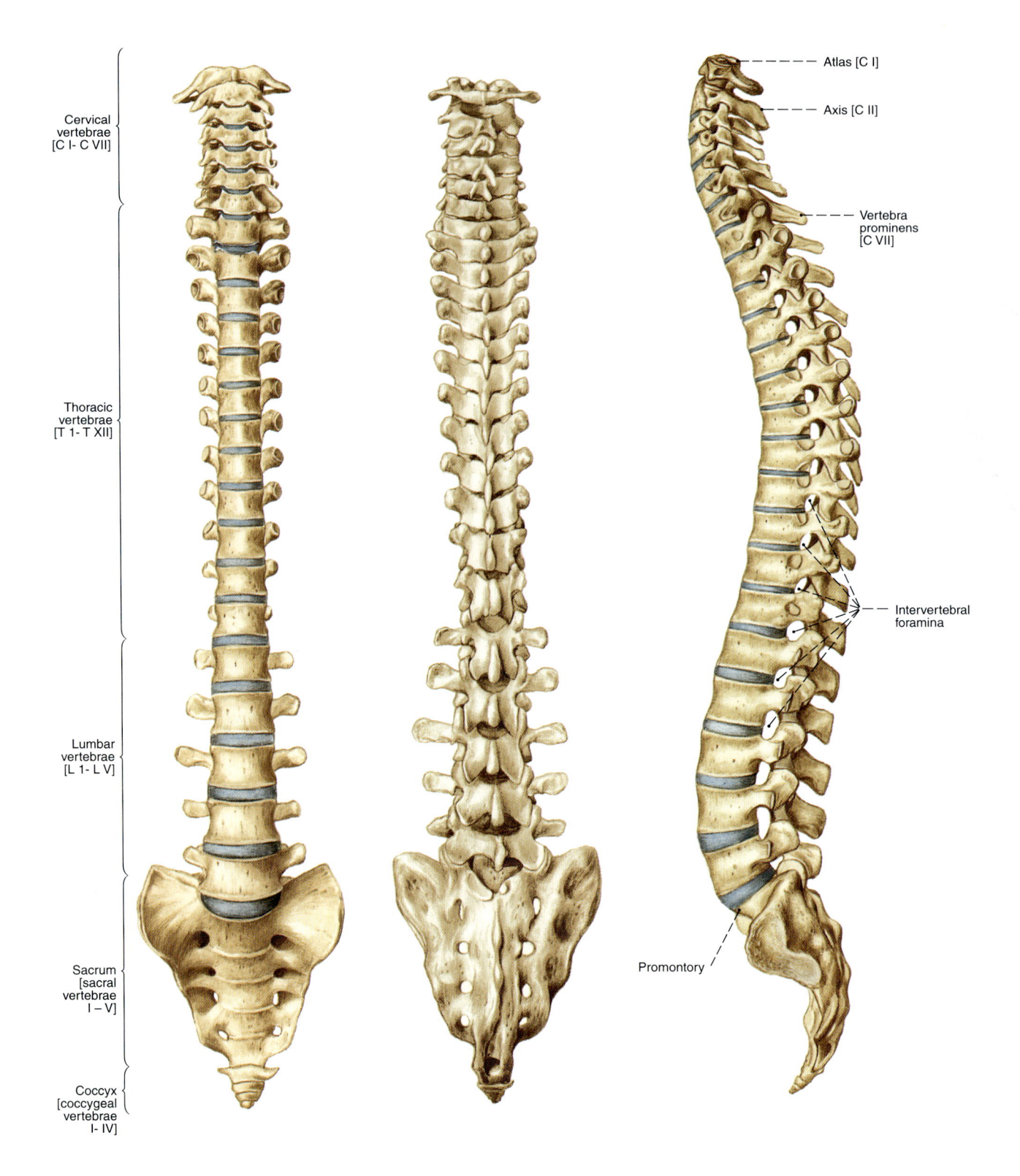

Fig. 708 Vertebral column, intervertebral discs in blue color; ventral aspect (30%).

Fig. 709 Vertebral column, dorsal aspect (30%).

Fig. 710 Vertebral column; intervertebral discs in blue color; left lateral aspect (30%).

Vetebral column 3

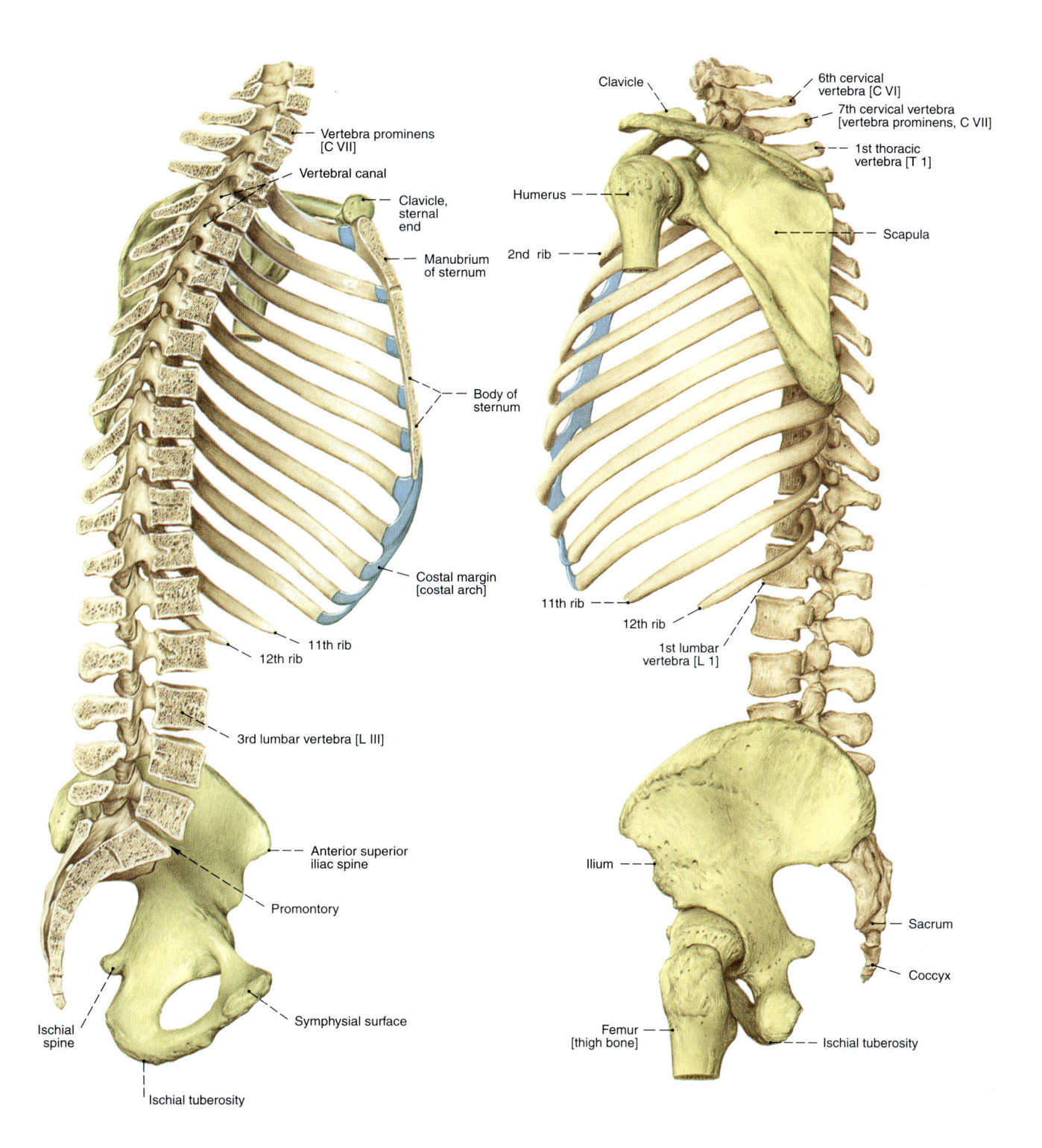

Fig. 711 Vertebral column; pectoral girdle [shoulder girdle]; pelvic girdle; vertebral column sectioned in the median plane; left medial aspect (25%).

Fig. 712 Vertebral column; pectoral girdle [shoulder girdle]; pelvic girdle; vertebral column sectioned in the median plane; left lateral aspect (25%).

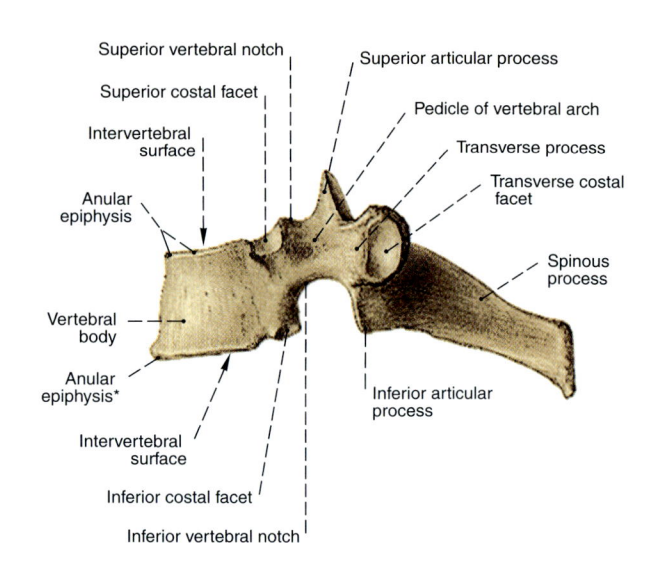

Fig. 713 Vertebra; typical features for example in the 5th thoracic vertebra [T V]; lateral aspect (80%).

* Also: rim of vertebral body.

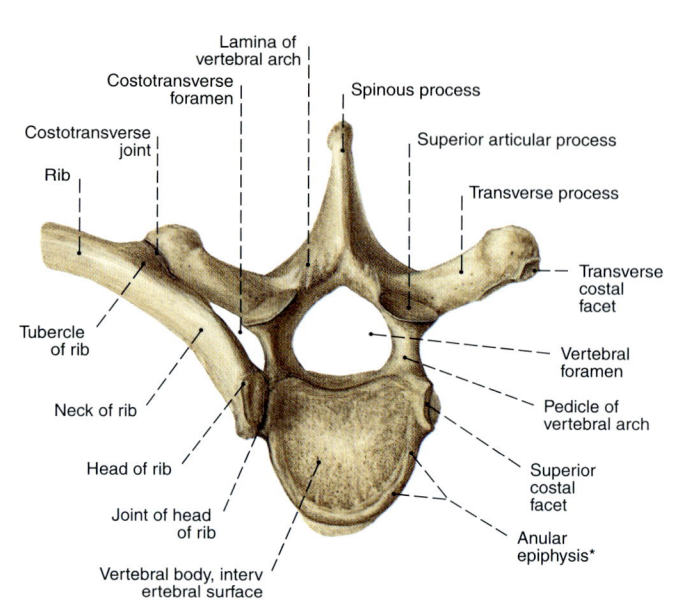

Fig. 714 Vertebra; typical features, for example, in the 5th thoracic vertebra [T V]; cranial aspect (80%).

* Also: rim of vertebral body.

Features of typical vertebrae (excluding atlas and axis)

	7 cervical vertebrae [CI–C VII]	12 thoracic vertebrae [TI–TXII]	5 lumbar vertebrae [LI–LV]	Sacrum [sacral vertebrae I–V]
Intervertebral surfaces of vertebral bodies	Rectangular, small with uncus of body [uncinate process] on cranial surface	Basically triangular, caudal vertebrae rounded	Bean-shaped, large	
Vertebral foramen	Large, triangular	Round	Small, triangular	Sacral canal, oval
Articular processes	Oblique dorsal inclination	Frontal, dorsal inclination	Lateral part : sagittal ; medial part : frontal	Fused to intermediate sacral crest
Transverse processes	Comprise an anterior and a posterior tubercle, a groove for spinal nerve and a foramen transversarium	Club-shaped with costal facets	Mammillary and accessory processes	Fused to lateral sacral crest
Spinous processes	Horizontal, short, bifurcated	Different steep downward direction	Horizontal, laterally flattened, massive	Fused to median sacral crest
Costal elements	Ventral part of transverse process and dorsal tubercle	None, because there are ribs	Costal processes	Lateral parts
Characteristic feature	Foramen transversarium	Superior and inferior costal facets	Mammillary and accessory processes	Synostotic fusion of vertebrae

Vertebrae 5

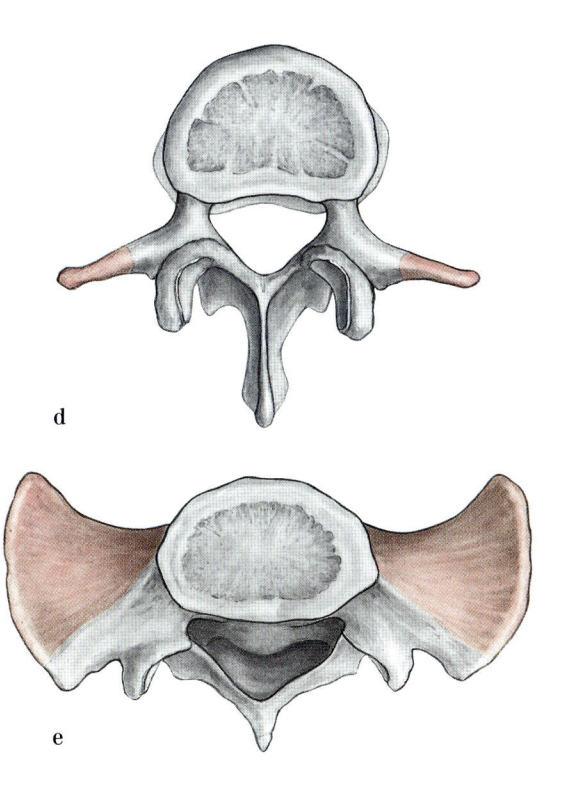

Fig. 715 a-e Regional characteristic features of vertebrae. The material derived from the embryonic costal processes (pink) form ribs only in the thoracic region.

a 1st cervical vertebra [atlas, C I]
b 4th cervical vertebra [C IV]
c 1st thoracic vertebra [T I], respective ribs and sternum
d 3rd lumbar vertebra [L III]
e Sacrum [sacral vertebrae I- V]

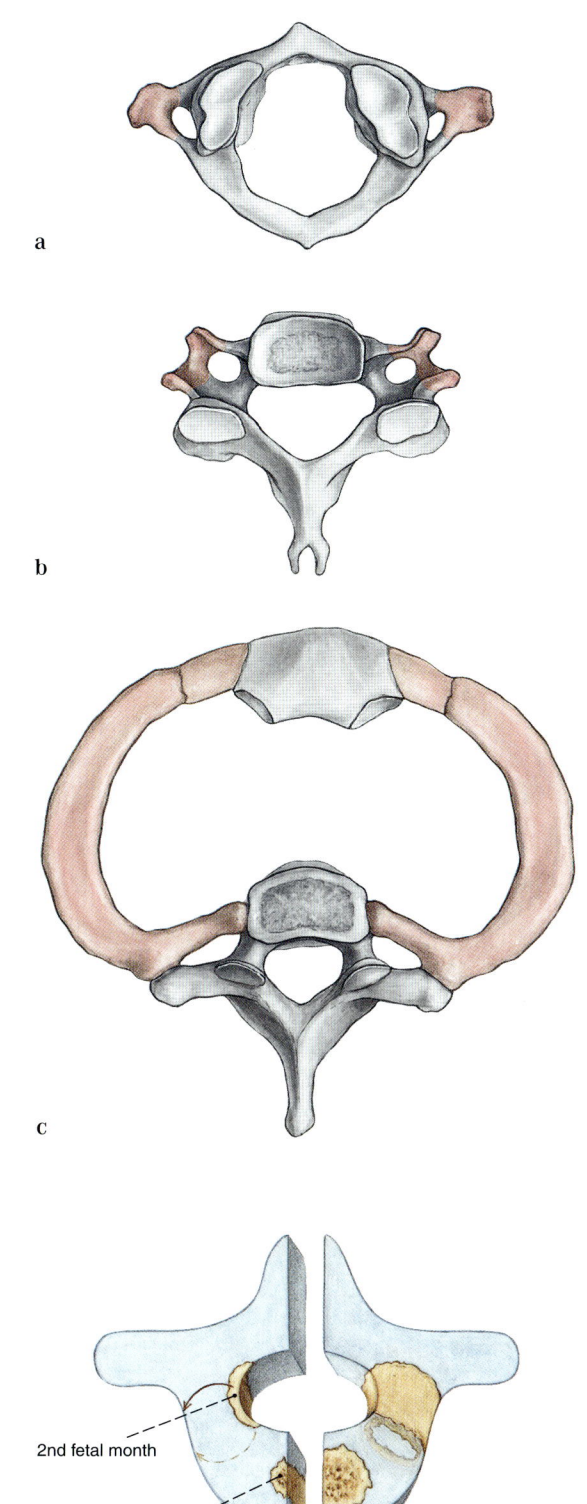

Fig. 716 Vertebral development.
Appearance of primary ossification centers (pedicle, 2nd fetal month; body, 3rd-6th fetal months) in a lumbar vertebra. Synostosis of ossification centers of vertebral arch with those of vertebral body occurs between 3rd and 6th year of life.

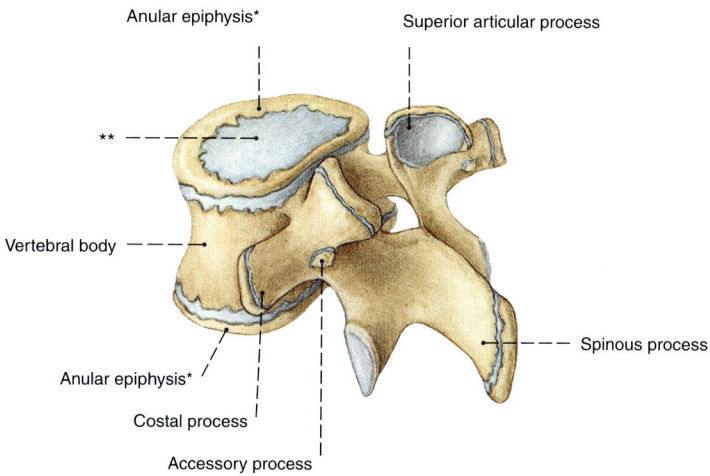

Fig. 717 Vertebral development.
In the epiphyses of vertebral bodies ring-shaped ossification centers (rims*) appear during the 8th year of life and fuse with the vertebral bodies until the 18th year of life. The central parts of epiphyses remain as hyaline cartilaginous plates (**) throughout life. Secondary ossification centers (apophyses) form on the processes.

6 Back

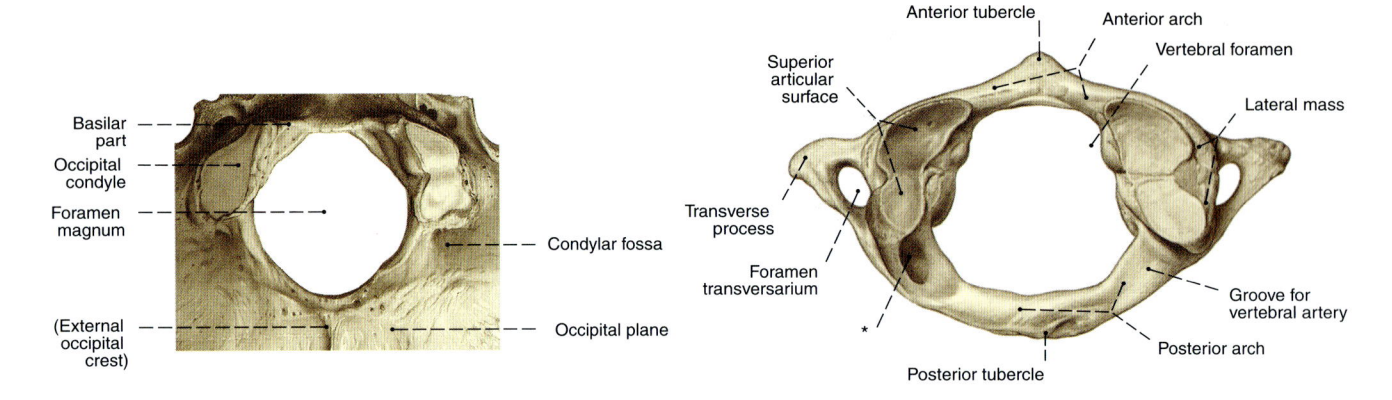

Fig. 718 Occipital bone; part showing foramen magnum and articular processes of atlanto-occipital joint; caudal aspect (80%).

Fig. 719 1st cervical vertebra [atlas, C I]; cranial aspect (85%).
The superior articular surfaces of atlas are frequently divided.
* Variation: canal for vertebral artery.

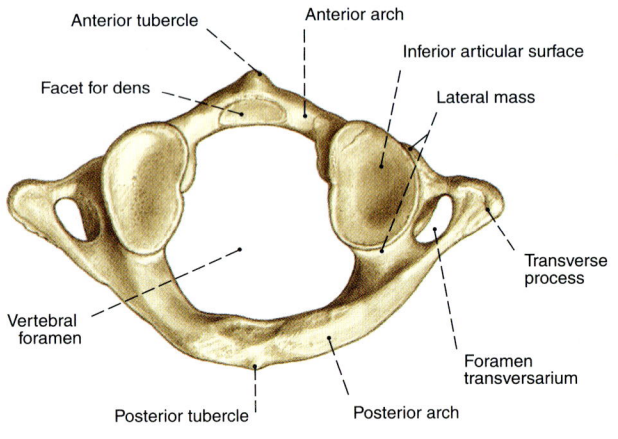

Fig. 720 1st cervical vertebra [atlas, C I]; caudal aspect (85%).

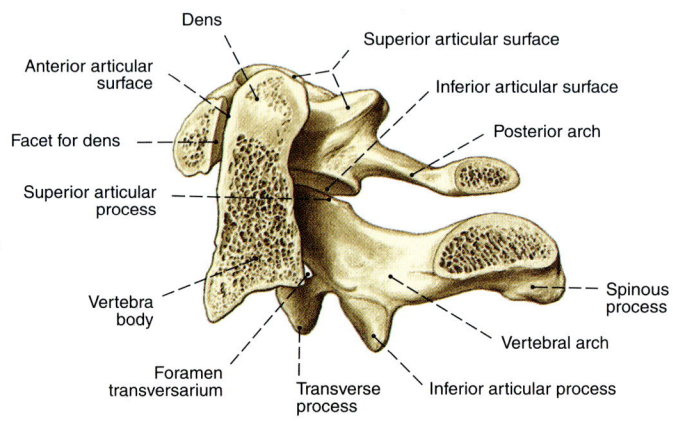

Fig. 721 1st and 2nd cervical vertebrae [atlas and axis, C I, C II]; median section, medial aspect (90%).

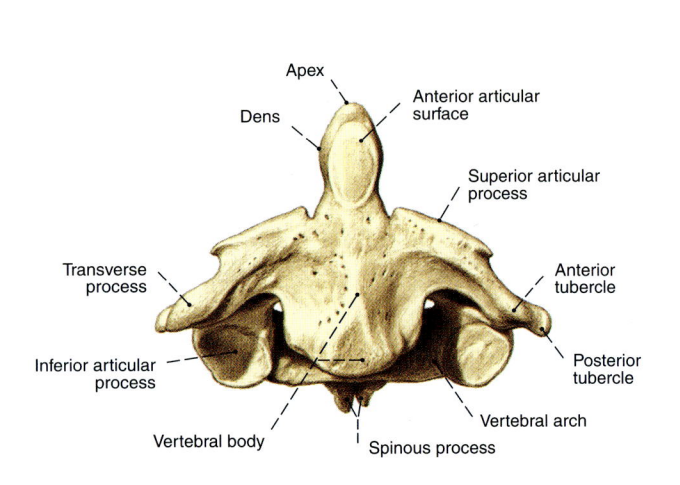

Fig. 722 2nd cervical vertebra [axis, C II]; ventral aspect (90%).

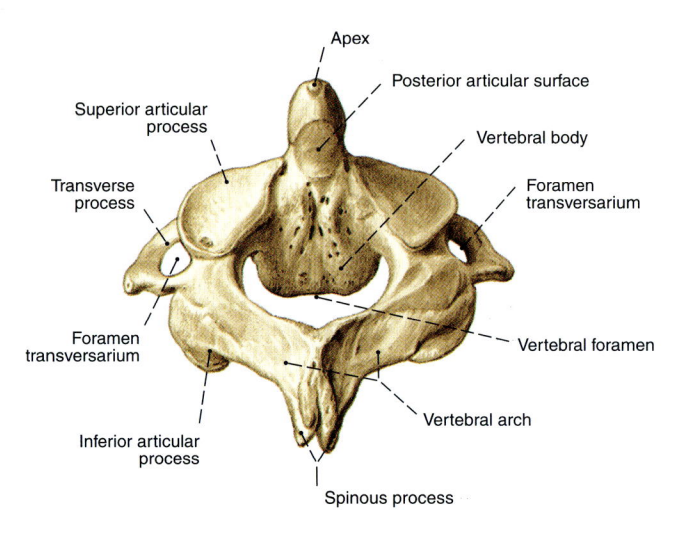

Fig. 723 2nd cervical vertebra [axis, C II]; dorsocranial aspect (90%).

Vertebrae

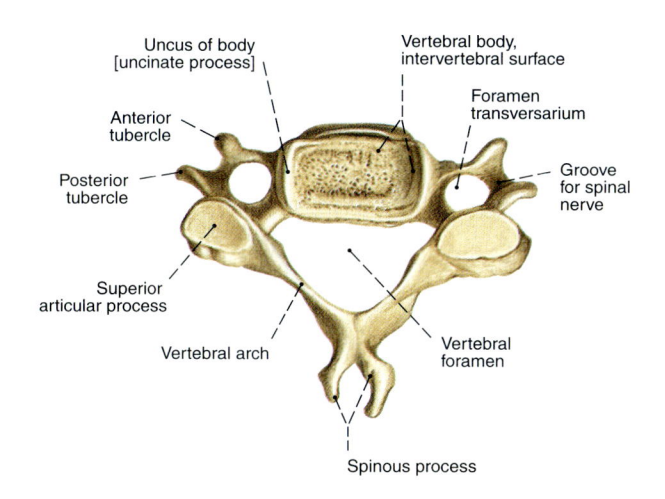

Fig. 724 5th cervical vertebra [C V]; cranial aspect (100%).
The spinous processes of the 2nd–6th cervical vertebrae are usually bifurcated.

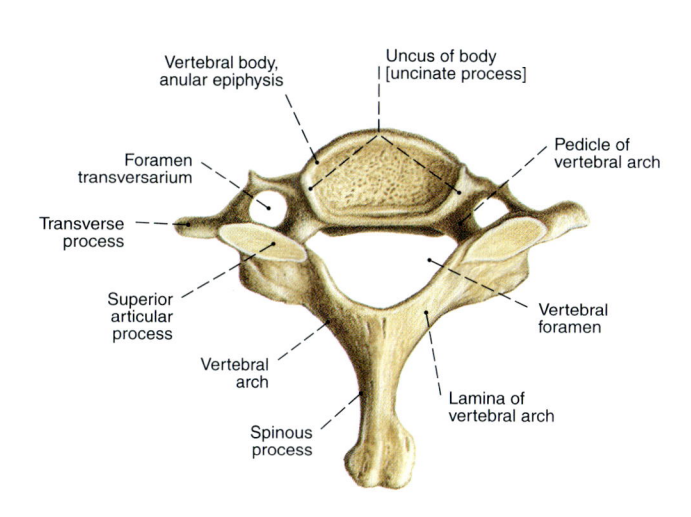

Fig. 725 7th cervical vertebra [C VII]; cranial aspect (100%).
The 7th cervical vertebra, also called vertebra prominens, is usually easy to identify due to its prominent spinous process. However, the spinous process of the 1st thoracic vertebra is usually even longer.

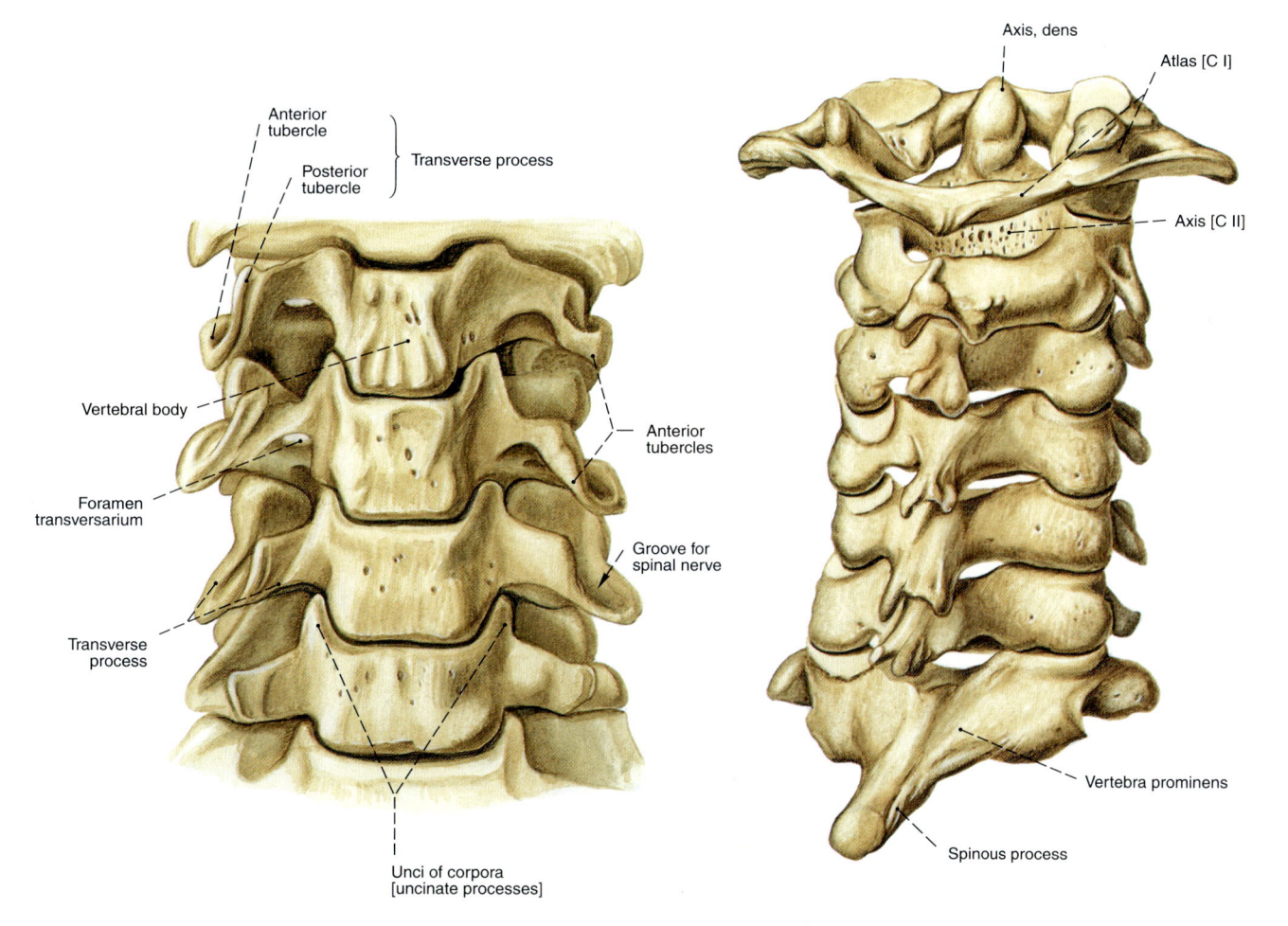

Fig. 726 2nd–7th cervical vertebrae [C II–C VII]; ventral aspect (120%).

Fig. 727 1st–7th cervical vertebrae [C I–C VII]; dorsolateral aspect (110%).

8 Back

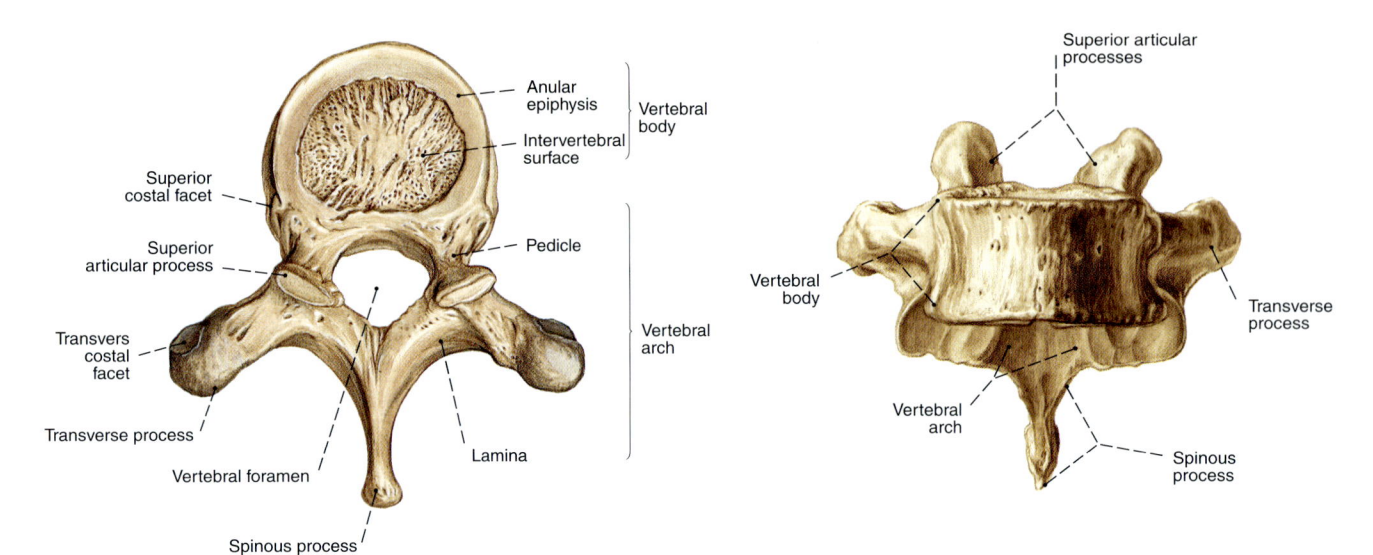

Fig. 728 10th thoracic vertebra [T X]; cranial aspect (90%).

Fig. 729 10th thoracic vertebra [T X]; ventral aspect (90%).

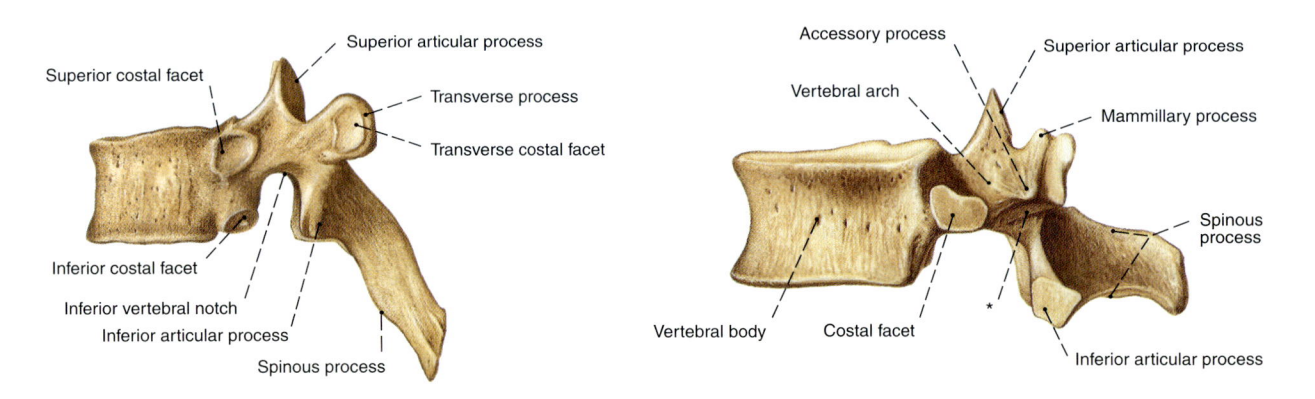

Fig. 730 6th thoracic vertebra [T VI]; left lateral aspect (90%).

Fig. 731 12th thoracic vertebra [T XII]; left lateral aspect (80%).

* Region of vertebral arch between superior and inferior articular processes (so-called "isthmus" = intra-articular portion).

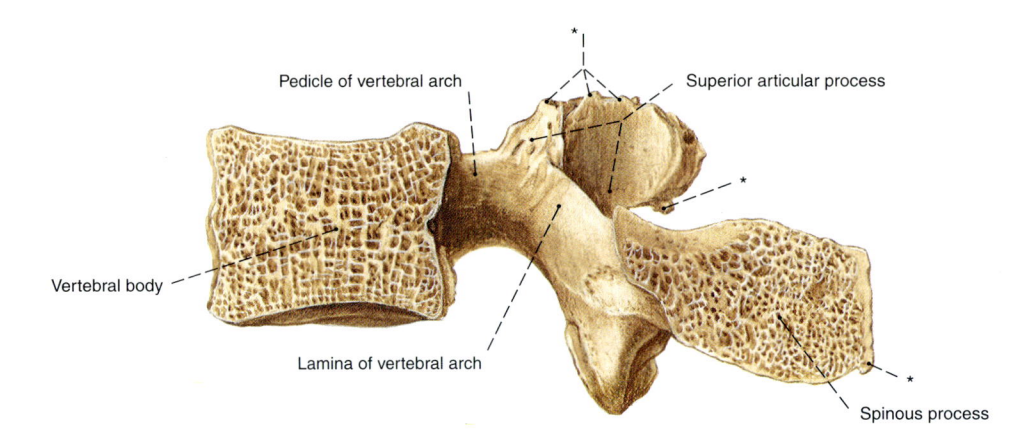

Fig. 732 3rd lumbar vertebra [L III]; median section; specimen of older person; medial aspect (110%).

* Ossified ligamentous insertions.

Vertebrae 9

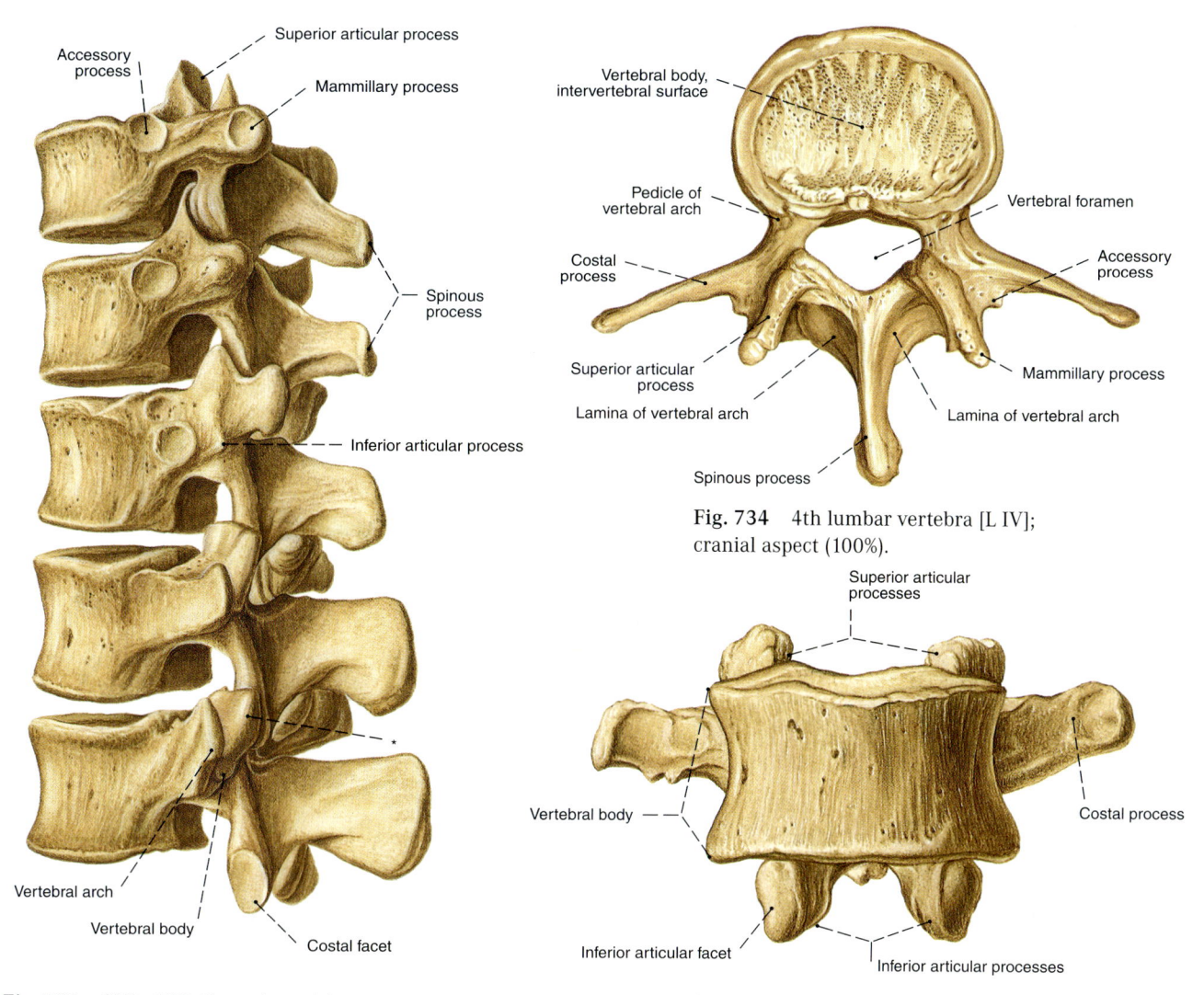

Fig. 733 10th–12th thoracic vertebrae [T X–T XII] and 1st–2nd lumbar vertebrae [L I–L II]; dorsolateral aspect (70%).

Fig. 734 4th lumbar vertebra [L IV]; cranial aspect (100%).

Fig. 735 4th lumbar vertebra [L IV]; ventral aspect (100%).

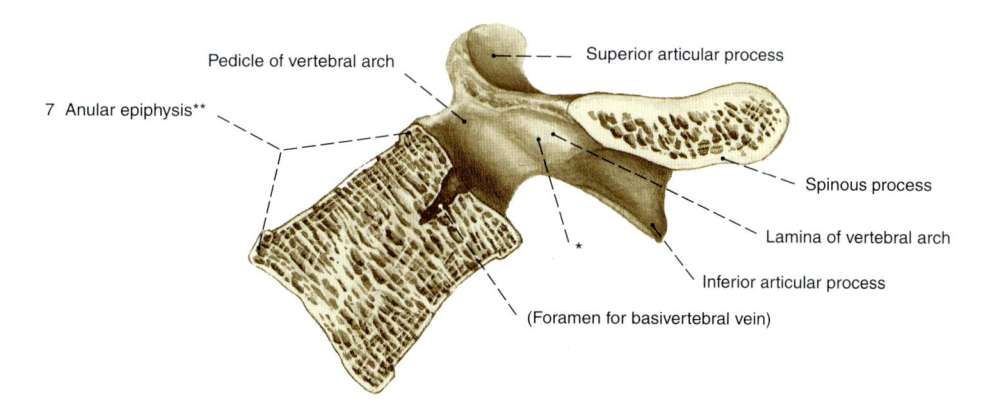

Fig. 736 5th lumbar vertebra [L V]; median section; medial aspect (100%). Note the characteristic wedge shape of the body of the 5th lumbar vertebra.

* Region of vertebral arch between superior and inferior articular processes. Here, in the 5th, rarely also in the 4th lumbar vertebrae, a cleft bridged by connective tissue (spondylolysis) may occur, probably due to excessive local flexion stress. Subsequently the cranial vertebra may slide (olisthesis) from the top of the caudal vertebra (spondylolisthesis).

** In this specimen the anterior border is pathologically oblique.

10 Back

Fig. 737 Sacrum; dorsal aspect (60%).

Fig. 738 Sacrum; ventrocaudal aspect (60%).

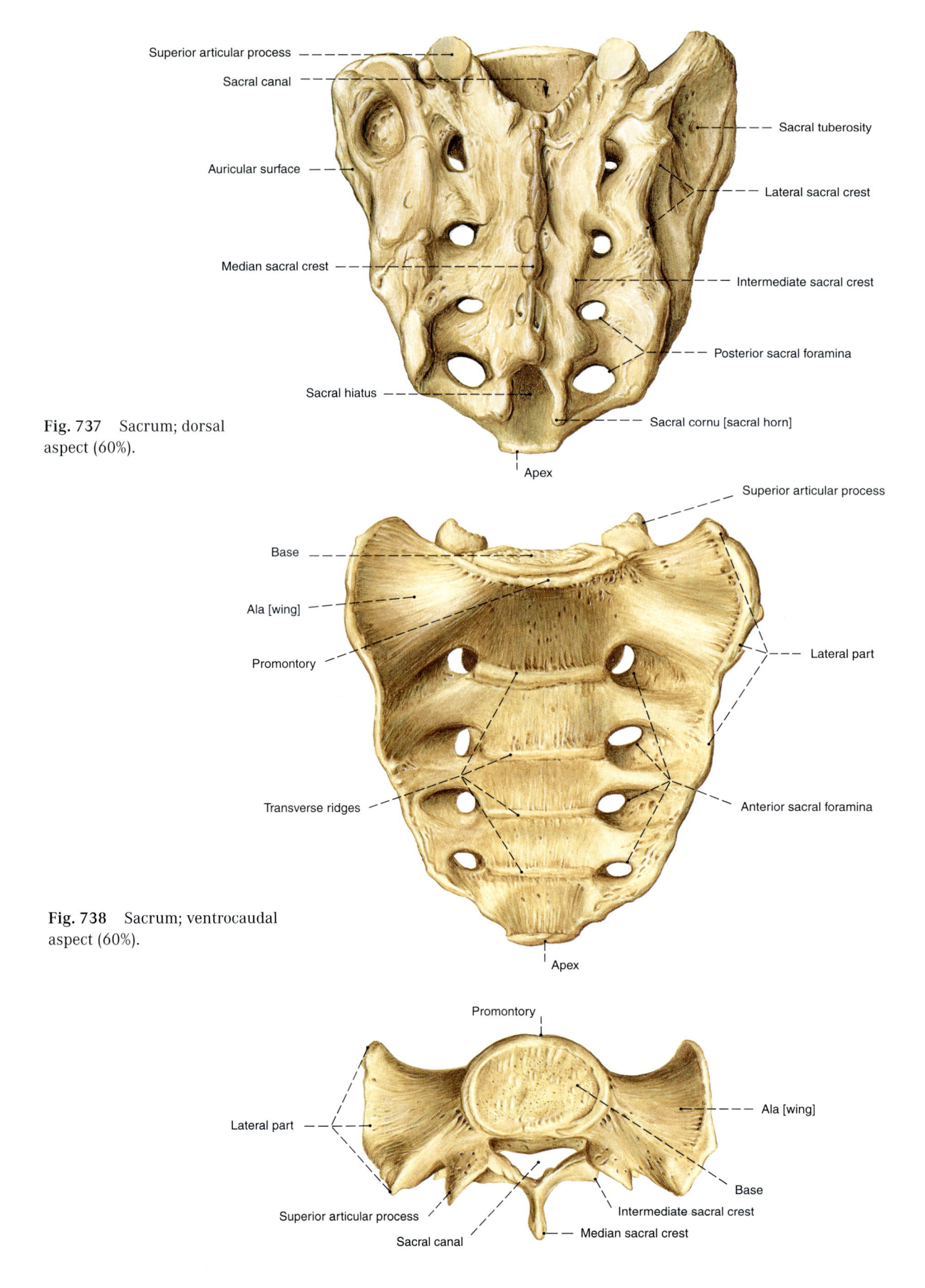

Fig. 739 Sacrum; cranial aspect (55%).

Sacrum and coccyx 11

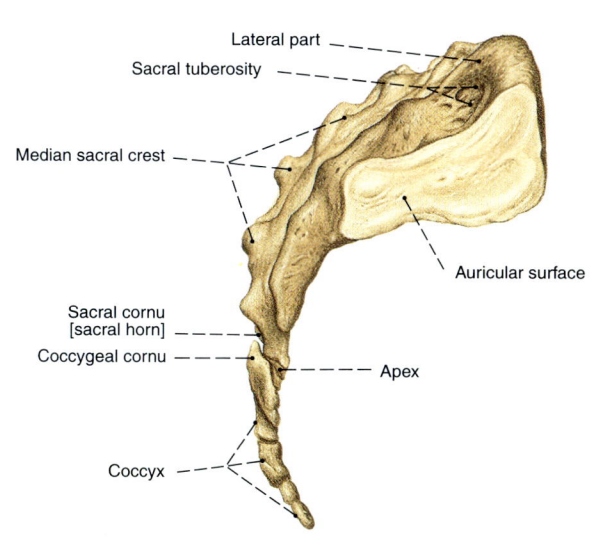

Fig. 740 Sacrum; right lateral aspect (45%).

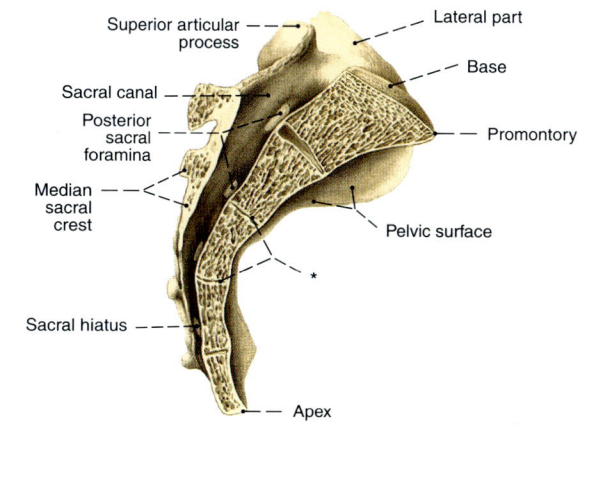

Fig. 741 Sacrum, median section; medial aspect (45%).

* Remnants of the intervertebral discs also remain in the adult.

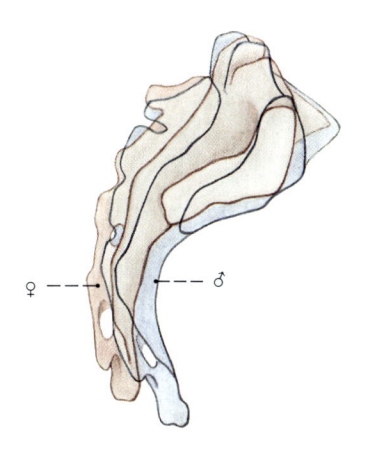

Fig. 742 Sacrum; sex differences; lateral aspect.

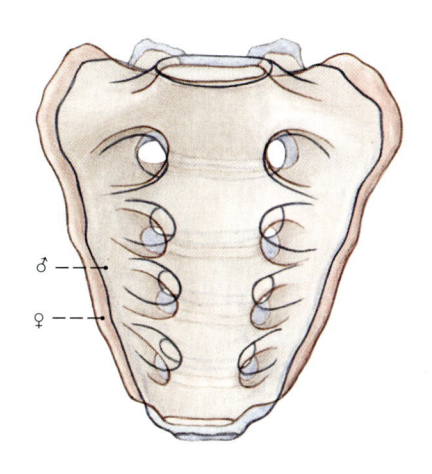

Fig. 743 Sacrum; sex differences; ventral aspect.

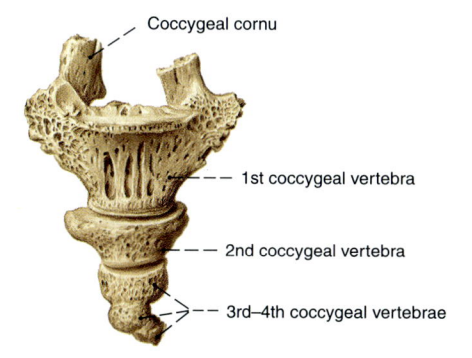

Fig. 744 Coccyx; ventrocranial aspect (105%). Despite variations in the development of intervertebral discs, the entire postsacral vertebral rudiments are called coccyx.

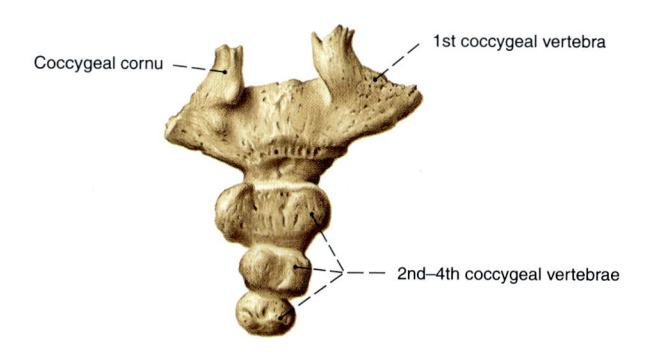

Fig. 745 Coccyx; dorsocaudal aspect (105%).

12 Back

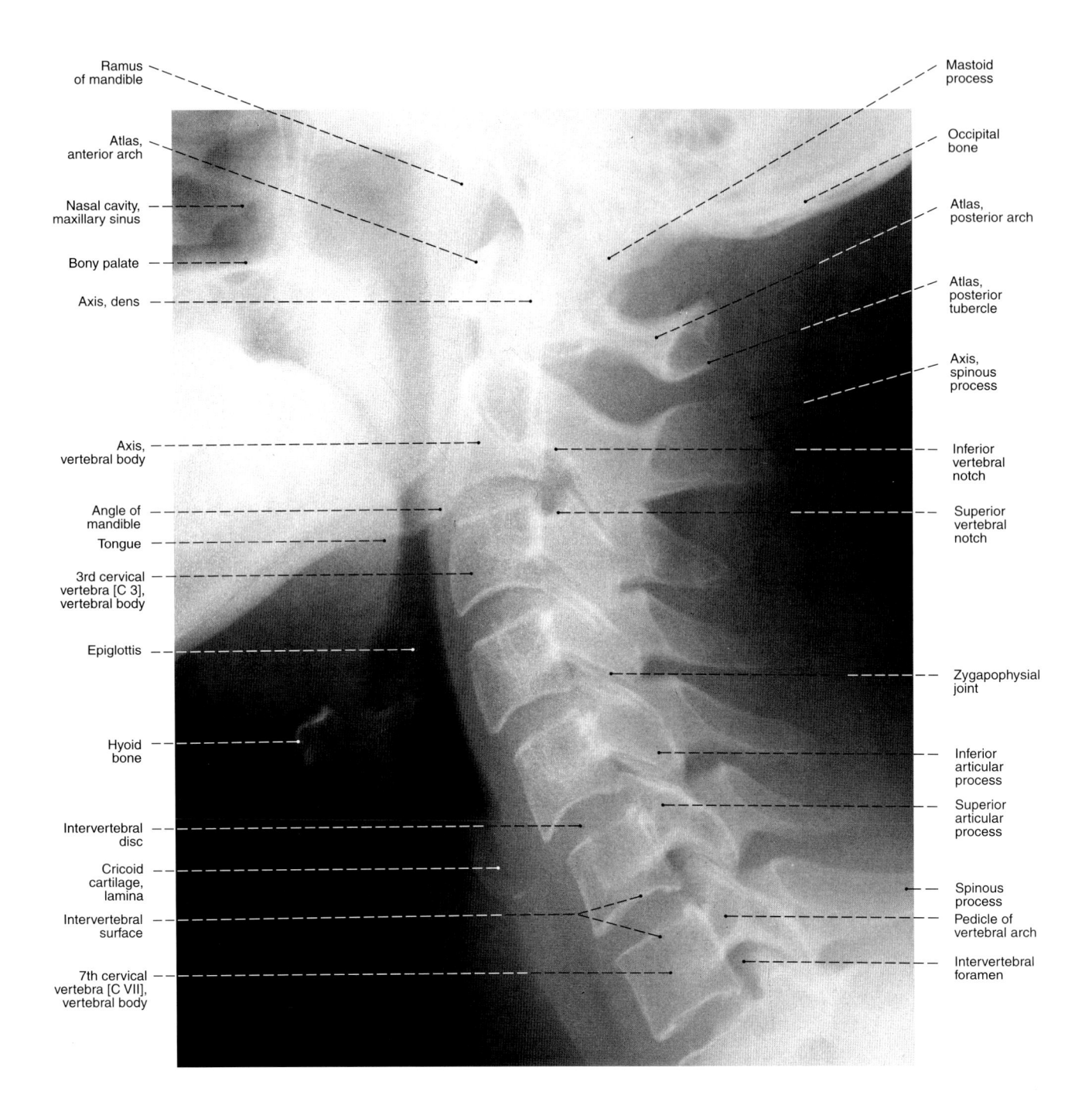

Fig. 746   Cervical vertebrae; lateral radiograph of cervical vertebral column in upright position; central beam directed toward 3rd cervical vertebra; shoulders depressed.

Vetebral column 13

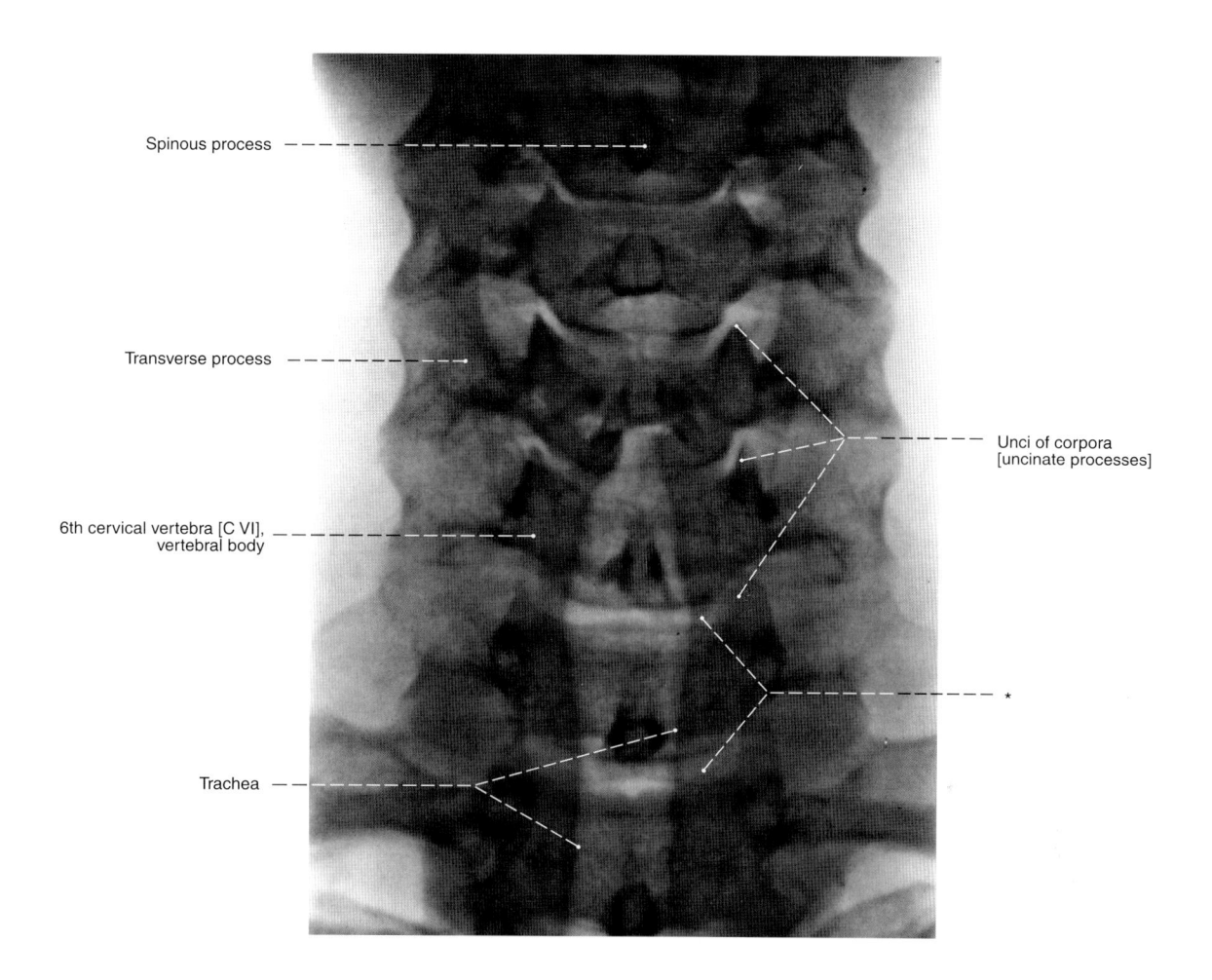

Fig. 747 Cervical vertebrae; AP radiograph of cervical vertebral column in upright position; central beam directed toward 3rd cervical vertebra.
* Spaces of intervertebral discs.

14 Back

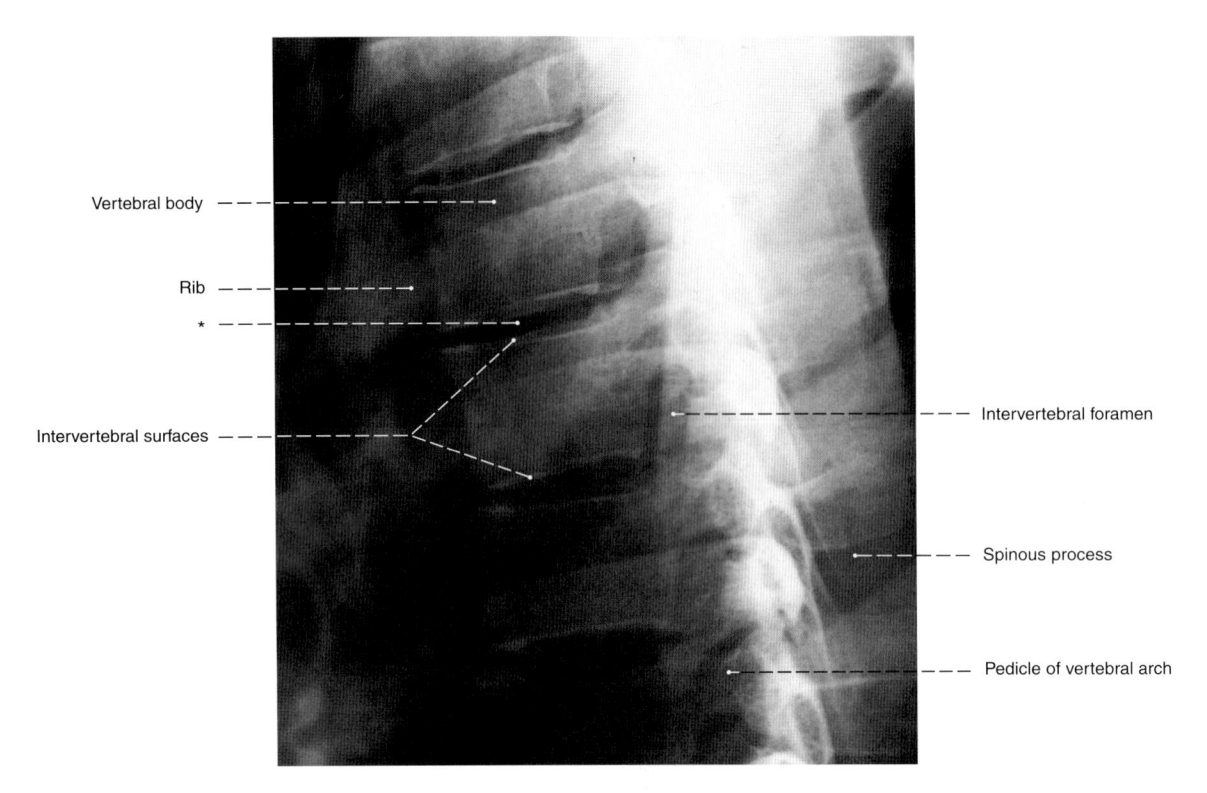

Fig. 748 Thoracic vertebrae; lateral radiograph of thoracic vertebral column in upright position; thorax in inspiration; central beam directed toward 6th thoracic vertebra.
* Space of intervertebral discs.

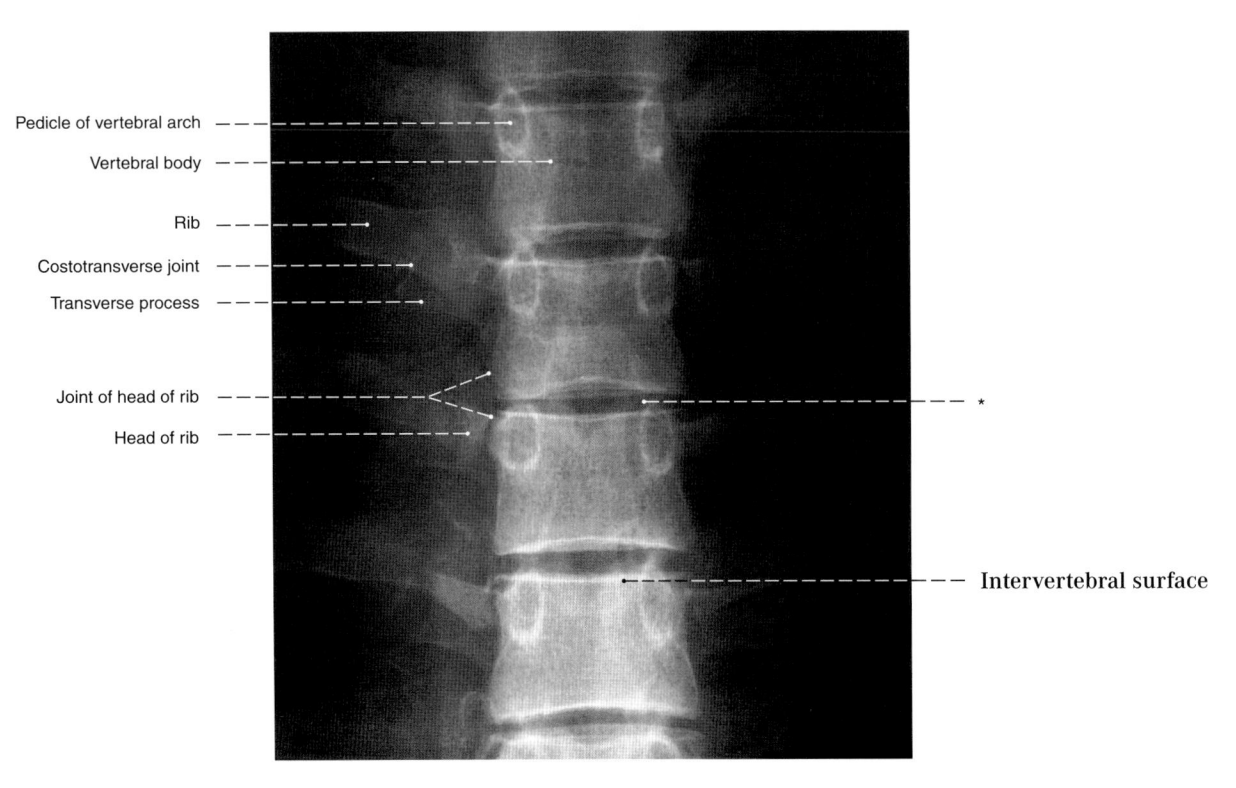

Fig. 749 Thoracic vertebrae; AP radiograph of thoracic vertebral column in upright position; thorax in inspiration; central beam directed toward 6th thoracic vertebra.
* Space of intervertebral discs.

Vertebral column 15

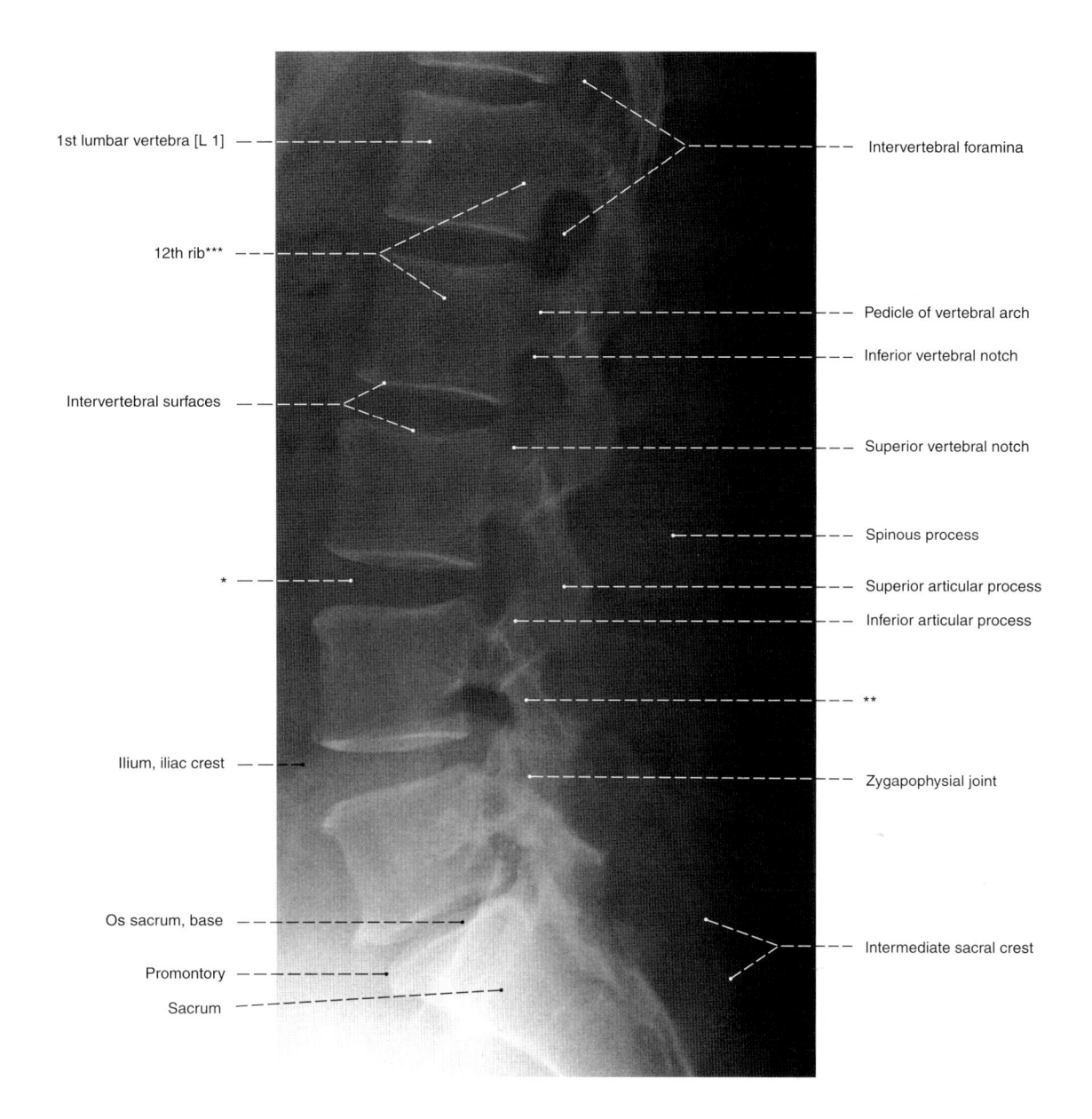

Fig. 750 Lumbar vertebrae; lateral radiograph of lumbar vertebral column in upright position; central beam directed toward 2nd lumbar vertebra.

The oblique anterior borders of the lower lumbar vertebrae are pathological alterations.

*   Space of intervertebral disc.
**   Region of vertebral arch between superior and inferior articular processes (so-called "isthmus" = intra-articular portion).
*** Ends of lines indicate the course of the hardly visible 12th rib.

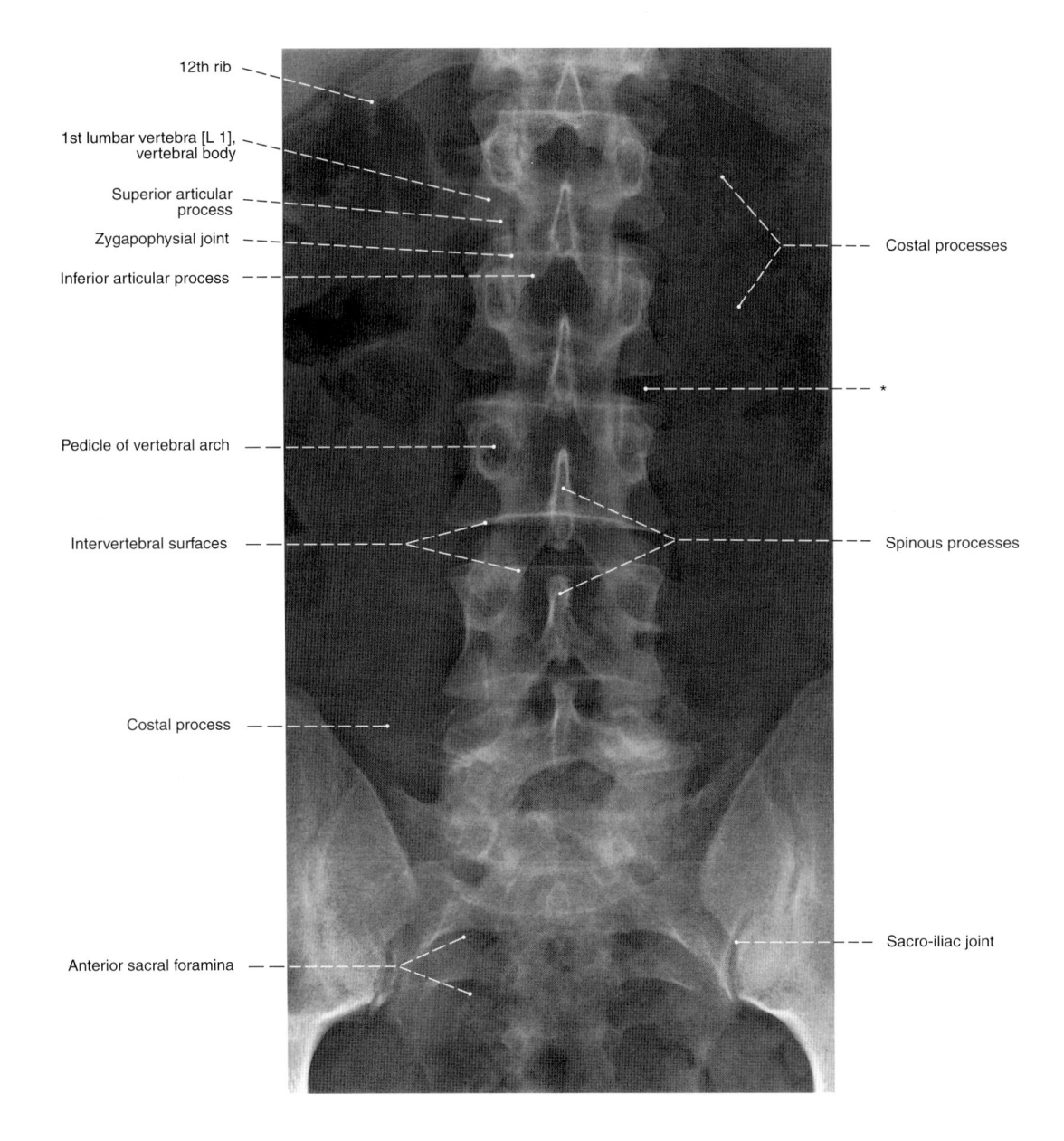

Fig. 751 Lumbar vertebrae; AP radiograph of lumbar vertebral column and sacrum in upright position; central beam directed toward 2nd lumbar vertebra. The oblique anterior borders of the lower lumbar vertebrae are pathological alterations.

* Space of intervertebral disc.

Craniocervical joints 17

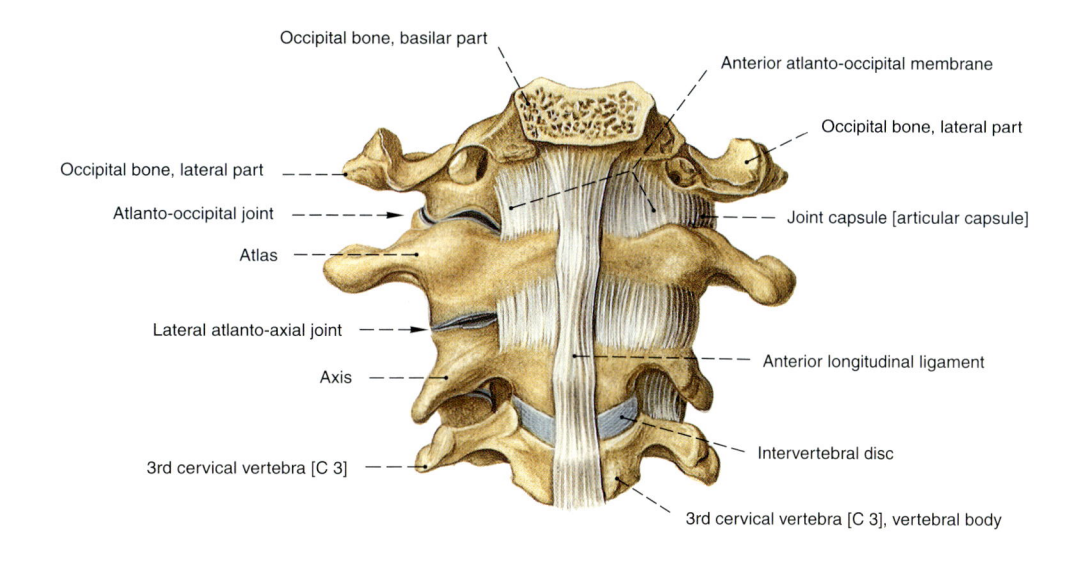

Fig. 752 Craniocervical joints and upper cervical vertebral column; joint capsules removed on the left; ventral aspect.

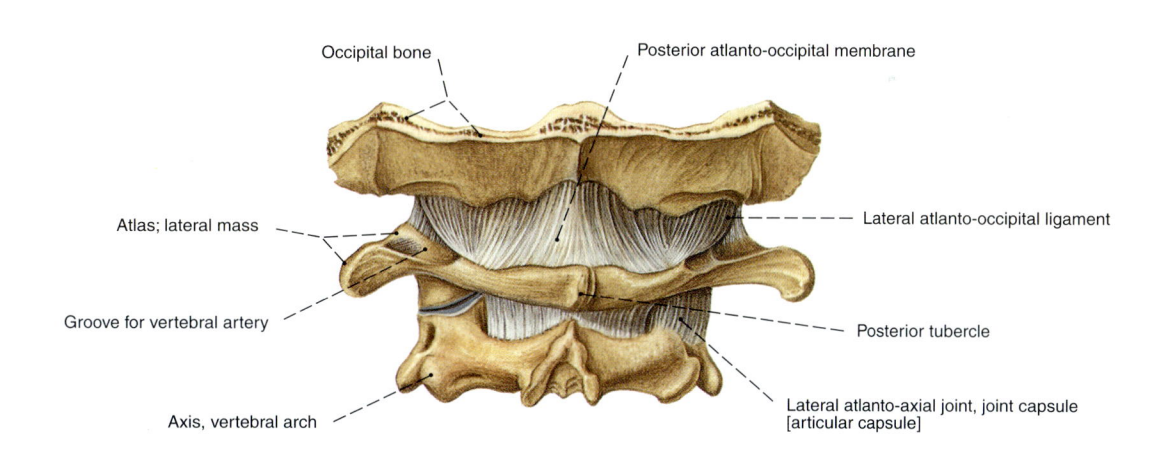

Fig. 753 Craniovertebral joints; joint capsules of lateral atlanto-axial joint removed on the left; dorsal aspect.

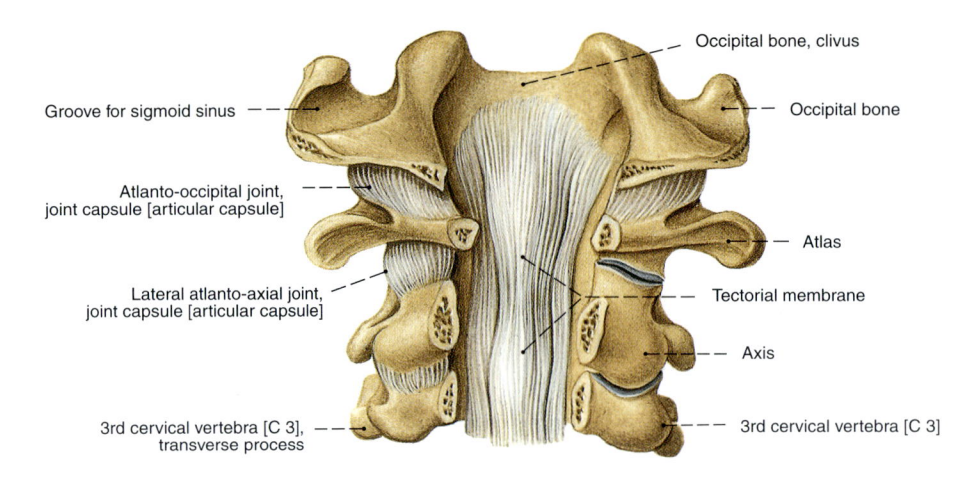

Fig. 754 Craniocervical joints, deep ligaments exposed after opening foramen magnum and vertebral canal; joint capsules partially removed on the right; dorsal aspect.

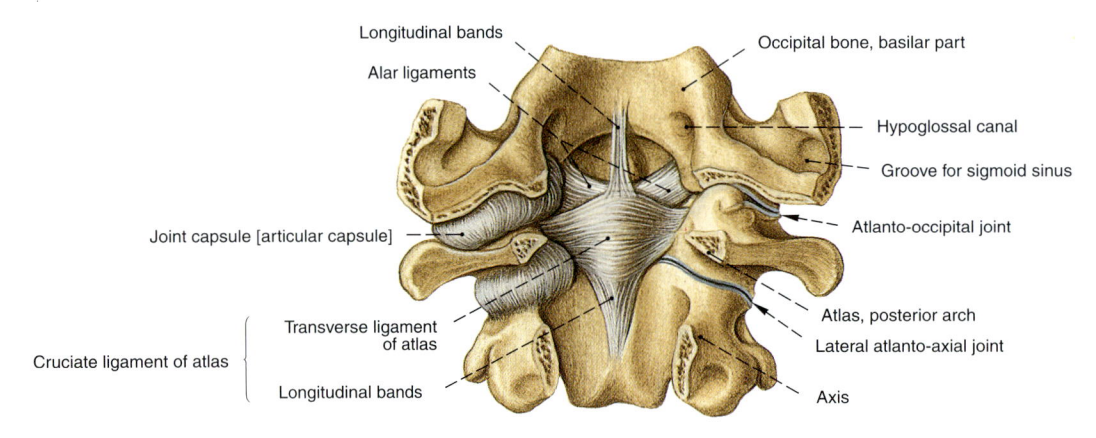

Fig. 755 Craniocervical joints, deep ligaments exposed after opening foramen magnum and vertebral canal; joint capsules partially removed on the right; dorsal aspect.

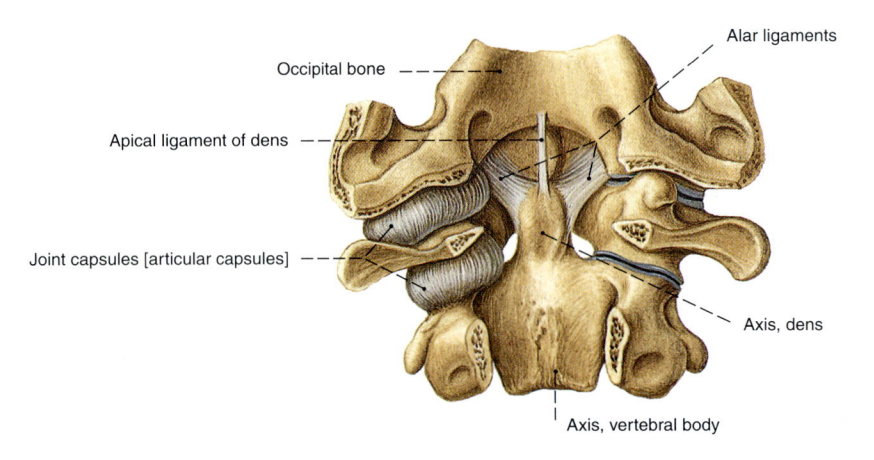

Fig. 756 Craniocervical joints, deep ligaments exposed after opening foramen magnum and vertebral canal; joint capsules removed on the right; dorsal aspect. The alar ligaments frequently insert also at the lateral masses of atlas.

Craniocervical joints 19

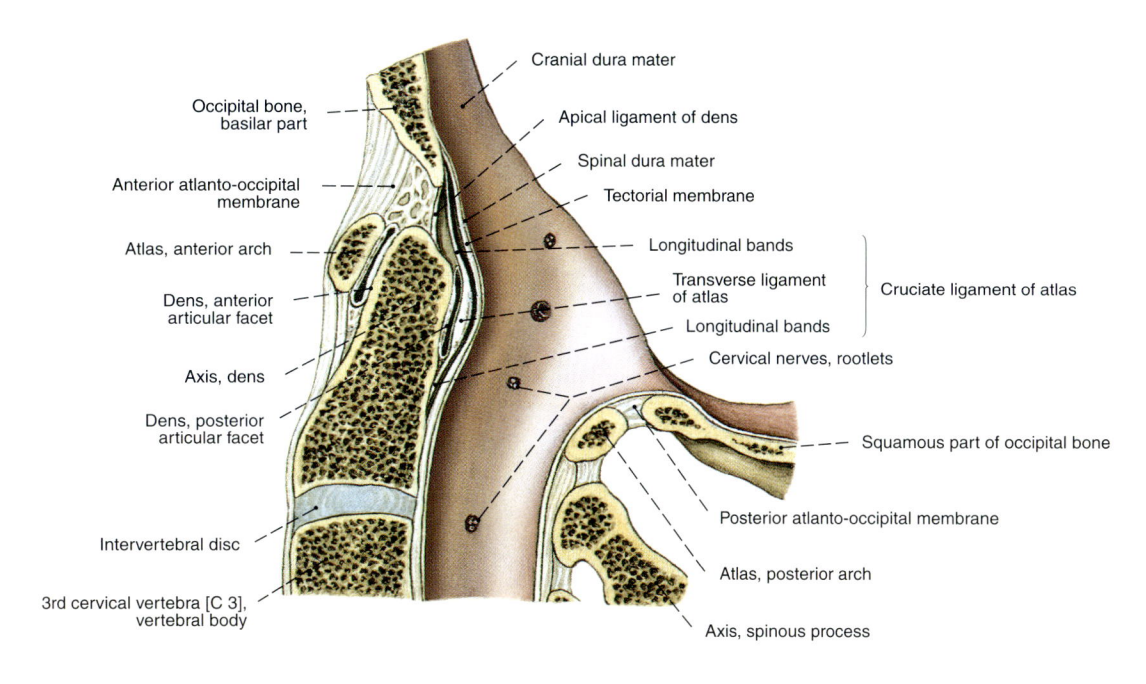

Fig. 757 Craniocervical joints; median section; medial aspect.

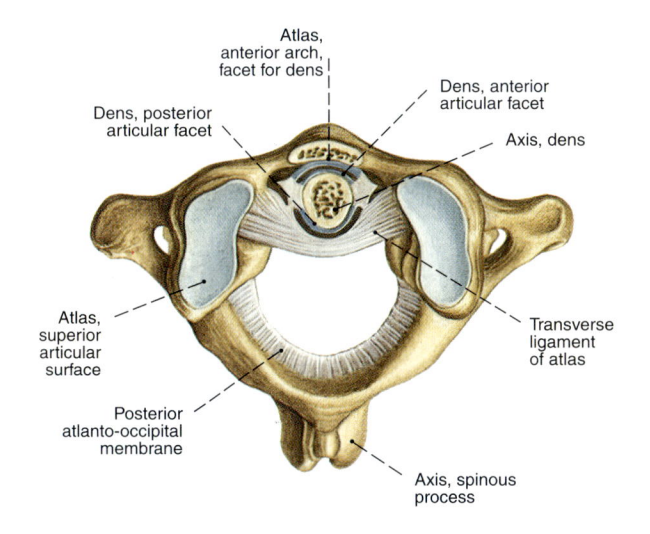

Fig. 758 Craniocervical joints; occipital bone removed; cranial aspect.

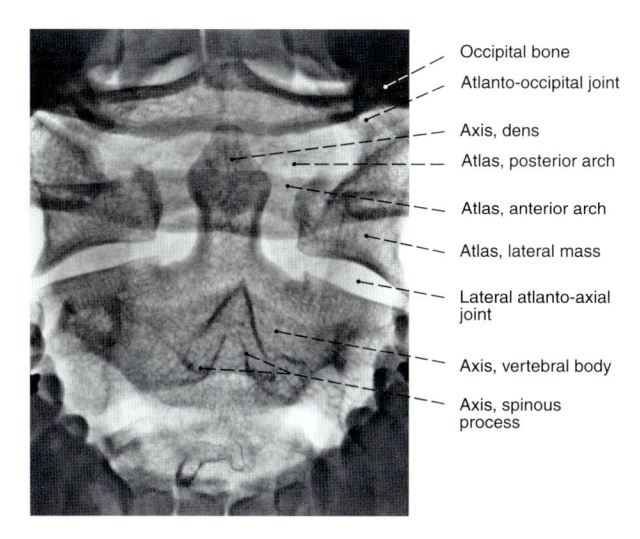

Fig. 759 Craniocervical joints, AP radiograph; open mouth view.

20 Back

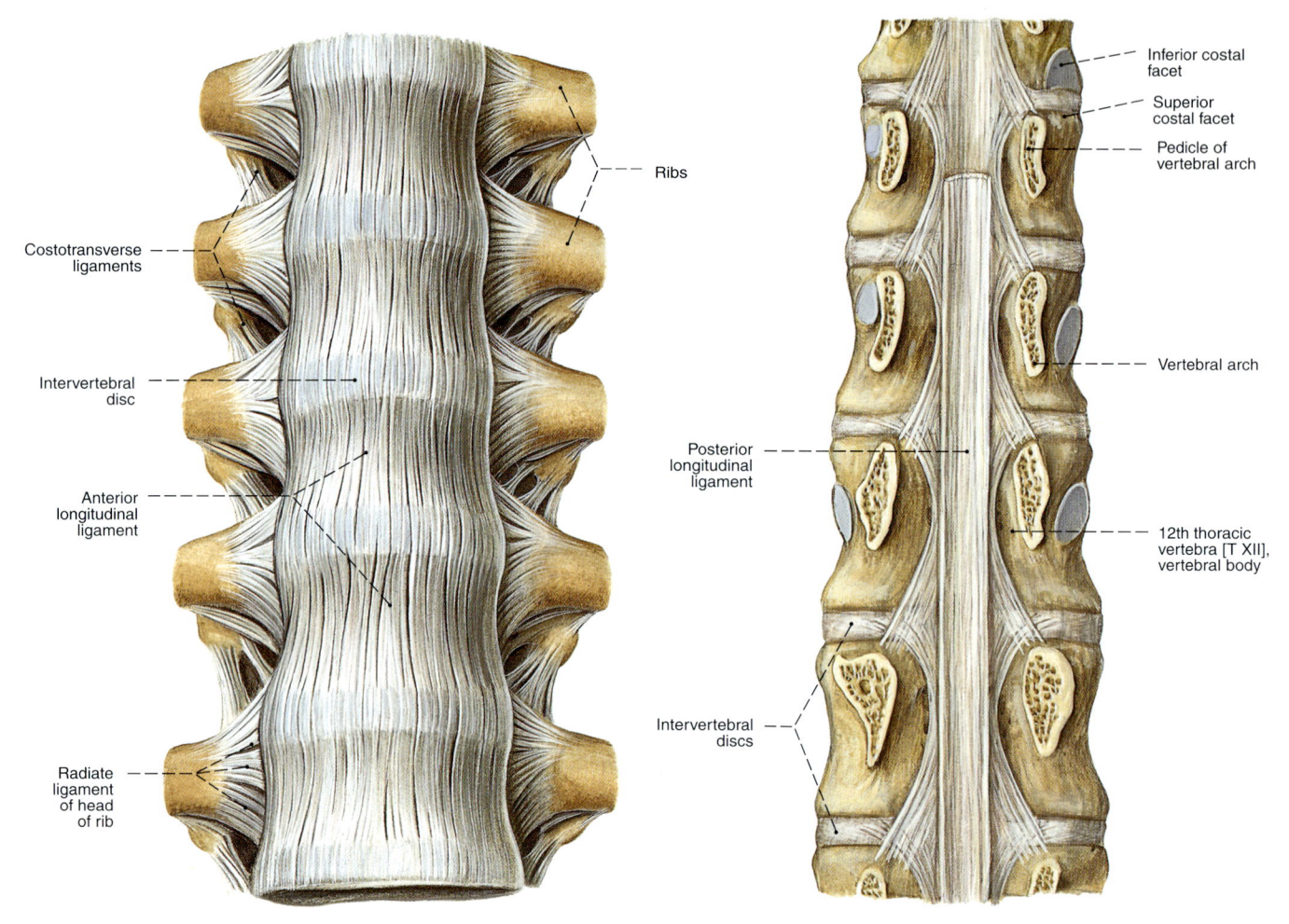

Fig. 760 Ligaments of vertebral column; e.g. in the lower thoracic vertebral column; ventral aspect.

Fig. 761 Ligaments of vertebral column; e.g. in the lower thoracic and the upper lumbar vertebral column; vertebral canal opened by a frontal section through pedicles; dorsal aspect.

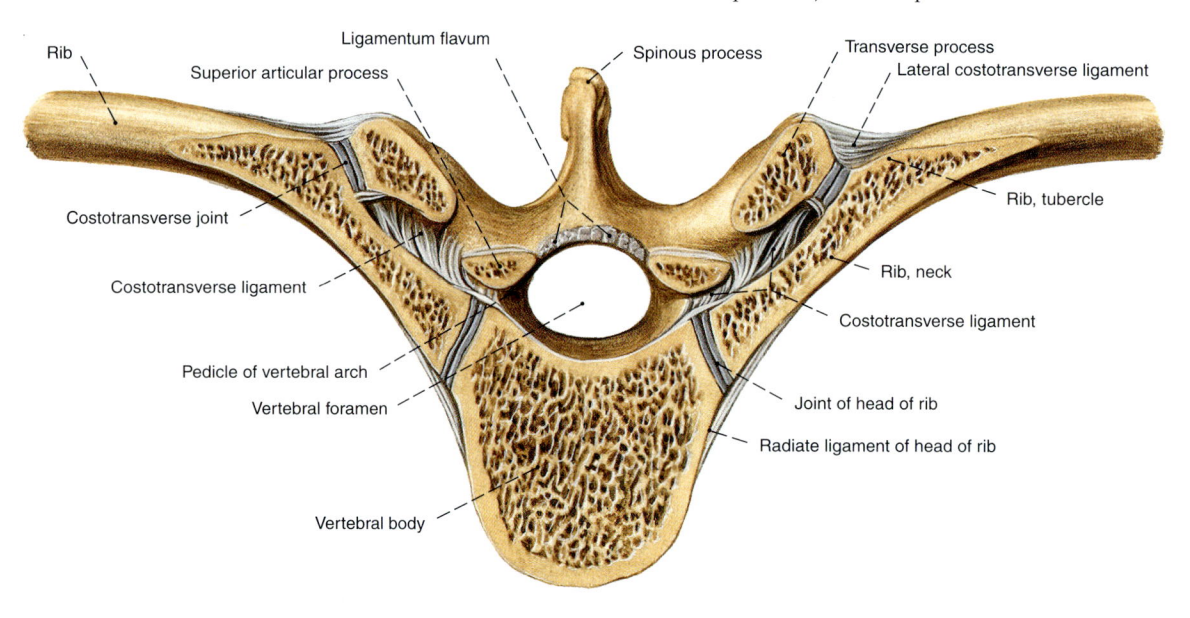

Fig. 762 Costovertebral joints; horizontal section at level of lower part of joint of head of rib; cranial aspect.

Ligaments of vertebral column 21

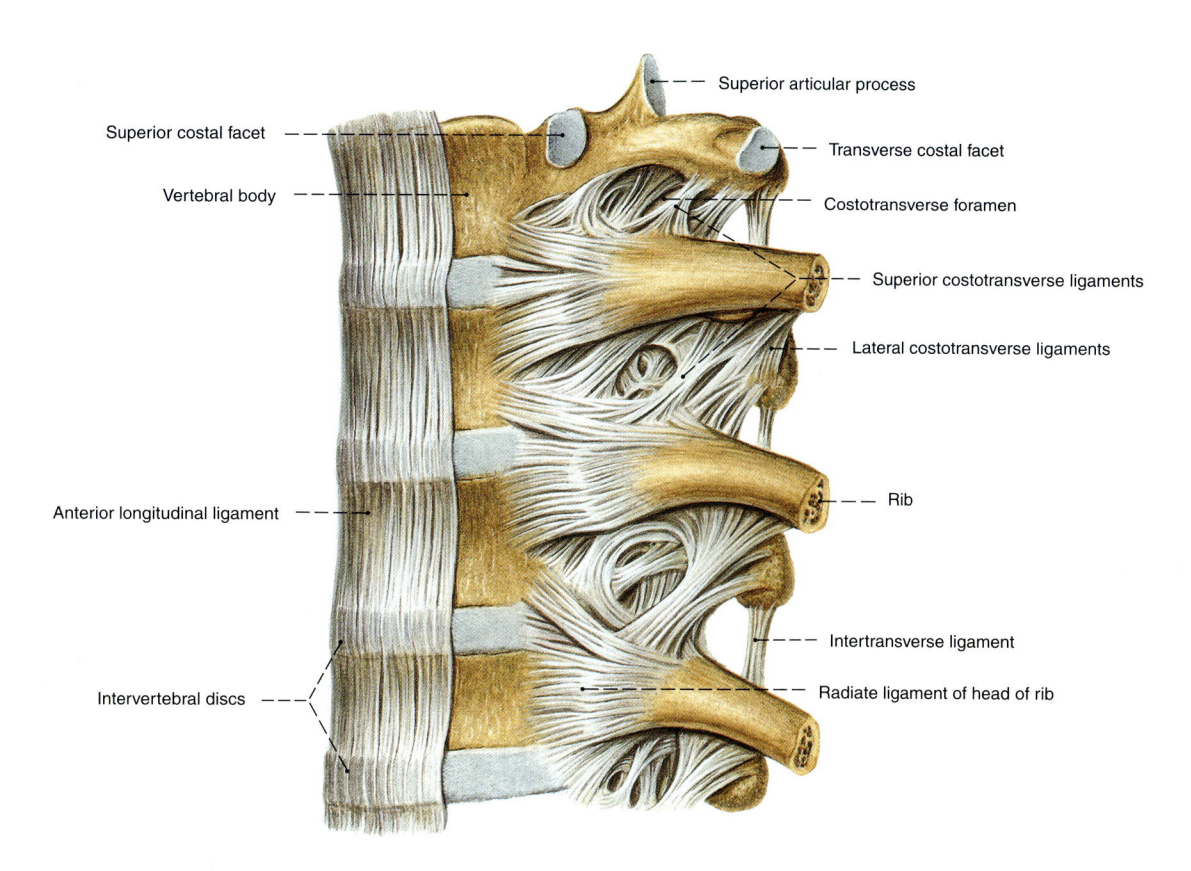

Fig. 763 Ligaments of vertebral column and costovertebral joints; lateral parts of anterior longitudinal ligament removed; left lateral aspect.

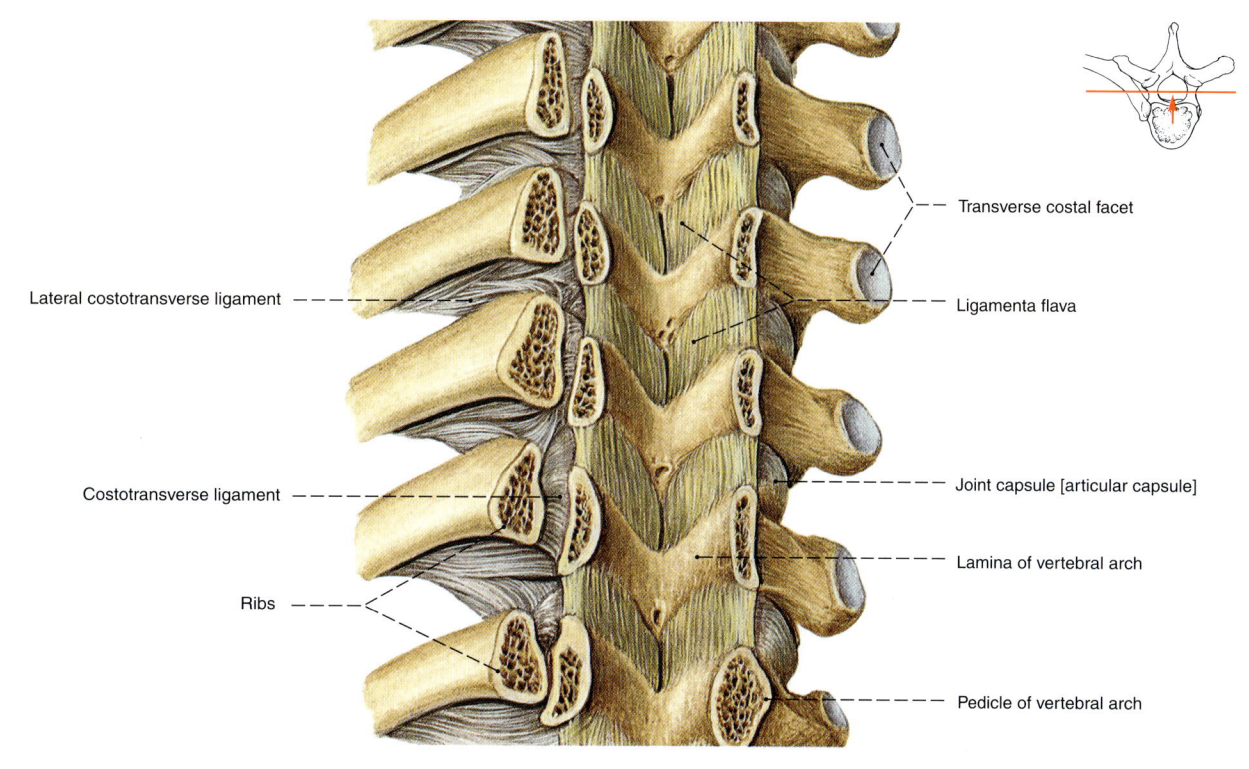

Fig. 764 Ligaments of vertebral arches; vertebral canal opened by a frontal section through pedicles; ventral aspect.

The ligamenta flava of the lumbar vertebra lie ventral to the zygapophysial joints, thus forming the posterior wall of the intervertebral foramina.

22 Back

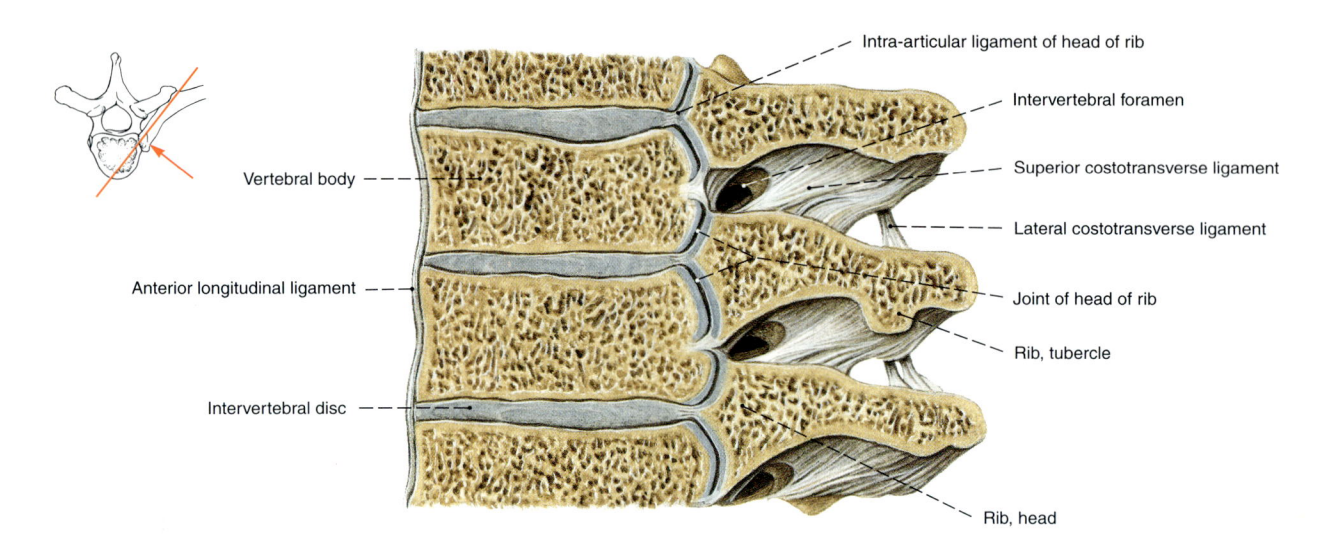

Fig. 765 Costovertebral joints; oblique vertical section through joints of heads of ribs; left lateral aspect.

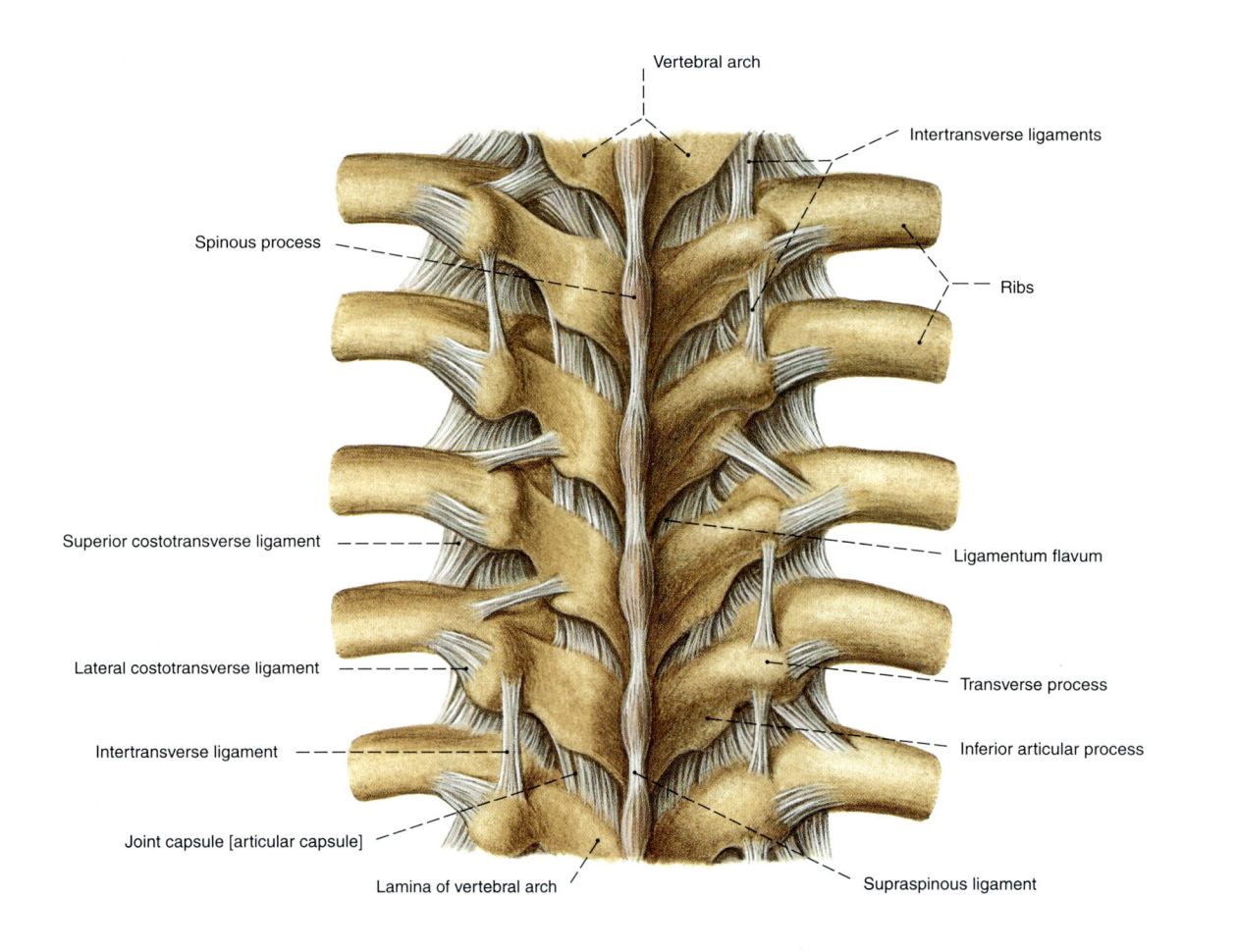

Fig. 766 Ligaments of vertebral arches and costovertebral joints; dorsal aspect.

Ligaments of vertebral column

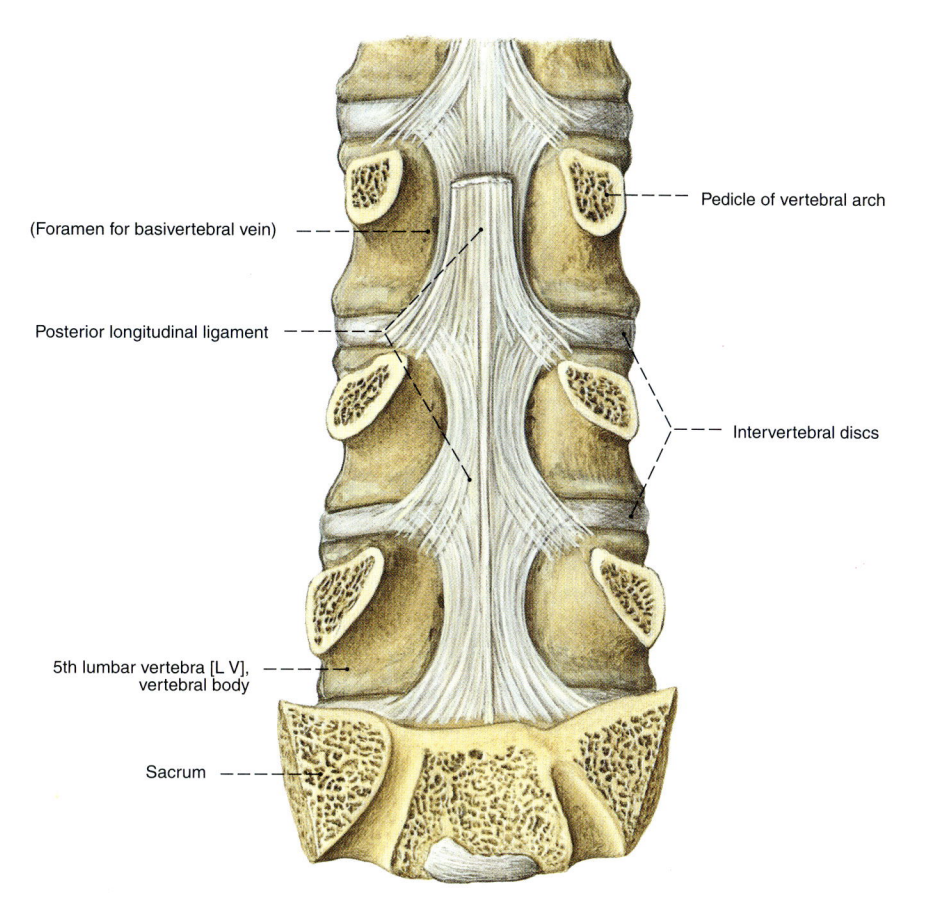

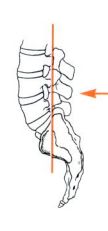

Fig. 767 Ligaments of lumbar vertebral column; vertebral canal opened; dorsal aspect.

Below the 2nd–3rd lumbar vertebrae the superficial layer of the posterior longitudinal ligament becomes a thin band, whereas the deep layer merges into the anulus fibrosus.

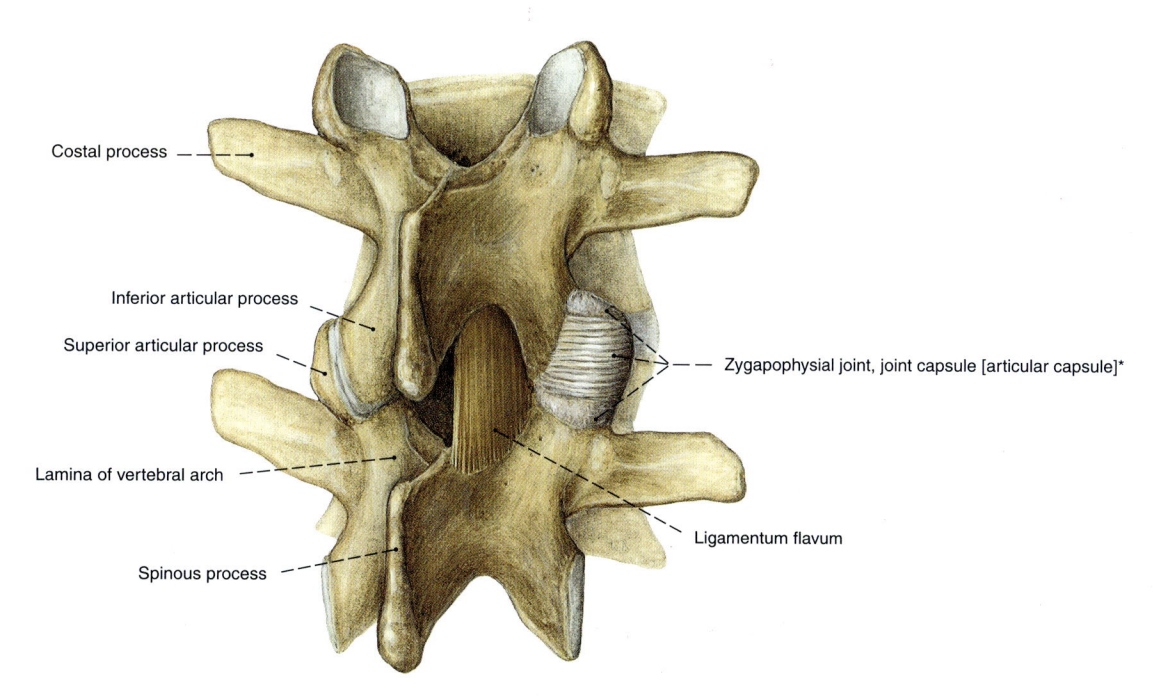

Fig. 768 Lumbar zygapophysial joints; ligamentum flavum removed on the left; right dorsal aspect.

* Only in the lumbar vertebral column are the zygapophysial joints strengthened by transverse running fibers ("transverse ligaments").

24 Back

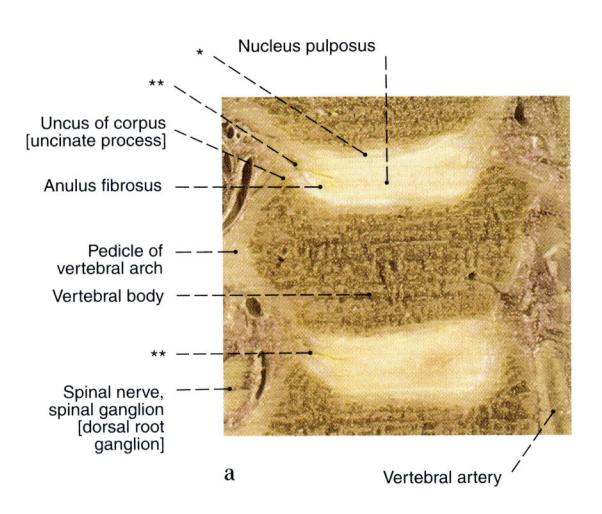

Fig. 769 a, b Intervertebral discs.
a Cervical intervertebral disc; frontal section at level of middle of vertebral body; ventral aspect (115%).
b Lumbar intervertebral disc; median section (115%).

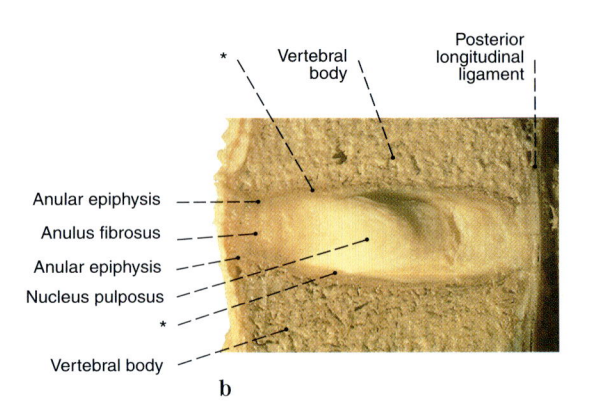

* Hyaline cartilaginous covers of end plates of vertebral bodies as non-ossified part of the epiphyses.
** Already in the first decade of life, clefts—the so-called "uncovertebral clefts"— develop in the lateral parts of the intervertebral discs. These clefts individually progress further medially in the following decades.

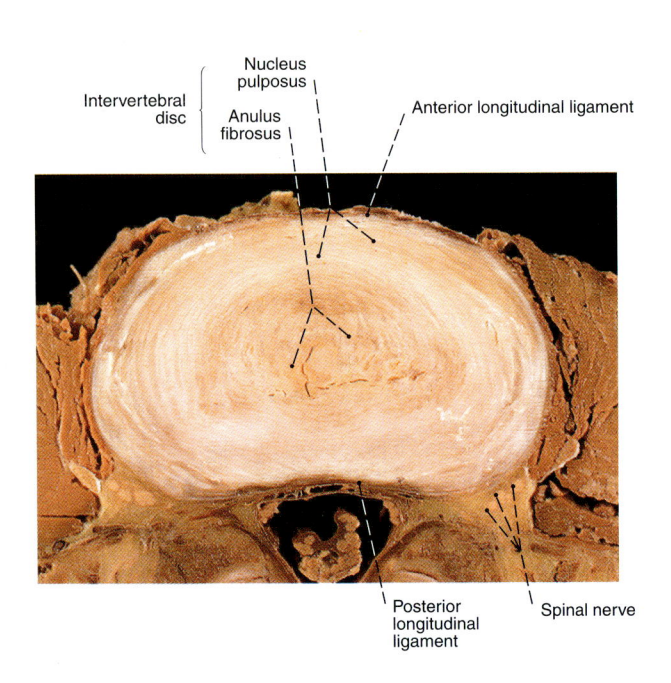

Fig. 770 Lumbar intervertebral disc; ventrocranial aspect (115%).

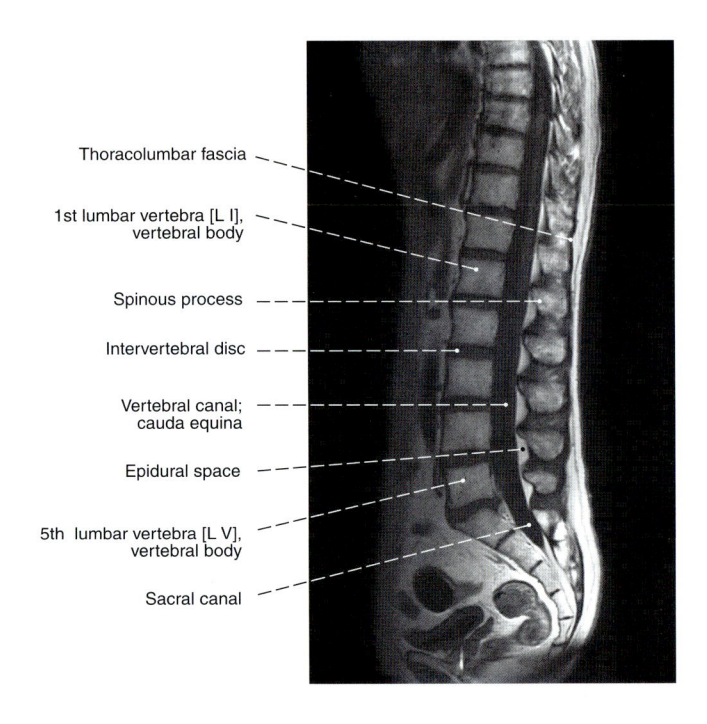

Fig. 771 Lumbar vertebral column; MRI; median section.

Intervertebral joints 25

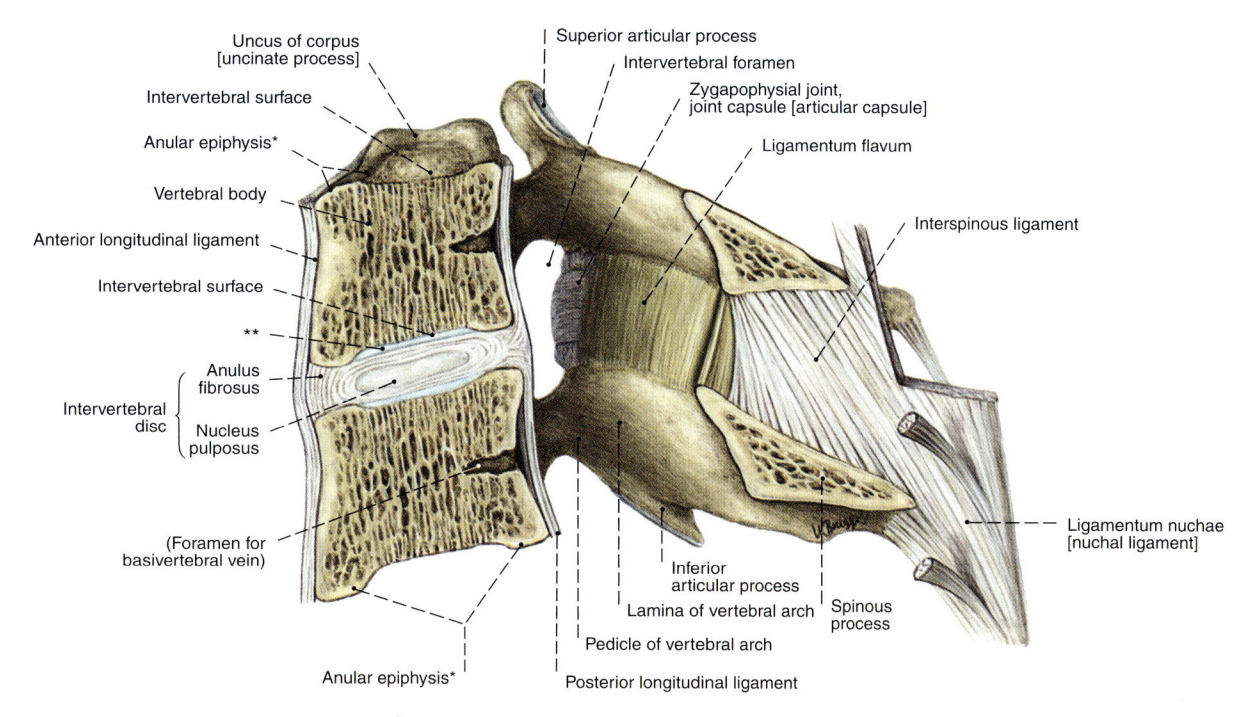

Fig. 772 Cervical intervertebral joints; diagram, median section (160%).

* Also: rim of vertebral body.
** Hyaline cartilaginous covers of end plates of vertebral bodies as non-ossified part of the epiphyses.

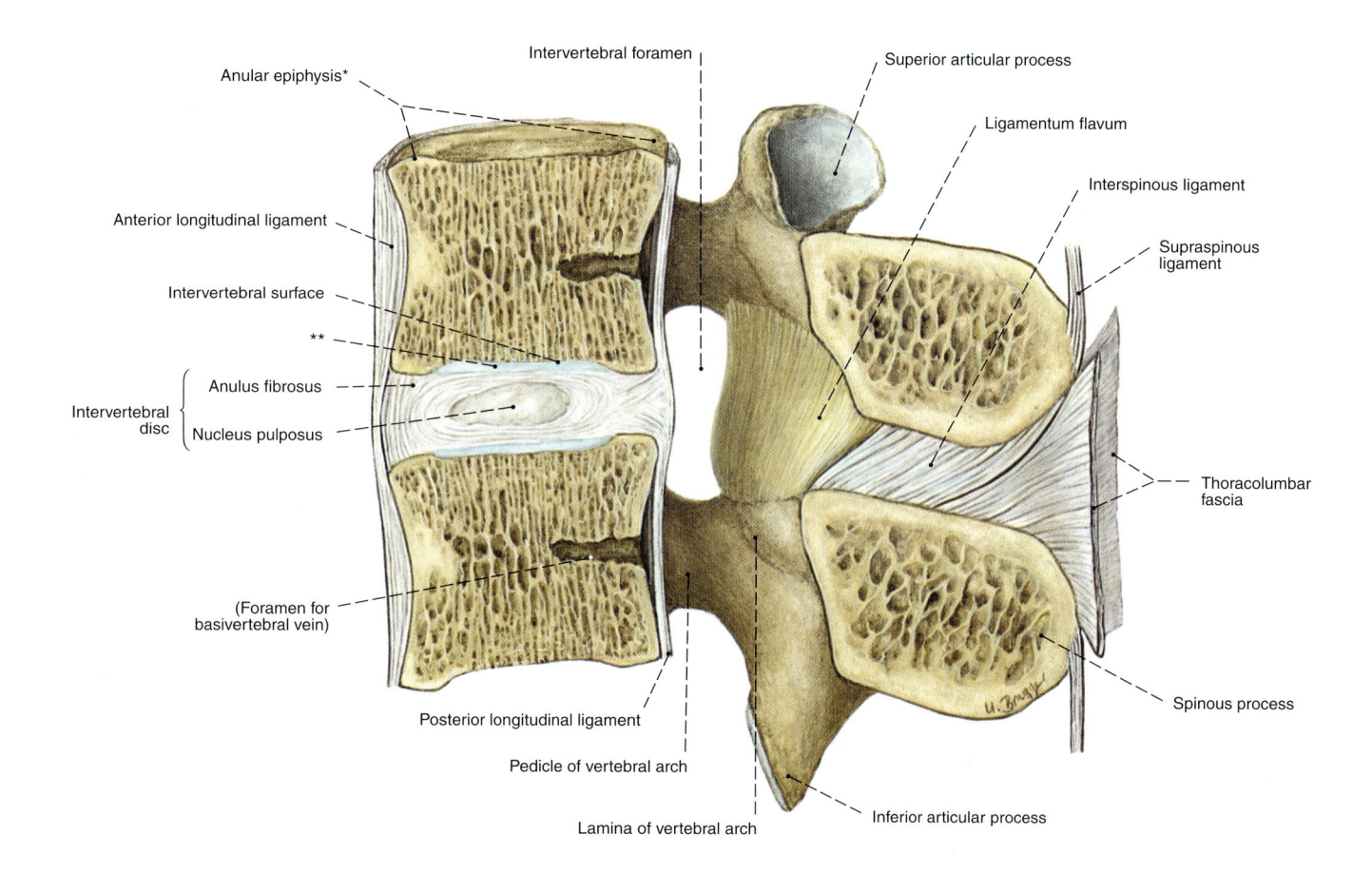

Fig. 773 Lumbar intervertebral joints; diagram, median section (120%).

* Also: rim of vertebral body.
** Hyaline cartilaginous covers of end plates of vertebral bodies as non-ossified part of the epiphyses.

26 Back

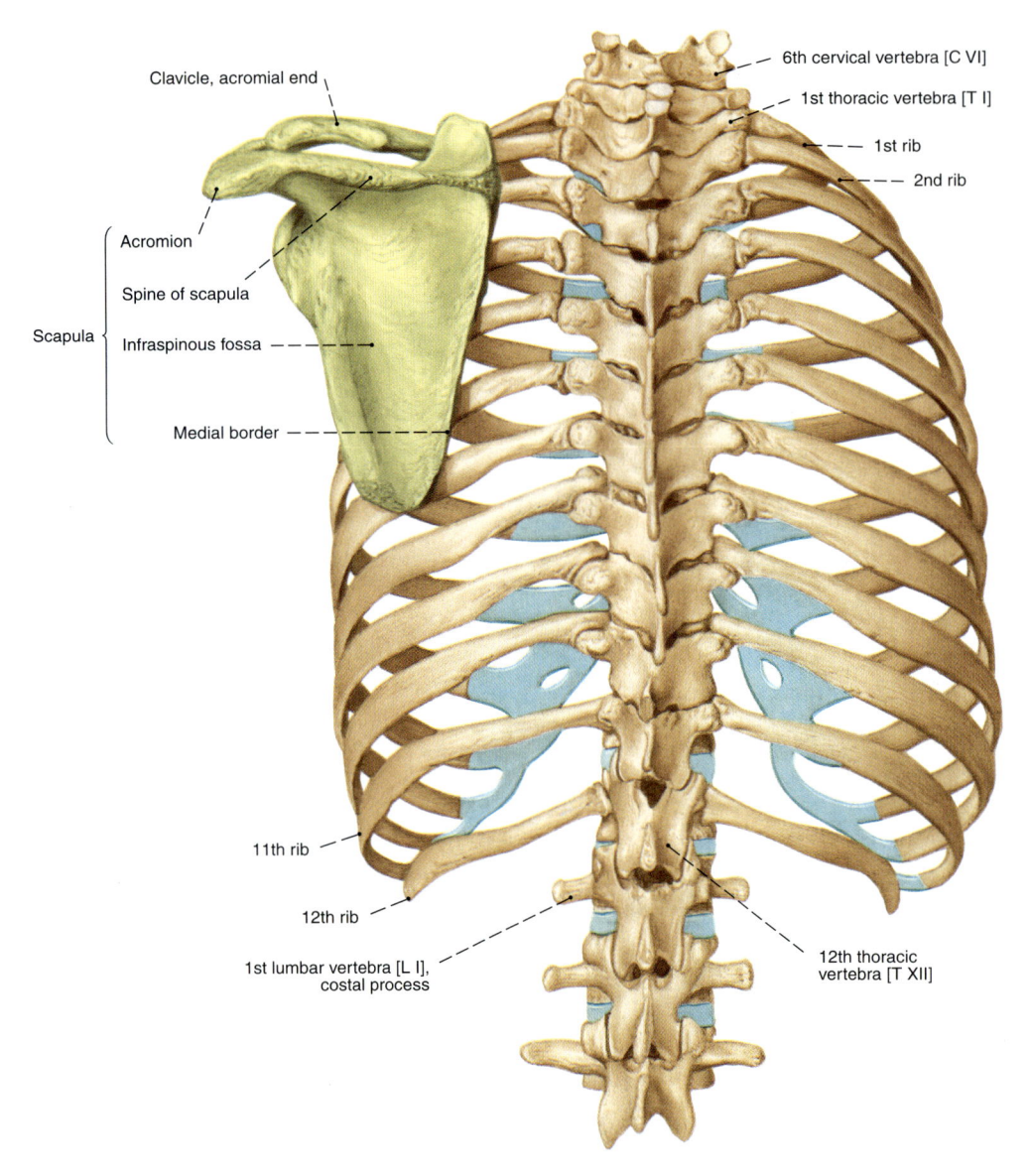

Fig. 774 Thoracic cage and left pectoral girdle [shoulder girdle]; dorsal aspect.

Trunk–pectoral girdle muscles (Figs. 775, 776)

The dorsal muscles of this group, trapezius, levator scapulae, rhomboid major, and rhomboid minor belong to the superficial muscles of the back according to their position; according to their development and innervation they are called immigrated muscles of the back. Serratus anterior muscle is located on the lateral thoracic wall and is hidden under the scapula when it courses dorsally.
The pectoralis minor and subclavius originate from the anterior thoracic wall. Both muscles are dealt with in the ventral muscles group of the shoulder.

Muscle *Innervation*	Origin	Insertion	Functions
1. Trapezius *Accessory nerve [XI] and direct branches from cervical plexus* In the area of origin between the middle and lower thoracic vertebrae a characteristic aponeurosis is developed.	**Descending part [superior part]:** squamous part of occipital bone (between highest and superior nuchal lines), spinous processes of upper cervical vertebrae (above ligamentum nuchae [nuchal ligament]) **Transverse part [middle part]:** spinous processes of lower cervical and upper thoracic vertebrae **Ascending part [inferior part]:** spinous processes of middle and lower thoracic vertebrae	**Descending part [superior part]:** clavicle (acromial third) **Transverse part [middle part]:** acromion **Ascending part [inferior part]:** spine of scapula	**Pectoral girdle [shoulder girdle]:** <u>Descending part [superior part]:</u> carry weight of shoulder girdle and arm (e.g. carrying a suitcase), elevation (e.g. inspiration) and upward rotation of scapula (for raising the arm above 90° - serratus anterior); when shoulder is fixed, rotation of head to contralateral side, both muscles together extend the cervical vertebral column <u>Transverse part [middle part]:</u> retraction of scapula <u>Ascending part [inferior part]:</u> depression of scapula and medial rotation <u>Vertebral column:</u> Transverse and ascending part of both sides together decrease thoracic kyphosis

Continued → S. 28

Muscles of back 27

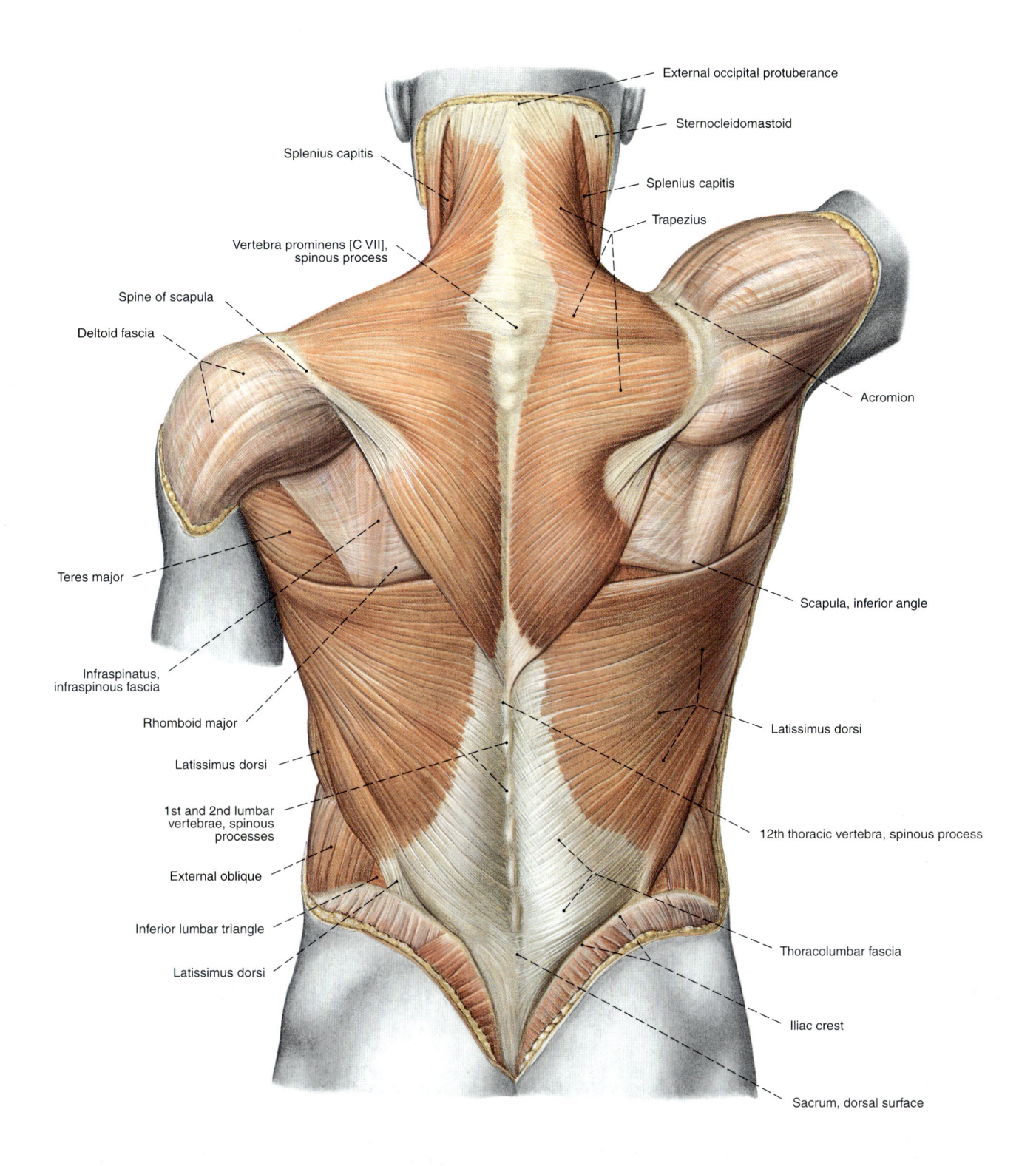

Fig. 775 Muscles of back; superficial layer of trunk-arm and trunk-pectoral girdle muscles; dorsal aspect.

Trunk – pectoral girdle muscles (continued)

Muscle *Innervation*	Origin	Insertion	Function
2. **Levator scapulae** *Direct branches from cervical plexus and dorsal scapular nerve (brachial plexus, supraclavicular part)*	Posterior tubercles of transverse processes of 1st-4th cervical vertebrae [C I-C IV]	Superior angle and immediate adjacent borders of scapula	**Pectoral girdle [shoulder girdle]:** elevation and medial rotation of scapula
3. **Rhomboid major** *Dorsal scapular nerve (brachial plexus, supraclavicular part)*	Spinous process of four upper thoracic vertebrae	Medial border of scapula (caudal to spine of scapula)	**Pectoral girdle [shoulder girdle]:** together with rhomboid minor retraction and elevation of scapula; together with serratus anterior fixation of scapula to trunk
4. **Rhomboid minor** *Dorsal scapular nerve (brachial plexus, supraclavicular part)*	Spinous process of 6th and 7th thoracic vertebrae	Medial border of scapula (cranial to spine of scapula)	**Pectoral girdle [shoulder girdle]:** together with rhomboid major, retraction and elevation of scapula; together with serratus anterior, fixation of scapula to trunk
5. **Serratus anterior** *Long thoracic nerve (brachial plexus, supraclavicular part)*	**Superior part:** 1st and 2nd ribs (slightly convergent) **Middle part:** 2nd-4th ribs (divergent) **Inferior part:** 5th-8th (9th) ribs (much convergent)	**Superior part:** superior angle of scapula **Middle part:** medial border of scapula **Inferior part:** inferior angle of scapula	**Pectoral girdle [shoulder girdle]:** All parts: protraction of scapula; together with rhomboid fixation of scapula to trunk (scapula alata or winged scapula when one part is paralyzed) Superior part: elevation Middle part: depression Inferior part: depression, lateral rotation (for elevation of arm above 90°) **Thorax:** When scapula is fixed elevation of ribs (inspiration)

Trunk – arm muscles (Fig. 775)

This group comprises the latissimus dorsi and pectoralis major muscles. Both originate from the trunk and course to the arm. Because of the position of its muscle belly, the latissimus dorsi belongs to the superficial muscles of back; like them it has immigrated from ventral.

The pectoralis major originates from the thoracic wall and is dealt with among the other ventral muscles of the shoulder.

Muscle *Innervation*	Origin	Insertion	Function
Latissimus dorsi *Thoracodorsal nerve (brachial plexus, supraclavicular part)*	Spinous processes of six lower thoracic vertebrae, all lumbar vertebrae (via thoracolumbar fascia), dorsal surface of sacrum, outer lip of iliac crest (dorsal third), (9th) 10th-12th rib; frequently from inferior angle of scapula	Crest of lesser tubercle [medial lip] (with a flat tendon spiraling around the teres major tendon; the two tendons separated by the subtendinous bursa of latissimus dorsi)	**Glenohumeral joint [shoulder joint]:** Adduction, medial rotation, extension **Pectoral girdle [shoulder girdle]:** Retraction and depression of scapula

Spinocostal muscles (Fig. 776)

The spinocostal muscles, serratus posterior superior and serratus posterior inferior lie superficial to the deep muscles of back.

Muscle *Innervation*	Origin	Insertion	Function
1. **Serratus posterior superior** *Ventral rami of cervical nerves [C 6] to thoracic nerve [T 2]*	Spinous process of 6th and 7th cervical and 1st and 2nd thoracic vertebrae	2nd-5th rib (lateral to angle of rib)	Elevation of 2nd-5th ribs (inspiration)
2. **Serratus posterior inferior** *Ventral rami of thoracic nerves [T 11] to lumbar nerve [L 2]*	Spinous process of 11th and 12th thoracic and 1st and 2nd lumbar vertebrae	9th-12th rib (caudal border)	Depression of 9th-12th rib (expiration); counteracts the diaphragm also in forced inspiration

Muscles of back 29

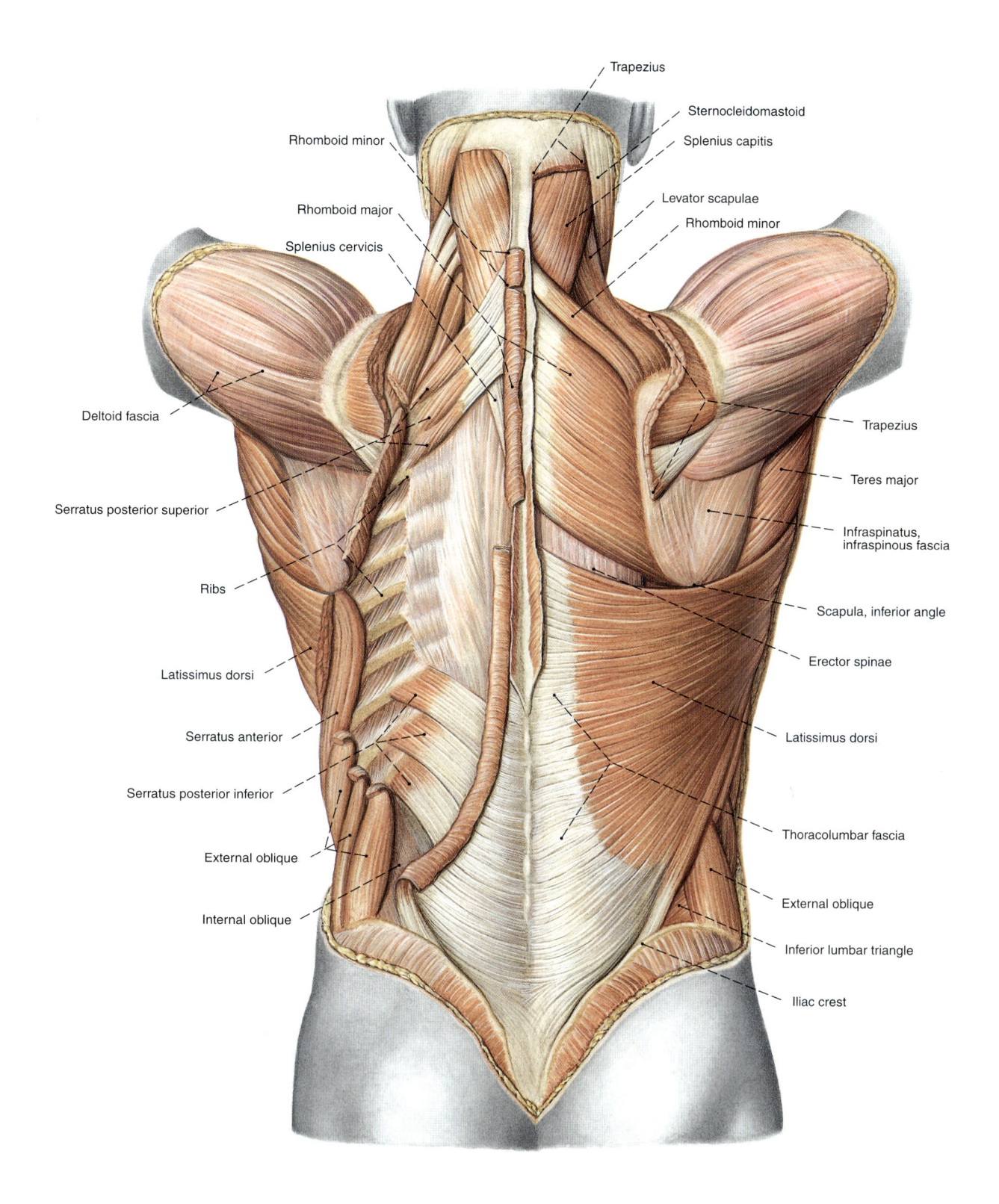

Fig. 776   Muscles of back; deep layer of trunk-arm and trunk-pectoral girdle muscles after extensive removal of superficial muscles on the left; dorsal aspect.

Back

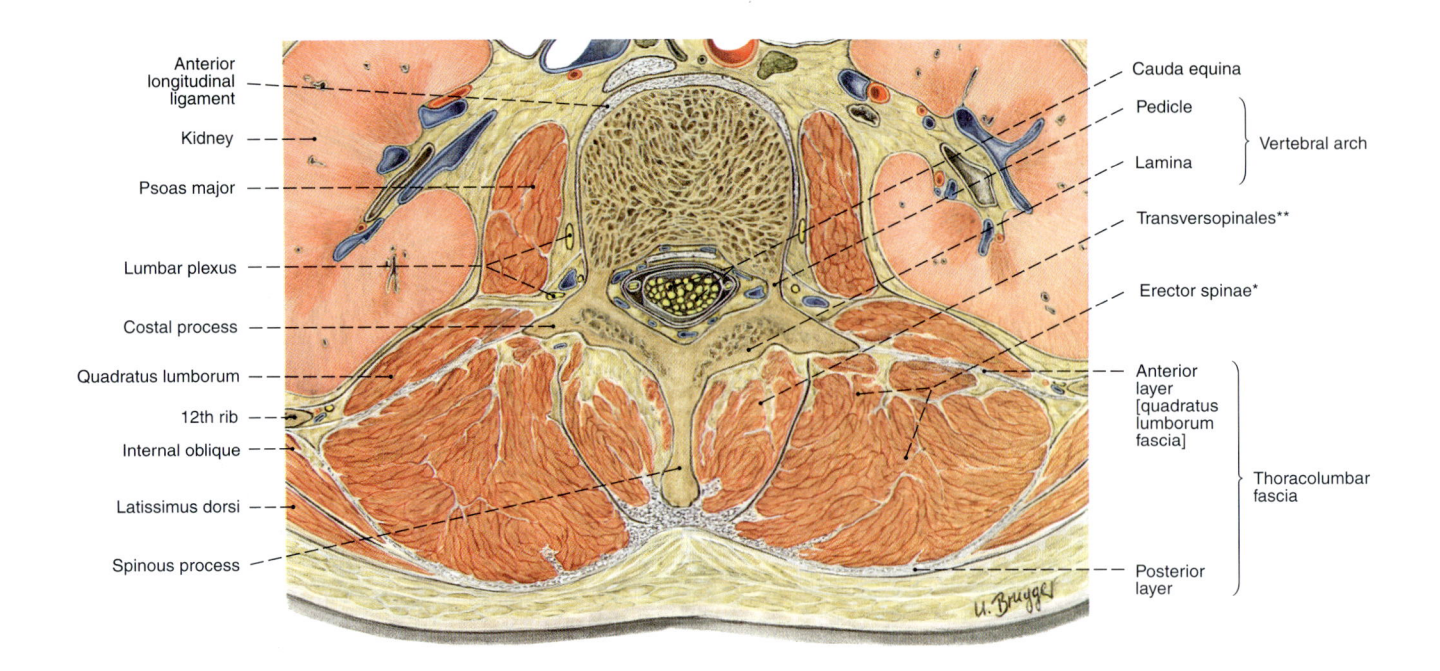

Fig. 777 Muscles of back; horizontal section at level of 2nd lumbar vertebra; caudal aspect.

The muscles of back proper lie in an osseofibrous tube, which is formed by dorsal parts of the vertebrae and by the thoracolumbar fascia. The muscles are grouped into a lateral* and medial tract**.

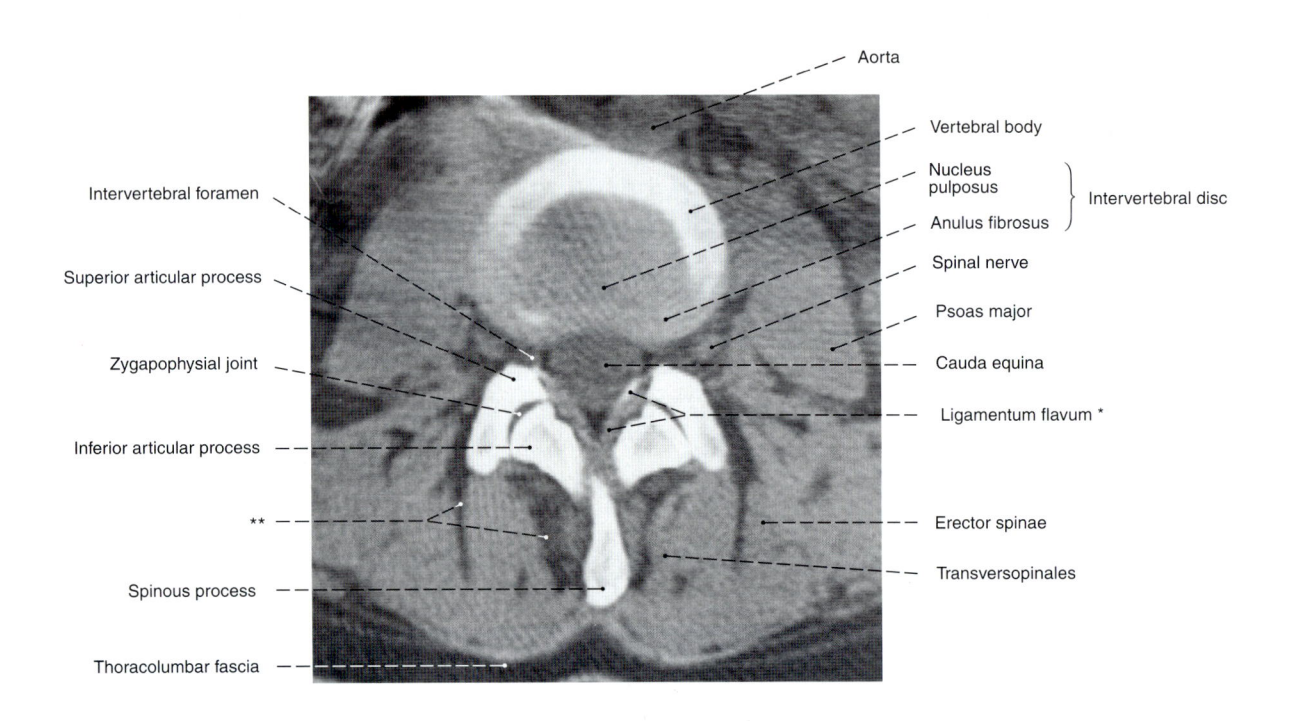

Fig. 778 Muscles of back; horizontal CT section at level of intervertebral disc between 3rd and 4th lumbar vertebrae; caudal aspect.

* Calcification or ossification at the sites of attachment of the ligamenta flava frequently occurs even in younger individuals.
** Fatty deposits.

Muscles of back 31

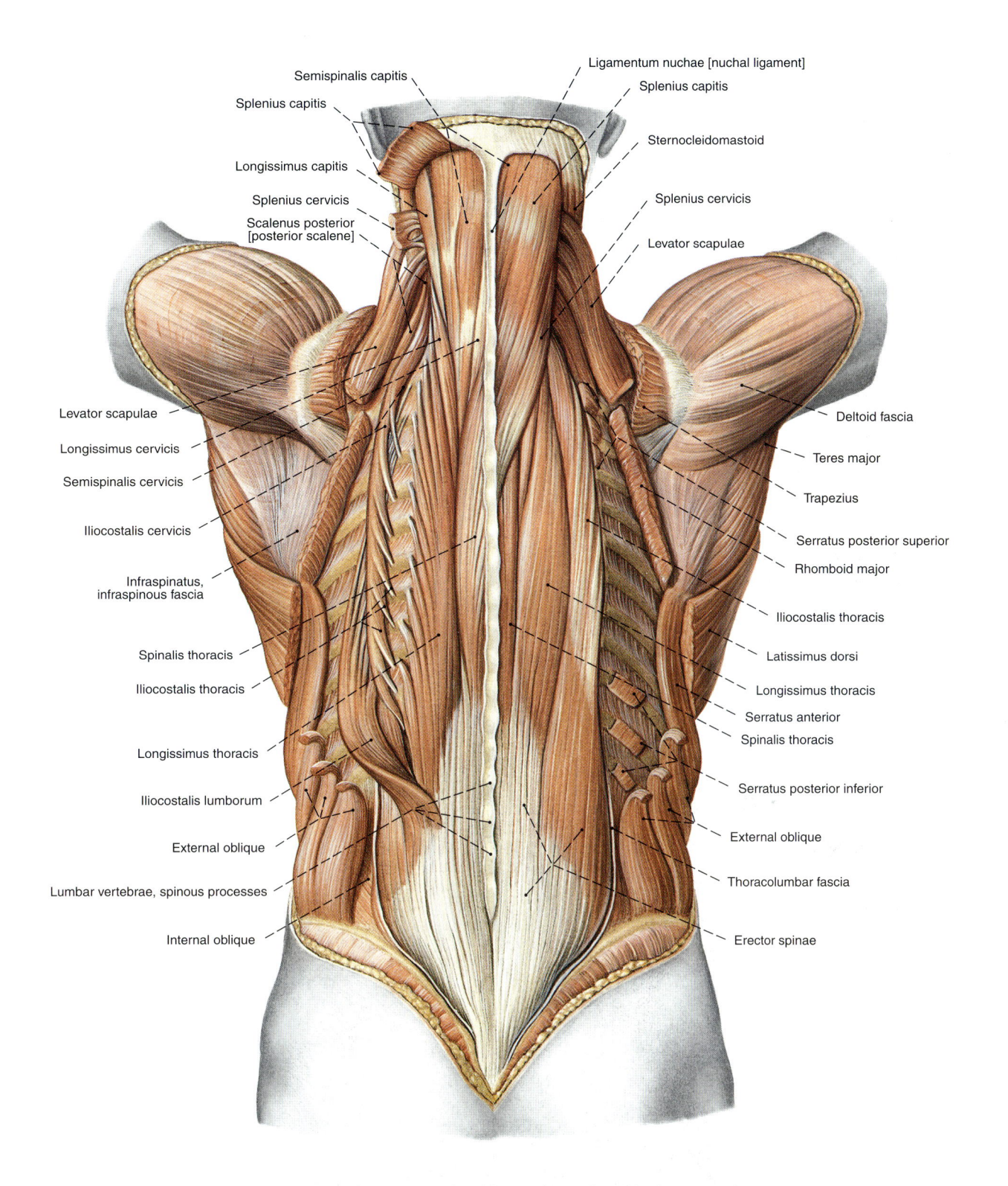

Fig. 779 Muscles of back; superficial layer of muscles of back proper after removal of posterior layer of thoracolumbar fascia and overlying trunk-arm and trunk-pectoral girdle muscles; dorsal aspect.

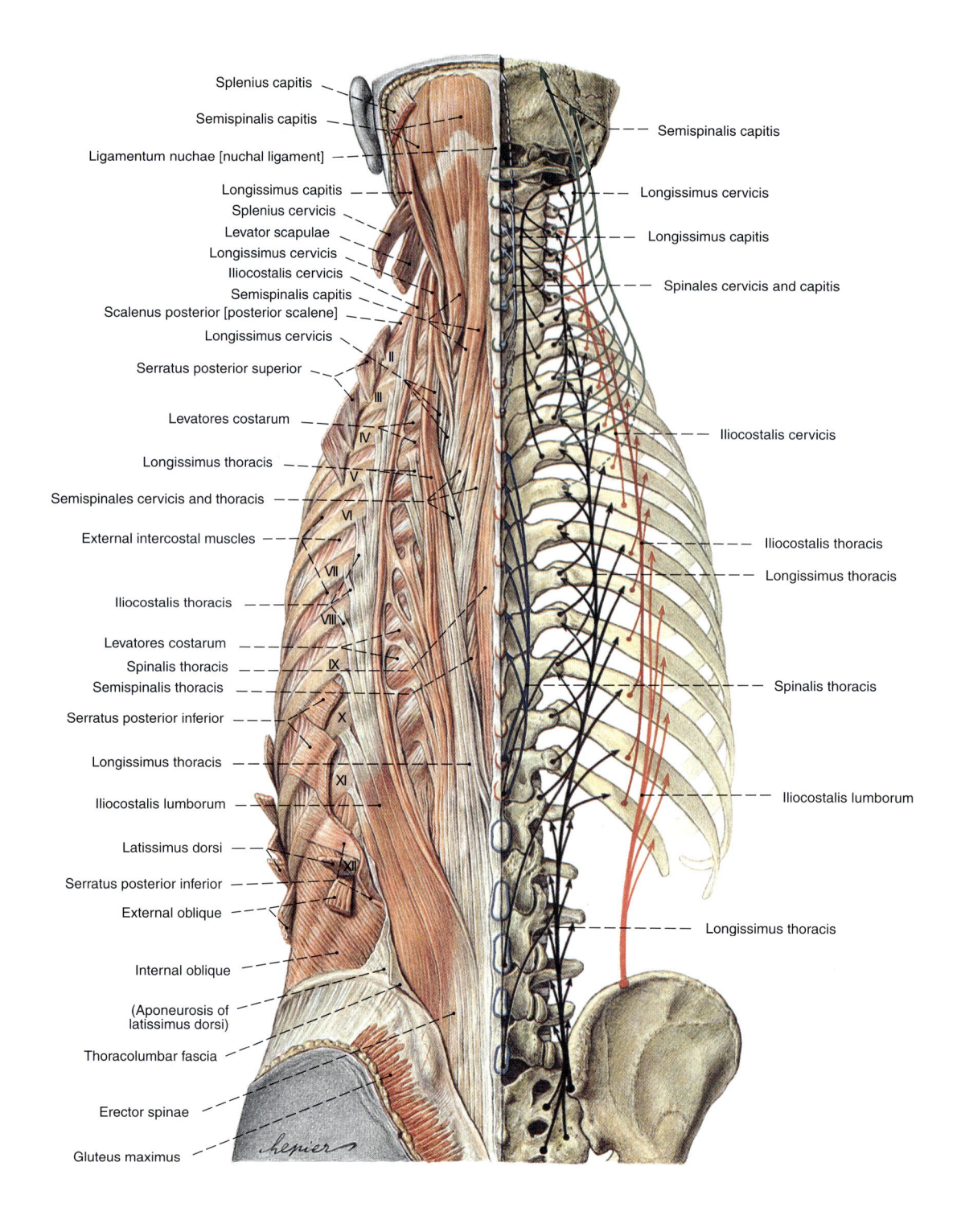

Fig. 780 Muscles of back; long parts of muscles of back proper after removal of posterior layer of thoracolumbar fascia and overlying trunk arm and trunk pectoral girdle muscles; schematic courses of muscles on the right; spinous processes of cervical vertebrae in green, of thoracic vertebrae in red, and of lumbar vertebrae in blue; II – XII = ribs; dorsal aspect.

33 Muscles of back

Muscles of back proper, lateral tract (Figs. 779, 780)

The lateral tract of muscles of back proper covers the medial tract and thus is also called the superficial part of the muscles of back proper. These comprise the straight running iliocostalis, longissimus, and intertransversarii. The splenius muscles diverge obliquely cranial (spinotransversales). The levatores costarum course obliquely caudal to the ribs.

Muscle/Innervation	Origin	Insertion	Function
1. **Iliocostalis lumborum** *Posterior rami [dorsal rami] of lumbar nerves*	Together with the longissimus thoracis from the spinous processes of lumbar vertebrae, dorsal surface of sacrum, iliac crest (dorsal third, thoracolumbar fascia	5th–12th ribs (at angle of rib)	
2. **Iliocostalis thoracis** *Posterior rami [dorsal rami] of thoracic nerves*	12th–7th ribs (medial to angle of rib)	(6th)7th–1st ribs (at angle of rib)	
3. **Iliocostalis cervicis** *Posterior rami [dorsal rami] of spinal nerves* The longissimus thoracic blends with longissimus cervicis and spinalis.	7th–(4th) 3rd ribs (medial to angle of rib)	Posterior tubercles of transverse processes of 6th–(4th) 3rd cervical vertebrae	
4. **Longissimus thoracis** *Posterior rami [dorsal rami] of spinal nerves*	Together with iliocostalis lumborum from spinous processes of lumbar vertebrae, dorsal surface of sacrum; frequently from mammillary processes of 2nd and 1st lumbar vertebrae and transverse processes of 12th–6th thoracic vertebrae	Medial part: mammillary processes of 5th lumbar vertebra, accessory processes of 4th–1st lumbar vertebrae, transverse processes of thoracic vertebrae; Lateral part: costal processes of 4th–1st lumbar vertebrae, thoracolumbar fascia (anterior layer [quadratus lumborum fascia]), 12th–2nd ribs (medial to angle of rib)	
5. **Longissimus cervicis** *Posterior rami [dorsal rami] of spinal nerves*	Transverse processes of 6th–1st thoracic and 7th–3rd cervical vertebrae	Posterior tubercle of transverse processes of 5th–2nd cervical vertebrae	Acting unilateral: lateral flexion Acting bilateral: extension
6. **Longissimus capitis** *Posterior rami [dorsal rami] of spinal nerves*	Transverse processes of 3rd thoracic–3rd cervical vertebrae	Mastoid process (posterior border)	
7. **Lateral lumbar intertransversarii** *Posterior and anterior rami [dorsal and ventral rami] of spinal nerves*	Iliac tuberosity, costal and accessory processes of 5th–1st lumbar vertebrae, transverse process of 12th thoracic vertebra	Costal process of 5th lumbar vertebra, transverse process of 12th thoracic vertebra	
8. **Medial lumbar intertransversarii** *(see no. 7)*	Accessory processes of 4th–1st lumbar vertebrae	Mammillary processes of 4th–2nd lumbar vertebrae	
9. **Thoracic intertransversarii** *(see no. 7)*	Transverse processes of 12th–10th lumbar vertebrae.	Accessory and mammillary processes of 1st lumbar vertebra up to transverse process of 11th thoracic vertebra	
10. **Posterior cervical intertransversarii** *(see no. 7)*	Posterior tubercles of transverse processes of 6th–1st cervical vertebrae	Posterior tubercles of transverse processes of 7th–2nd cervical vertebrae	
11. **Anterior cervical intertransversarii** *(see no. 7)*	Anterior tubercles of transverse processes of 6th–1st cervical vertebrae	Anterior tubercles of transverse processes of 7th–2nd cervical vertebrae	
12. **Splenius cervicis** *Posterior rami [dorsal rami] of cervical nerves*	Spinous processes of 3rd thoracic up to 7th cervical vertebrae, ligamentum nuchae [nuchal ligament] (from 3rd cervical vertebra)	Posterior tubercles of transverse processes of (3rd)2nd–1st cervical vertebra	Acting unilateral: lateral flexion, rotation of cervical vertebral column and head to ipsilateral side;
13. **Splenius capitis** *Posterior rami [dorsal rami] of cervical nerves*	Spinous processes of 6th to 3rd cervical vertebrae, supraspinous ligament	Mastoid process, superior nuchal line	Acting bilateral: extension of cervical vertebral column
14. **Levatores costarum** *Posterior rami [dorsal rami] of 8th cervical nerve [C 8] and of thoracic nerves* Levatores costarum longi are missing in the middle thoracic region.	Transverse processes of 11th thoracic to 7th cervical vertebrae (levatores costarum longi extend over two ribs, levatores costarum breves insert in the next caudal rib)	12th–1st ribs (lateral to angle of rib)	Elevation of ribs; lateral flexion and rotation of vertebral column

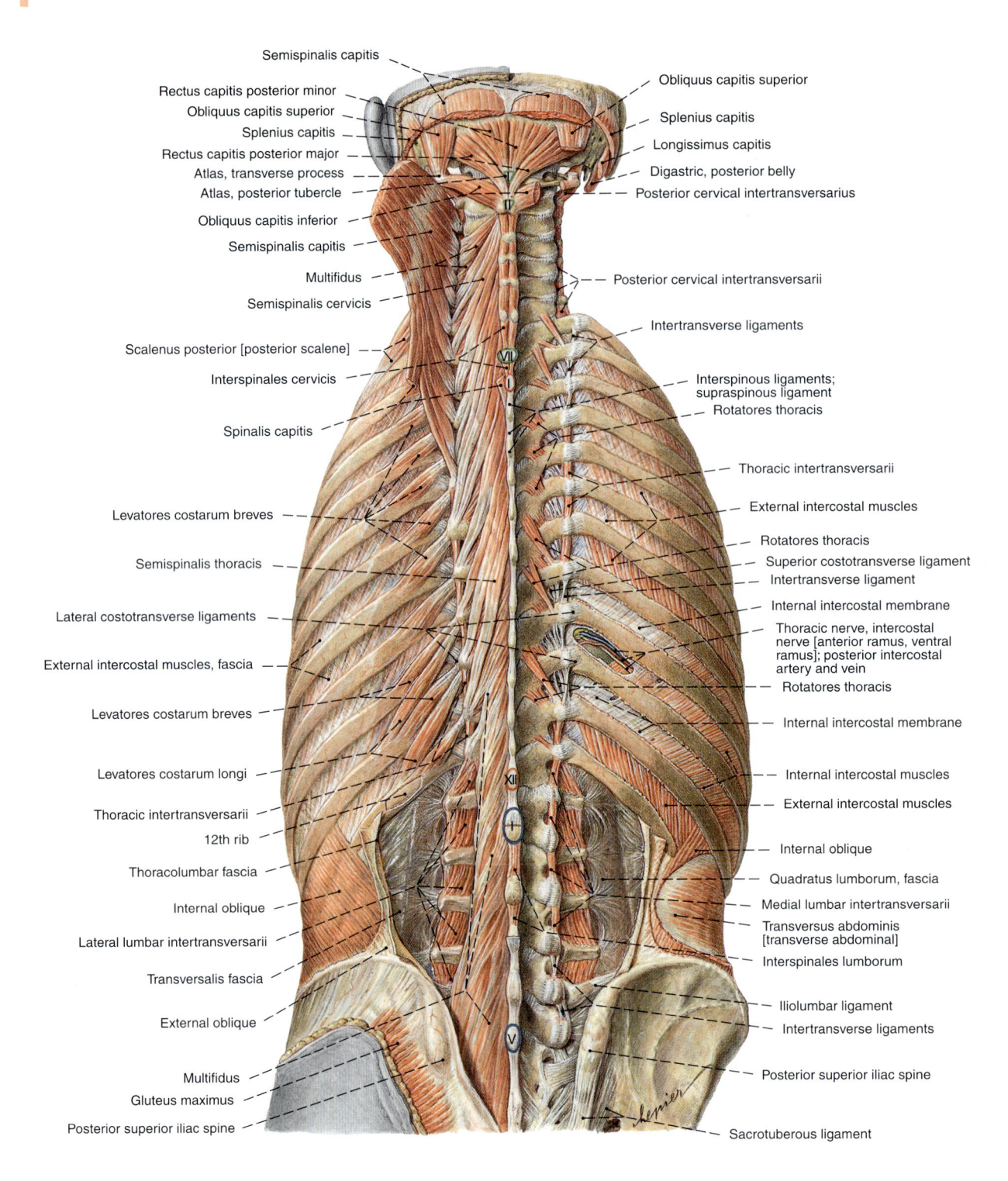

Fig. 781 Muscles of back and suboccipital muscles; deep layer after removal of all superficial muscles and thoracolumbar fascia; 9th intercostal space partially opened; dorsal aspect. Roman numerals indicate spinous processes of respective vertebrae.

Muscles of back proper, medial tract (Figs. 780, 781)

The medial tract of muscles of back lies deep to the lateral tract and thus is also called the deep part of the muscles of back proper. These comprise the straight running interspinales and spinalis. The rotatores, multifidus, and semispinalis converge obliquely cranial (transversospinales).

Muscle *Innervation*	Origin	Insertion	Function
1. **Interspinales lumborum** *Posterior rami [dorsal rami] of spinal nerves*	Spinous processes of 5th–1st lumbar vertebrae	Median sacral crest (superior border), spinous process of 5th–2nd lumbar vertebrae	Segmental extension
2. **Interspinales thoracis** *Posterior rami [dorsal rami] of spinal nerves*	Spinous processes of (12th)11th–2nd (1st) thoracic vertebrae	Spinous process of (1st lumbar) 12th–3rd (2nd) thoracic vertebrae	
3. **Interspinales cervicis** *Posterior rami [dorsal rami] of spinal nerves*	Spinous processes of 7th–2nd cervical vertebrae	Spinous process of 1st thoracic –3rd cervical vertebrae	
4. **Spinalis thoracis** *Posterior rami [dorsal rami] of spinal nerves*	Spinous processes of (3rd) 2nd, 1st lumbar and 112th–10th thoracic vertebrae (blends with longissimus thoracis)	Spinous process of (10th) 9th–2nd thoracic vertebrae (blends with multifidus)	
5. **Spinalis cervicis** *Posterior rami [dorsal rami] of spinal nerves*	Spinous processes of (4th)3rd–1st thoracic and 7th–6th cervical vertebrae	Spinous process of 6th (5th)–2nd cervical vertebrae	Acting unilateral: lateral flexion; Acting bilateral: extension
6. **Spinalis capitis** *Posterior rami [dorsal rami] of spinal nerves* *(inconstant muscle)*	Spinous processes of 3rd–1st thoracic and 7th–6th cervical vertebrae	Squamous part of occipital bone (between highest and superior nuchal lines near to external occipital protuberance)	
7. **Rotatores** *Posterior rami [dorsal rami] of spinal nerves* The rotatores comprise: rotatores cervicis, rotatores thoracis, and rotatores lumborum (inconstant)	Mammillary processes of lumbar vertebrae, transverse processes of thoracic vertebrae, inferior articular processes of cervical vertebrae (rotatores longi extend over two vertebrae, rotatores breves insert in the next cranial vertebra)	Spinous process (roots) of 3rd–1st lumbar, 12th–1st thoracic, and 7th–2nd cervical vertebrae	Acting unilateral: segmental lateral flexion, rotation Acting bilateral: extension
8. **Multifidus** *Posterior rami [dorsal rami] of spinal nerves*	Dorsal surface of sacrum, posterior sacroiliac ligament, iliac crest (dorsal part), mammillary processes of lumbar vertebrae, inferior articular processes of 7th–4th cervical vertebrae (fibers extend over two-four vertebrae)	Spinous process of 5th–1st lumbar, 12th–1st thoracic, and 7th–2nd cervical vertebrae	
9. **Semispinalis thoracis** *Posterior rami [dorsal rami] of spinal nerves*	Transverse processes of (12th) 11th–7th (6th) thoracic vertebrae	Spinous processes of 3rd thoracic–6th cervical vertebrae	
10. **Semispinalis cervicis** *Posterior rami [dorsal rami] of spinal nerves*	Transverse processes of (7th) 6th thoracic–7th cervical vertebrae	Spinous processes of 6th–2nd cervical vertebrae	Acting unilateral: rotation of vertebral column and head to contralateral side
11. **Semispinalis capitis** *Posterior rami [dorsal rami] of spinal nerves*	Transverse processes of (8th) 7th thoracic–3rd cervical vertebrae	Squamous part of occipital bone (between highest and superior nuchal lines, medial part)	Acting bilateral: extension

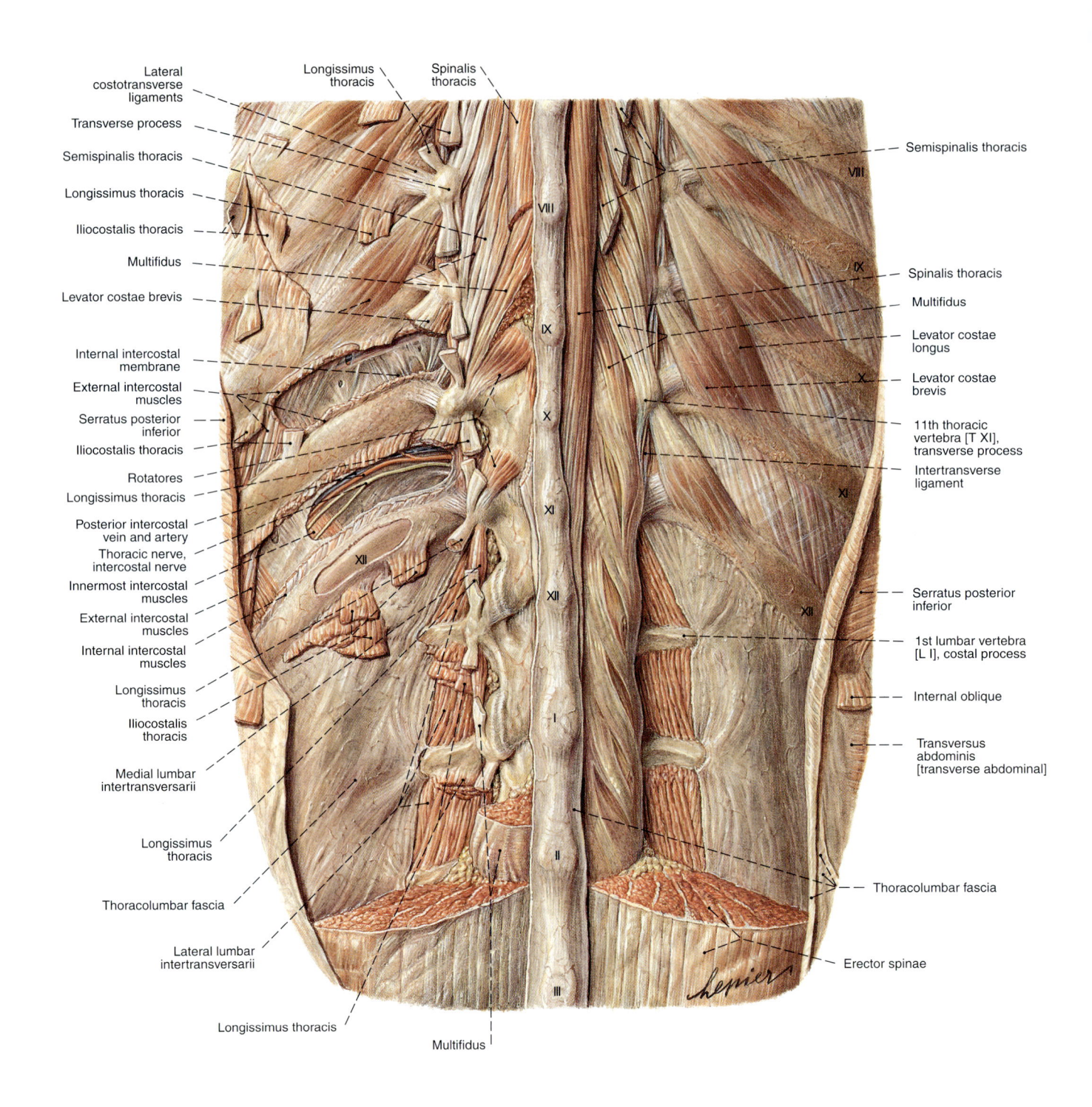

Fig. 782 Muscles of back; stepwise exposure of muscles of back proper and muscles of trunk between 8th and 12th thoracic vertebrae (VIII–XII) and 1st to 3rd lumbar vertebrae (I–III); 11th intercostal space partially opened; dorsal aspect.

Muscles of back 37

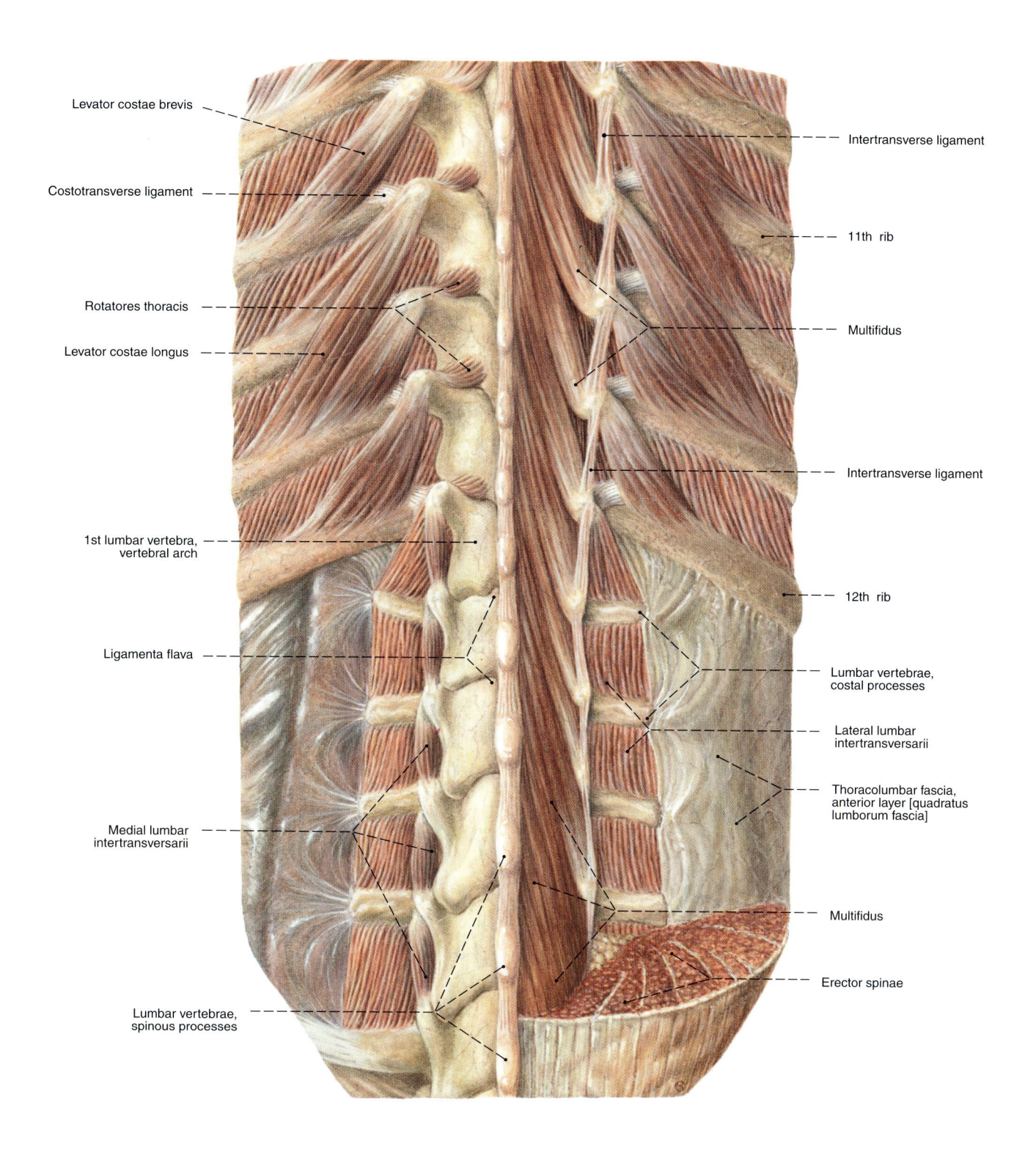

Fig. 783 Muscles of back; deepest layer in the region of lower thoracic and upper lumbar vertebrae after removal of thoracolumbar fascia; dorsal aspect.

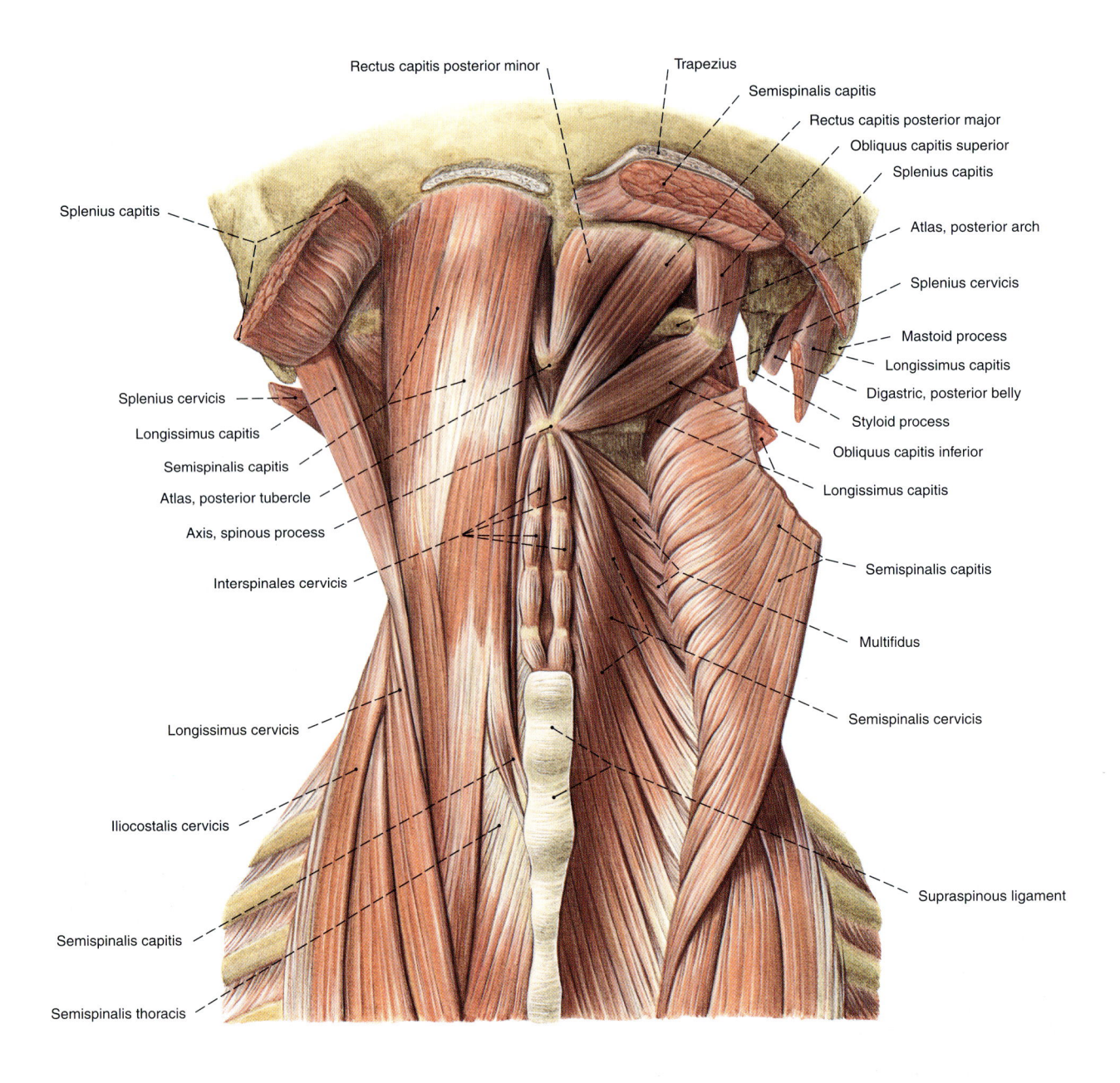

Fig. 784 Muscles of back and suboccipital muscles; after removal of some superficial muscles; dorsal aspect.

Muscles of back 39

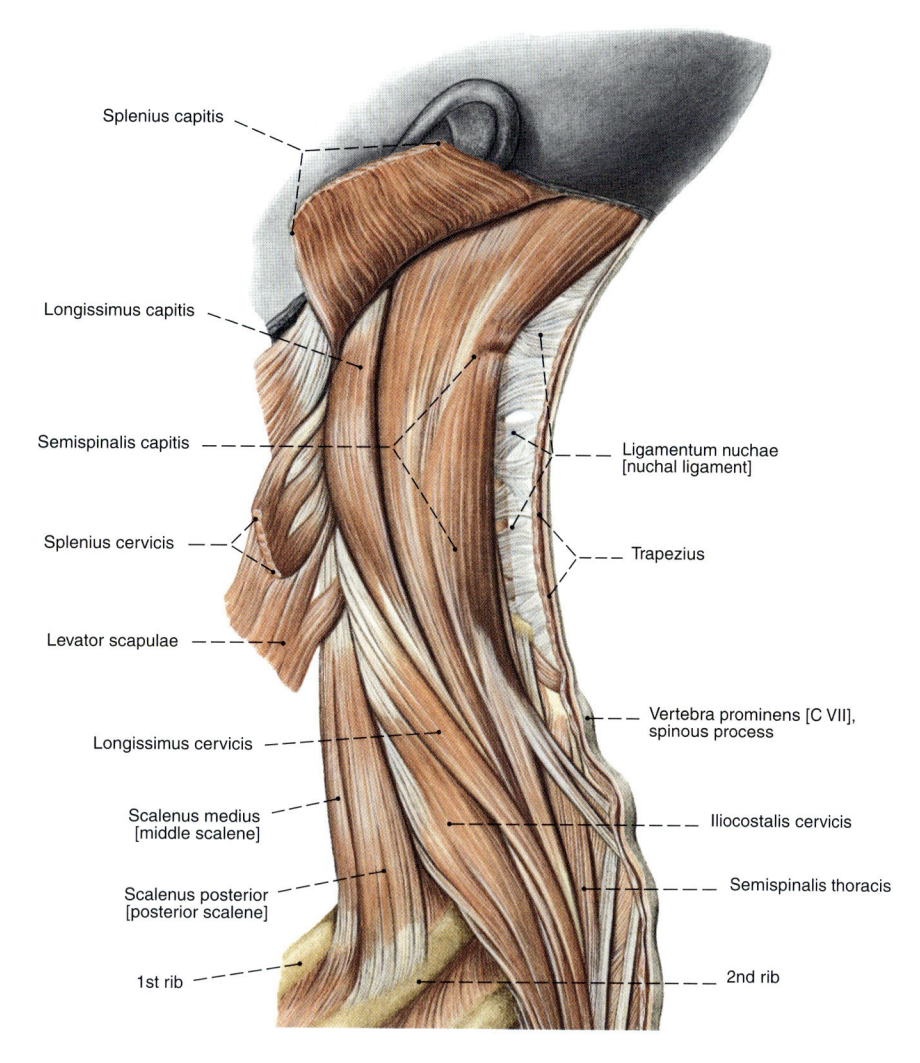

Fig. 785 Muscles of back and neck; after removal of superficial muscles of back; left lateral aspect.

Suboccipital muscles (Figs. 784, 786)

The medial tract of the muscles of back proper comprise the rectus capitis posterior minor and major, and the obliquus capitis superior and inferior, the rectus capitis lateralis belongs to the lateral tract.

Muscle/*Innervation*	Origin	Insertion	Function
1. **Rectus capitis posterior major** *Suboccipital nerve (dorsal ramus of 1st cervical nerve [C 1]*	Spinous process of axis	Inferior nuchal line (medial third)	They act together in fine control of position and kinematics of craniocervical joints
2. **Rectus capitis posterior minor** *Suboccipital nerve (see no. 1)*	Posterior tubercle of posterior arch of atlas	Inferior nuchal line (medial third)	
3. **Obliquus capitis superior** *Suboccipital nerve (see no. 1)*	Posterior tubercle of transverse process of atlas	Inferior nuchal line (lateral third)	
4. **Obliquus capitis inferior** *Suboccipital nerve (see no. 1)*	Spinous process of axis	Transverse process of atlas (posterior border)	
5. **Rectus capitis lateralis** *Cervical nerve (ventral ramus of 1st cervical nerve [C 1]*	Transverse process of atlas (anterior border)	Jugular process of occipital bone	

40 Back

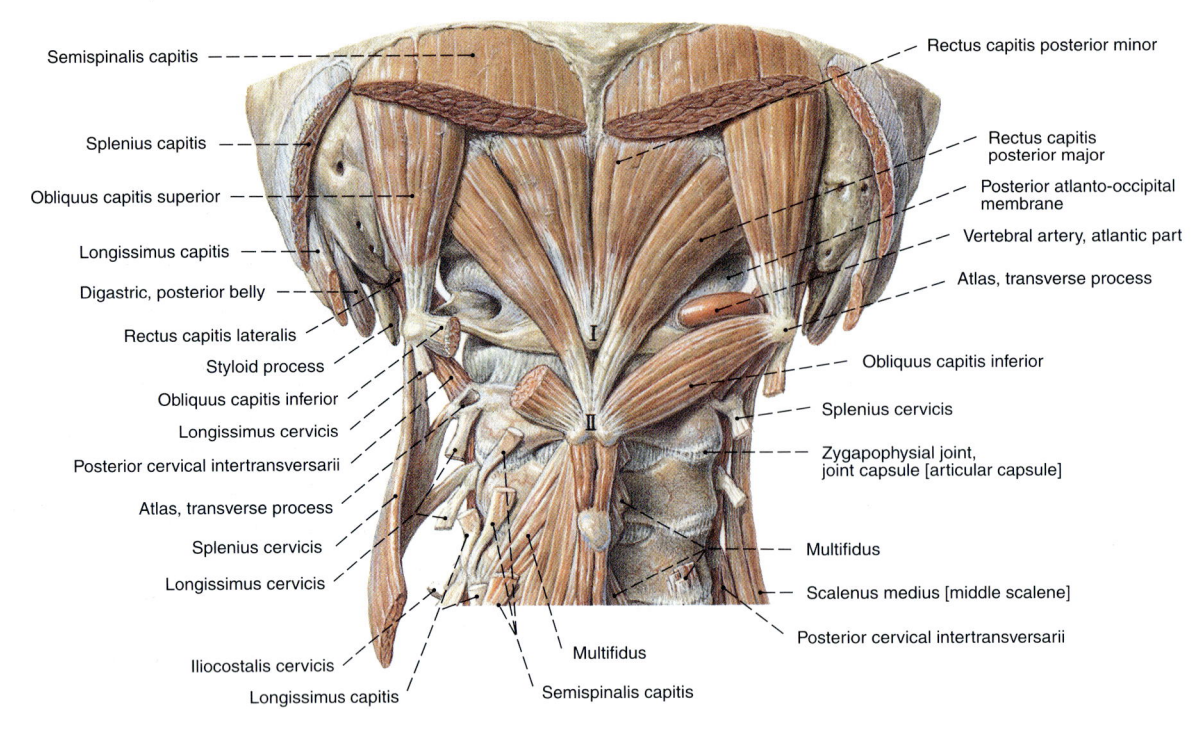

Fig. 786 Suboccipital muscles; dorsal aspect.
I = Posterior tubercle of atlas
II = Spinous process of axis

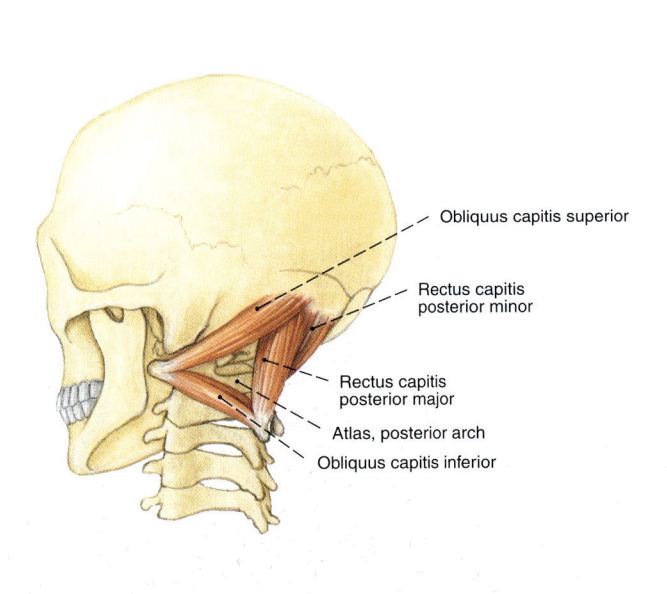

Fig. 787 Suboccipital muscles; semischematic diagram; dorsolateral aspect.

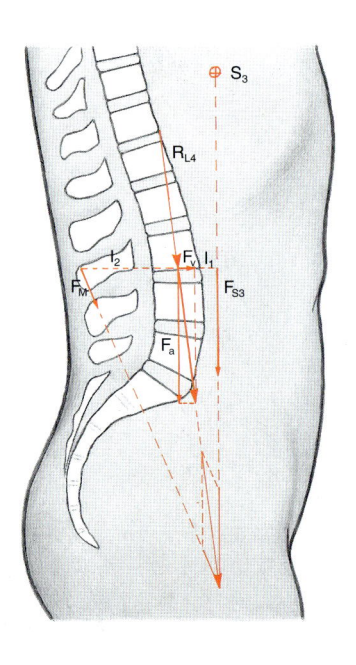

S_3 Center of gravity of 3/6 parts of body weight
F_{S3} Force of body weight effective in lumbar vertebral column
R_{L4} Resulting force effective in intervertebral joints L3/L4
F_M Force of muscles of back
F_V Ventral directed shear-stress effective in zygapophysial joints
F_a Axial pressure force effective in intervertebral disc and vertebral body
l_1 Lever arm of parts of body weight effective in lumbar vertebral column in upright position
l_2 Lever arm of muscles of back

Fig. 788 Load of lumbar vertebral column in upright position.

Horizontal sections through vertebral column 41

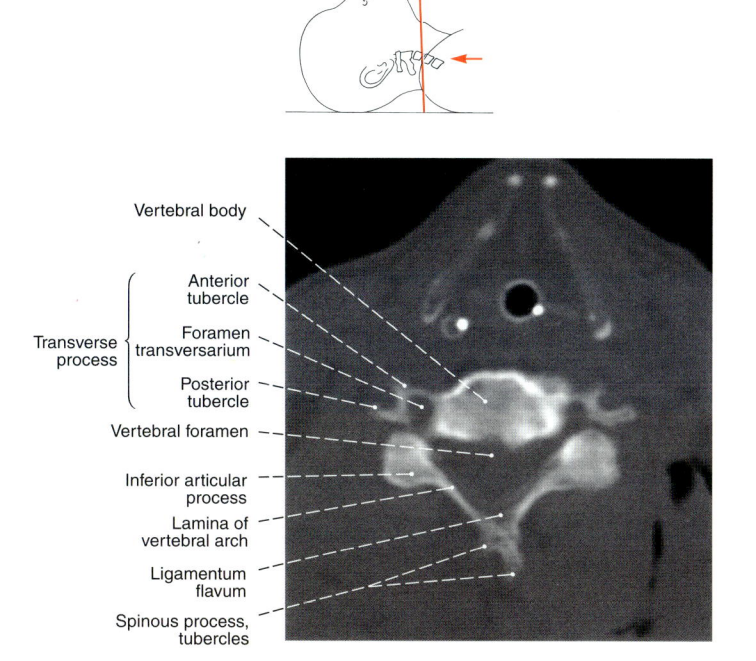

Fig. 789 Cervical vertebral column; computer tomographic horizontal section at level of intervertebral disc between 4th and 5th cervical vertebrae; caudal aspect.

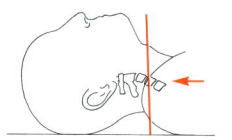

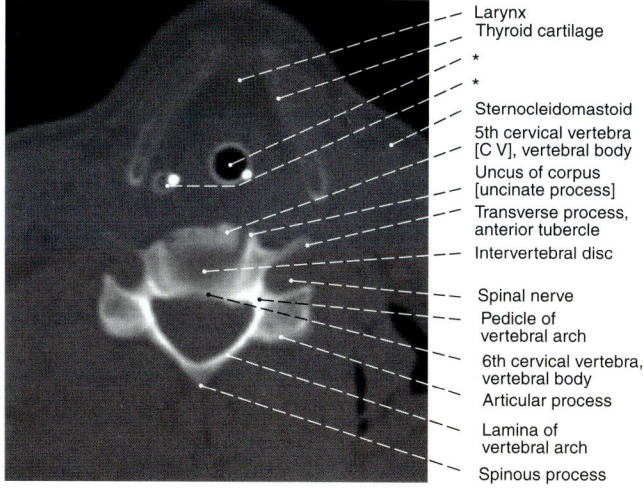

Fig. 790 Cervical vertebral column; computer tomographic horizontal section at level of 5th/6th cervical vertebrae; caudal aspect.

* Respiratory tube and endoscopic instrument.

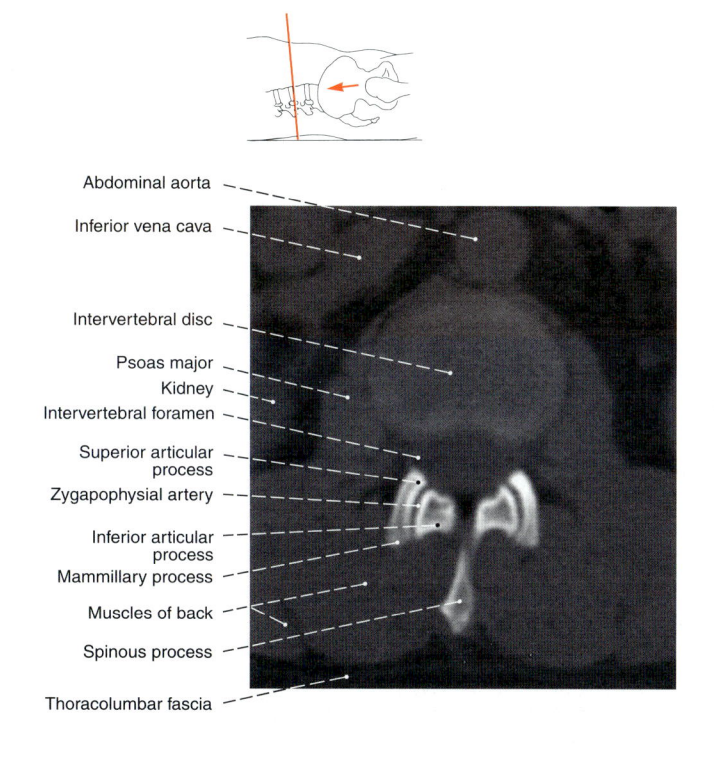

Fig. 791 Lumbar vertebral column; computer tomographic horizontal section at level of intervertebral disc between 2nd and 3rd lumbar vertebrae; caudal aspect.

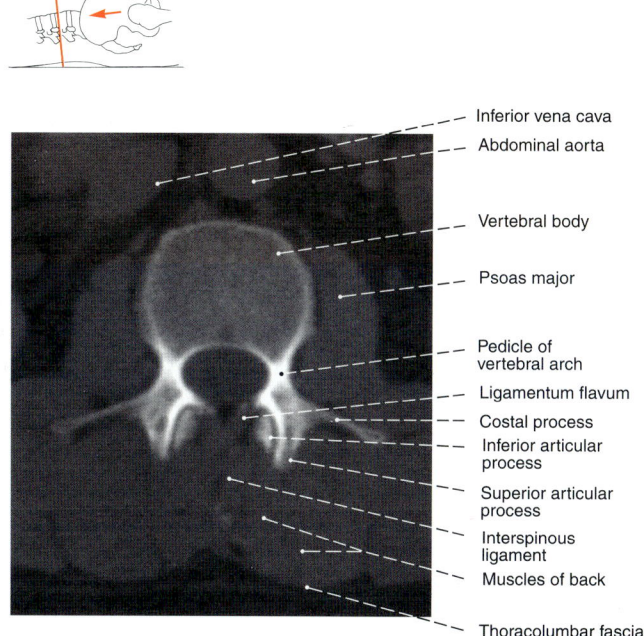

Fig. 792 Lumbar vertebral column; computer tomographic horizontal section at level of pedicles of 3rd lumbar vertebra; caudal aspect.

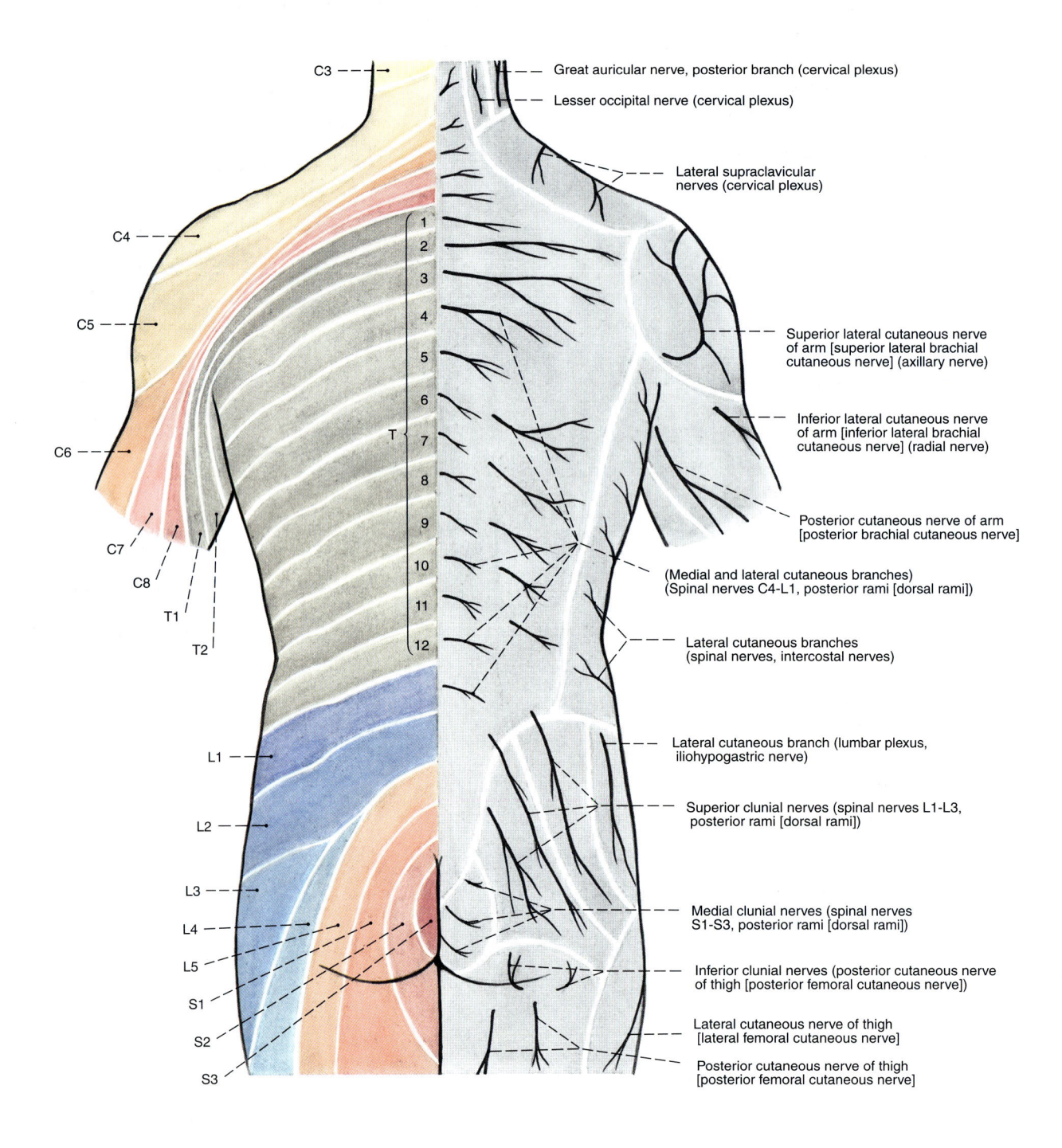

Fig. 793 Segmental innervation of skin (dermatomes) and cutaneous nerves of back; dorsal aspect.

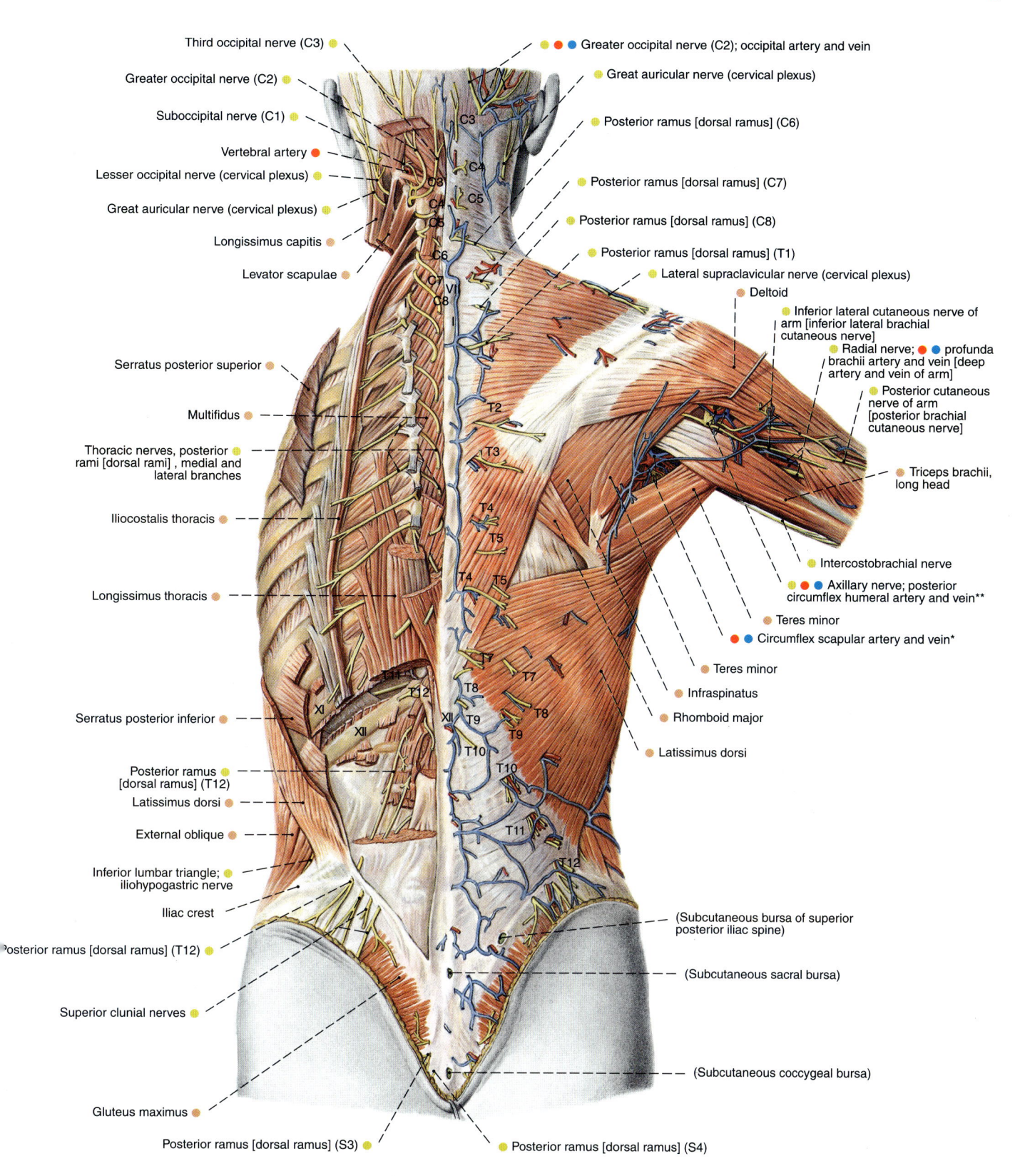

Fig. 794 Blood vessels and nerves of back; after removal of superficial muscles of shoulder girdle on the left; dorsal aspect.
* Blood vessels and nerves in triangular space.
** Blood vessels and nerves in quadrangular space.

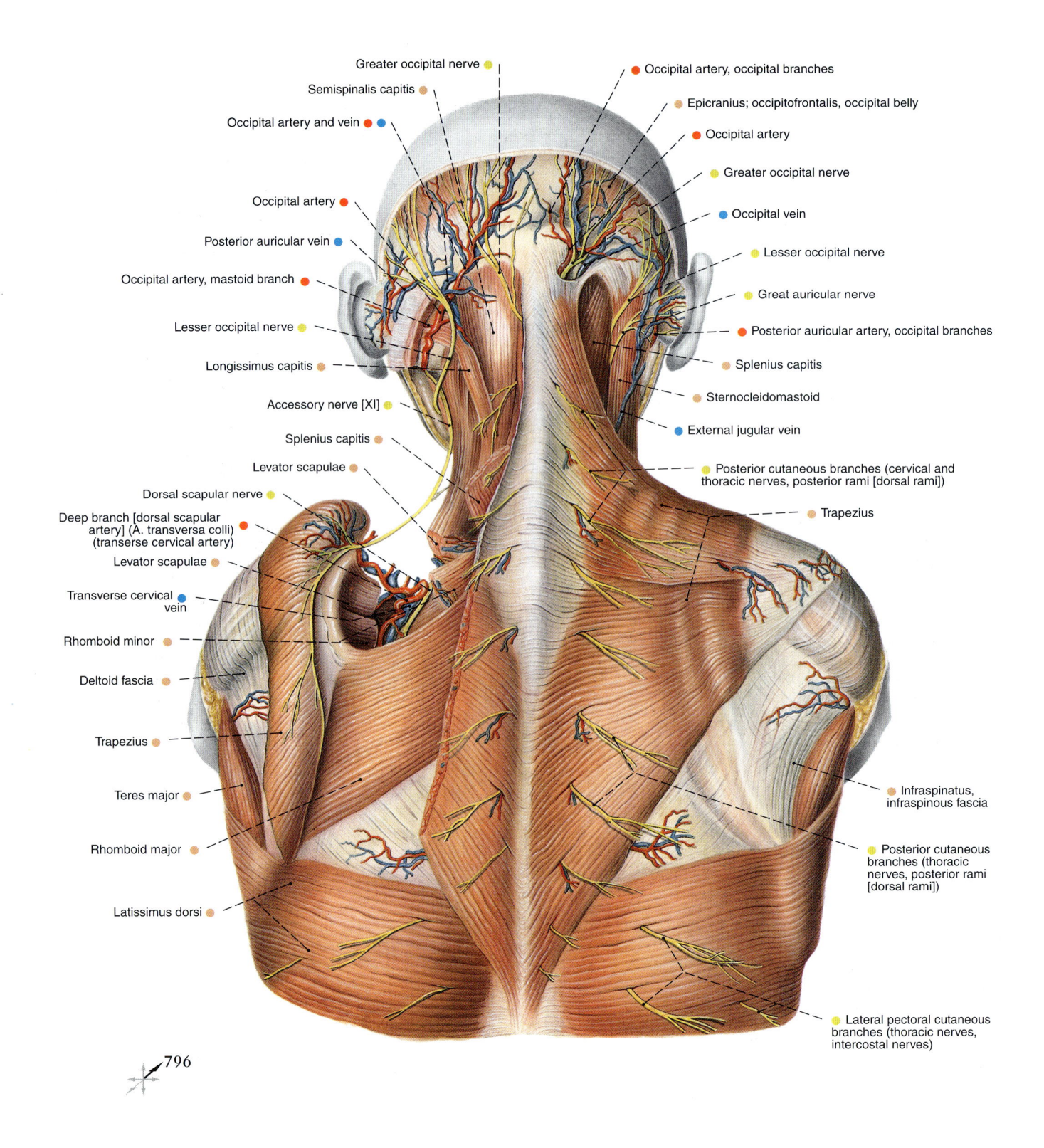

Fig. 795 Blood vessels and nerves of occipital and posterior cervical region and upper back; after partial removal of superficial muscles of back on the left; dorsal aspect.

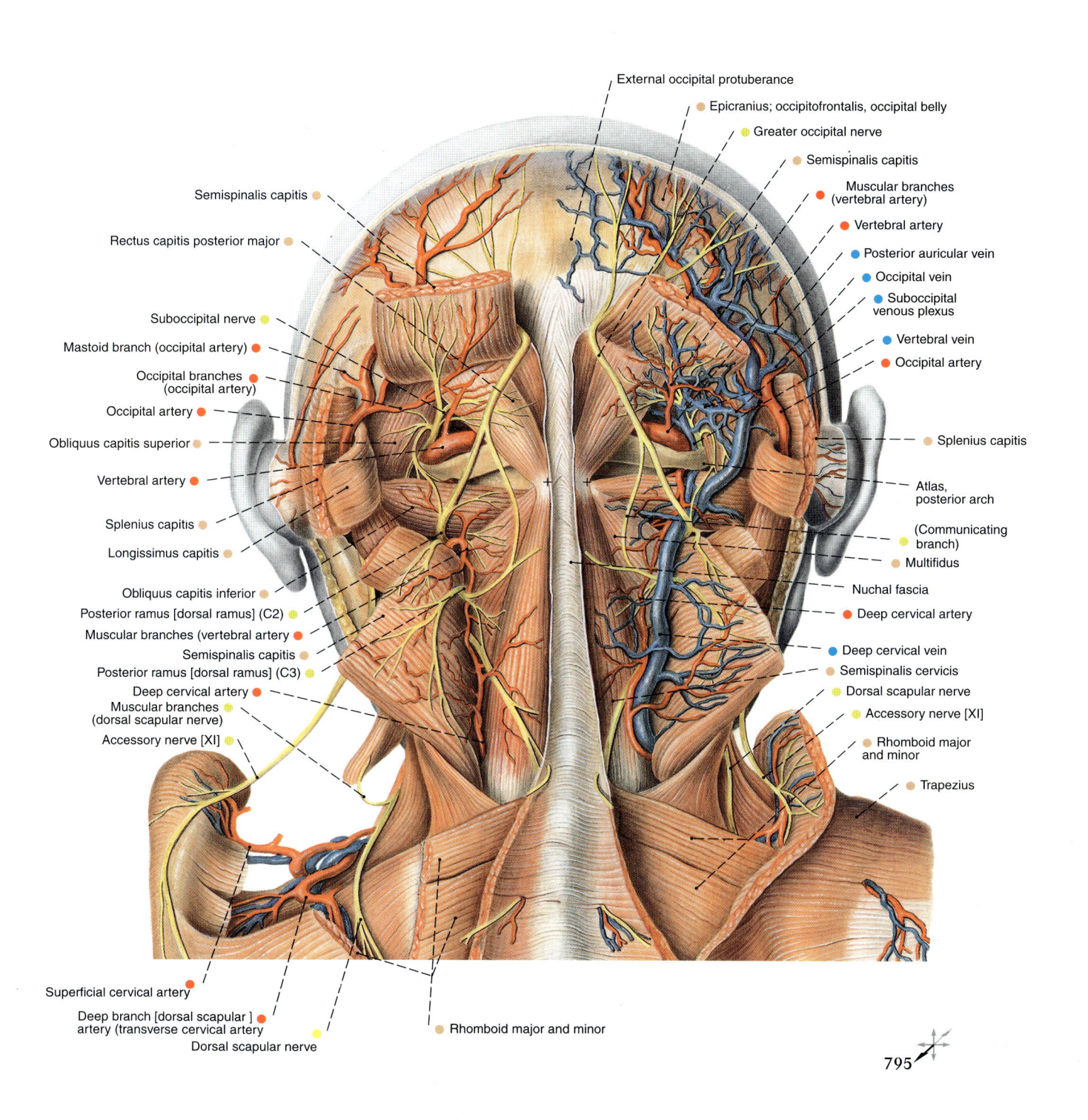

Blood vessels and nerves of occipital region 45

Fig. 796 Blood vessels and nerves of occipital and posterior cervical region; dorsal aspect.
* Tubercles of spinous process of axis.

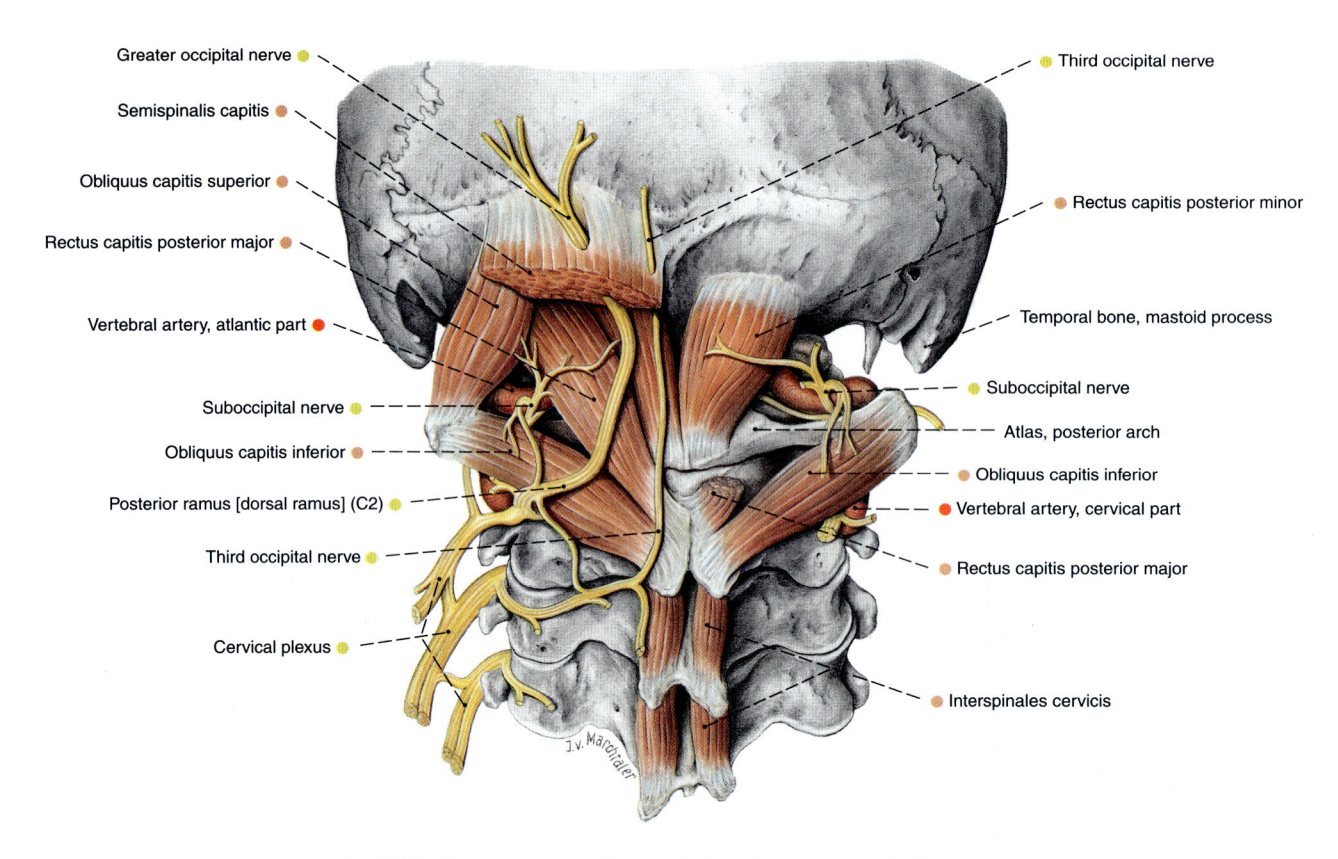

Fig. 797 Nerves of posterior cervical region and vertebral artery; dorsal aspect.

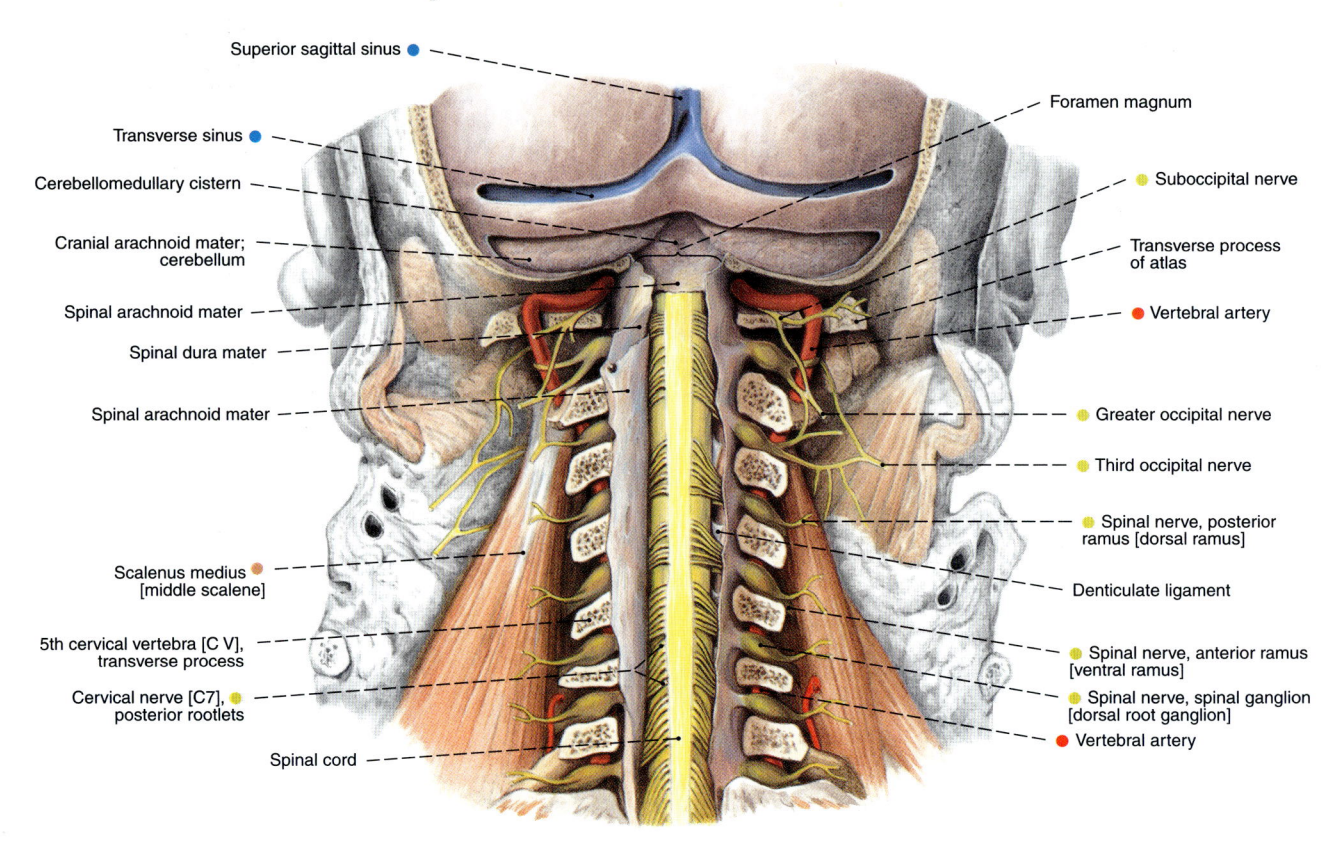

Fig. 798 Blood vessels and nerves of posterior cervical region and contents of vertebral canal; occipital bone partially and vertebral arches completely removed; stepwise exposure of meninges; dorsal aspect.

Blood vessels and nerves of vertebral canal 47

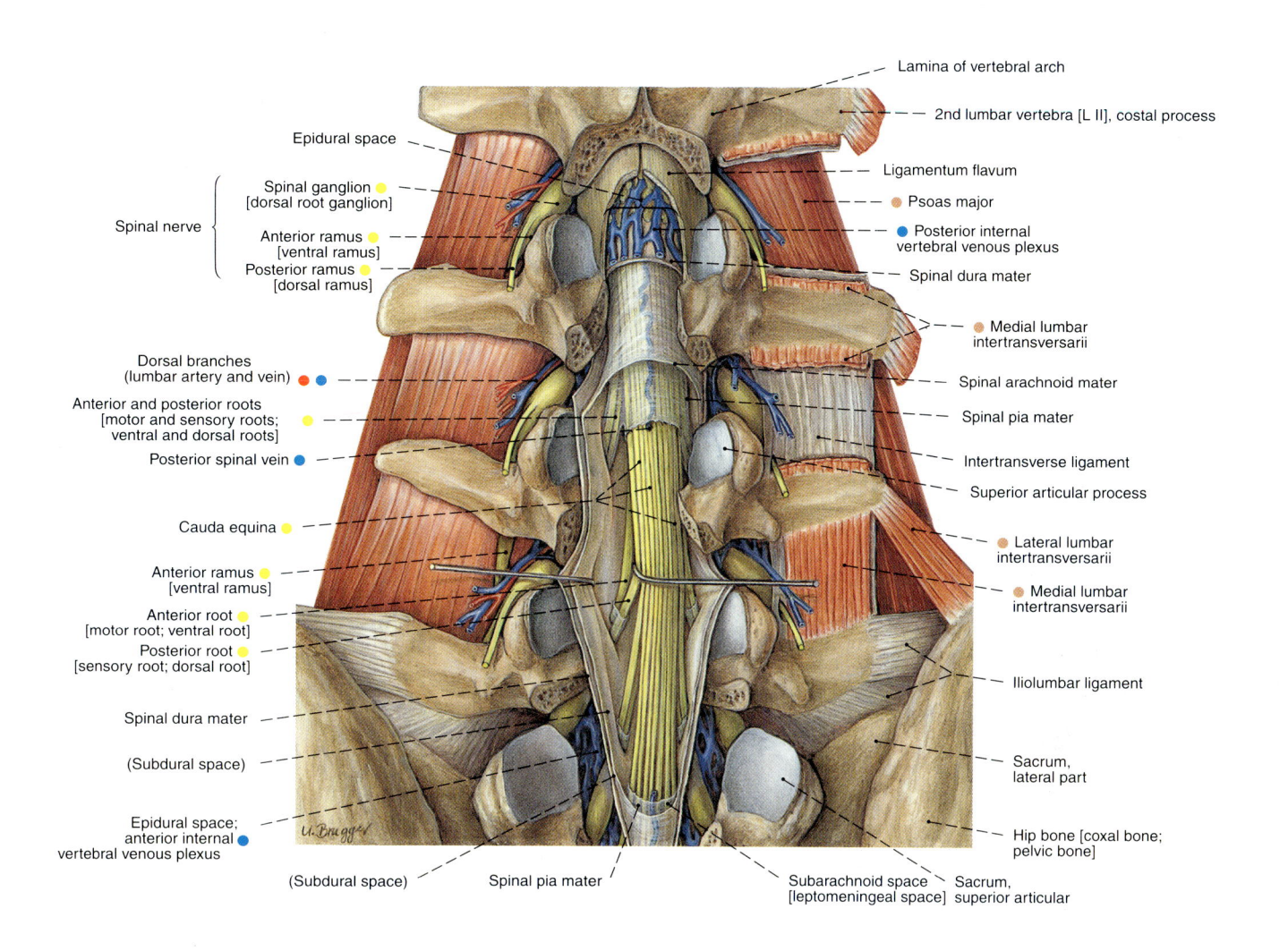

Fig. 799 Blood vessels and nerves of lumbar vertebral canal; vertebral arches removed; stepwise exposure of meninges; dorsal aspect.

48 Thoracic and abdominal walls

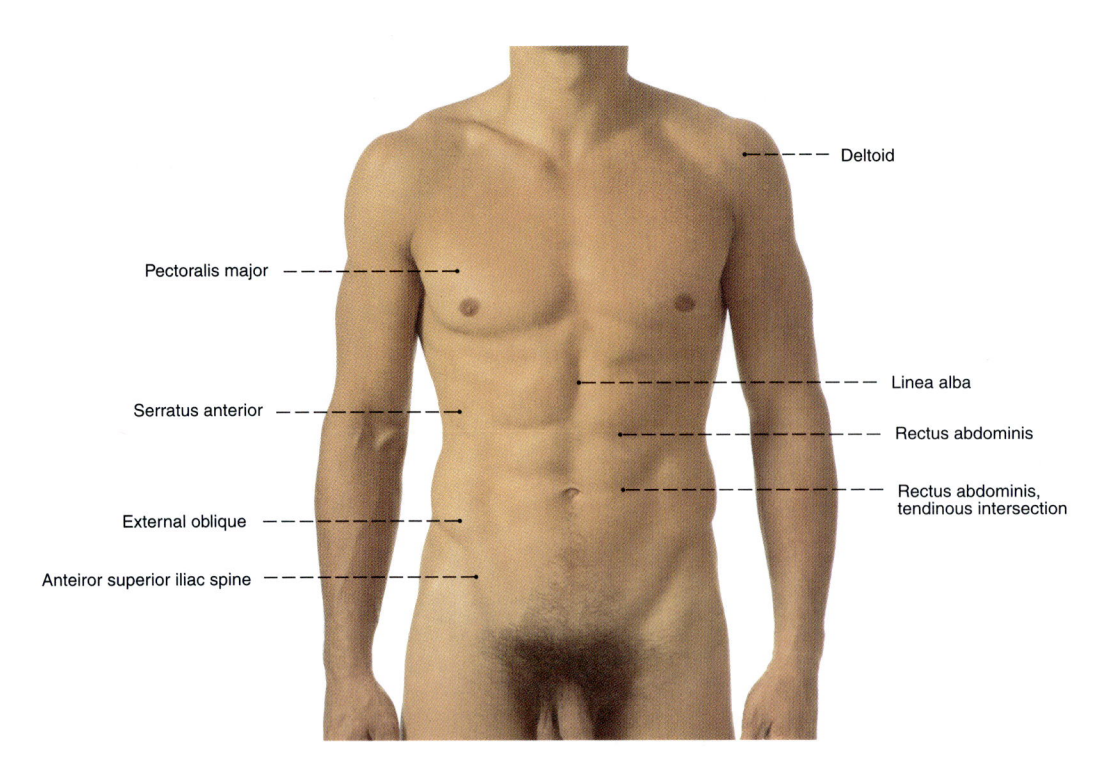

Fig. 800 Surface anatomy of thoracic and abdominal walls of a young male with prominent muscles indicated.
Note the upper border of pubic hair, which in the male extends triangularly to the umbilicus, whereas in the female it has a horizontal border (Fig. 801).
Regions of thoracic and abdominal walls are shown in Fig. 7.

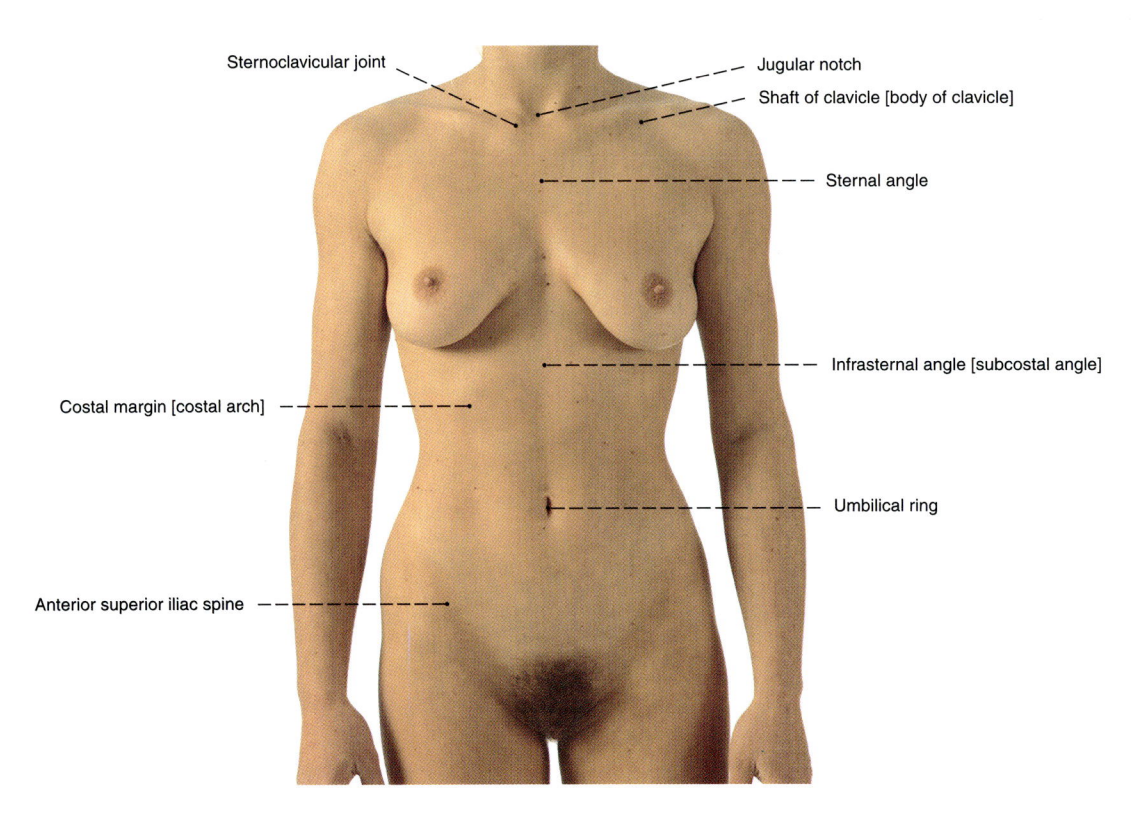

Fig. 801 Surface anatomy of thoracic and abdominal walls of a young female with prominent bones indicated.
Orientation lines of thoracic and abdominal walls are shown in Fig. 2.

Ribs 49

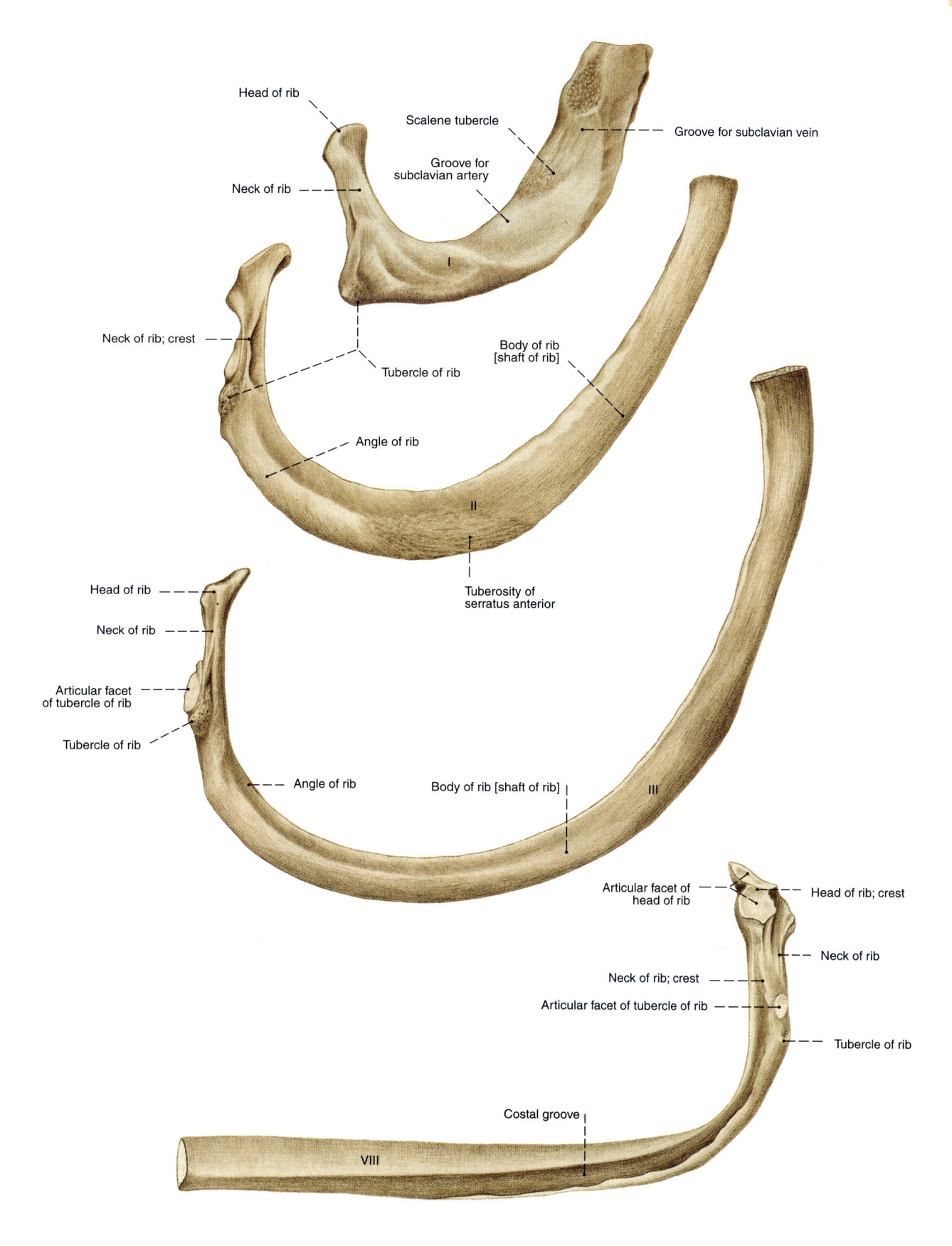

Fig. 802 Ribs;
Ribs I–III; superior aspect.
Rib VIII; inferior aspect.

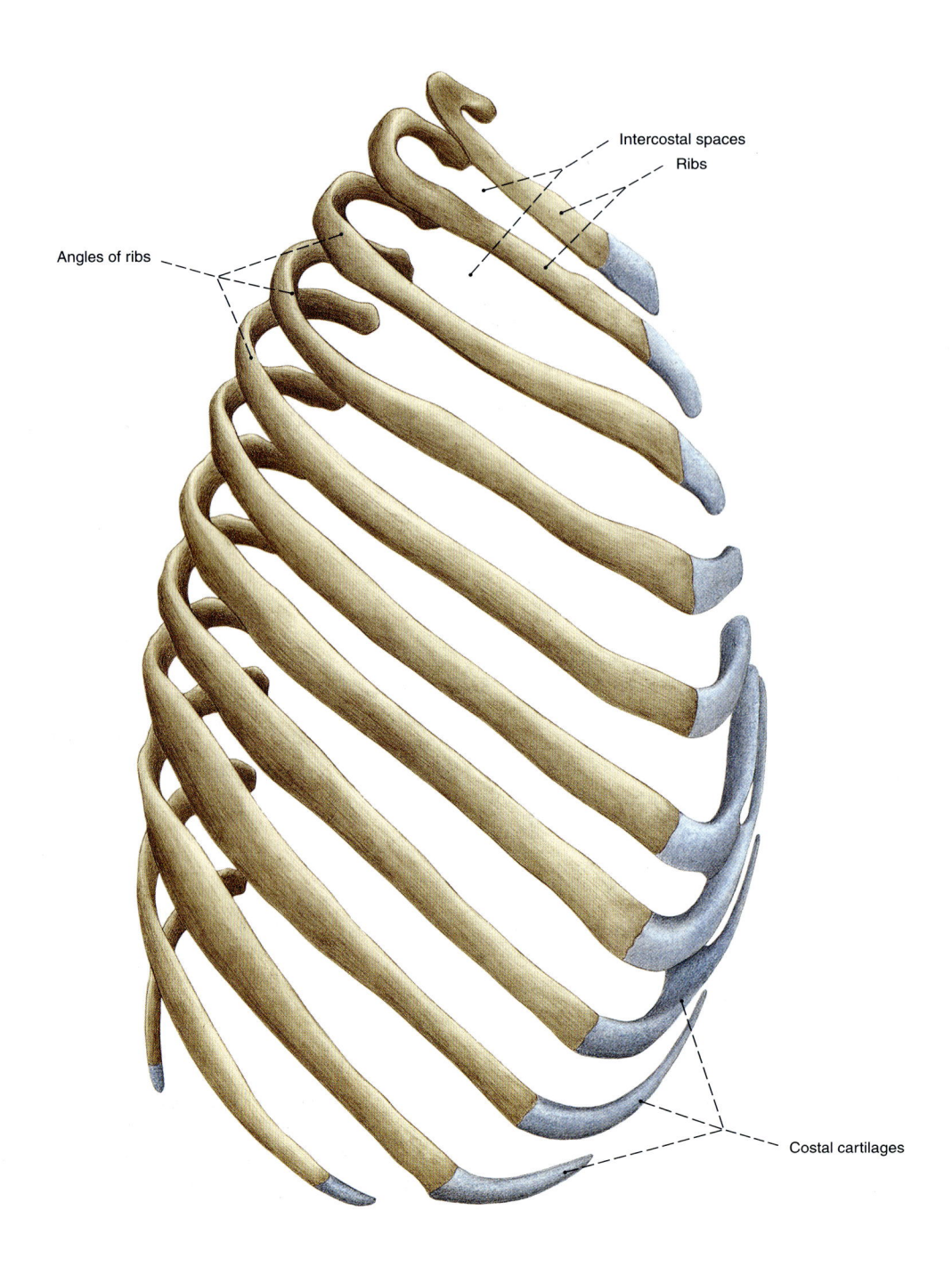

Fig. 803 Ribs; right aspect.
Ribs shown in their natural distance.

Sternum 51

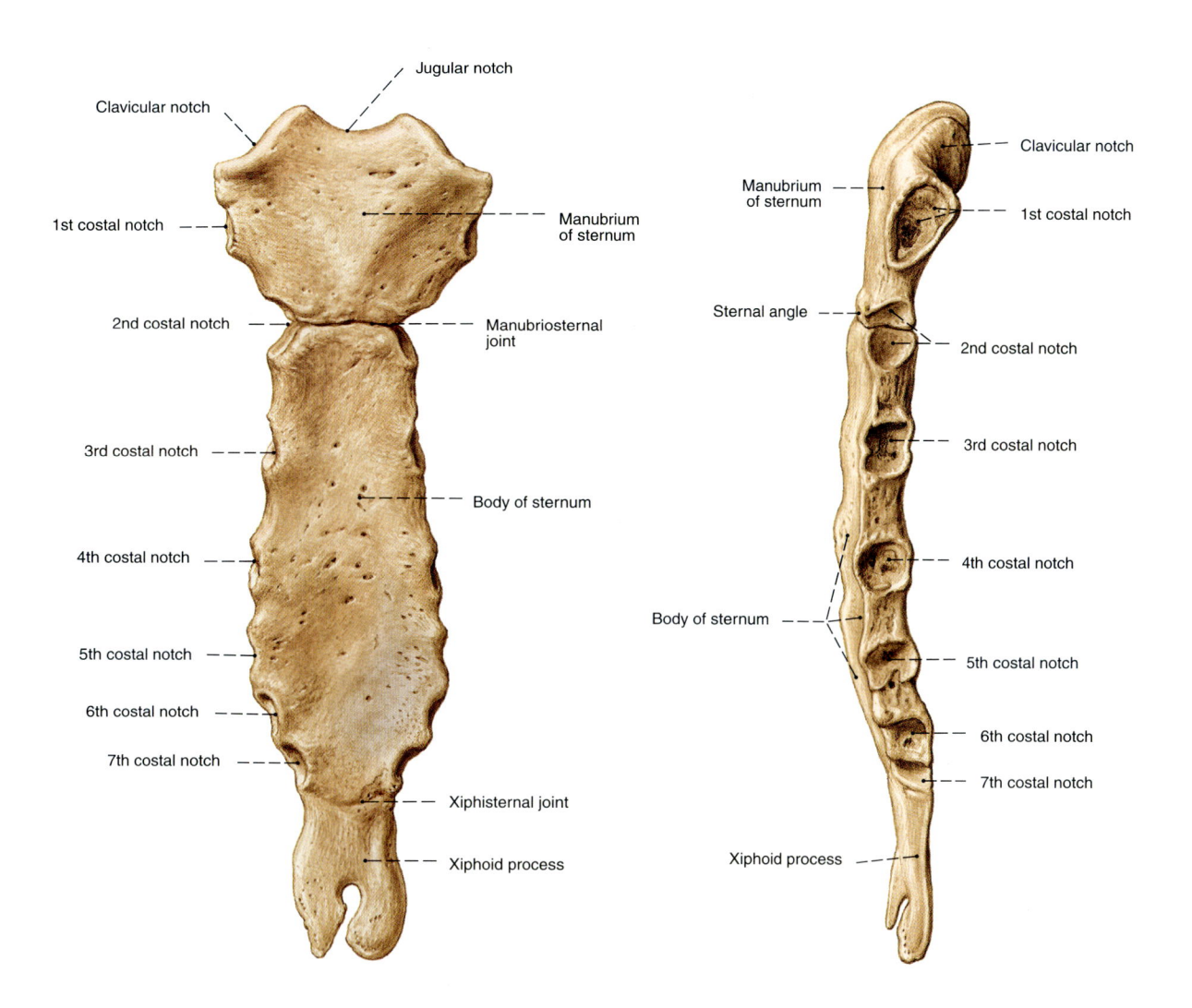

Fig. 804 Sternum; anterior aspect. Shape, length, and direction (dorsal or ventral) of xiphoid process vary considerably.

Fig. 805 Sternum; left lateral aspect. For counting ribs and intercostal spaces on the anterior thoracic wall the sternal angle, to which the 2nd rib is attached, is important

52 *Thoracic and abdominal walls*

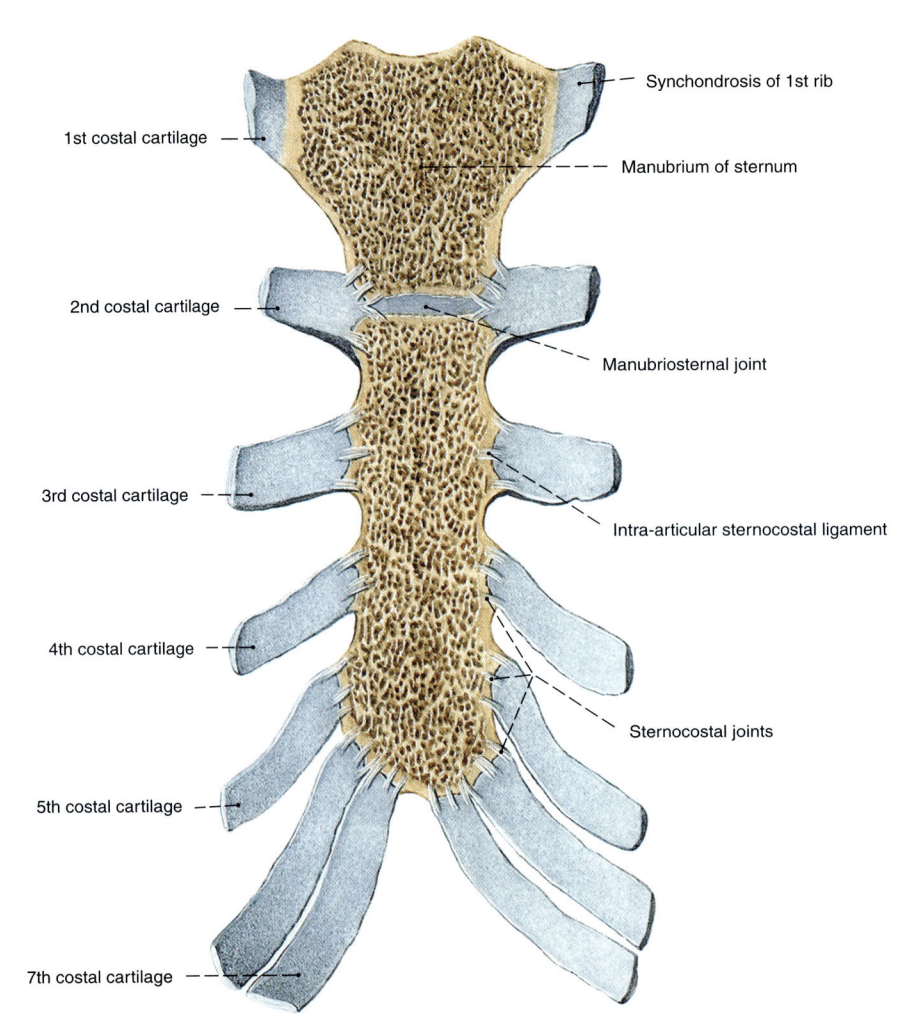

Fig. 806 Sternum; costal cartilages; frontal section; anterior aspect.

Note that the xiphoid process is not apparent, due to the curvature of the sternum.

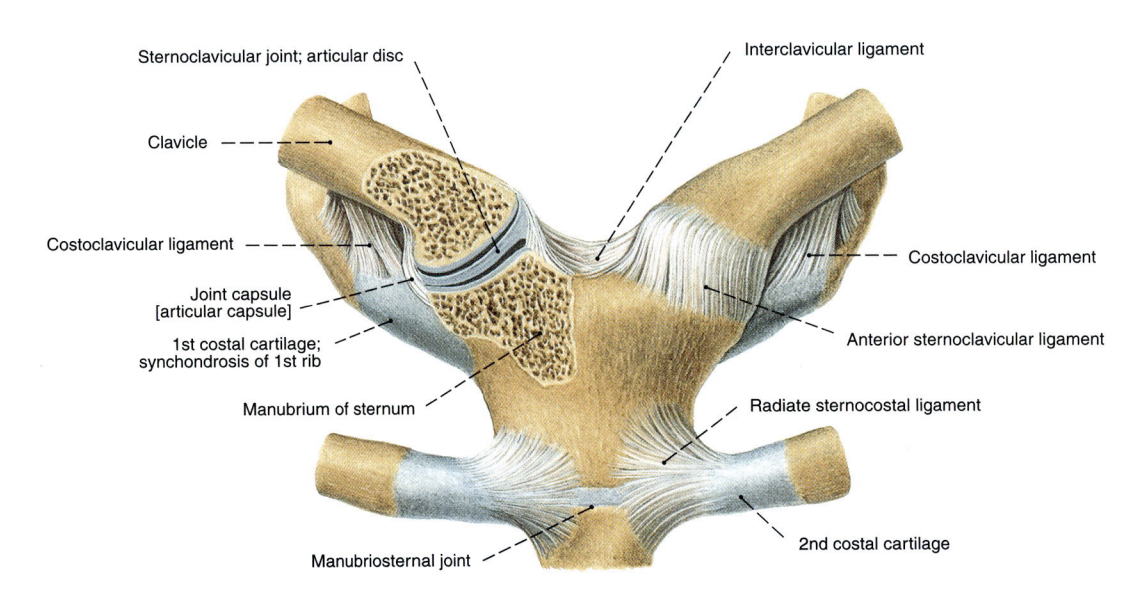

Fig. 807 Sternoclavicular joint; the right joint opened by a frontal section to expose the articular disc; anterior aspect.

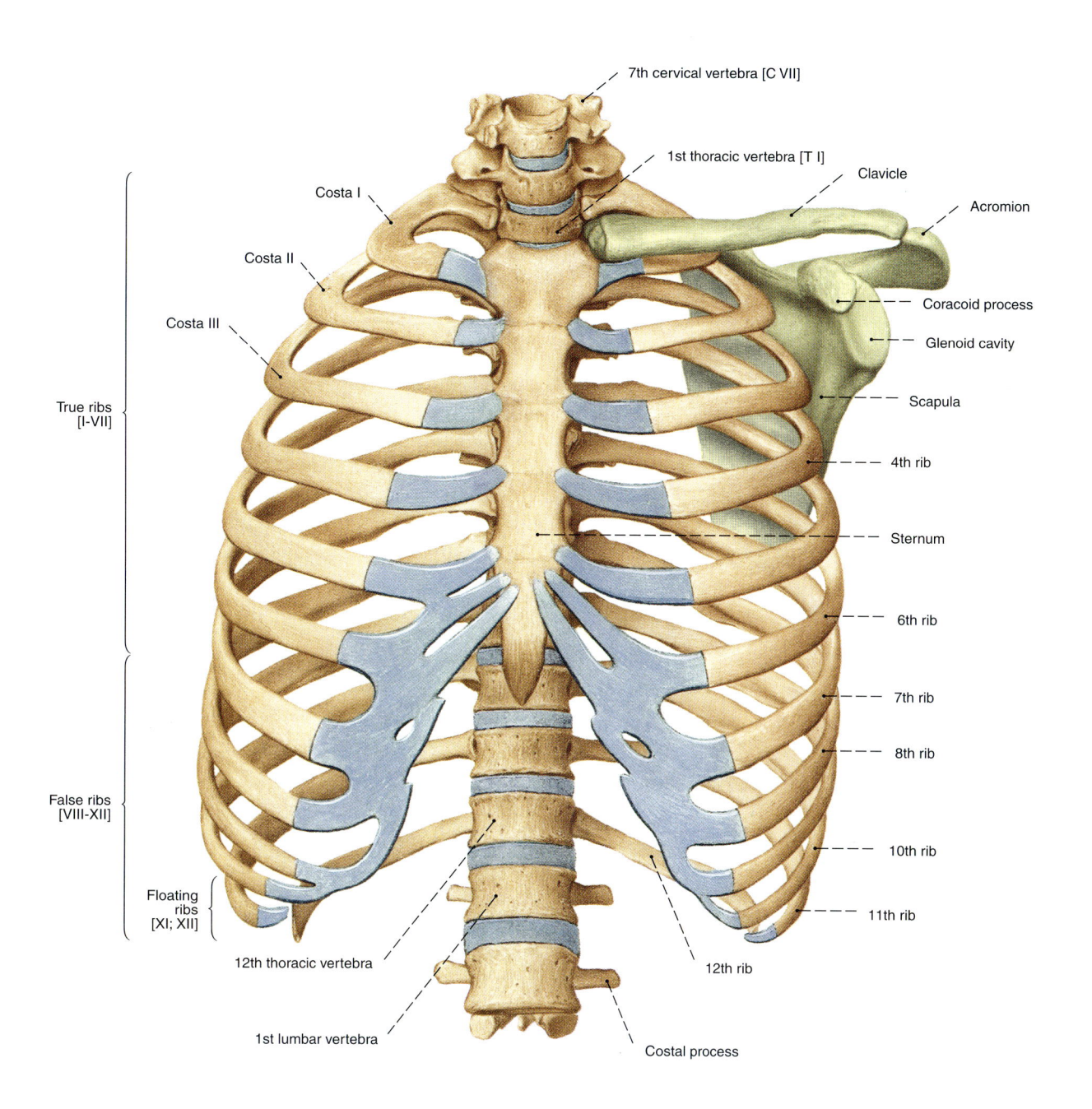

Thoracic cage 53

Fig. 808   Thoracic cage; left pectoral girdle [shoulder girdle]; anterior aspect.
The thoracic cage is shown in moderate inspiration. Bones of pectoral girdle [shoulder girdle] highlighted in green, cartilages in blue. Lengths of 11th and 12th ribs vary considerably.

54 Thoracic and abdominal walls

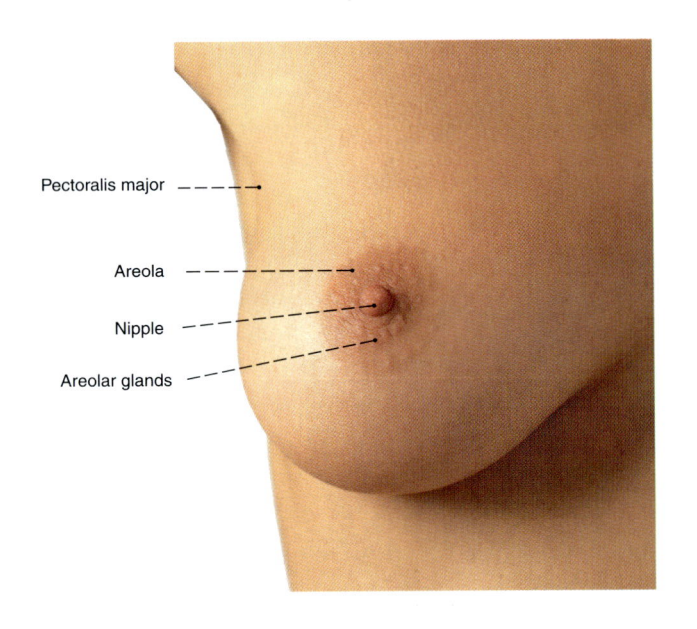

Fig. 809 Breast; anterior aspect.

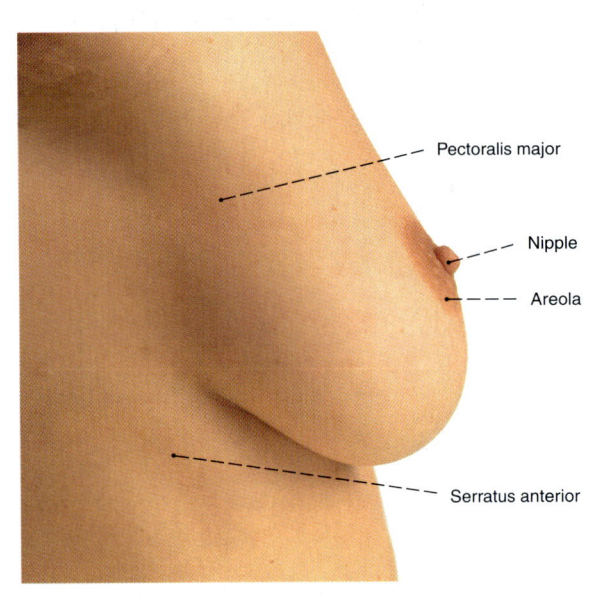

Fig. 810 Breast; right lateral aspect.

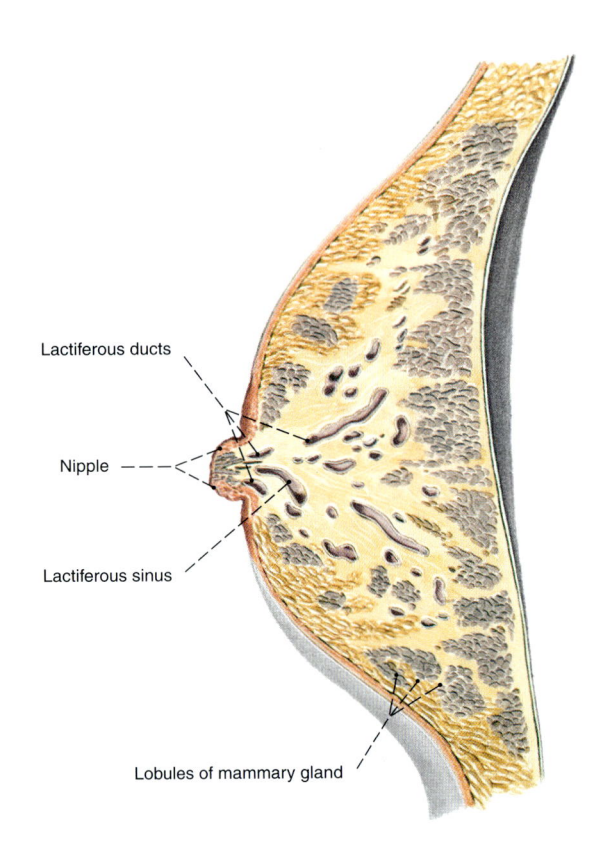

Fig. 811 Mammary gland of a pregnant woman; sectioned sagittally into halves; lateral aspect.

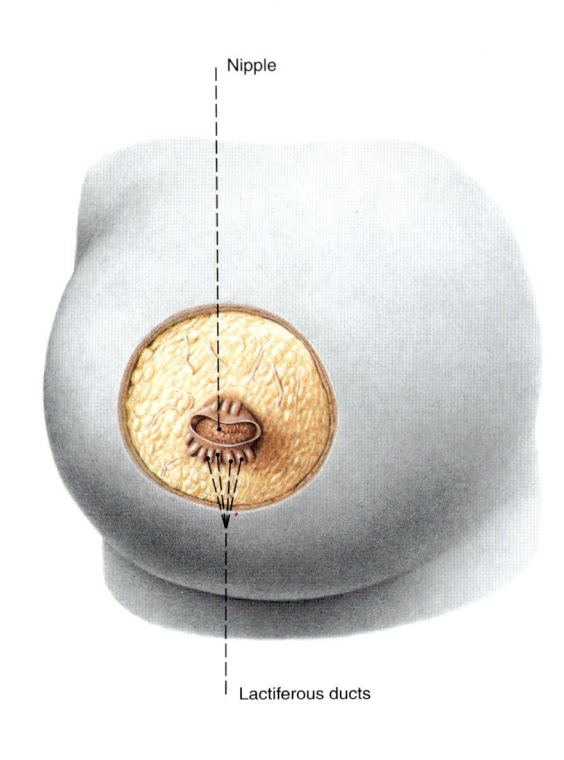

Fig. 812 Mammary gland of a pregnant woman; skin of areola removed and skin surrounding nipple reflected; anterior aspect.

Mammary gland 55

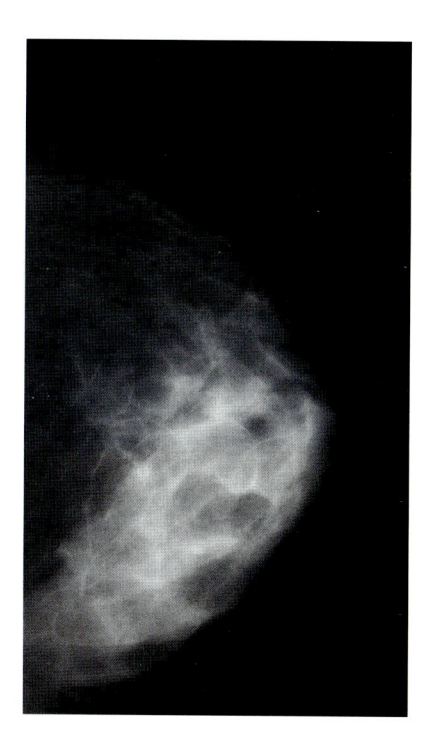

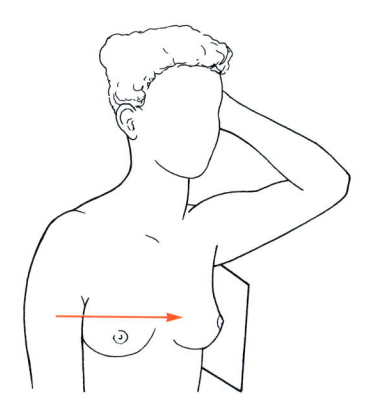

Fig. 813 Radiograph of mammary gland; lateral mammography of a 47-year-old woman.

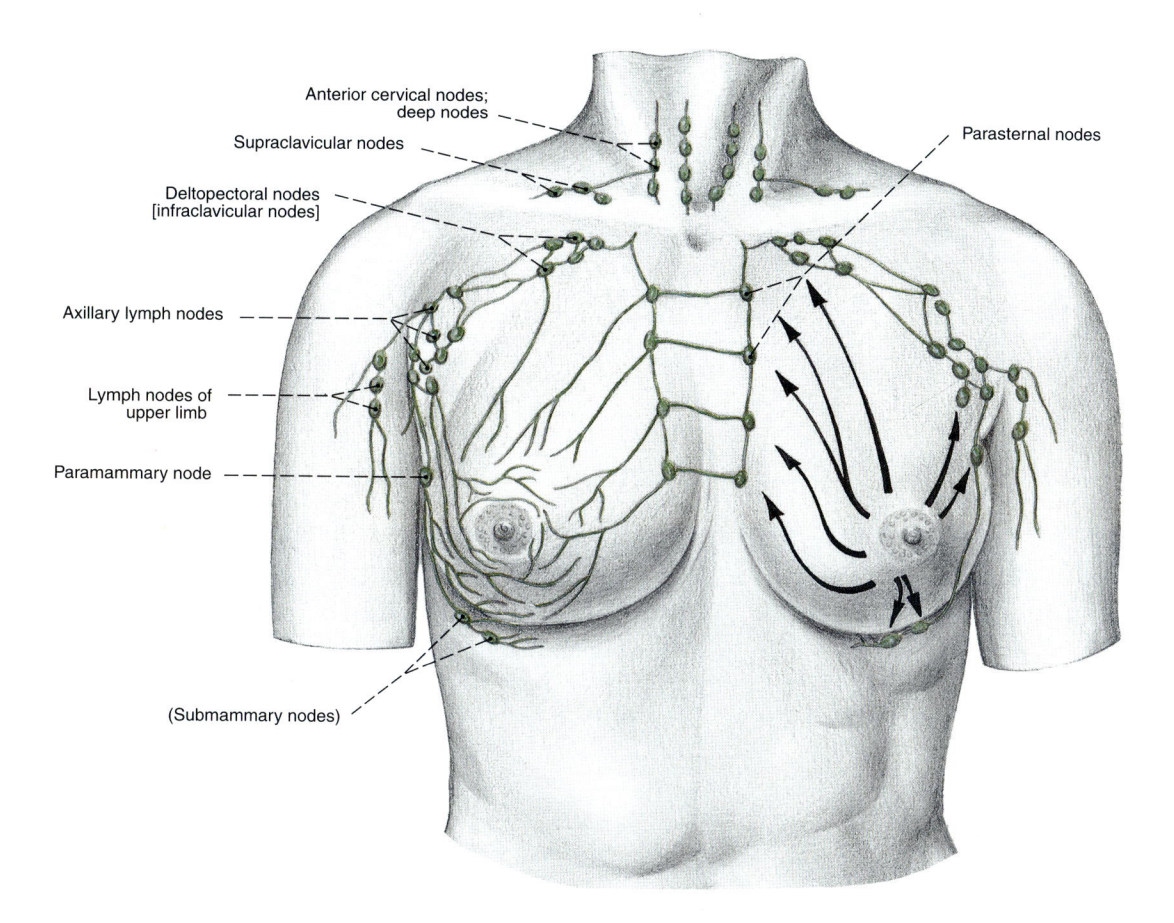

Fig. 814 Lymphatic drainage of female mammary gland and site of regional lymph nodes.
(From: BENNINGHOFF/ GOERTTLER: Lehrbuch der Anatomie des Menschen, vol. 2, 12th ed., Urban & Schwarzenberg, Munich 1979).

Note the communications of lymphatic vessels of both sides and lymphatic drainage into intrathoracic lymph nodes.

56 Thoracic and abdominal walls

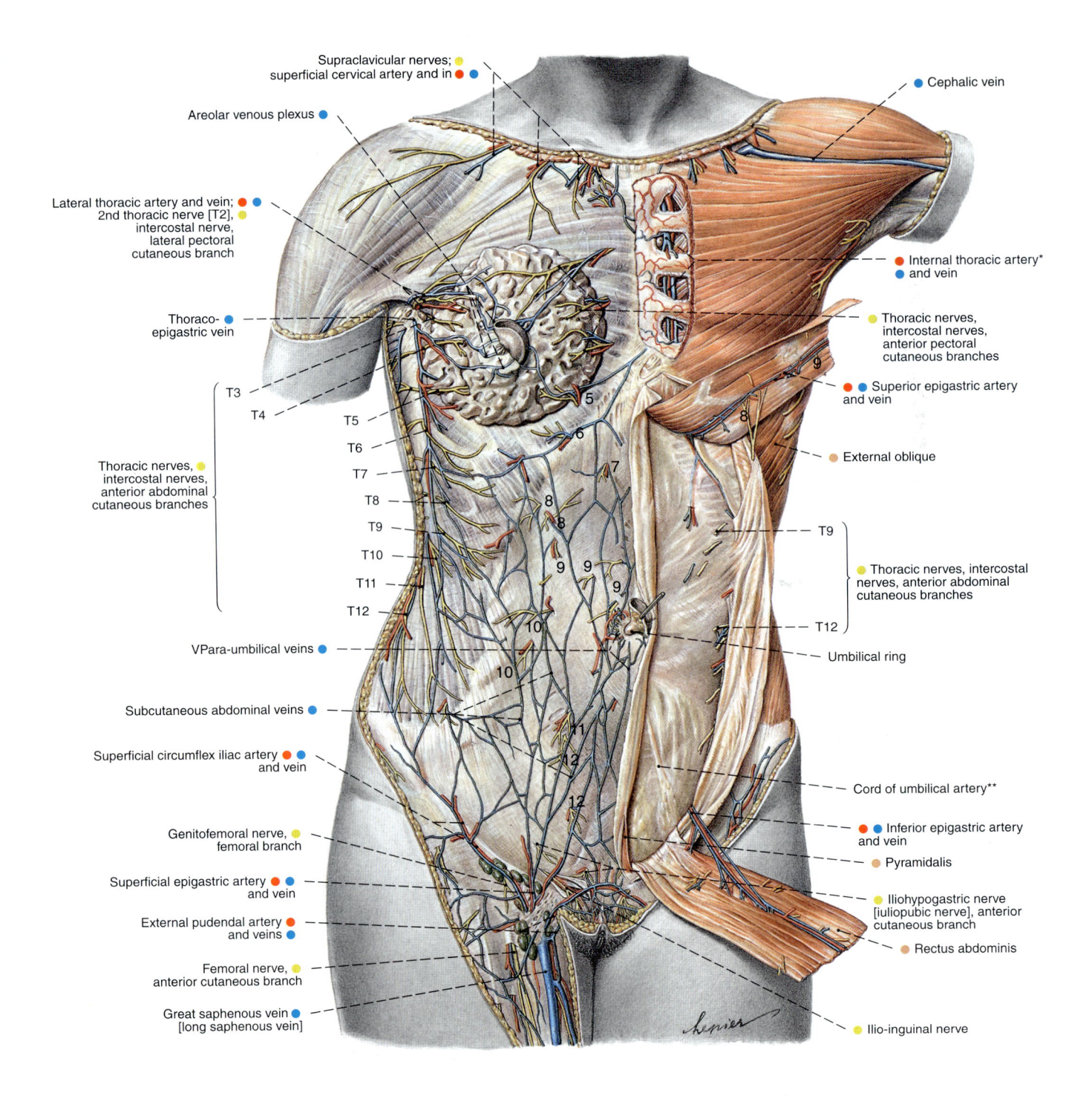

Fig. 815 Blood vessels and nerves of thoracic and abdominal walls; superficial layer shown on the right; anterior aspect. Arabic numerals indicate cutaneous branches of respective intercostal nerves.

* Clinically: internal mammary artery.
** The cord of umbilical artery causes the medial umbilical fold internally.

Segmental innervation 57

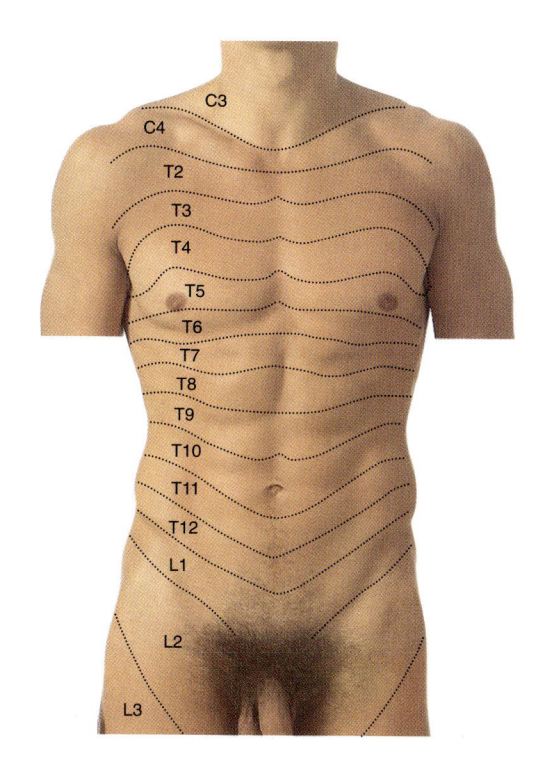

Fig. 816 Segmental sensory innervation of thoracic and abdominal walls (dermatomes).
Letters and numerals indicate respective spinal cord segments.

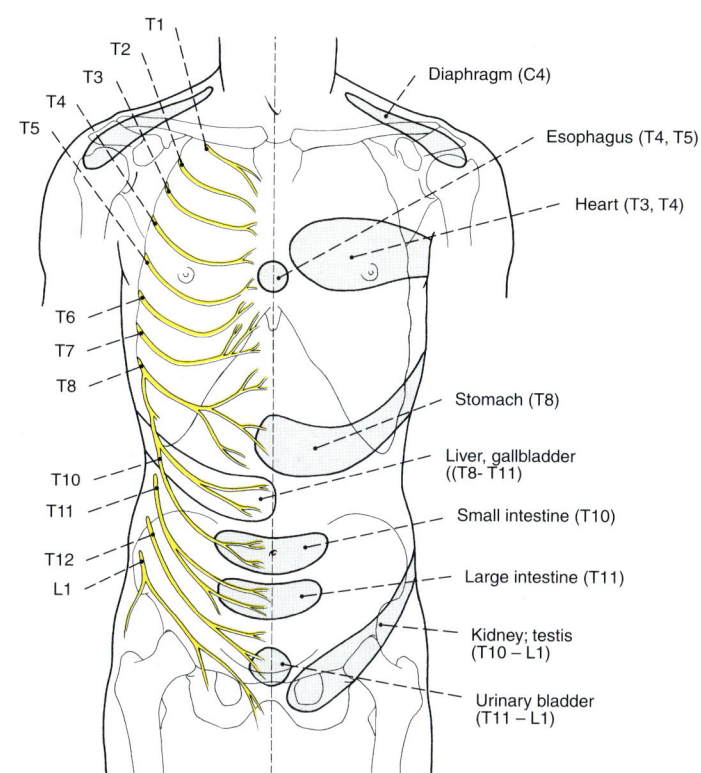

Fig. 817 Segmental sensory innervation of anterior thoracic and abdominal walls (dermatomes).
On the left side of the body regions of pain projection due to diseases of respective internal viscera (Head's zones) are indicated.

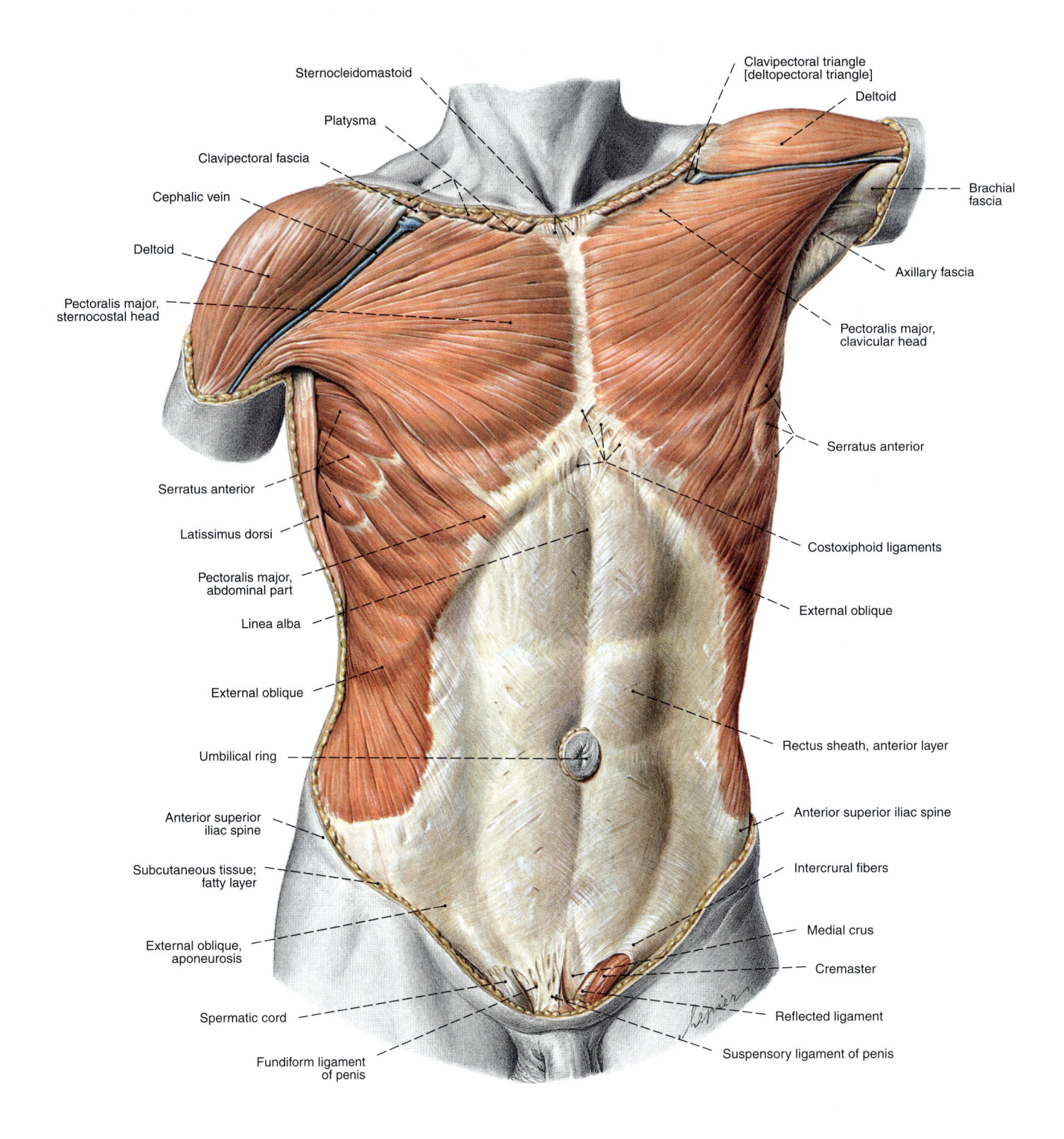

Fig. 818 Muscles of thoracic and abdominal walls; superficial layer; anterior aspect.

Muscles of thorax 59

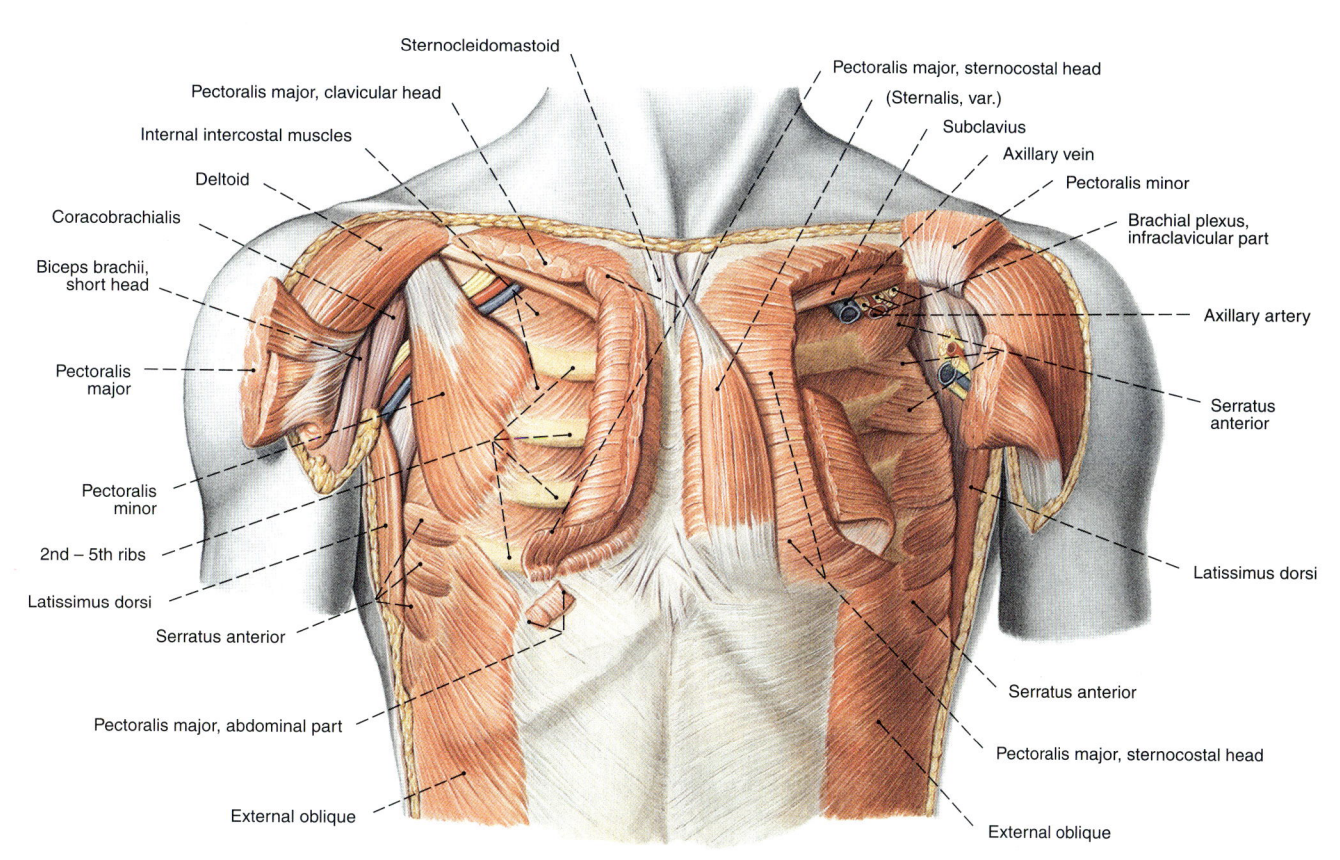

Fig. 819 Muscles of thorax; right pectoralis major partially removed, left pectoralis minor sectioned and reflected; external intercostal membrane removed; anterior aspect.

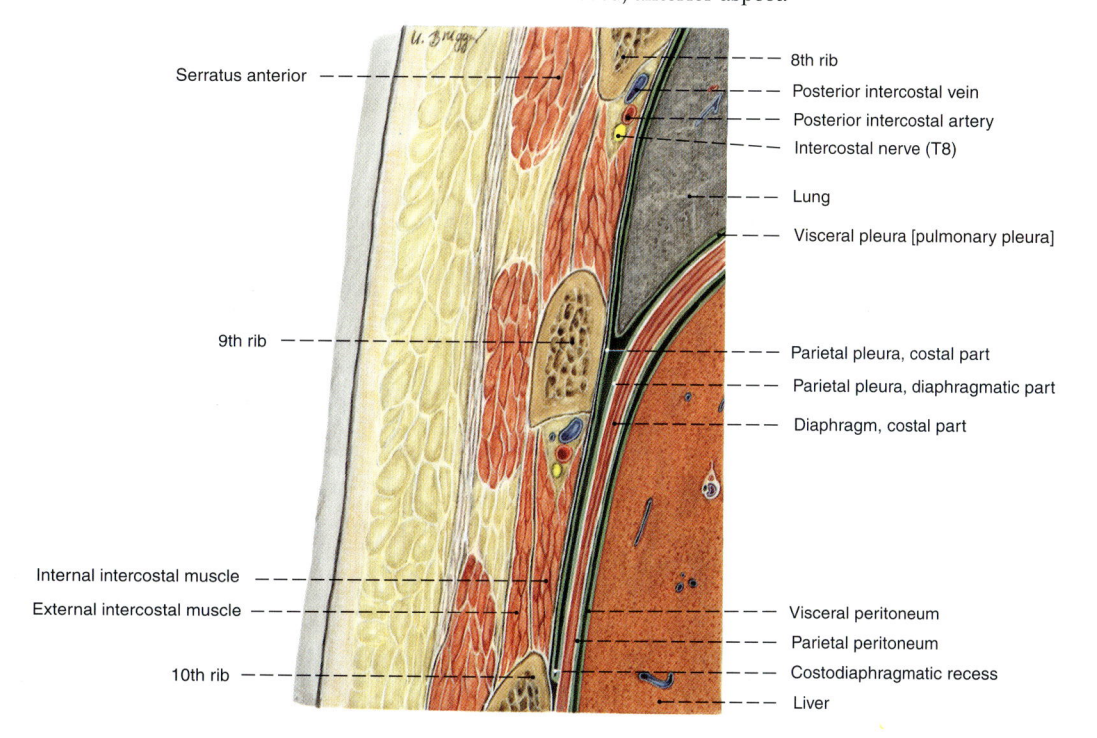

Fig. 820 Muscles of thorax; frontal section exposing thoracic wall, thoracic and abdominal cavity; right ventral aspect. During puncture for aspiration of fluid in the pleural cavity or during puncture of the liver, the course of intercostal nerves and blood vessels, the position of the diaphragm, and the expansion of the lung into the costodiaphragmatic recess must be considered.

Ventral muscles of shoulder (Figs. 818, 819)

The pectoralis major muscle is a trunk-arm muscle that forms the surface relief of the anterior upper thoracic wall. The pectoralis minor, a trunk-shoulder-girdle muscle, lies beyond it. The subclavius also is a trunk-shoulder-girdle muscle lying caudal to the clavicle. The deepest muscle, lying directly on the shoulder joint, is the subscapularis, which courses from the anterior surface of scapula to the humerus.

Muscle/*Innervation*	Origin	Insertion	Function
1. **Pectoralis major** *Medial and lateral pectoral nerves (brachial plexus, infra-/supraclavicular part)* The fibers converge to a wide tendon forming a flat pouch-like insertion.	**Clavicular head:** clavicle, (sternal half) **Sternocostal head:** manubrium and body of sternum, 1st–6th costal cartilages **Abdominal part:** rectus sheath (anterior layer)	Crest of greater tubercle [lateral lip]	**Glenohumeral joint [shoulder joint]:** Adduction (especially when arm is elevated), medial rotation clavicular part: flexion **Pectoral girdle [shoulder girdle]:** depression, anteversion (propulsion) **Thorax:** elevation of sternum, expands thorax (when arms are propped up it helps with deep inspiration)
2. **Pectoralis minor** *Medial and lateral pectoral nerves (brachial plexus, infra-/supraclavicular part)*	(2nd) 3rd–5th rib (near bone-cartilage junction)	Tip of coracoid process of scapula	**Pectoral girdle [shoulder girdle]:** depression, propulsion **Thorax:** elevates upper ribs, expands thorax (when arms are propped up and shoulder girdle is fixed it helps with deep inspiration)
3. **Subclavius** *Subclavius nerve (brachial plexus, supraclavicular part)*	1st rib (near bone-cartilage junction)	Clavicle (lateral third), fascia blends with adventitia of subclavian vein	**Pectoral girdle [shoulder girdle]:** Depression (limited), opposes lateral pull on clavicle
4. **Subscapularis** *Subscapular nerves (brachial plexus, infraclavicular part)*	Costal surface, subscapular fossa	Lesser tubercle and adjacent part of crest of lesser tubercle [medial lip] (below its insertion: subtendinous bursa of subscapularis)	**Glenohumeral joint [shoulder joint]:** Medial rotation, abduction in the plain of the scapula (cranial part), adduction in the plain of the scapula (caudal part)

Muscles of thoracic wall (Fig. 819)

The intercostal spaces are filled with the intercostal muscles. Medially the subcostales and the transversus thoracis cover the thoracic wall. Rarely a superficial sternalis muscle is found.
The muscle forming the surface relief of the anterior upper thoracic wall, the pectoralis major, is a trunk-arm muscle. It covers the pectoralis minor, a trunk-shoulder-girdle muscle. Both muscles are described in the group of ventral muscles of shoulder.

Muscle/*Innervation*	Origin	Insertion	Function
1. **Sternalis** *Branches from pectoral nerves (brachial plexus, supraclavicular part) or Intercostal nerves (thoracic nerves)* (inconstant muscle)	Border of sternum (from pectoralis fascia)	Blends with fascia	Contracts skin of thoracic wall
2. **External intercostal muscle** *Intercostal nerves (thoracic nerves)*	1st–11th rib (lower border, from tubercle to bone-cartilage junction)	2nd–12th rib (upper border of rib below)	Elevates ribs, braces intercostal spaces (inspiration)
3. **Internal intercostal muscle** *Intercostal nerves (thoracic nerves)*	2nd–12th rib (upper border, from sternal end of costal cartilage to angle)	Innermost intercostal muscles separated by posterior intercostal vessel and intercostal nerve	Lowers ribs, braces intercostal spaces (expiration)
4. **Subcostales** *Intercostal nerves (thoracic nerves)* (inconstant muscle)	Lower ribs (upper border, from tubercle to angle)	Lower ribs (lower border, second rib below)	Braces thoracic wall (expiration)
5. **Transversus thoracis** *Intercostal nerves (thoracic nerves)* (inconstant muscle)	Body of sternum, xiphoid process (dorsal lateral border), (6th) 7th costal cartilage	2nd–6th costal cartilage (near bone-cartilage junction)	

Muscles of thorax 61

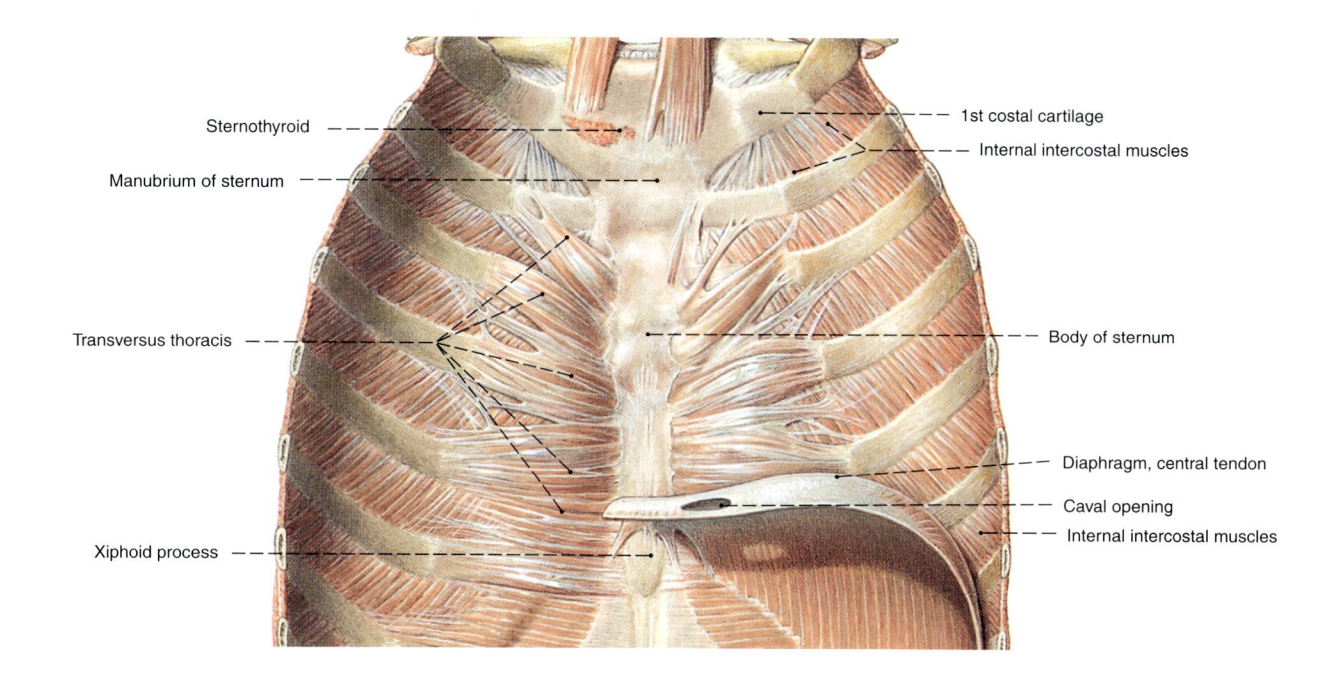

Fig. 821 Thoracic cage; anterior part with diaphragm on the right; posterior aspect.

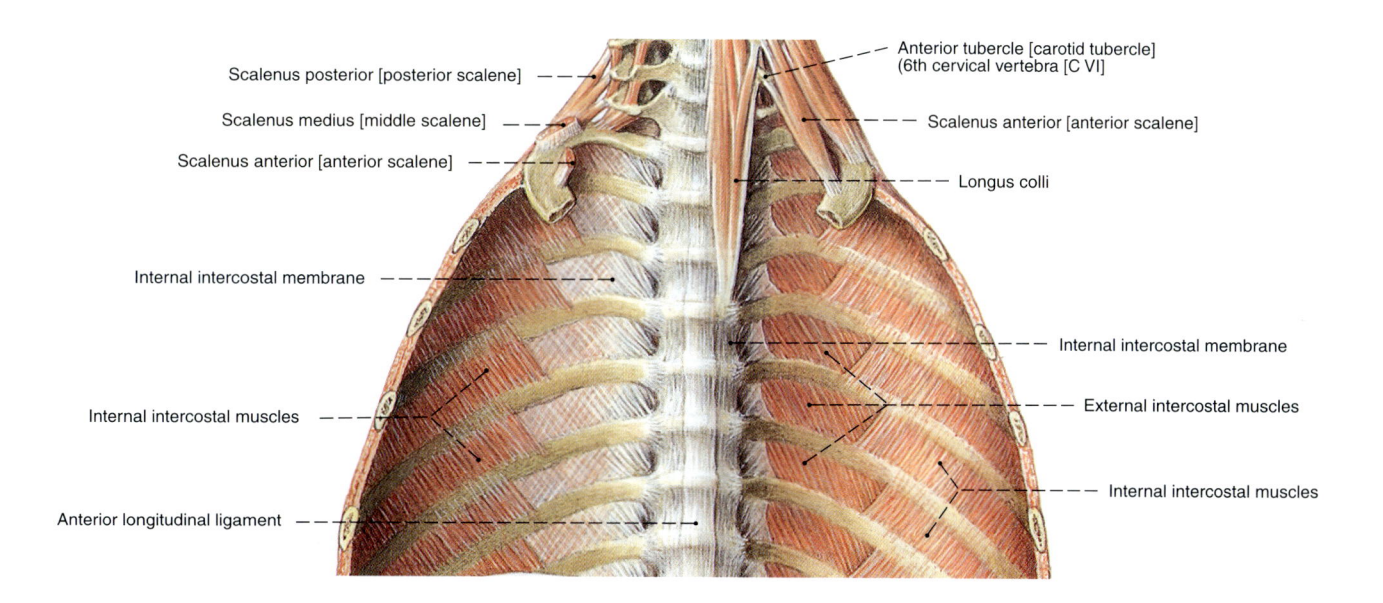

Fig. 822 Thoracic cage; posterior part seen in a frontal section; muscles of neck partially in situ; anterior aspect.

62 Thoracic and abdominal walls

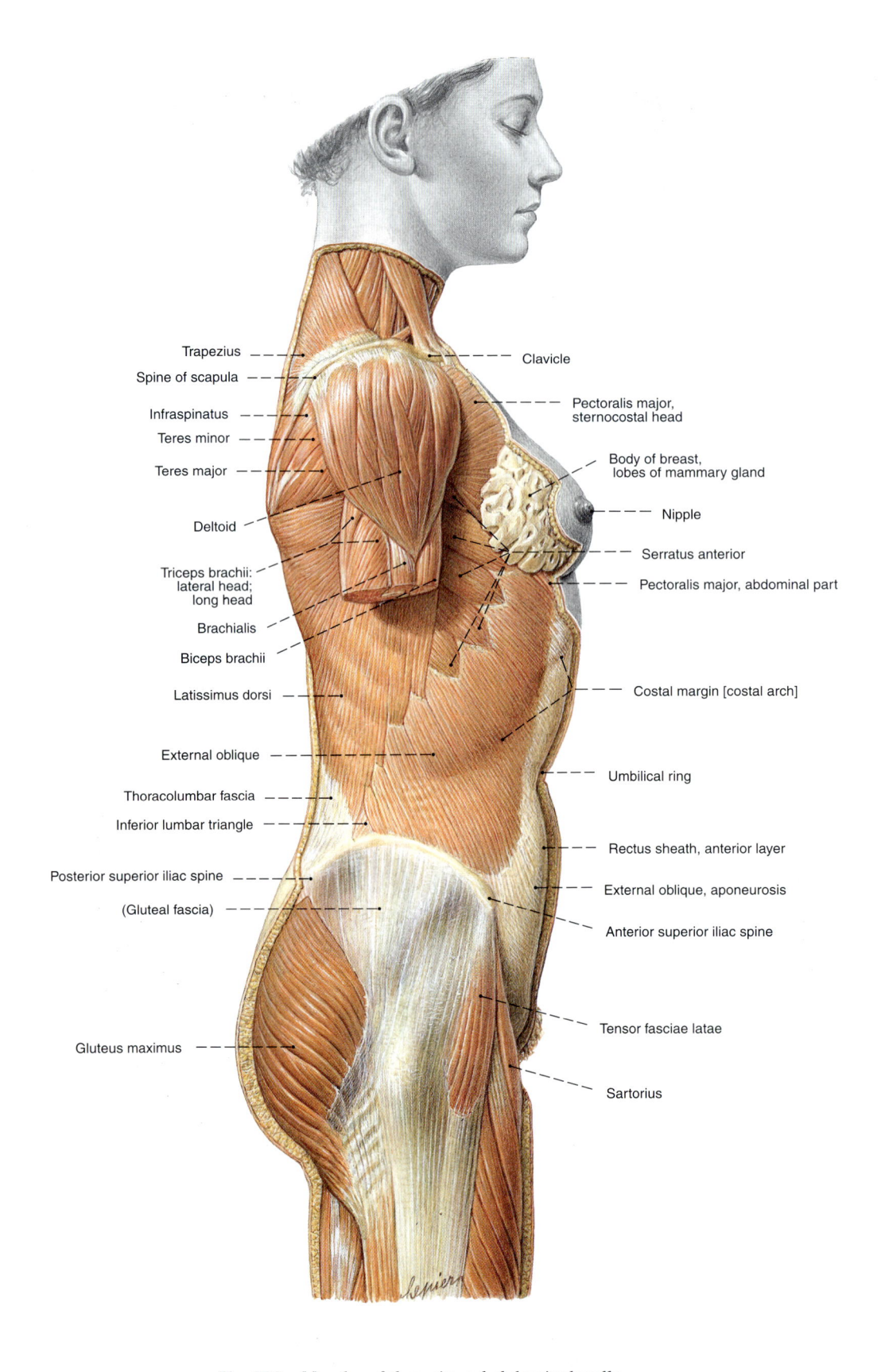

Fig. 823 Muscles of thoracic and abdominal walls; mammary gland dissected; lateral aspect.

Muscles of abdomen 63

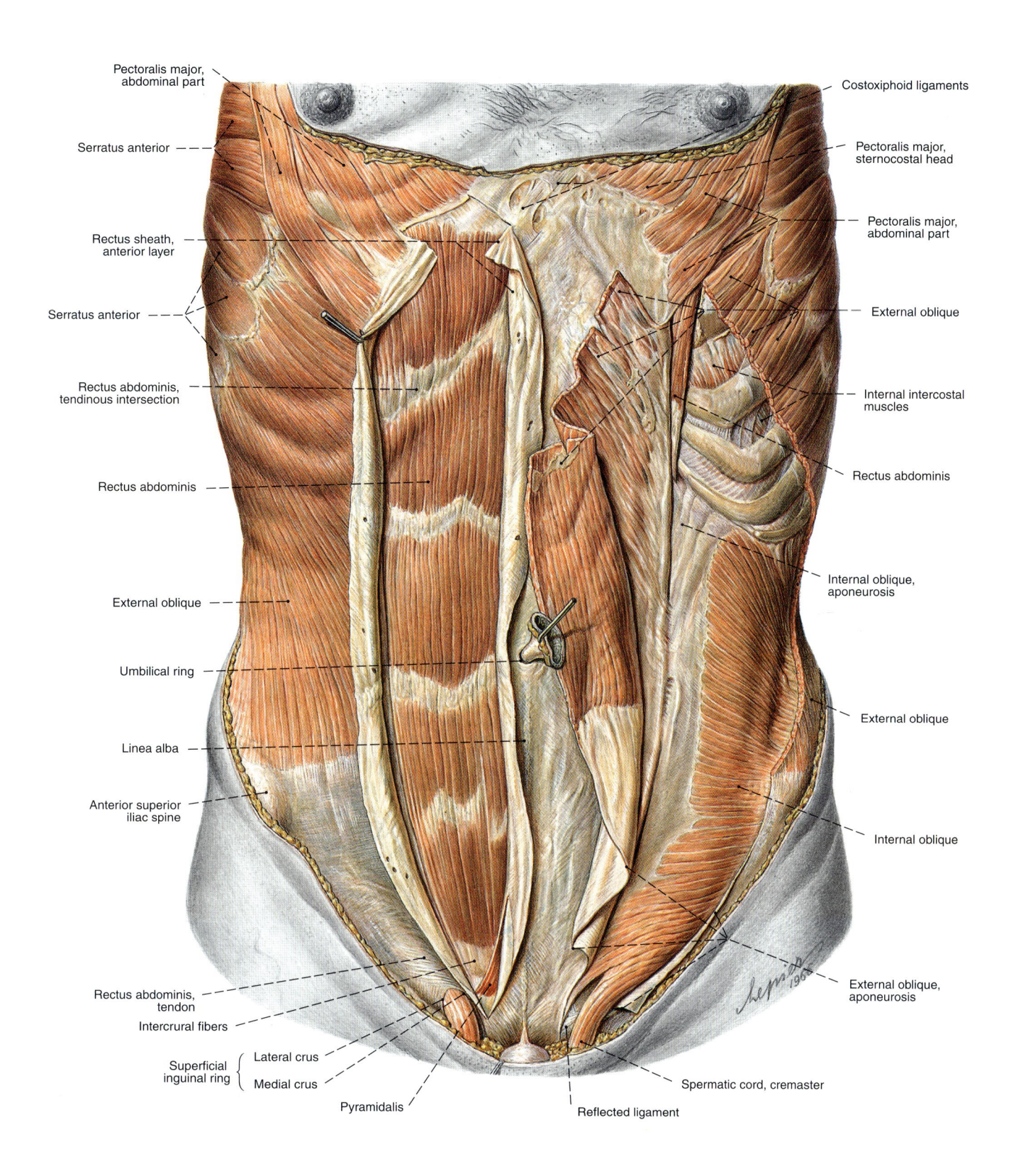

Fig. 824 Muscles of abdomen; anterior layer of rectus sheath split on the right to expose rectus abdominis and pyramidalis; external oblique sectioned on the left to expose internal oblique; anterior aspect.

64 Thoracic and abdominal walls

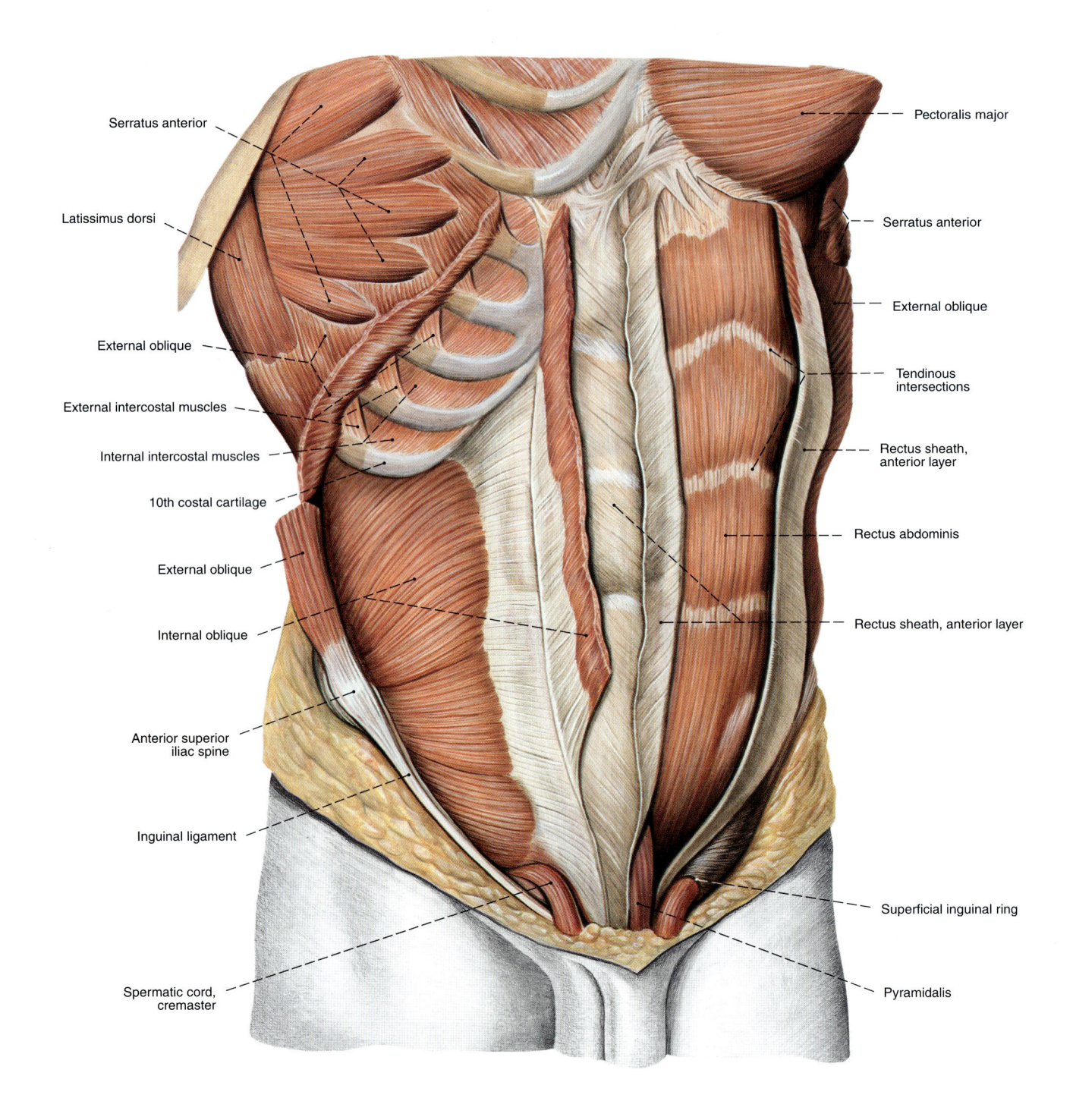

Fig. 825 Muscles of abdomen; anterior layer of rectus sheath opened on the right; external oblique sectioned on the left; external intercostal membrane removed; anterolateral aspect.

Muscles of abdomen

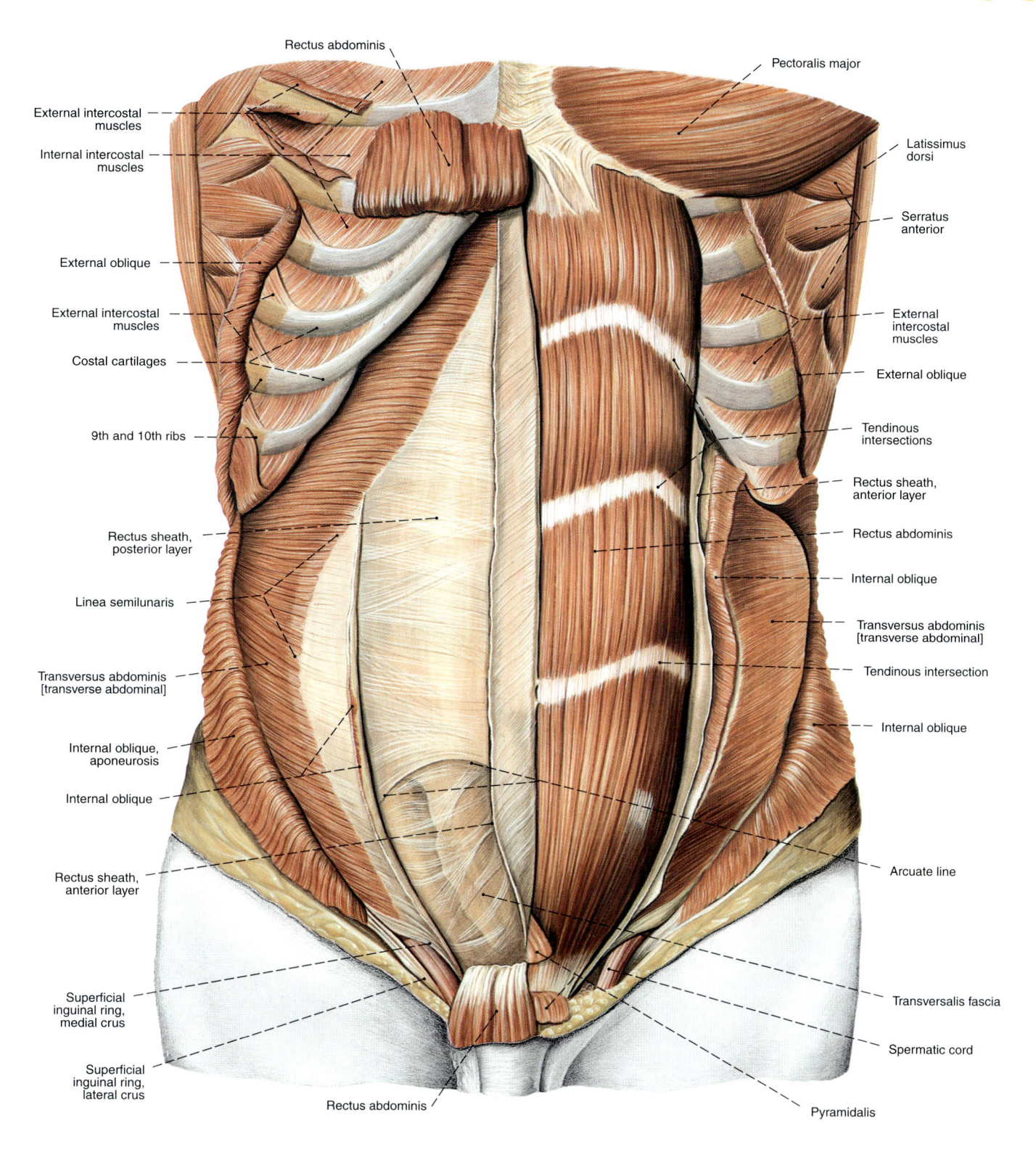

Fig. 826 Muscles of abdomen; pyramidalis sectioned on the left; rectus abdominis reflected upward and downward and external oblique opened on the right; anterior layer of rectus sheath reflected to the right over the midline; anterior aspect.

Thoracic and abdominal walls

Ventral muscles of abdominal wall (Fig. 826)

Both the anterior muscles of the abdominal wall, rectus abdominis, and pyramidalis lie within the rectus sheath.

Muscle *Innervation*	Origin	Insertion	Function
1. **Rectus abdominis** *Intercostal nerves (thoracic nerves); occasionally ventral rami of upper lumbar nerves*	5th – 7th costal cartilages (external surface), xiphoid process, costoxiphoid ligaments	Pubic crest, pubic symphysis	Flexes trunk toward pelvis, increases abdominal pressure, compresses abdomen in expiration
2. **Pyramidalis** *Caudal intercostal nerves (thoracic nerves) (inconstant muscle)*	Pubic crest, pubic symphysis (ventral of rectus abdominis)	Linea alba	Tenses linea alba

Lateral muscles of abdominal wall (Figs. 824, 826)

The lateral muscles of the abdominal wall comprise the external and internal oblique, and the transversus abdominis [transverse abdominal].
In the male the cremaster separates from the internal oblique and the transversus abdominis [transverse abdominal].

Muscle *Innervation*	Origin	Insertion	Function
1. **External oblique** *Caudal intercostal nerves (thoracic nerves), iliohypogastric nerve [iliopubic nerve; ilio-inguinal nerve; (lumbar plexus)*	5th–12th ribs (outer surface, interdigitations with serratus anterior)	Outer lip of iliac crest, inguinal ligament, pubic tubercle, pubic crest, linea alba (contributes to anterior layer of rectus sheath)	Acting unilateral: rotation of thorax to contralateral side, lateral flexion of vertebral column Acting bilateral: flexes trunk toward pelvis, increases abdominal pressure, compresses abdomen in expiration
2. **Internal oblique** *Caudal intercostal nerves (thoracic nerves), iliohypogastric nerve [iliopubic nerve; ilio-inguinal nerve; (lumbar plexus)*	Thoracolumbar fascia (posterior layer), intermediate zone of iliac crest, inguinal ligament (lateral 2/3)	(9th) 10th- 12th costal cartilage (lower border), linea alba (contributes to anterior and posterior layer of rectus sheath above arcuate line; below arcuate line all tendon fibers blend with the anterior layer). In the male the lowest fibers separate to form the cremaster, that continues in the spermatic cord.	Acting unilateral: rotation of thorax to ipsilateral side, lateral flexion of vertebral column Acting bilateral: flexes trunk toward pelvis, increases abdominal pressure, compresses abdomen in expiration Cremaster draws testis and sheaths upward.
3. **Transversus abdominis [transverse abdominal]** *Caudal intercostal nerves (thoracic nerves), iliohypogastric nerve [iliopubic nerve; ilio-inguinal nerve; genitofemoral nerve (lumbar plexus)*	(5th, 6th) 7th-12th costal cartilages (inner surface), costal processes of lumbar vertebrae (via anterior layer of thoracolumbar fascia), inner lip of iliac crest, inguinal ligament (lateral third)	Linea alba (contributes to posterior layer of rectus sheath above arcuate line and to the anterior layer below arcuate line). In the male the lowest fibers separate to form the cremaster, that continues in the spermatic cord.	Increases abdominal pressure, compresses abdomen in expiration

Posterior muscles of abdominal wall (Fig. 829)

The muscular base of the posterior abdominal wall is represented by the lumbar part of diaphragm superiorly and the quadratus lumborum inferiorly. This muscle is joined by the psoas major medially.

Muscle *Innervation*	Origin	Insertion	Function
1. **Quadratus lumborum** *Muscular branches (lumbar plexus); intercostal nerve (12th thoracic nerve)*	Outer lip of iliac crest (posterior third), iliolumbar ligament	12th rib (medial part), costal processes of 4th-1st lumbar vertebrae	Lowers ribs (expiration), lateral flexion of vertebral column

Inguinal canal 67

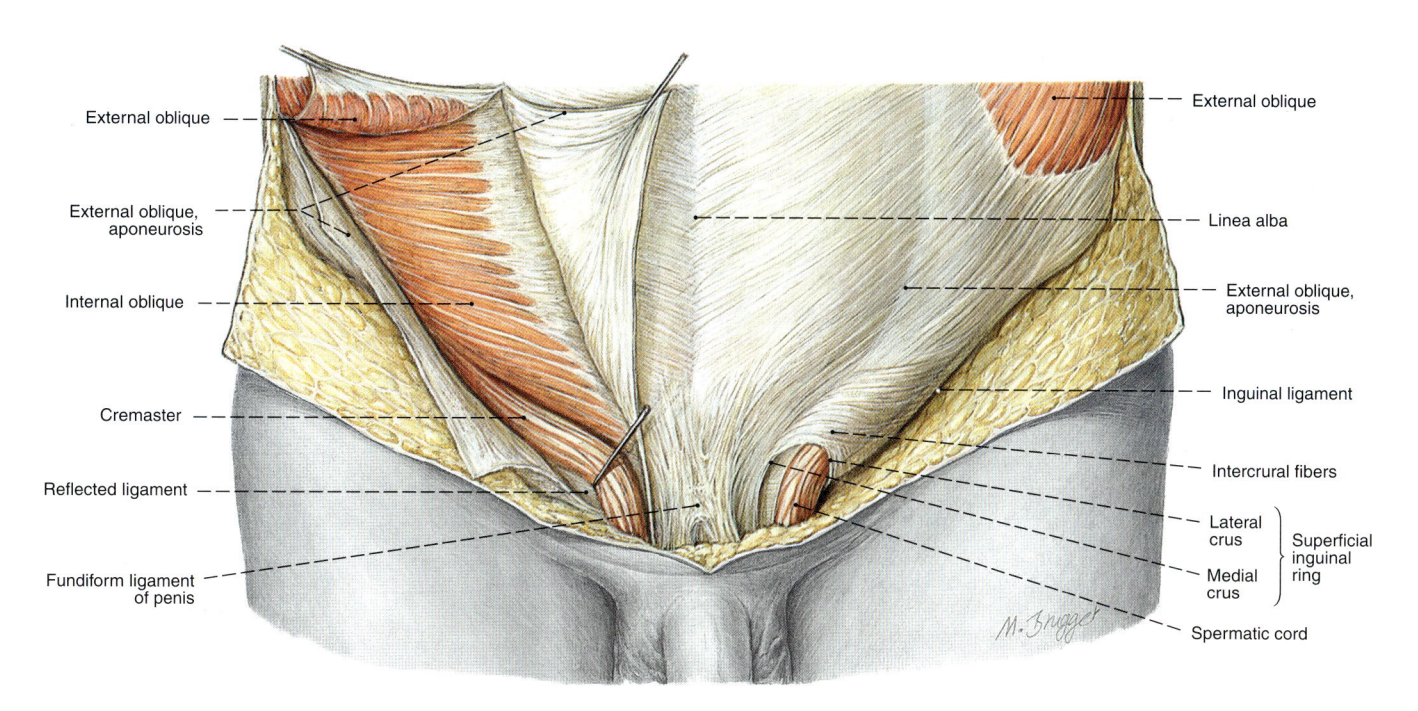

Fig. 827 Superficial inguinal ring; right spermatic cord retracted by a hook; aponeurosis of external oblique opened on the right; anterior aspect.
Compare Fig. 835.

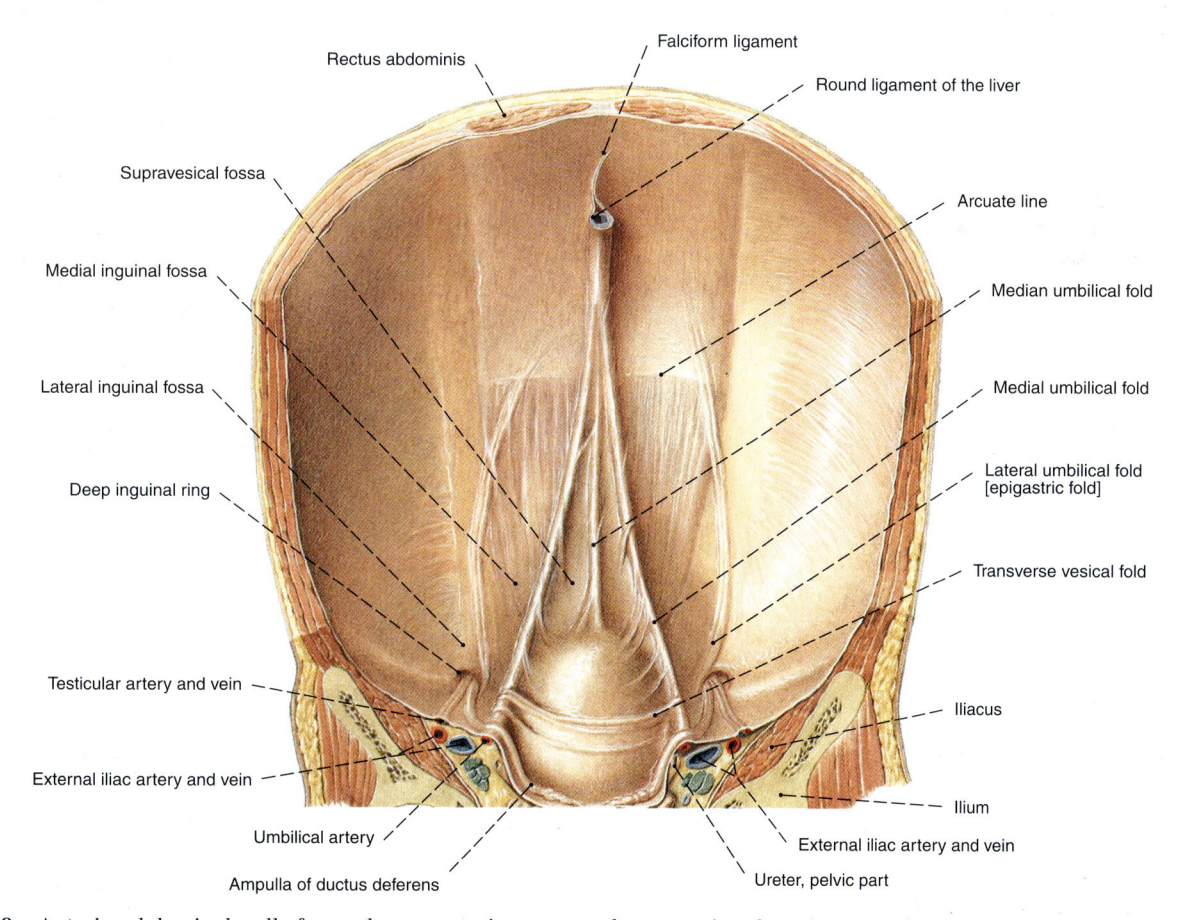

Fig. 828 Anterior abdominal wall of a newborn; posterior aspect.
The umbilical vein degenerates after birth. In cases of portal hypertension the vein may enlarge again. Compare Fig. 1029, portocaval anastomoses.

Thoracic and abdominal walls

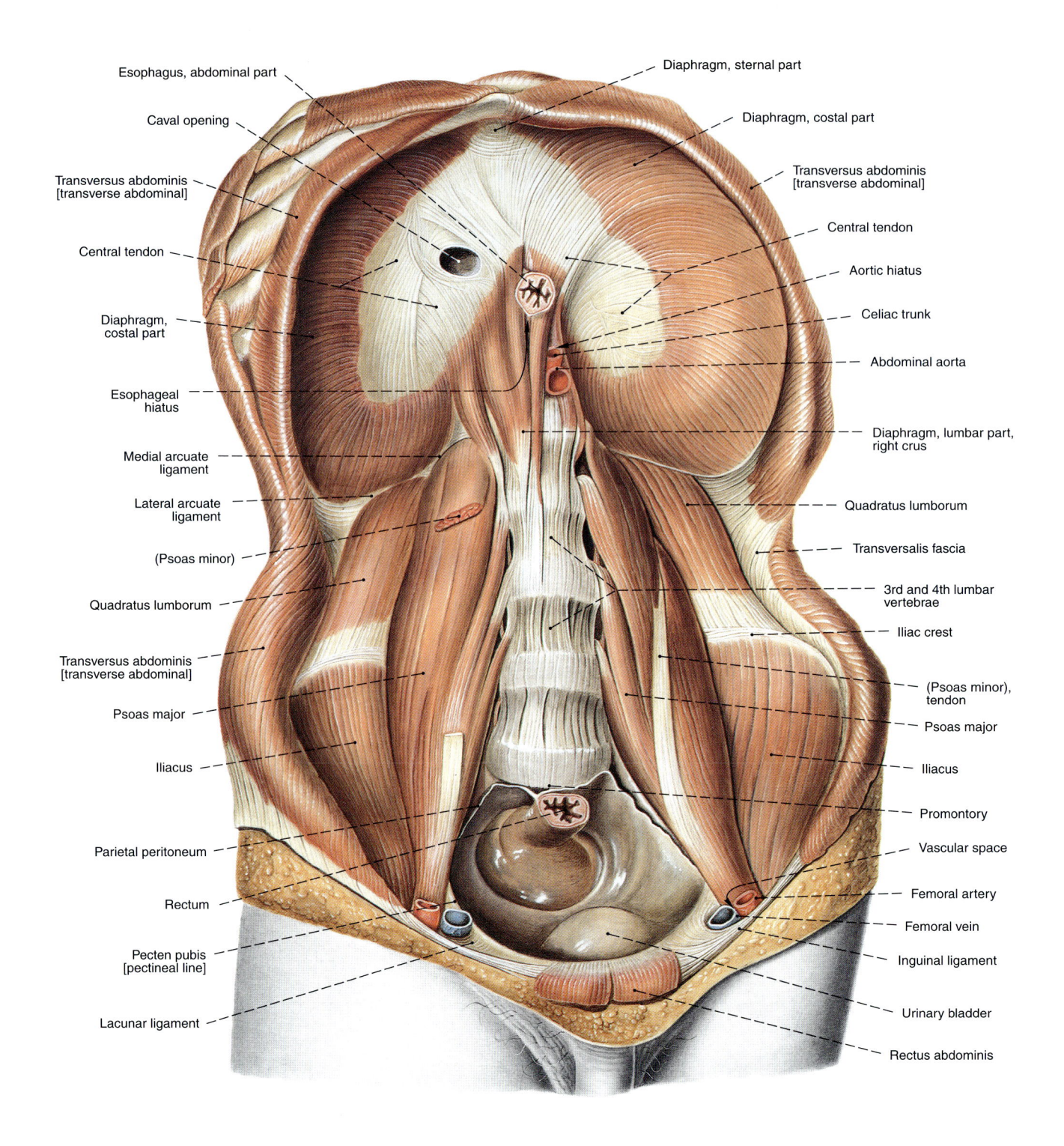

Fig. 829　Diaphragm; muscles of abdomen; anterior aspect.

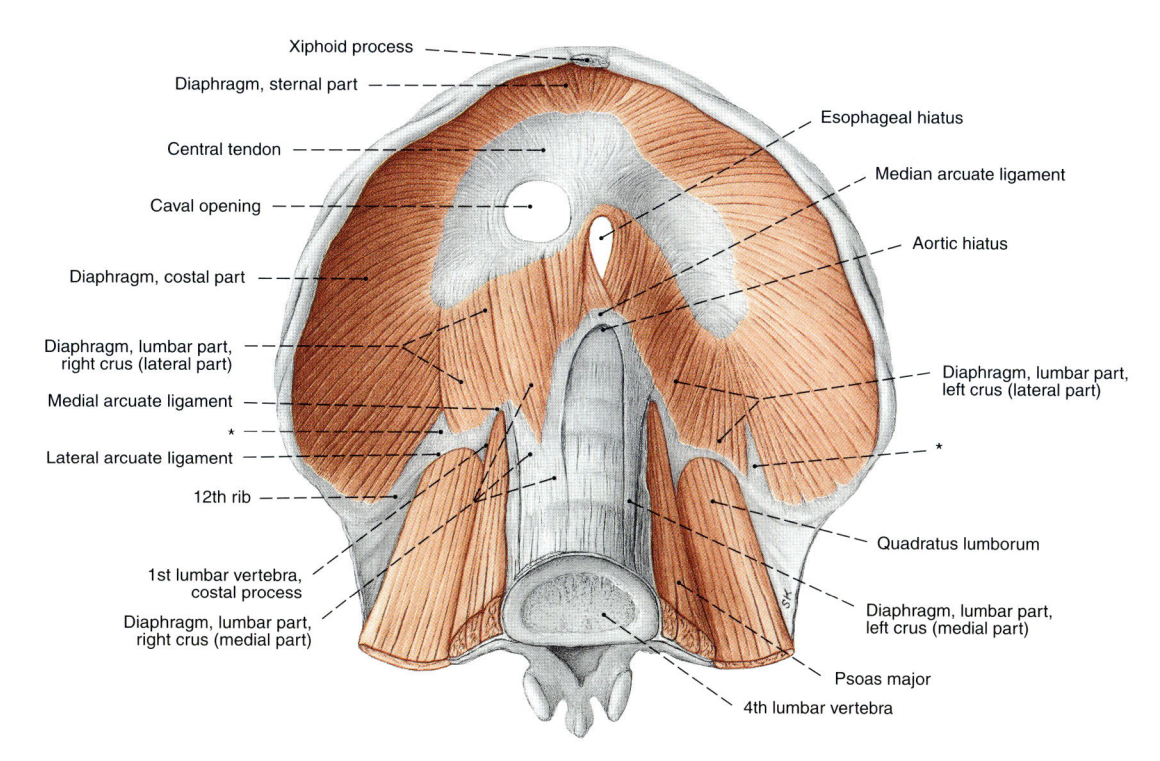

Diaphragm

Fig. 830 Diaphragm; and posterior abdominal wall; anterior aspect.

The right crus (medial part) frequently consists of three components and extends further distally than the left crus.
* Clinically: BOCHDALEK's triangle.

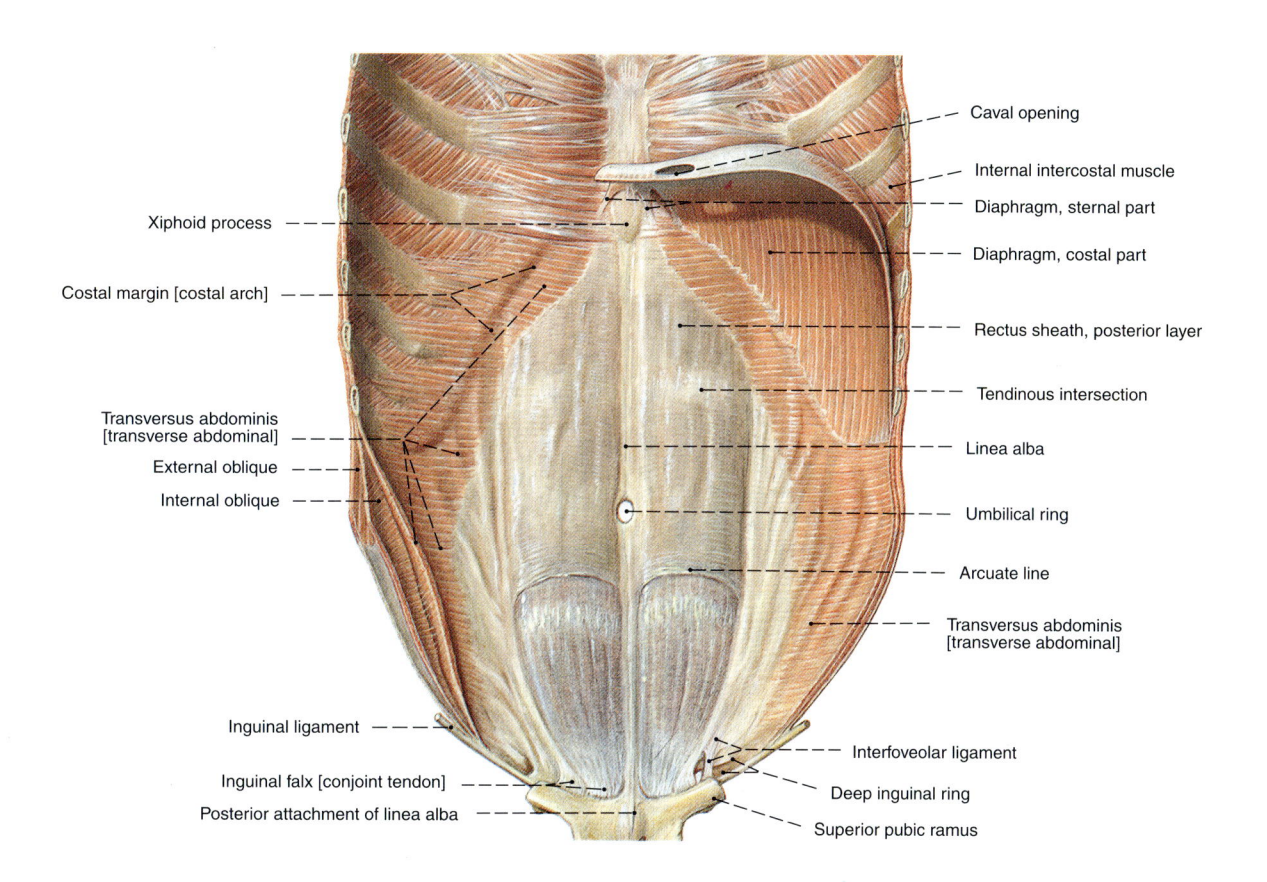

Fig. 831 Anterior abdominal wall and parts of diaphragm; posterior aspect.

Thoracic and abdominal walls

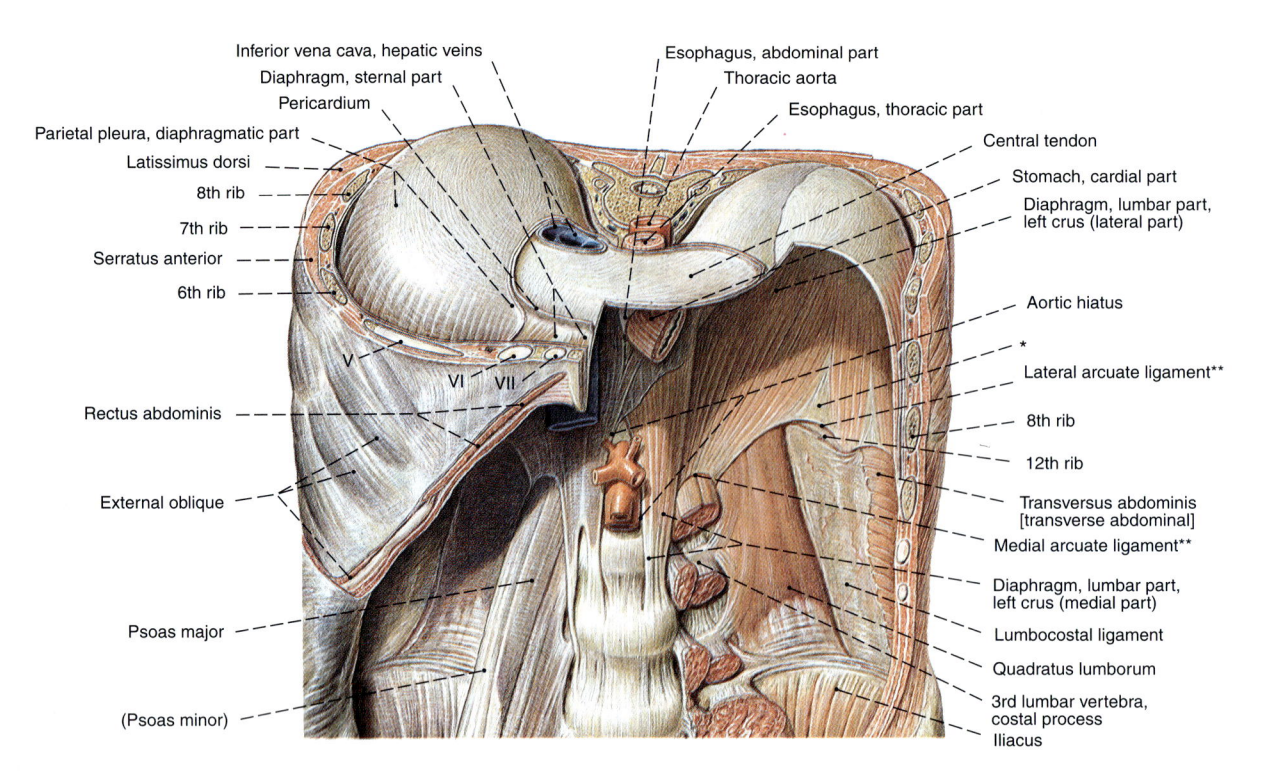

Fig. 832 Diaphragm with openings and muscles of posterior abdominal wall; trunk sectioned at level of 10th thoracic vertebra; anterior aspect.

* Clinically: BOCHDALEK's triangle, lumbocostal triangle, area without muscles.
** Also arches of psoas and quadratus, HALLER's arches.

Diaphragm (Fig. 832)

The diaphragm separates the thoracic and the abdominal cavities. Its dome forms the floor of the right and left pleural cavities. The lumbar part borders the retroperitoneal space and—strictly speaking—is part of the posterior abdominal wall.

Muscle *Innervation*	Origin	Insertion	Function
Diaphragm *Phrenic nerve (cervical plexus)*	**Sternal part:** xiphoid process (inner surface), rectus sheath (aponeurosis of transversus abdominis [transverse abdominal]) **Costal part:** 12th-6th costal cartilage (inner surface, interdigitates with origin of transversus abdominis [transverse abdominal]) **Lumbar part, right crus:** - Medial part: bodies of 1st-3rd lumbar vertebrae, intervertebral discs - Lateral part: medial and lateral arcuate ligaments **Lumbar part, left crus:** - Medial part: bodies of 1st-4th lumbar vertebrae, intervertebral discs - Lateral part: medial and lateral arcuate ligaments	All parts unite in the central tendon. Weak spaces and openings: sternocostal triangle, lumbocostal triangle, caval opening, aortic hiatus, esophageal hiatus	Diaphragmatic respiration (inspiration), increases abdominal pressure

Plexus lumbosacralis **71**

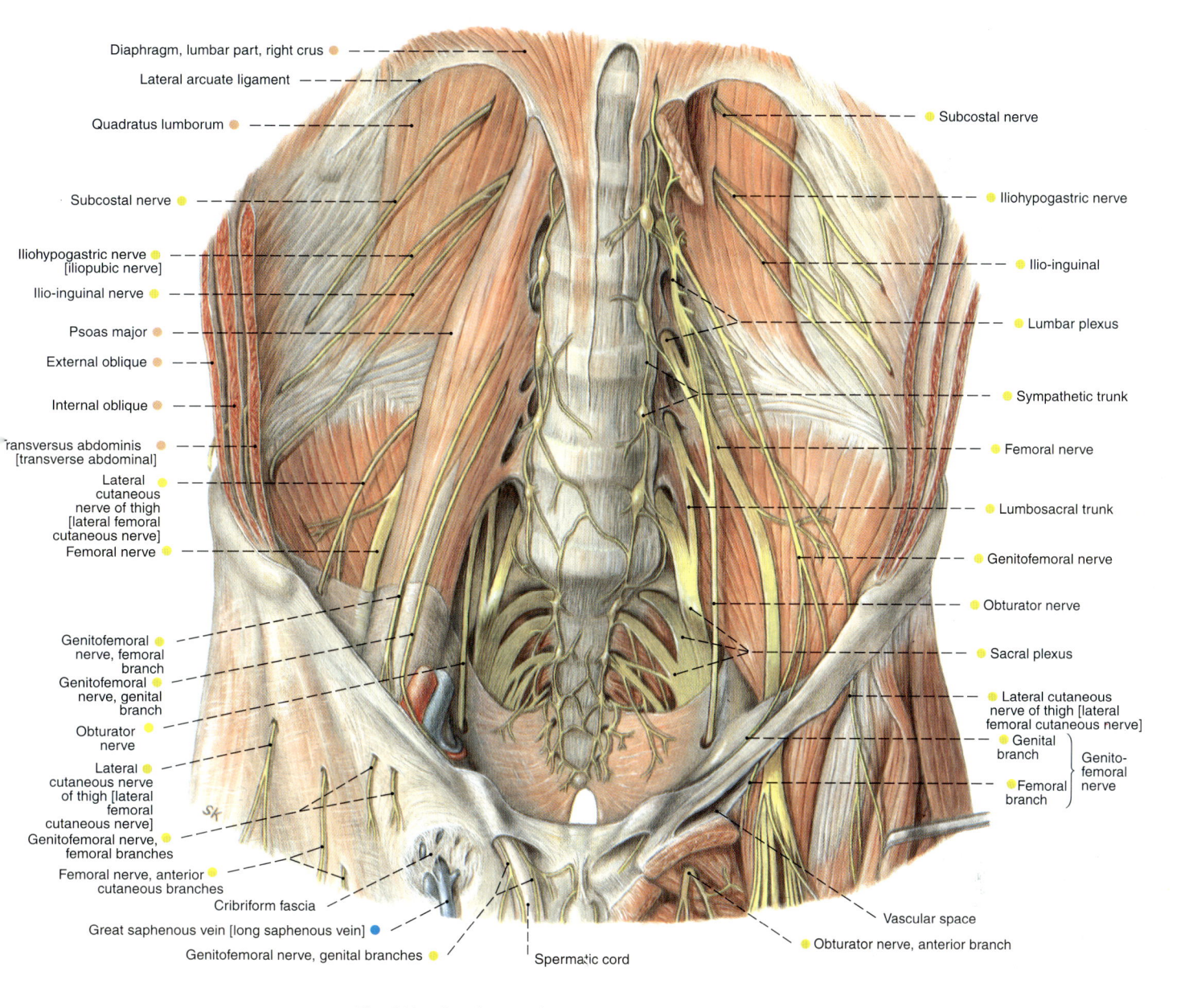

Fig. 833 Lumbosacral plexus;
after removal of psoas major, pectineus, and adductor longus on the left; anterior aspect.

Diaphragmatic openings

Name	Position	Structures
Aortic hiatus	Lumbar part, between right crus and left crus	Aorta; thoracic duct
Esophageal hiatus	Lumbar part, right crus	Esophagus; vagus nerves; phrenic nerve; left phrenico-abdominal branch
Caval opening	Central tendon	Inferior vena cava; phrenic nerve; right phrenico-abdominal branch
LARREY's cleft [triangle of MORGAGNI]	Between sternal part and costal part	Superior epigastric artery and vein
Unnamed	Lumbar part, right/left crus, (medial part)	Greater and lesser splanchnic nerves; azygos vein; hemi-azygos vein [inferior hemi-azygos vein]
Unnamed	Lumbar part, between medial part and lateral part	Sympathetic trunk

Thoracic and abdominal walls

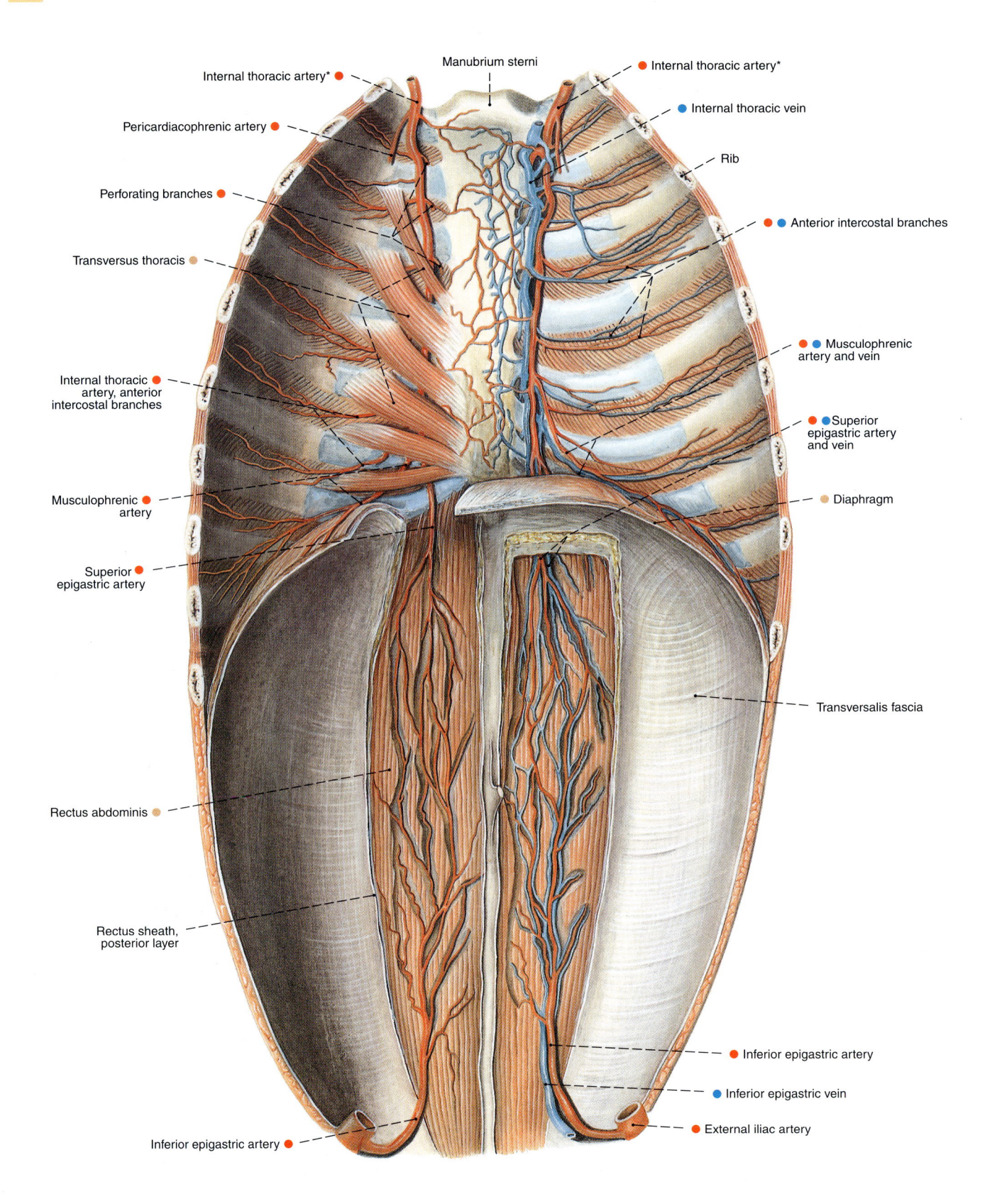

Fig. 834 Blood vessels of anterior thoracic and abdominal walls; transversus thoracis removed on the right; posterior aspect.

* Clinically: internal mammary artery.

Anterior abdominal wall and inguinal canal 73

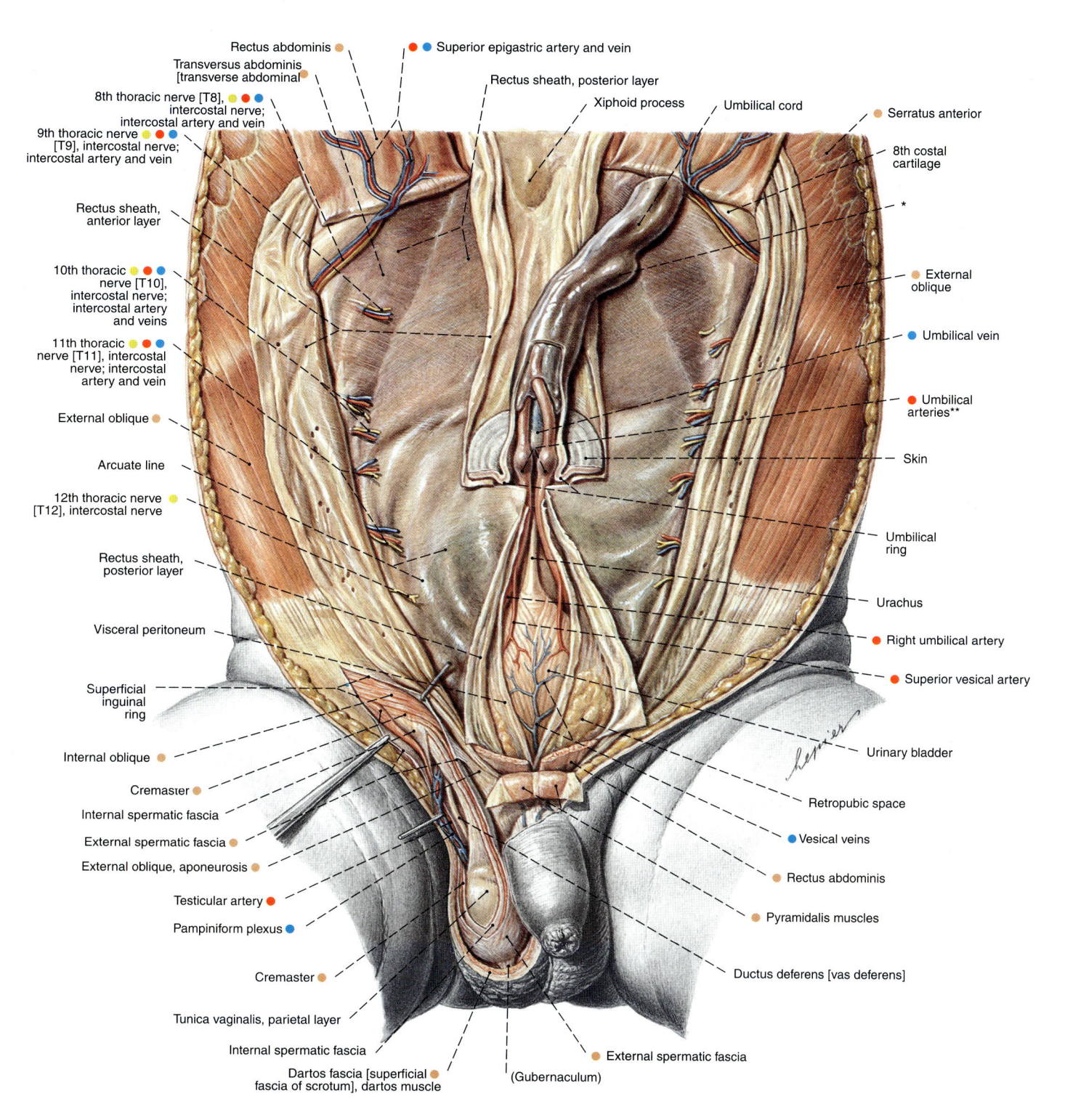

Fig. 835 Anterior abdominal wall of a newborn; rectus abdominis muscles reflected upward and abdominal cavity opened in the median plane to expose urinary bladder and urachus; inguinal canal dissected on the right; anterior aspect.

* Thickening formed by loops of umbilical blood vessels (false umbilical cord knot).
** Thrombus in umbilical arteries.

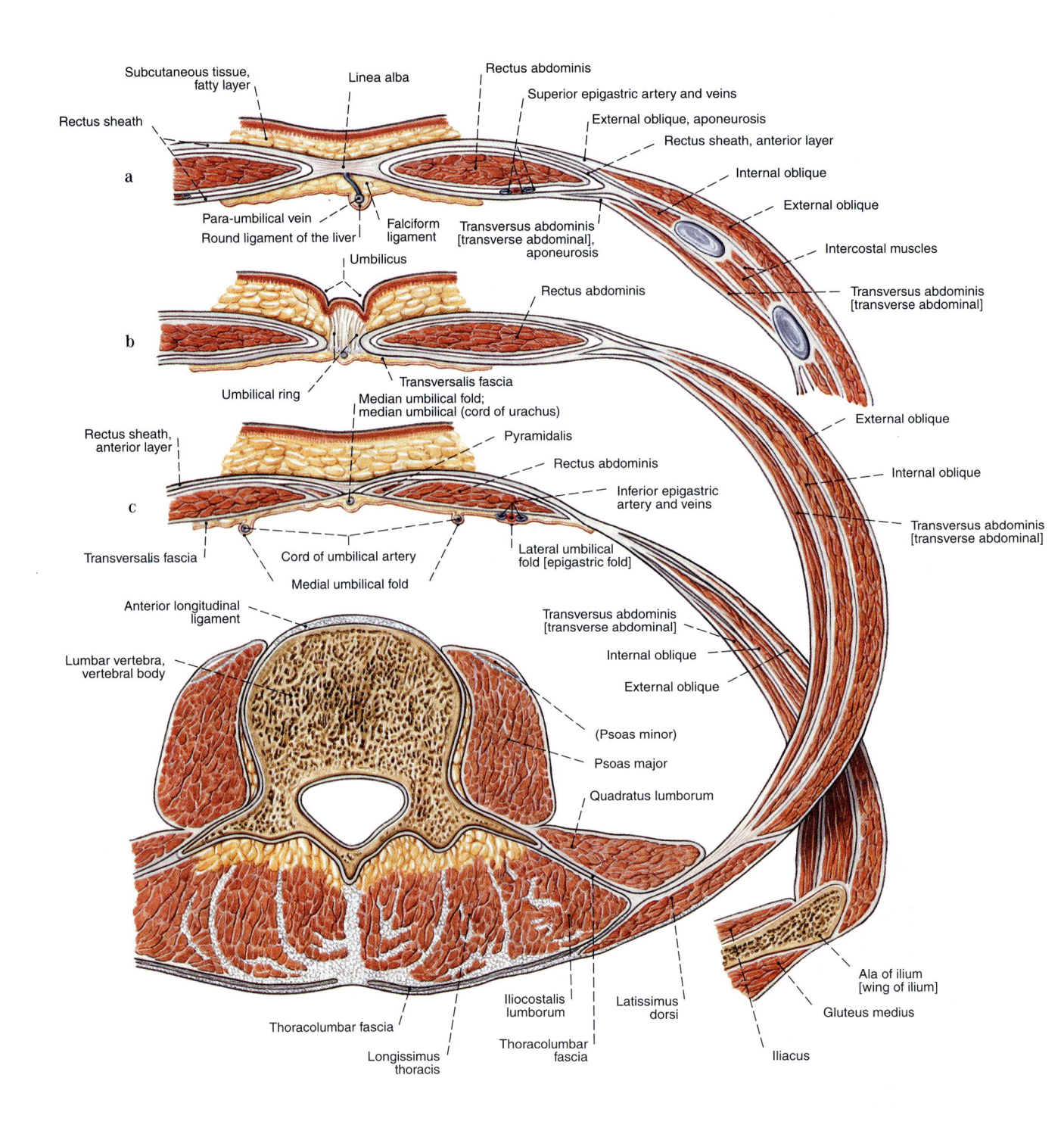

Fig. 836 a–c Muscles of abdomen; horizontal sections.

a   Above umbilicus
b   At level of umbilicus
c   Below umbilicus and arcuate line

Muscles of abdomen

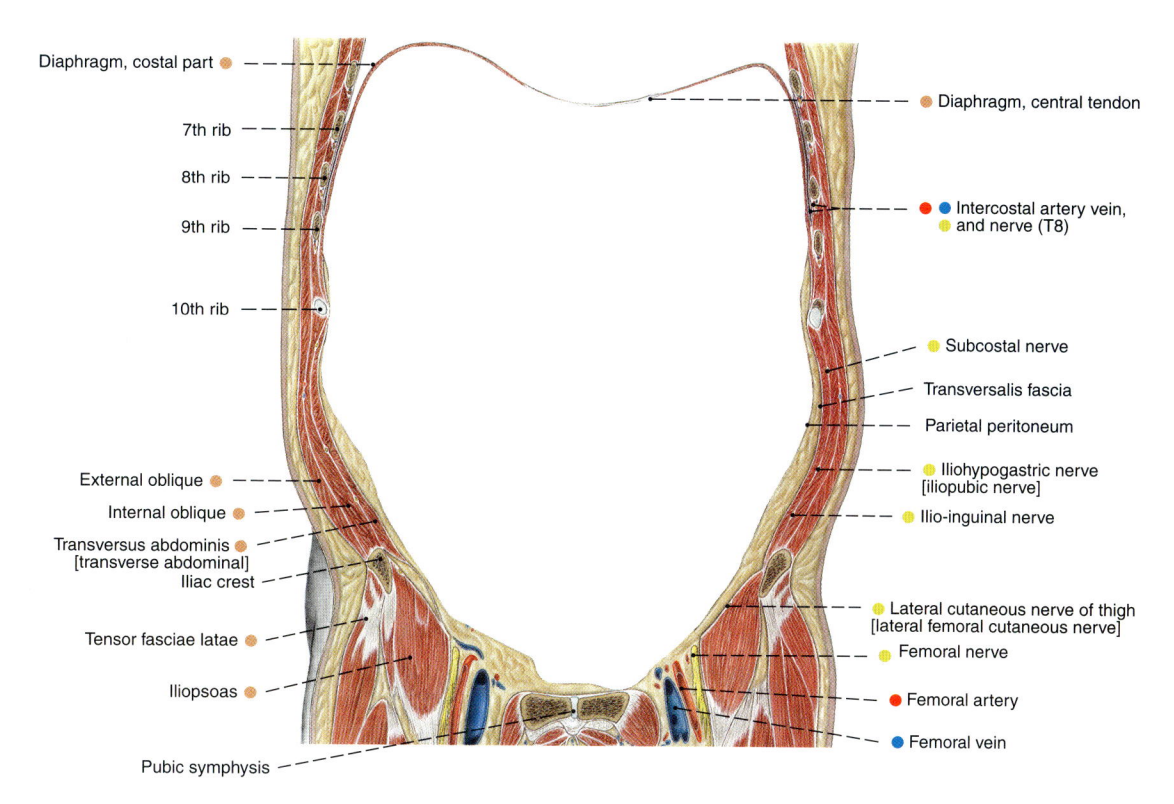

Fig. 837 Muscles of abdomen; frontal section; ventral aspect. Compare Fig. 1134.

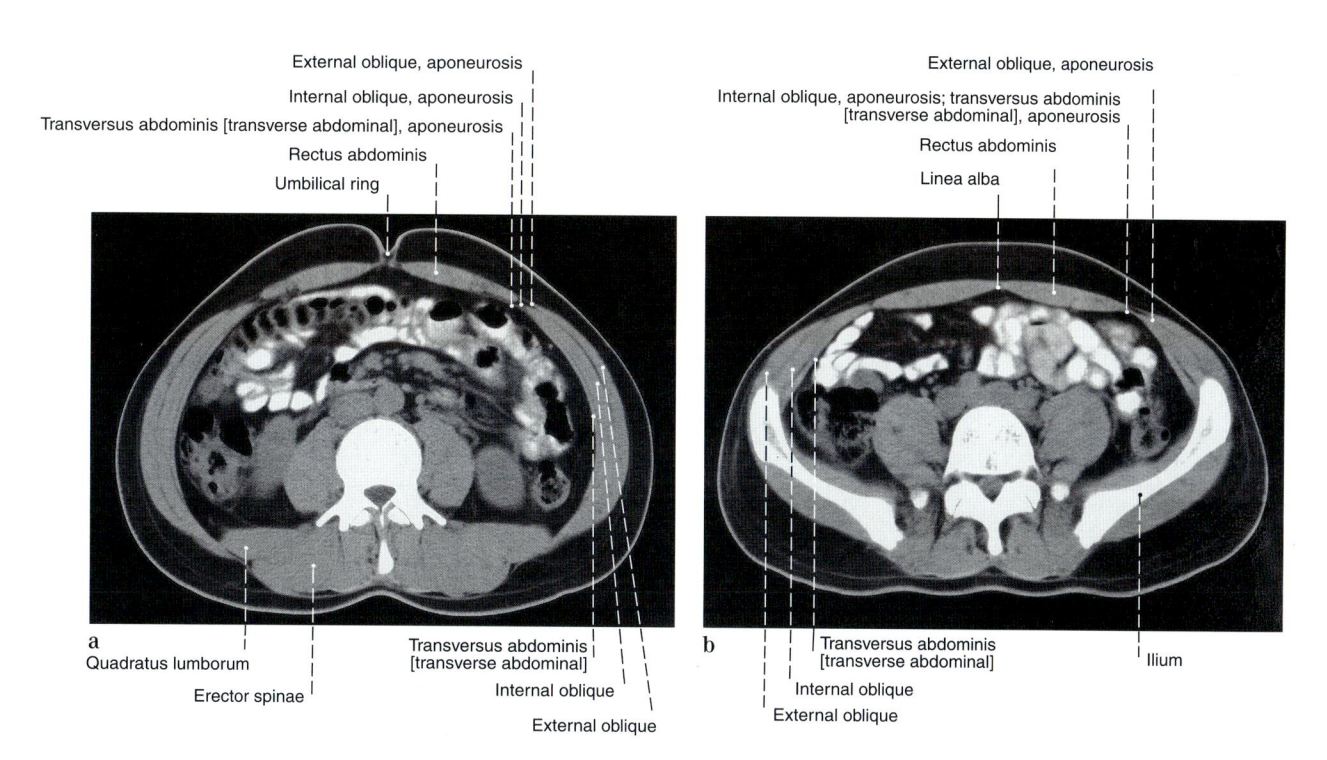

Fig. 838 a, b Muscles of abdomen; computer tomographic horizontal sections.
a At level of umbilicus
b At level of 5th lumbar vertebra

The contribution of aponeuroses to the rectus sheath is clearly visible (compare Figs. 837 and 1148).

Thoracic viscera

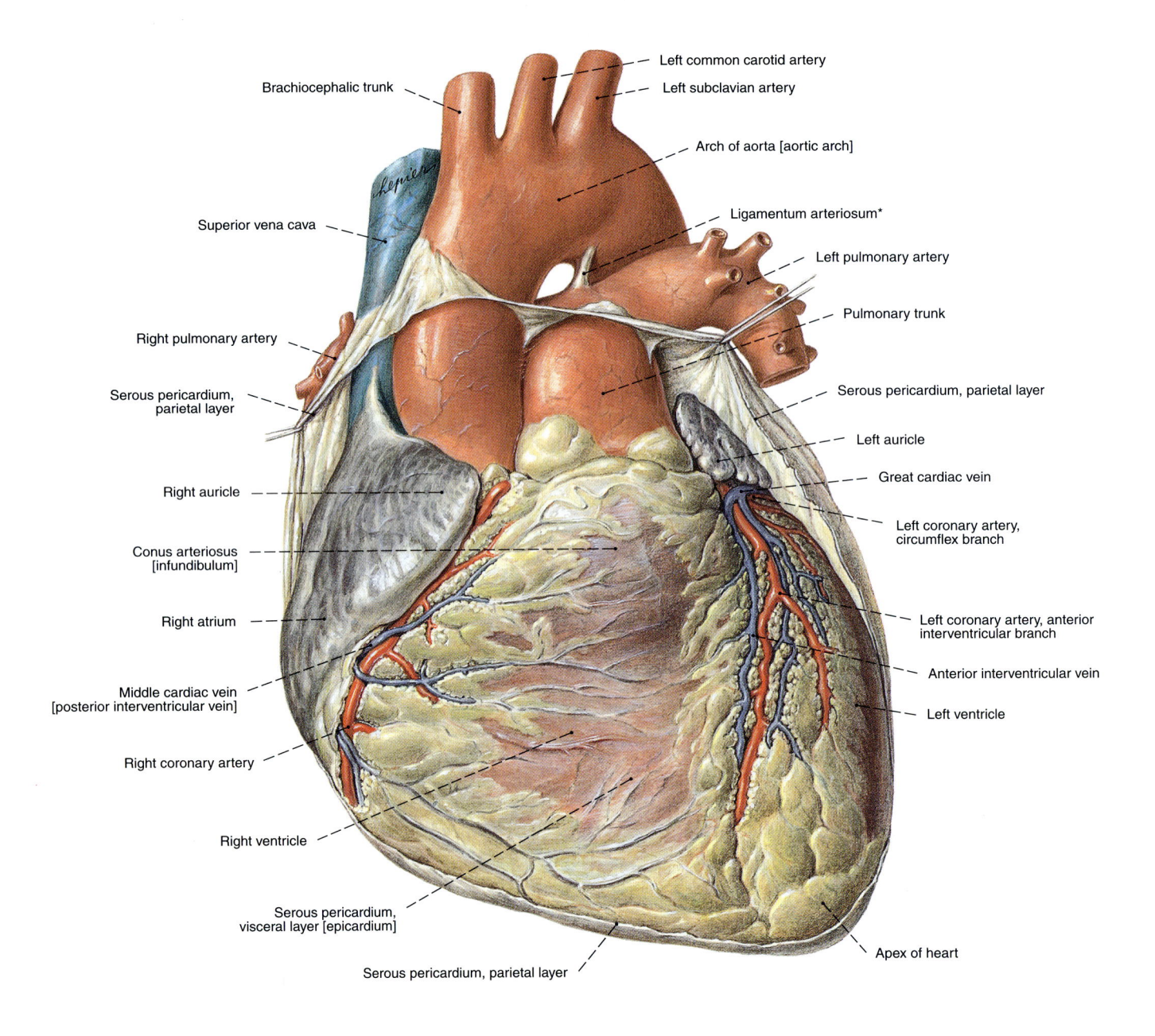

Fig. 839 Heart; pericardium opened and parietal layer mostly removed; larger branches of coronary blood vessels dissected; visceral layer [epicardium] not shown on descending aorta and pulmonary trunk; ventral aspect.

* BOTALLO's ligament formed from the remnants of the fetal ductus arteriosus [BOTALLO's duct].

Fibrous pericardium	
Serous pericardium	Pericardium
Parietal layer	
Visceral layer	= Epicardium

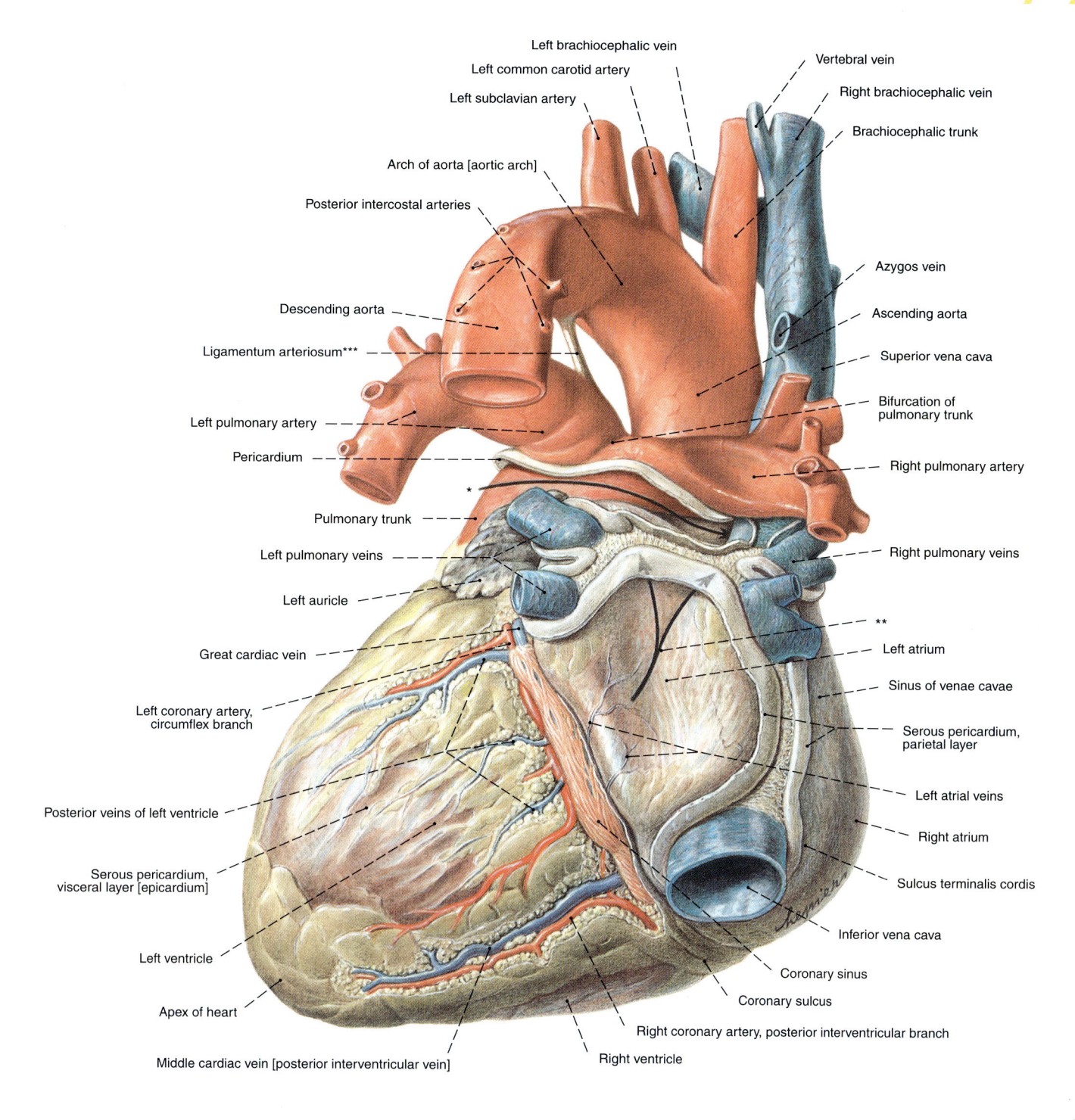

Fig. 840 Heart and great blood vessels; pericardium severed next to the great blood vessels; larger branches of coronary blood vessels dissected; dorsal aspect.

* Arrow in transverse pericardial sinus.
** Double arrows in oblique pericardial sinus.
*** BOTALLO's ligament formed from the remnants of the fetal ductus arteriosus [BOTALLO's duct].

78 *Thoracic viscera*

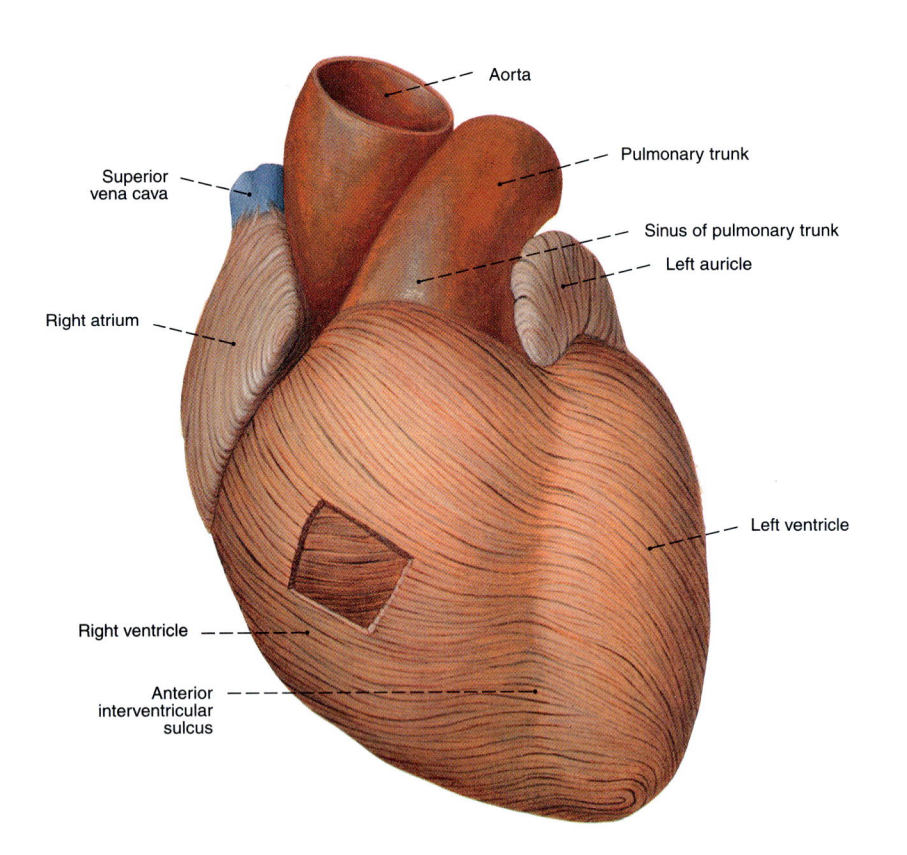

Fig. 841 Myocardium; parts of the superficial muscle layer of the right ventricle removed to expose the deep layer; ventral aspect.

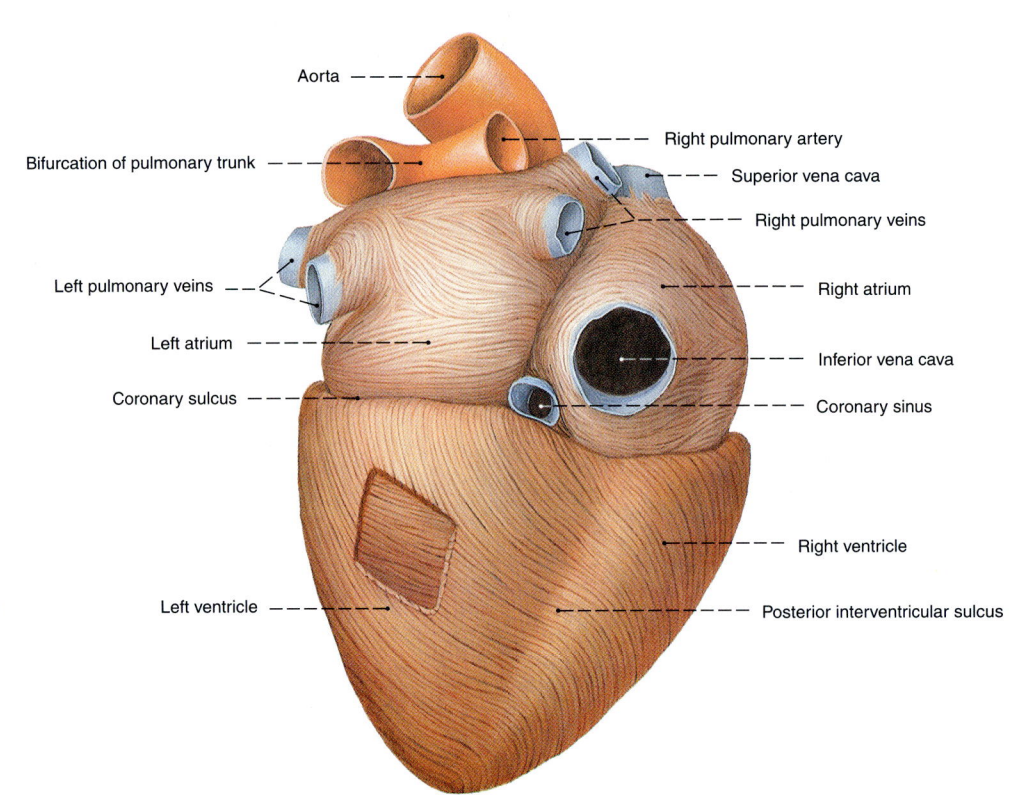

Fig. 842 Myocardium; parts of the superficial muscle layer of the left ventricle removed to expose the deep layer; the intersection of myocardium after removal of coronary sinus is not shown; dorsocaudal aspect.

Heart 79

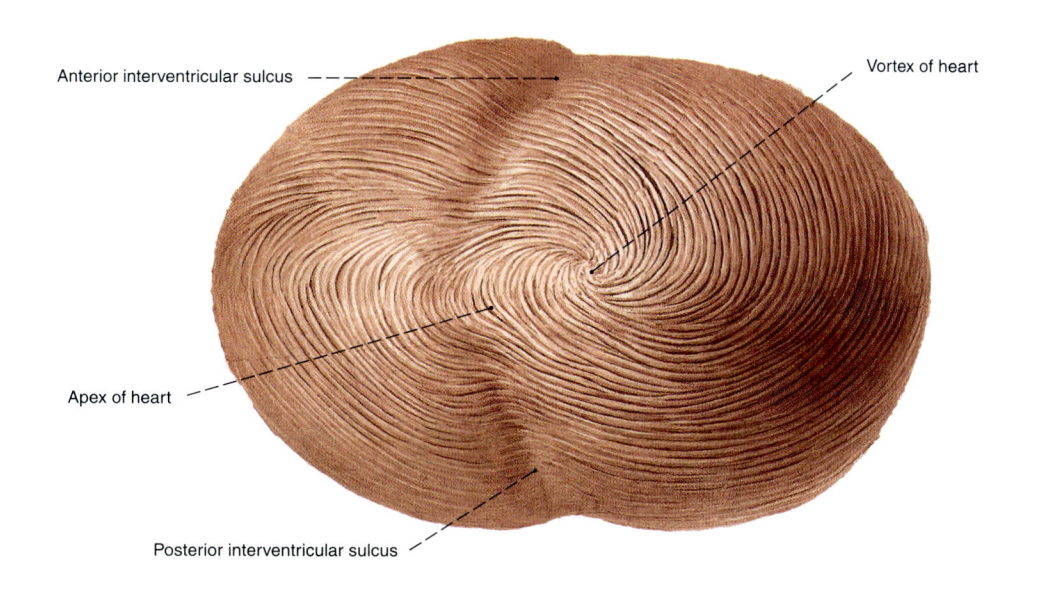

Fig. 843 Myocardium; viewed from the apex.

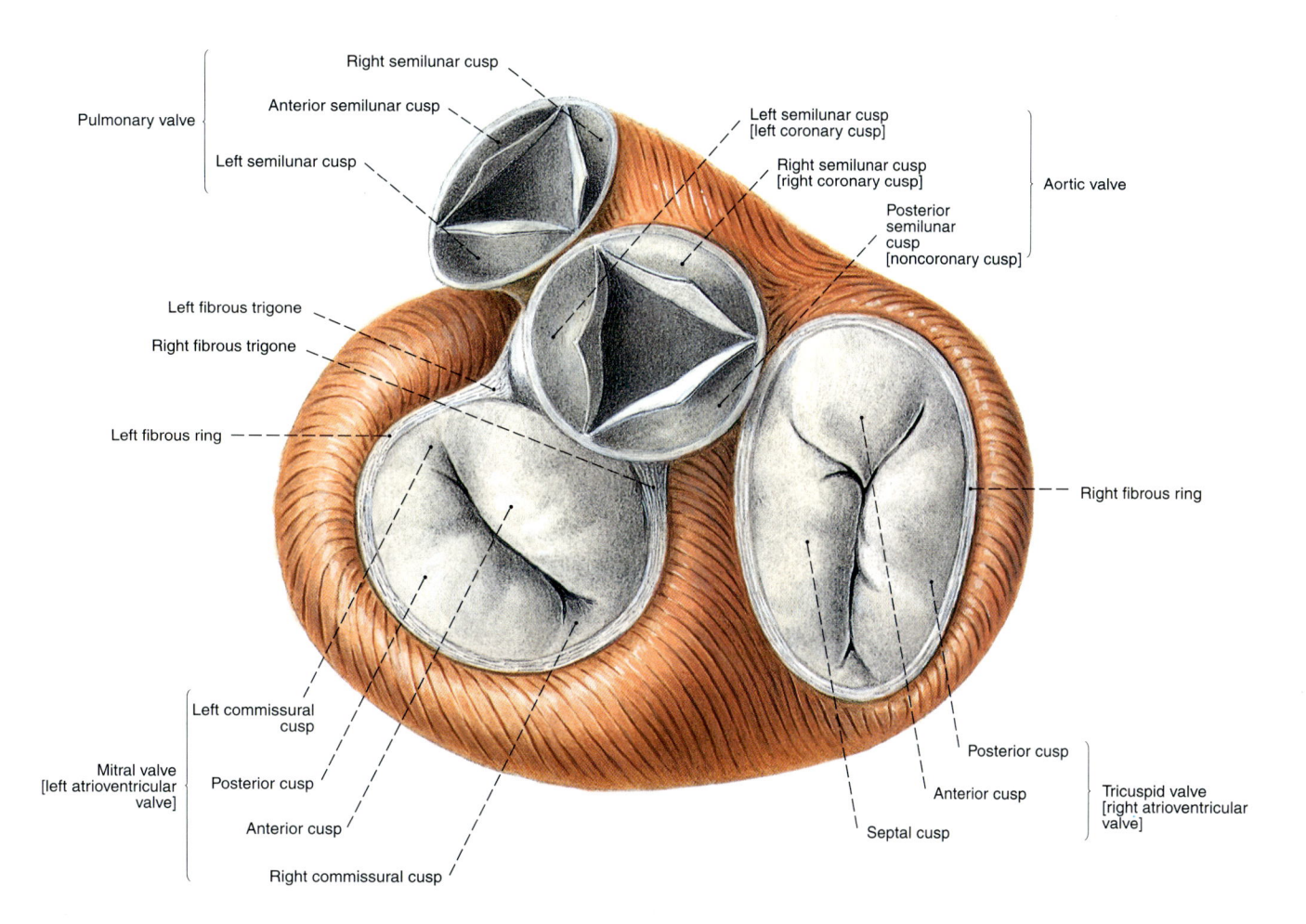

Fig. 844 Myocardium; cardiac valves; surface of cut interatrial septum and opening for bundle of HIS not shown; systolic phase with open arterial and closed atrioventricular valves; cranial aspect.

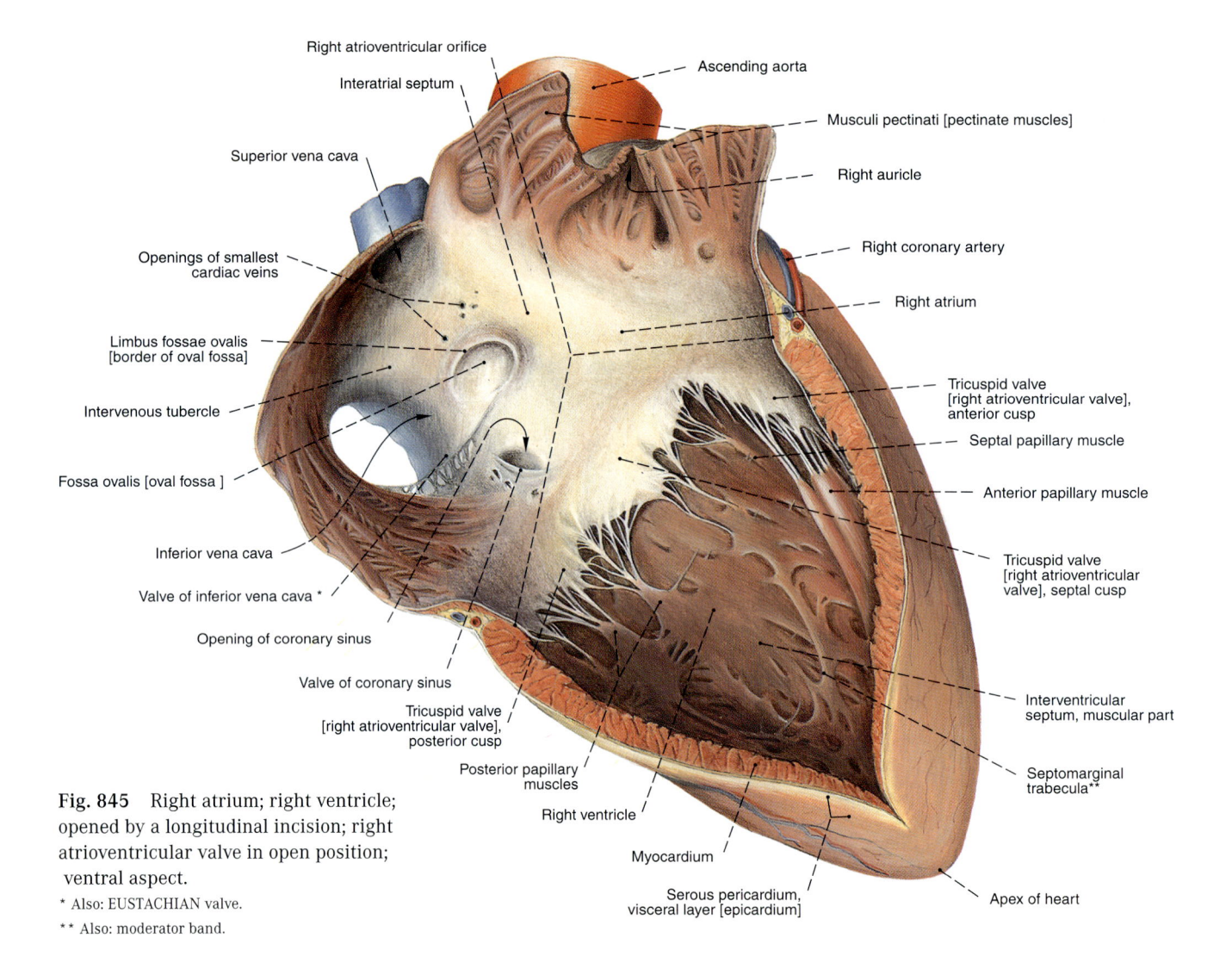

Thoracic viscera

Fig. 845 Right atrium; right ventricle; opened by a longitudinal incision; right atrioventricular valve in open position; ventral aspect.

* Also: EUSTACHIAN valve.
** Also: moderator band.

Fig. 846 Right atrium of a newborn; anterior wall of atrium reflected to expose foramen ovale; right ventral aspect.
For the significance of the foramen ovale before birth see Fig. 41.

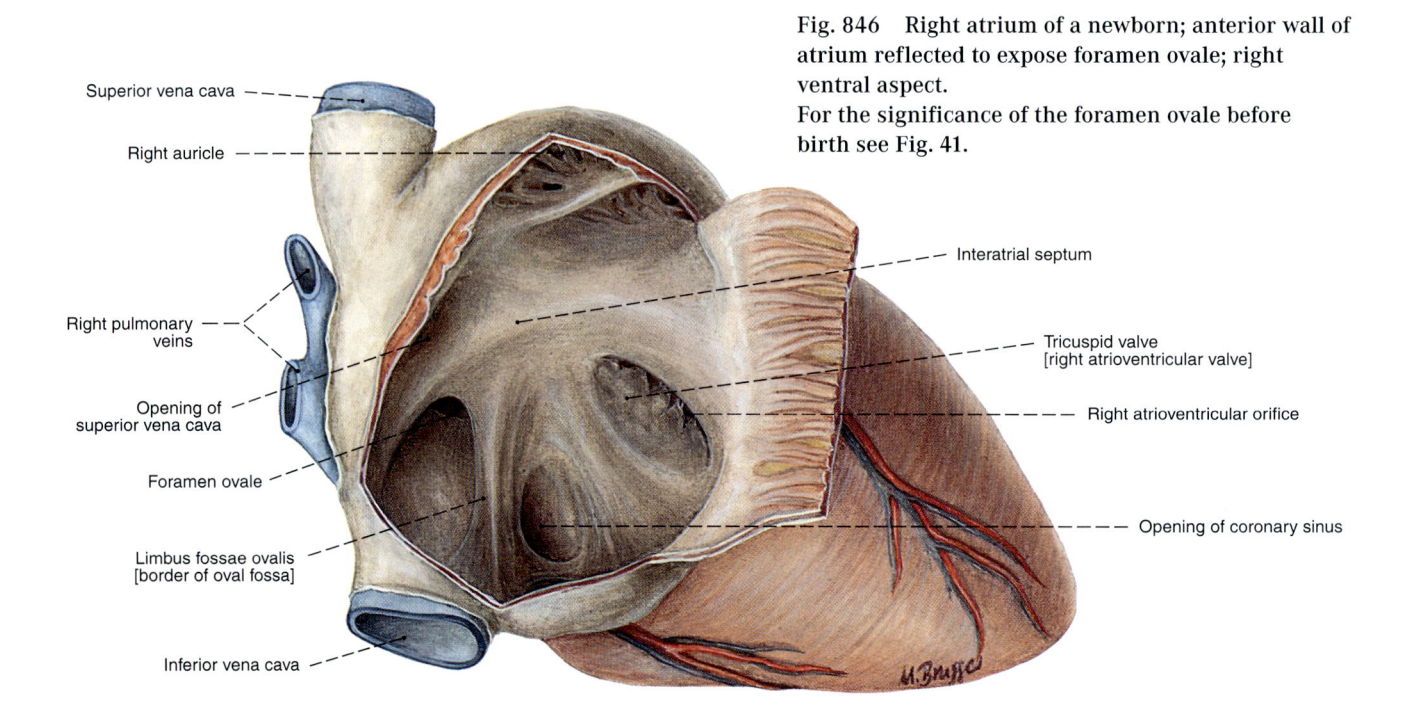

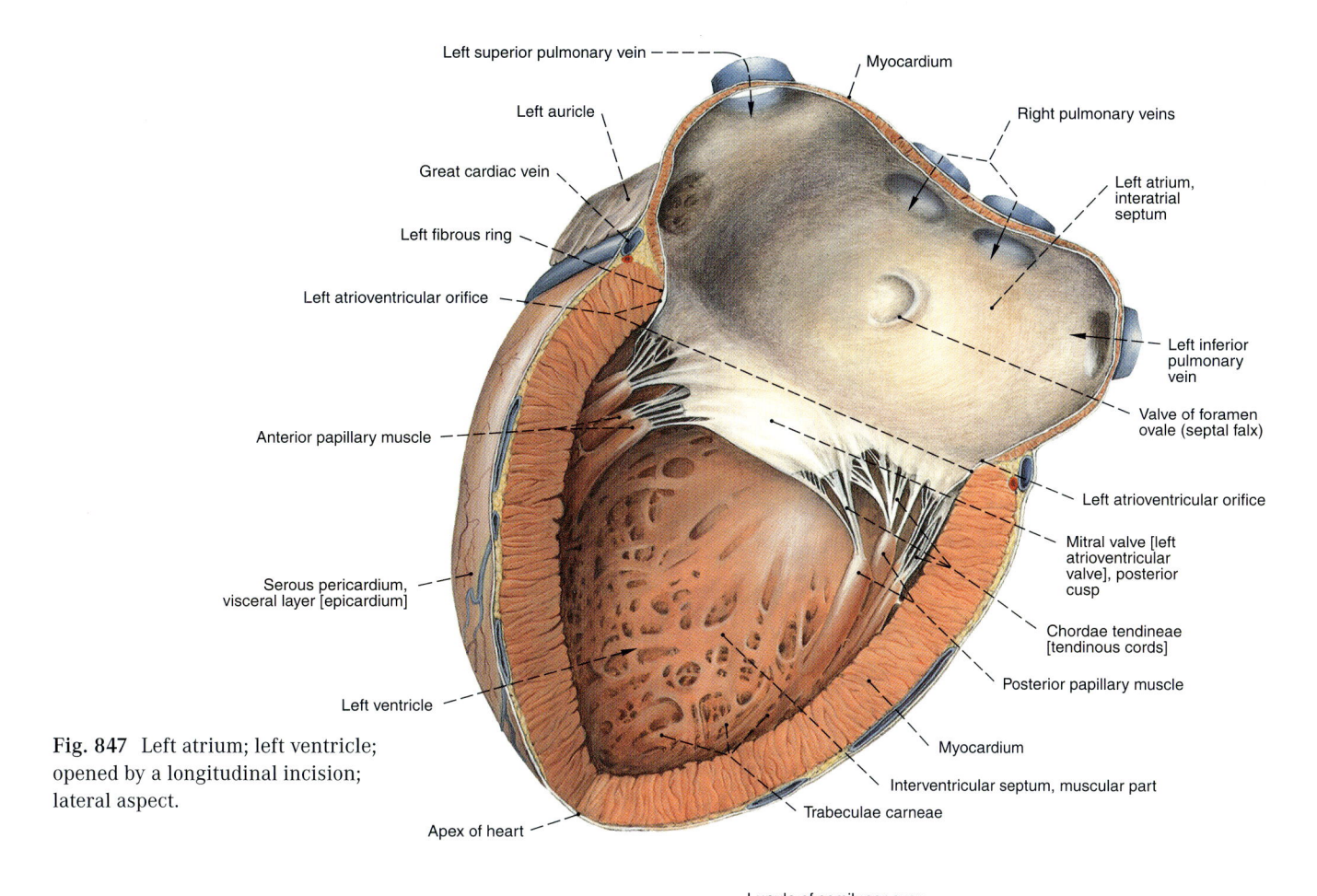

Heart 81

Fig. 847 Left atrium; left ventricle; opened by a longitudinal incision; lateral aspect.

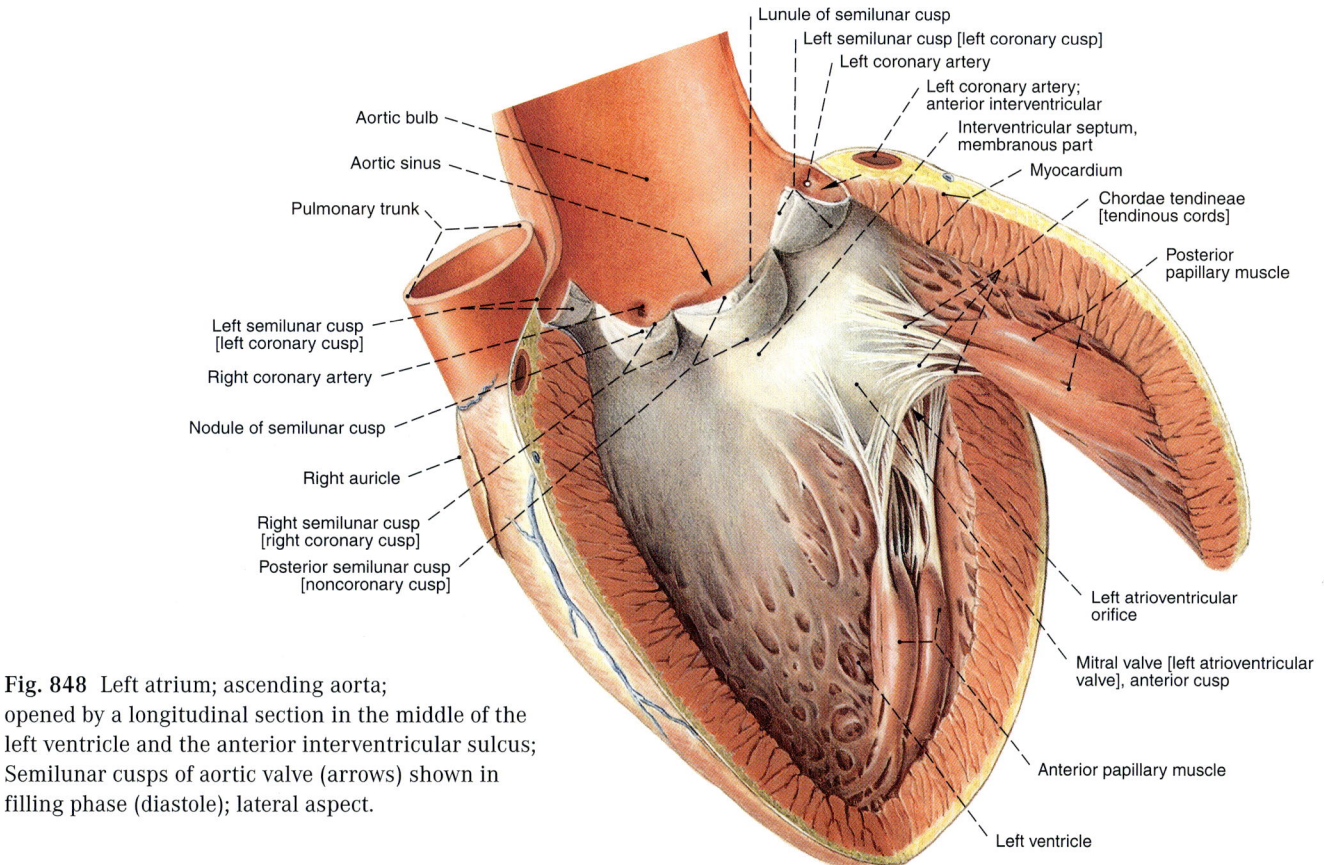

Labels: Left superior pulmonary vein; Myocardium; Left auricle; Right pulmonary veins; Great cardiac vein; Left atrium, interatrial septum; Left fibrous ring; Left atrioventricular orifice; Left inferior pulmonary vein; Valve of foramen ovale (septal falx); Anterior papillary muscle; Left atrioventricular orifice; Mitral valve [left atrioventricular valve], posterior cusp; Serous pericardium, visceral layer [epicardium]; Chordae tendineae [tendinous cords]; Posterior papillary muscle; Left ventricle; Myocardium; Interventricular septum, muscular part; Trabeculae carneae; Apex of heart

Fig. 848 Left atrium; ascending aorta; opened by a longitudinal section in the middle of the left ventricle and the anterior interventricular sulcus; Semilunar cusps of aortic valve (arrows) shown in filling phase (diastole); lateral aspect.

Labels: Lunule of semilunar cusp; Left semilunar cusp [left coronary cusp]; Left coronary artery; Aortic bulb; Left coronary artery; anterior interventricular; Aortic sinus; Interventricular septum, membranous part; Pulmonary trunk; Myocardium; Chordae tendineae [tendinous cords]; Left semilunar cusp [left coronary cusp]; Posterior papillary muscle; Right coronary artery; Nodule of semilunar cusp; Right auricle; Right semilunar cusp [right coronary cusp]; Posterior semilunar cusp [noncoronary cusp]; Left atrioventricular orifice; Mitral valve [left atrioventricular valve], anterior cusp; Anterior papillary muscle; Left ventricle

82 *Thoracic viscera*

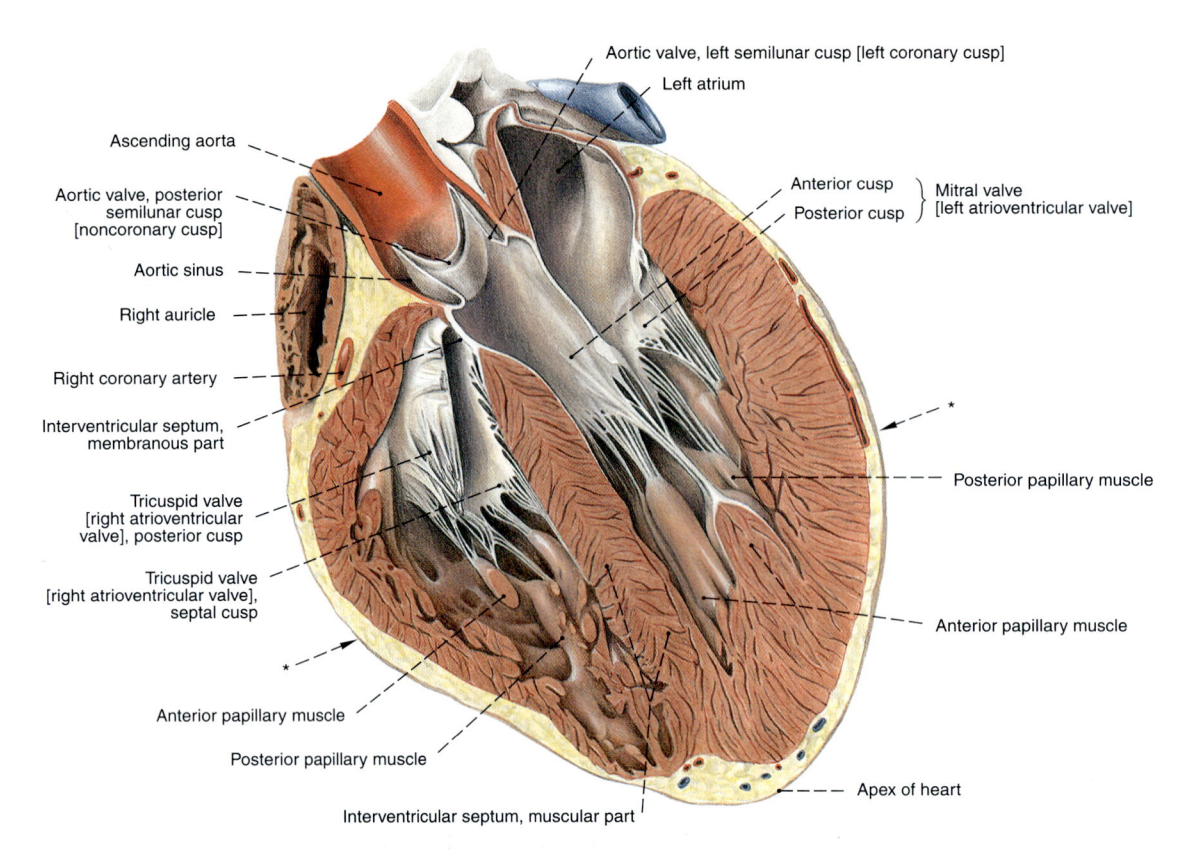

Fig. 849 Left and right ventricles; opened by a longitudinal section along the axis of the heart; left lateral ventral aspect. Note the differences in thickness of myocardium between right and left ventricles.
* Plane of section of Fig. 850.

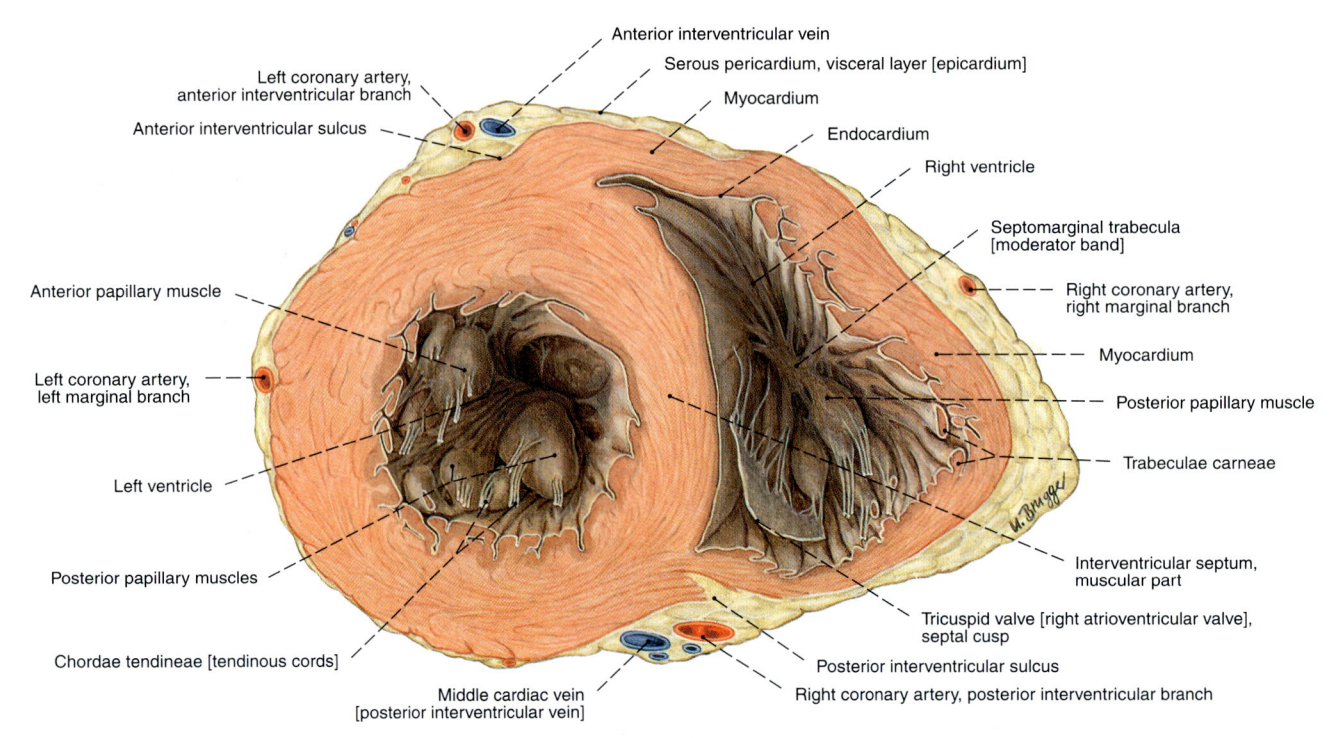

Fig. 850 Left and right ventricles; cross-section perpendicular to axis of the heart; superior aspect. Note the differences in thickness of myocardium of right and left ventricles.

Heart 83

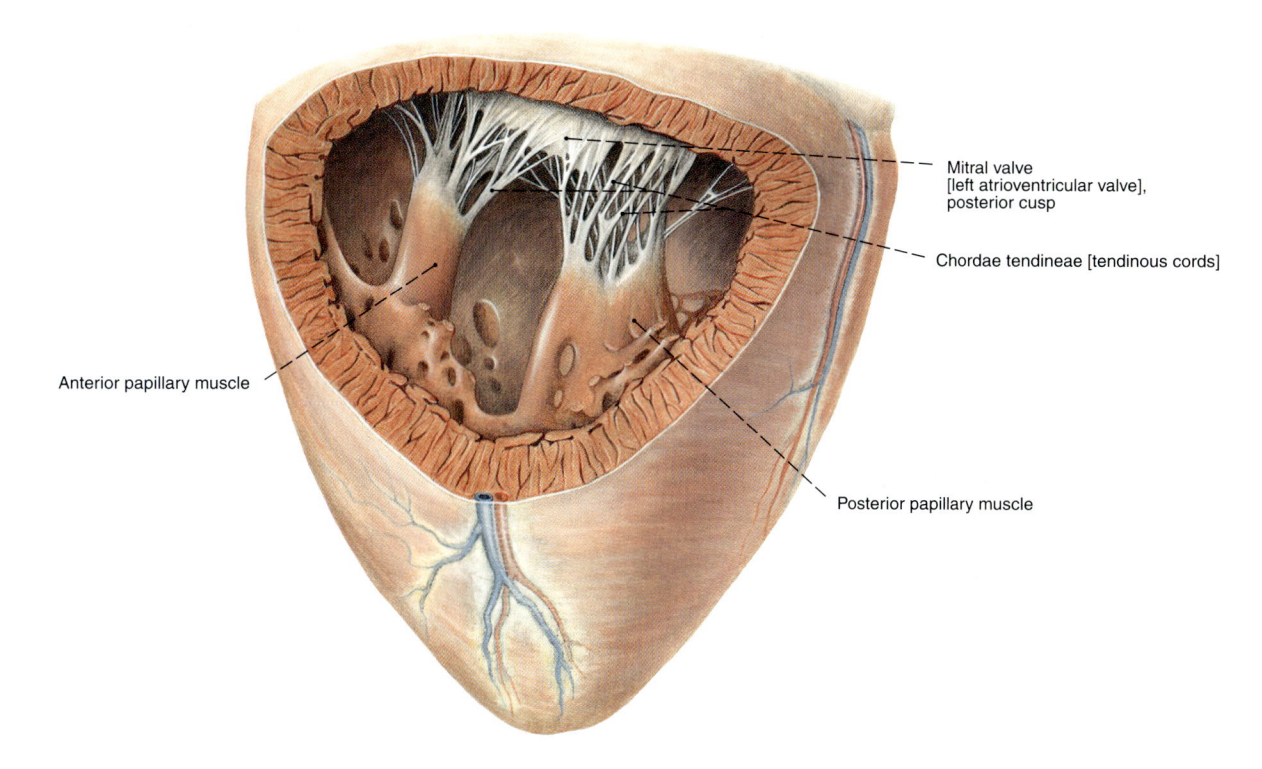

Fig. 851 Left ventricle; window view of papillary muscles and chordae tendineae [tendinous cords]; left ventral caudal aspect.

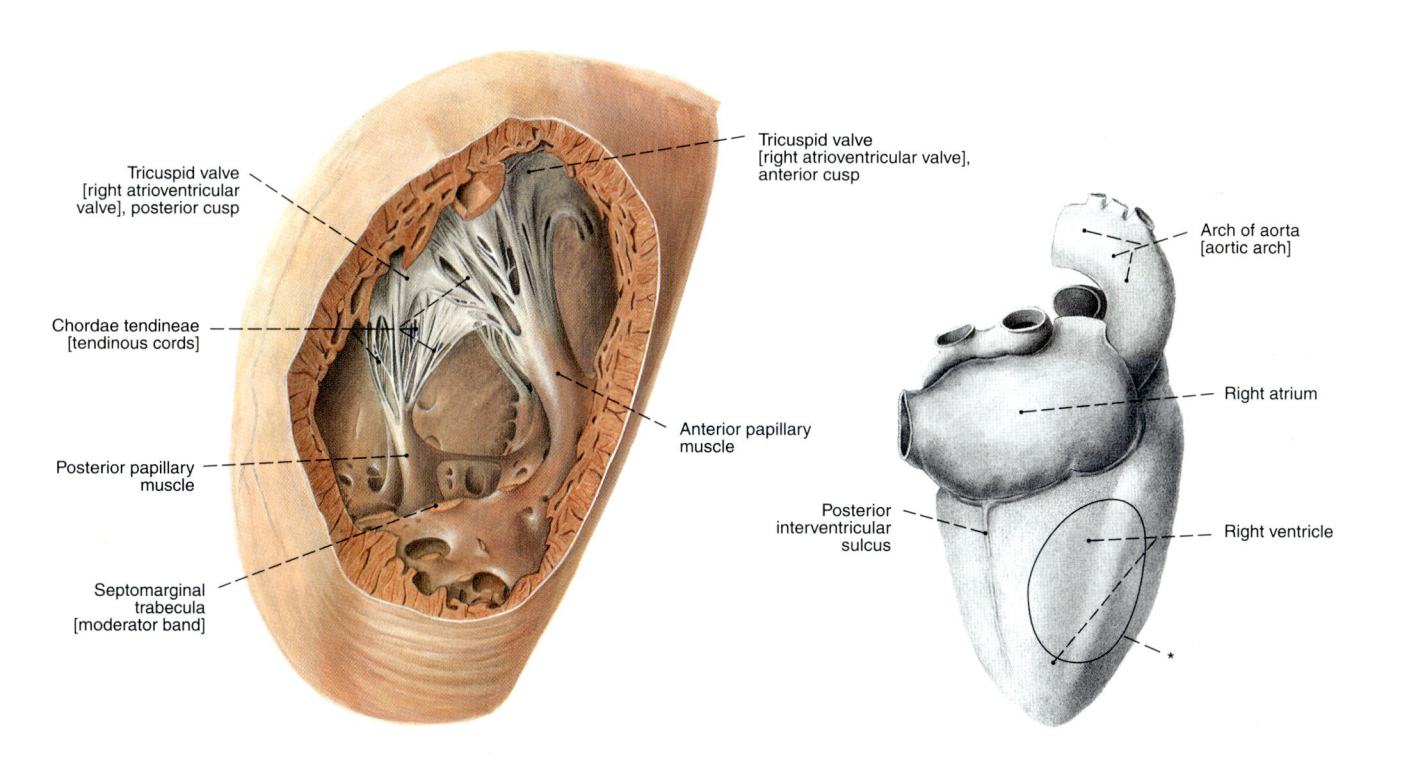

Fig. 852 Right ventricle; window view of papillary muscles and chordae tendineae [tendinous cords]; dorsal aspect.
* Contour of window.

84   *Thoracic viscera*

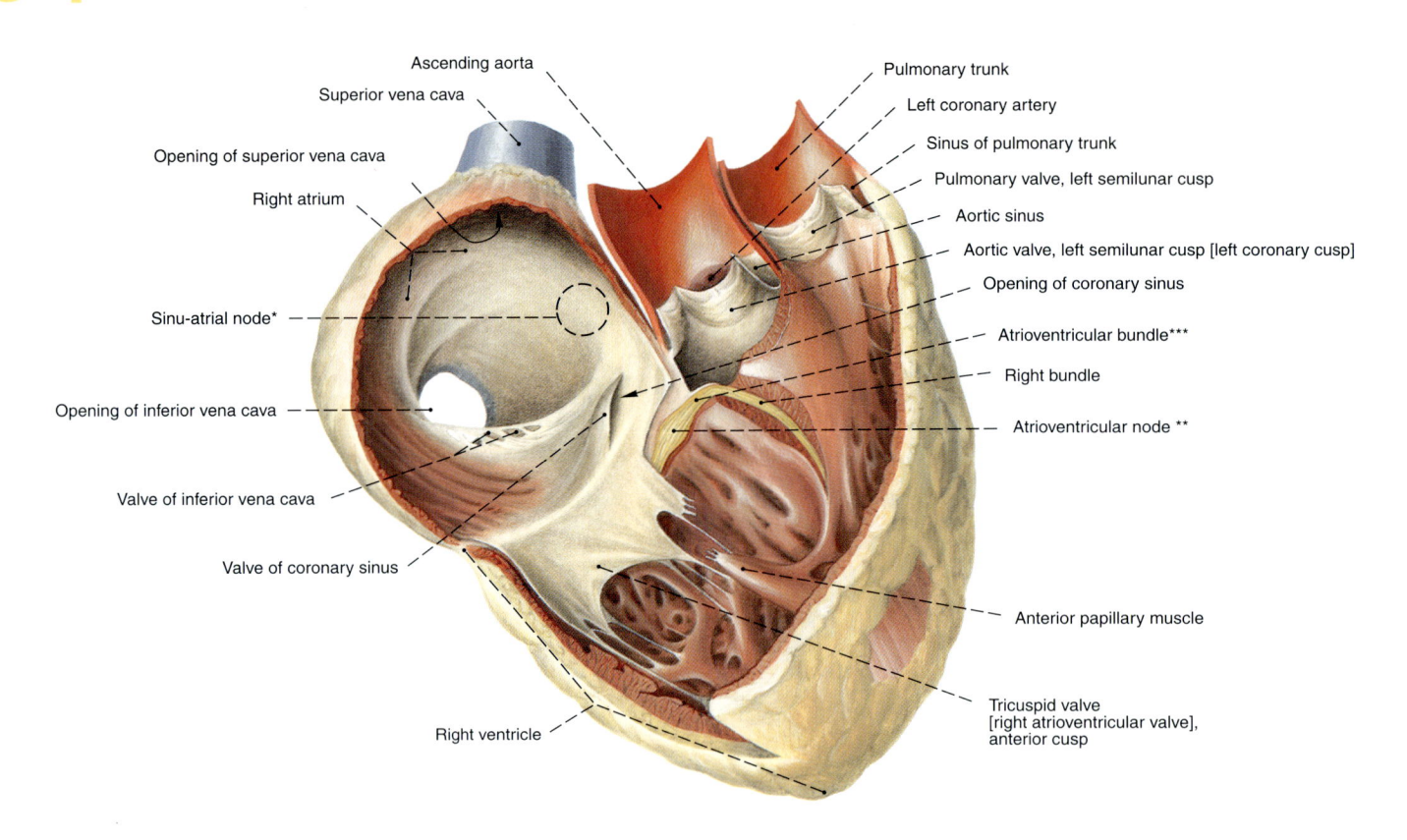

Fig. 853 Right atrium, right ventricle with conducting system of heart; atrium, ventricle, and arteries opened; conducting system of heart highlighted in yellow; ventral aspect.

* Clinically: node of KEITH-FLACK.
** Clinically: node of TAWARA [ASCHOFF-TAWARA node].
*** Clinically: bundle of HIS.

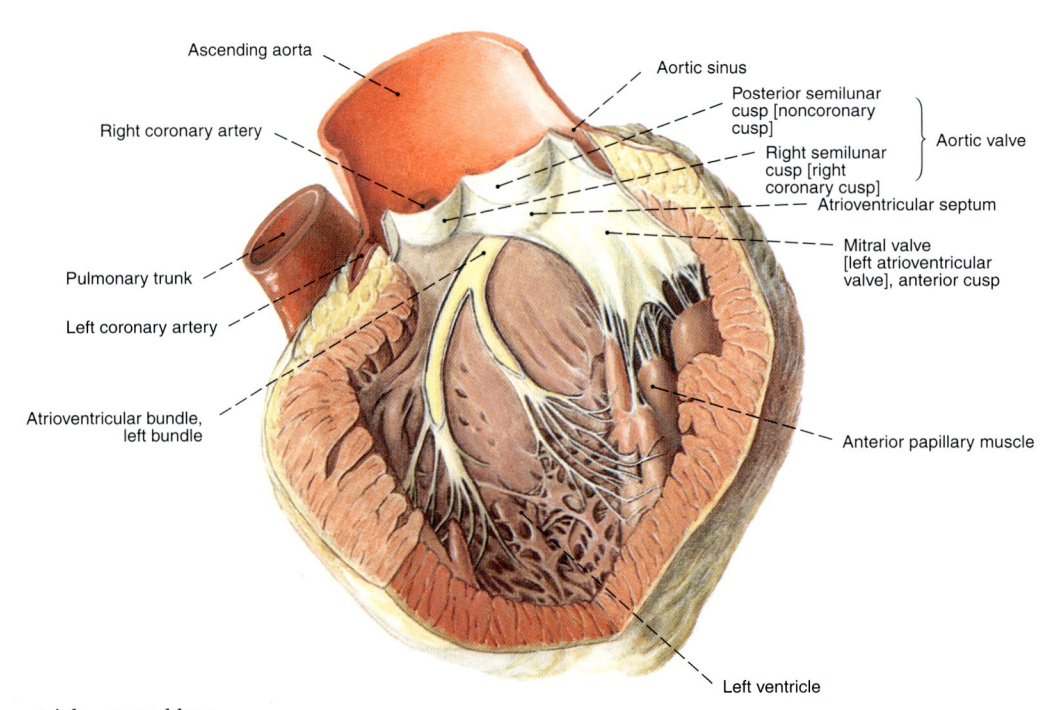

Fig. 854 Left ventricle; opened by a longitudinal section; left bundle highlighted in yellow; left ventral aspect.

Heart 85

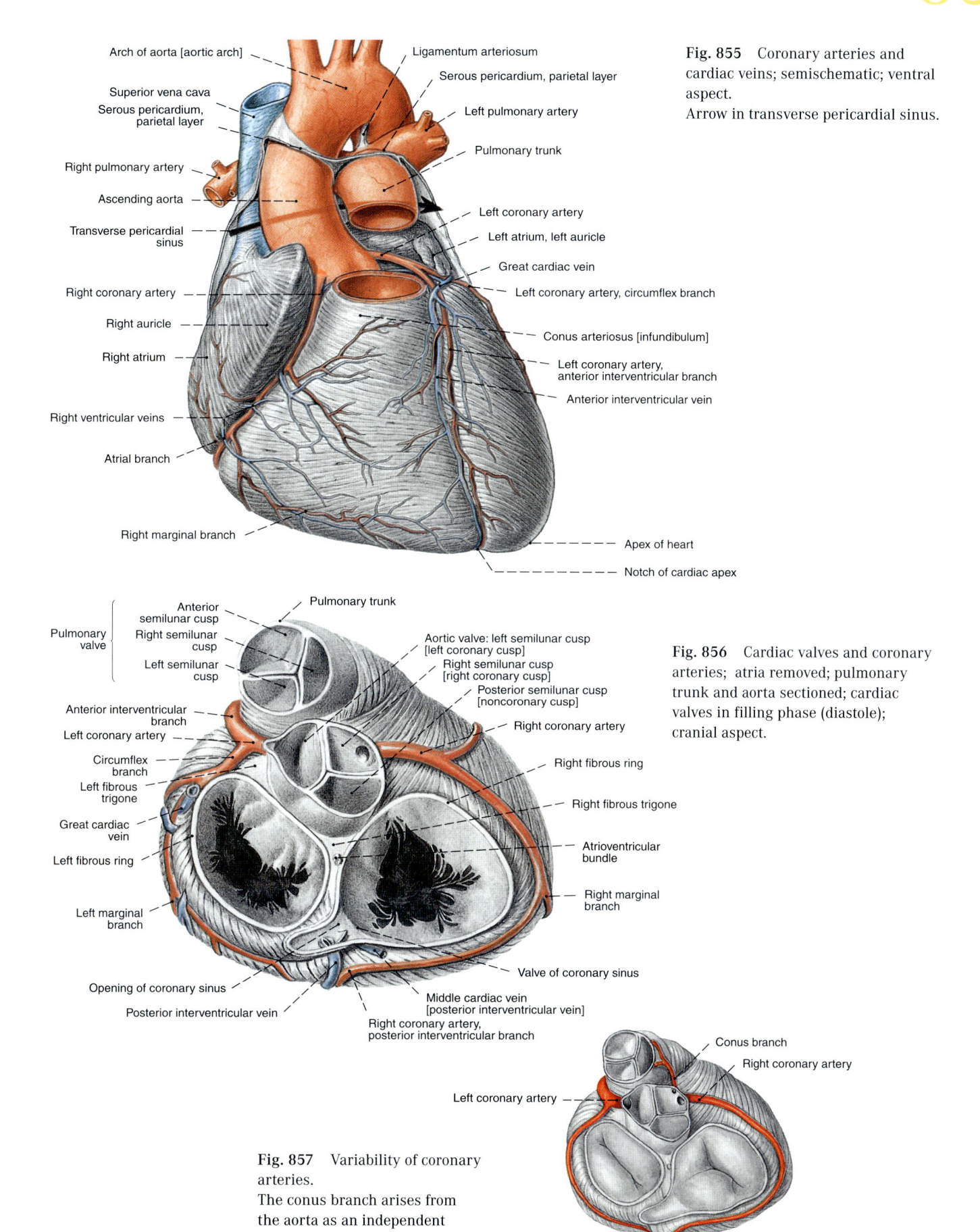

Fig. 855 Coronary arteries and cardiac veins; semischematic; ventral aspect.
Arrow in transverse pericardial sinus.

Fig. 856 Cardiac valves and coronary arteries; atria removed; pulmonary trunk and aorta sectioned; cardiac valves in filling phase (diastole); cranial aspect.

Fig. 857 Variability of coronary arteries.
The conus branch arises from the aorta as an independent artery in approximately 37%.

Thoracic viscera

Fig. 858 Coronary arteries; dorsal blood vessels in lighter shade; the posterior interventricular branch arises from the right coronary artery (balanced coronary artery distribution); ventral aspect. Compare Fig. 861 a.

Fig. 859 Coronary arteries; the posterior interventricular branch arises from the left coronary artery (dominant left coronary artery distribution); ventral aspect. Compare Fig. 861 b.

Fig. 860 Coronary arteries; the posterior wall of ventricles is mainly supplied by branches from the right coronary artery (dominant right coronary artery distribution); ventral aspect. Compare Fig. 861 c.

1 Left coronary artery, circumflex branch
2 Left coronary artery, posterior left ventricular branch
3 Right coronary artery, posterior interventricular branch
4 Right coronary artery

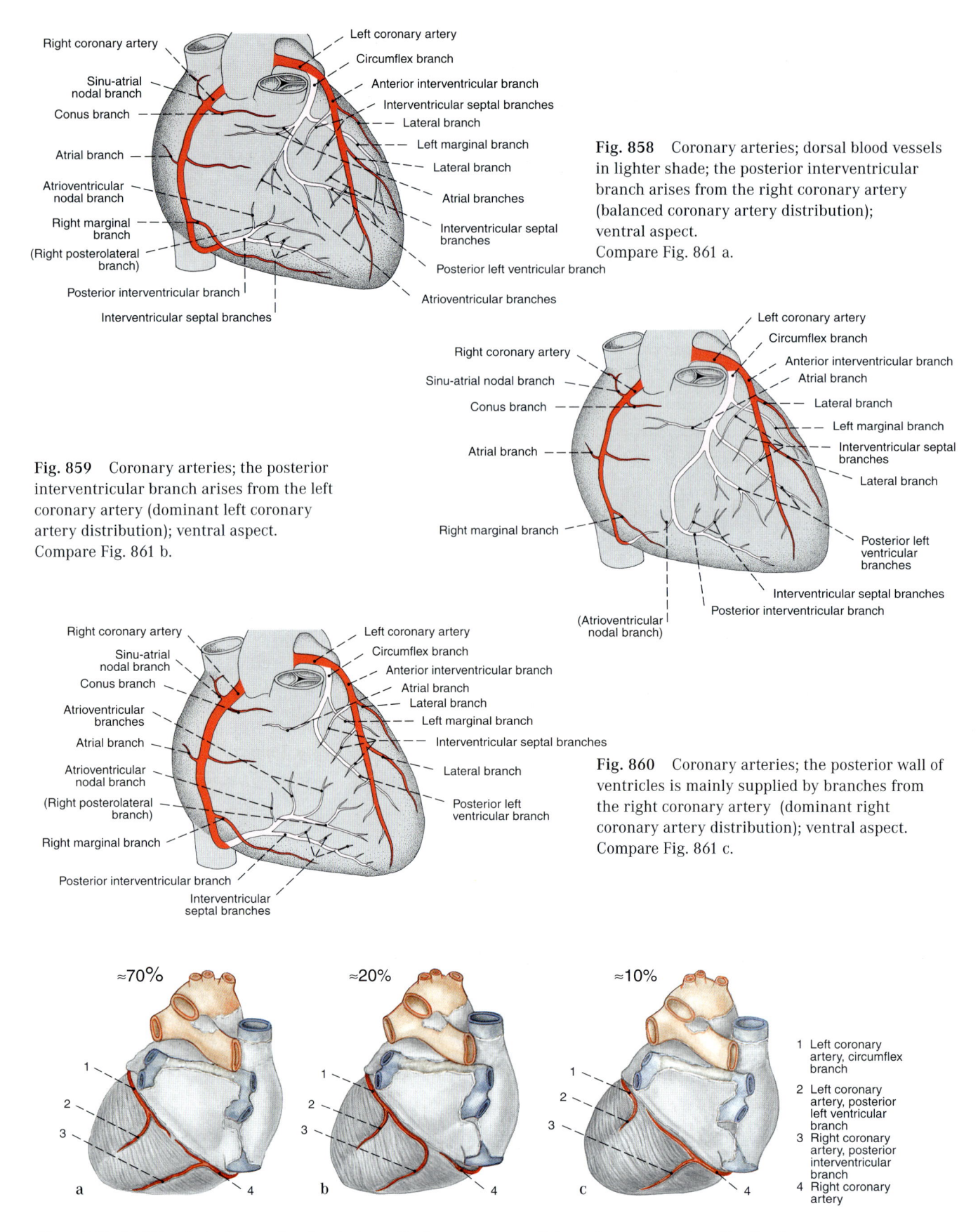

Fig. 861 Variability of arterial supply of posterior wall of heart; dorsal aspect.

a Balanced coronary artery distribution
b Dominant left coronary artery distribution
c Dominant right coronary artery distribution

Heart 87

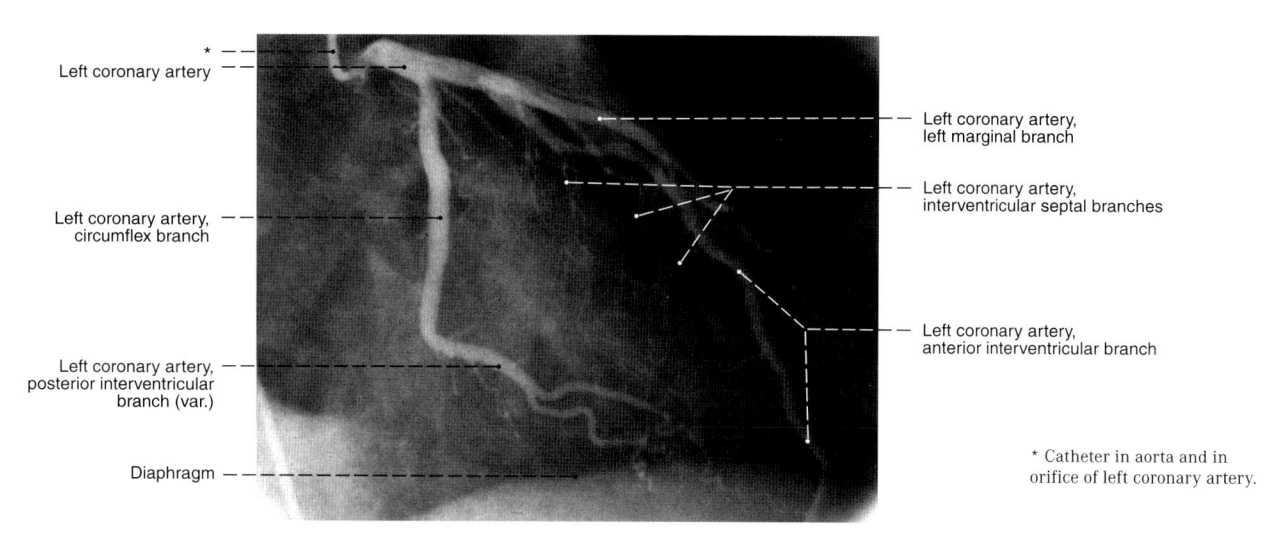

Fig. 862 Left coronary artery; coronary angiography (radiograph after selective injection of contrast medium); right anterior oblique view (RAO), beam from right anterior to left posterior.

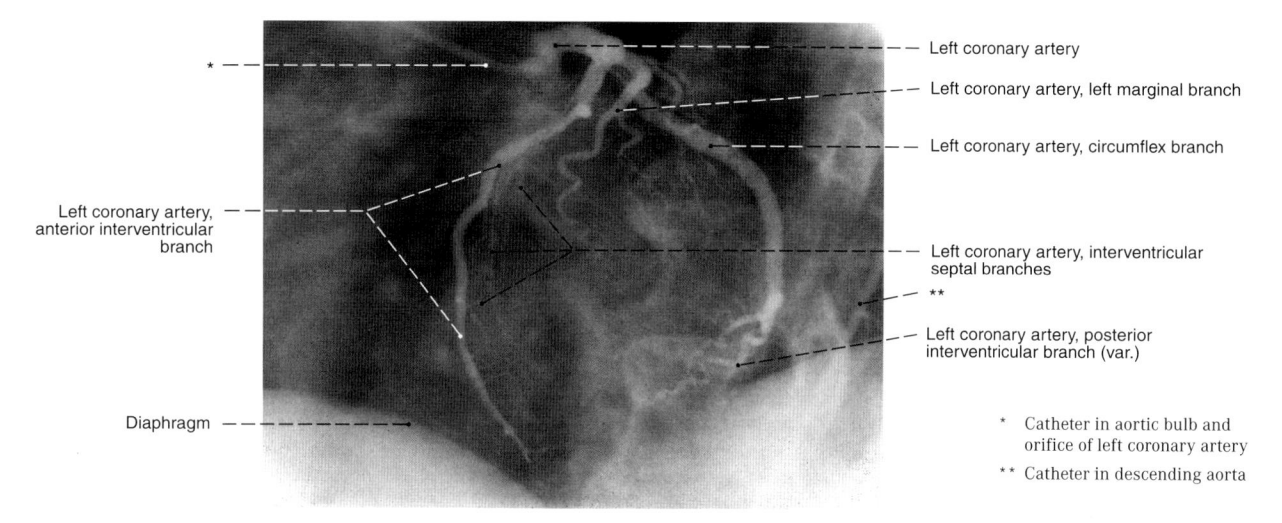

Fig. 863 Left coronary artery; coronary angiography (radiograph after selective injection of contrast medium); left anterior oblique view (LAO), beam from left anterior to right posterior. Same patient as in Fig. 862.

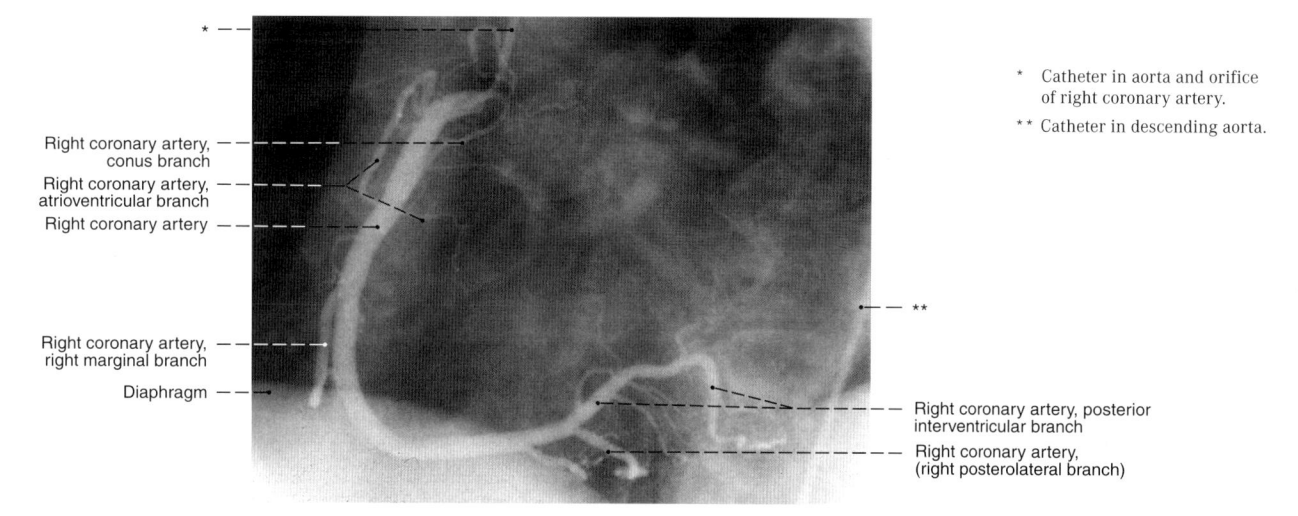

Fig. 864 Right coronary artery; coronary angiography (radiograph after selective injection of contrast medium); left anterior oblique view (LAO), beam from left anterior to right posterior. Same patient as in Figs. 862 and 863.

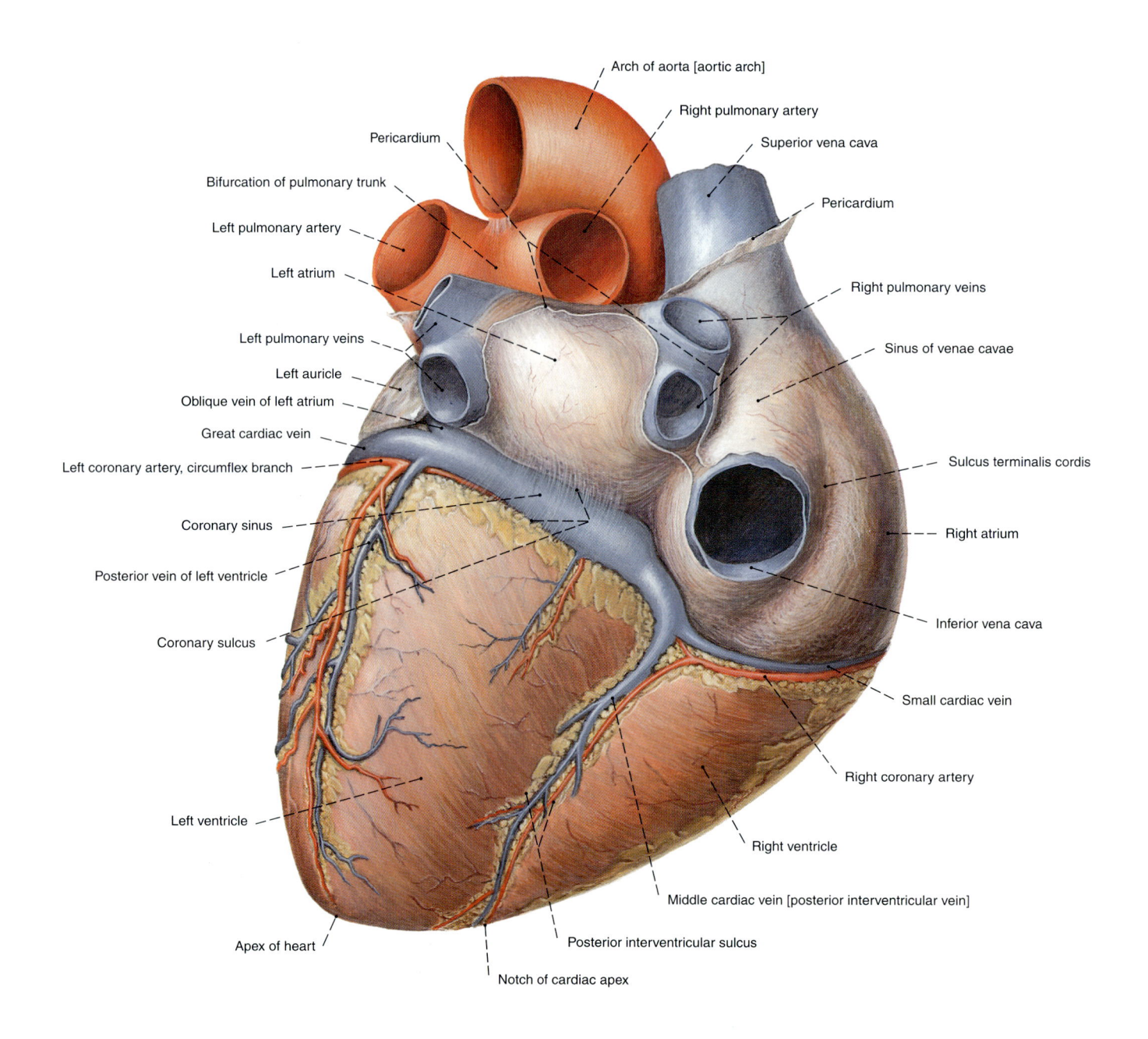

Fig. 865   Cardiac veins; pericardium removed up to the great blood vessels; dorsocaudal aspect.
The coronary sinus is frequently covered with thin muscular fibers (compare Fig. 840).

Heart 89

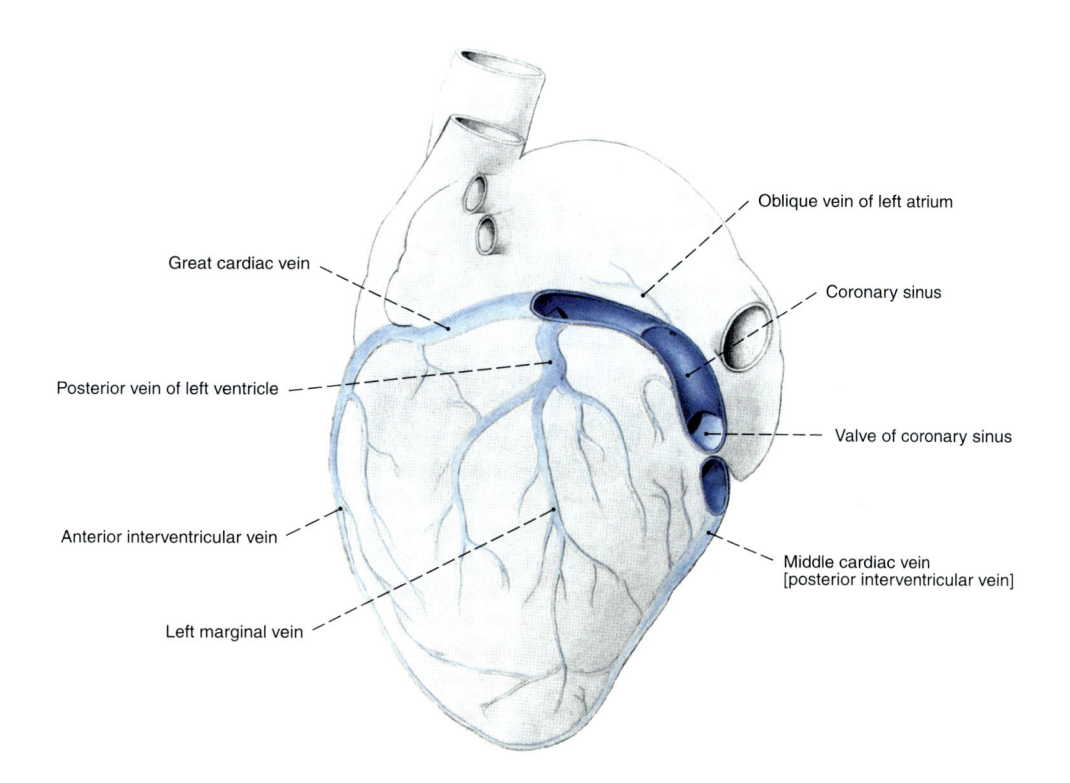

Fig. 866 Cardiac veins; branches of large cardiac veins schematically (from VON LÜDINGHAUSEN); left caudal aspect.
Size and course of cardiac veins vary considerably.

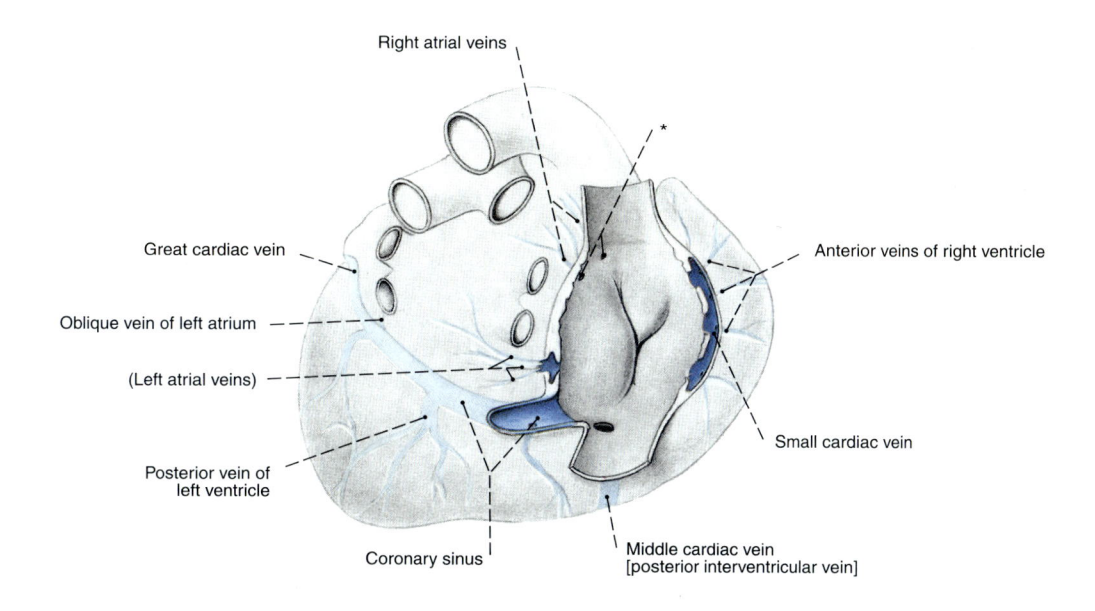

Fig. 867 Cardiac veins; right atrium removed to expose orifices of cardiac veins (from VON LÜDINGHAUSEN); cranial aspect.

* Orifices of anterior atrial veins (LANNELONGUE's crypts). Orifices of cardiac veins vary considerably.

90 Thoracic viscera

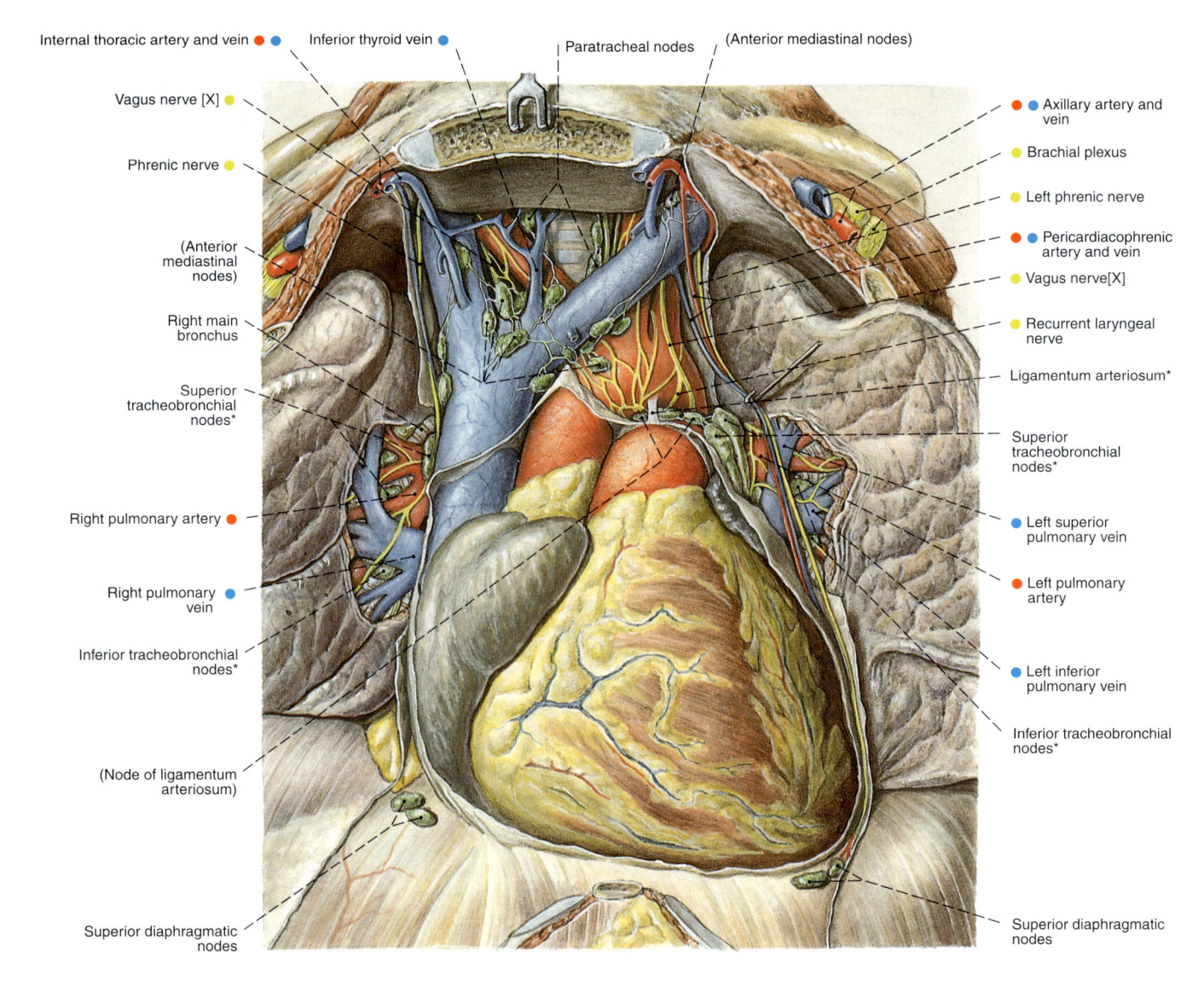

Fig. 868 Position of heart in thorax; thymus removed; manubrium of sternum retracted cranially; pericardium partially removed and hilum of lung dissected to expose mediastinal lymph nodes; ventral aspect.
* Clinically: hilar lymph nodes.
** Clinically: BOTALLO's ligament formed from the remnants of the fetal ductus arteriosus [BOTALLO's duct].

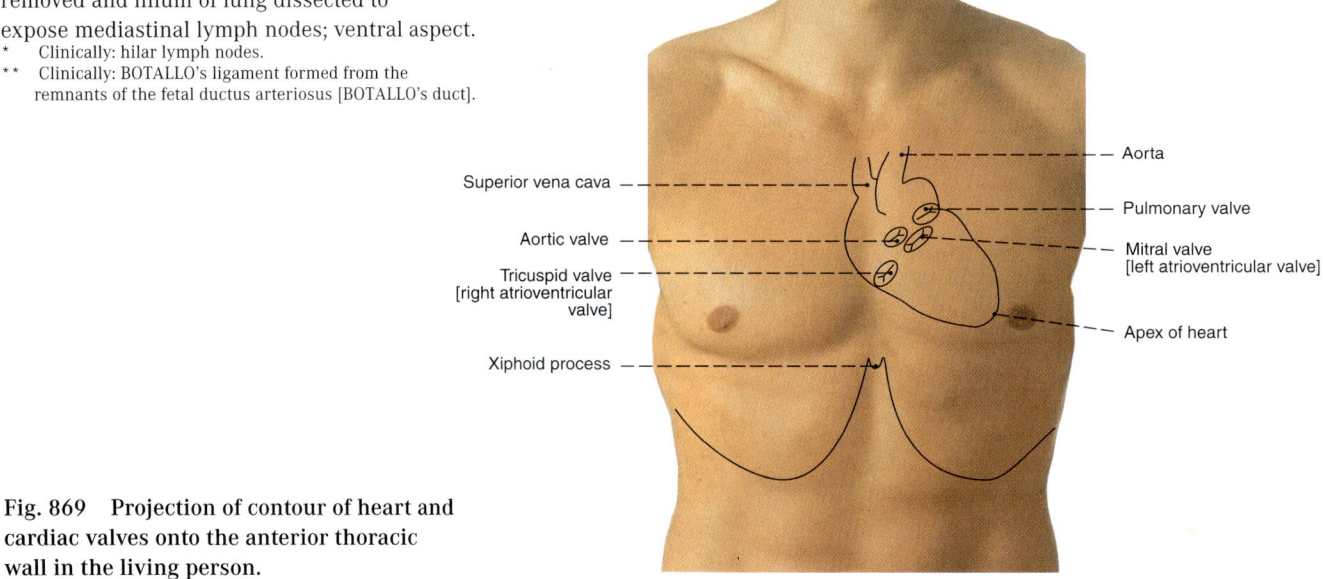

Labels (left): Internal thoracic artery and vein; Vagus nerve [X]; Phrenic nerve; (Anterior mediastinal nodes); Right main bronchus; Superior tracheobronchial nodes*; Right pulmonary artery; Right pulmonary vein; Inferior tracheobronchial nodes*; (Node of ligamentum arteriosum); Superior diaphragmatic nodes.

Labels (top): Inferior thyroid vein; Paratracheal nodes; (Anterior mediastinal nodes).

Labels (right): Axillary artery and vein; Brachial plexus; Left phrenic nerve; Pericardiacophrenic artery and vein; Vagus nerve [X]; Recurrent laryngeal nerve; Ligamentum arteriosum*; Superior tracheobronchial nodes*; Left superior pulmonary vein; Left pulmonary artery; Left inferior pulmonary vein; Inferior tracheobronchial nodes*; Superior diaphragmatic nodes.

Fig. 869 Projection of contour of heart and cardiac valves onto the anterior thoracic wall in the living person.

Labels: Superior vena cava; Aortic valve; Tricuspid valve [right atrioventricular valve]; Xiphoid process; Aorta; Pulmonary valve; Mitral valve [left atrioventricular valve]; Apex of heart.

Heart 91

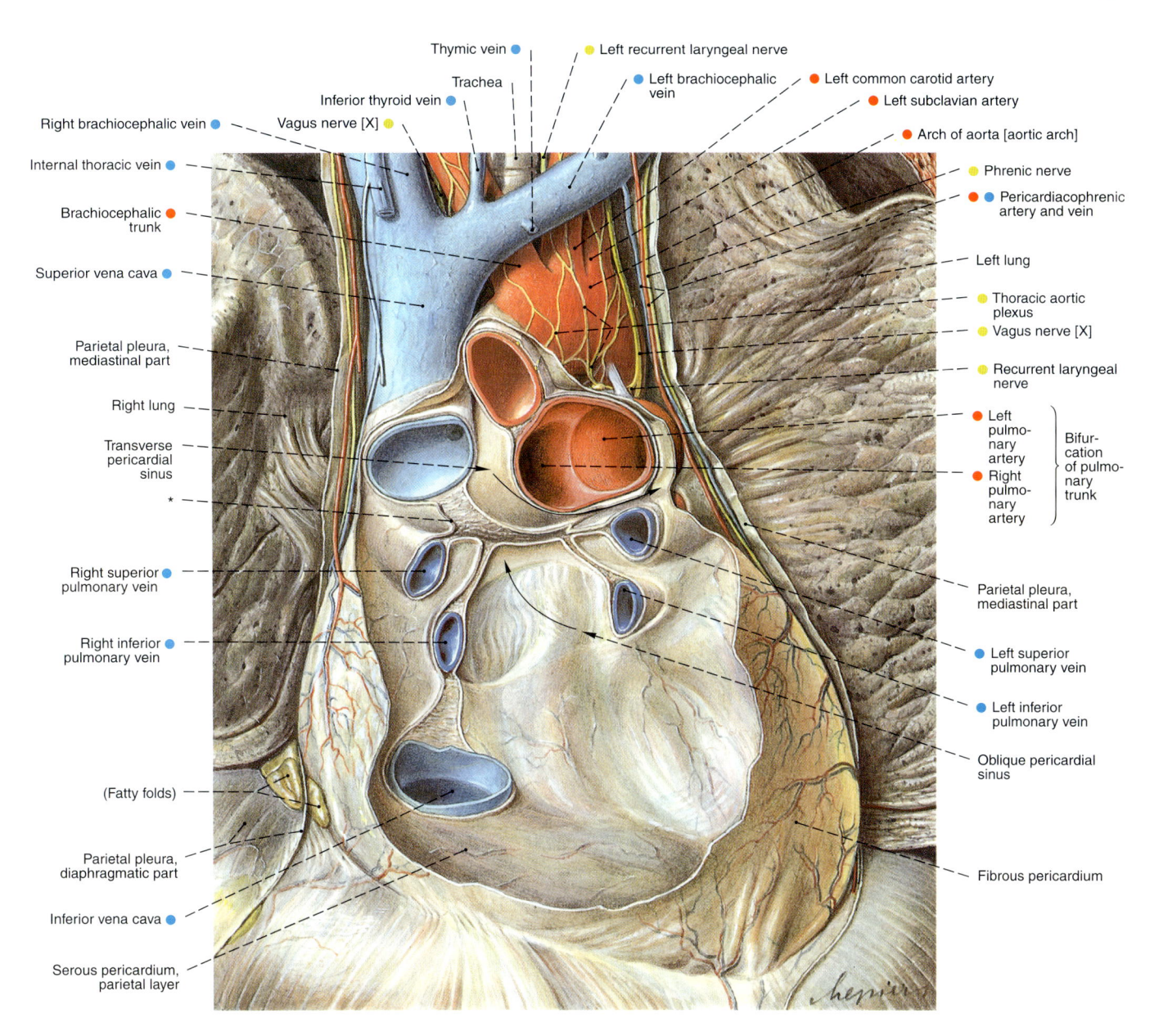

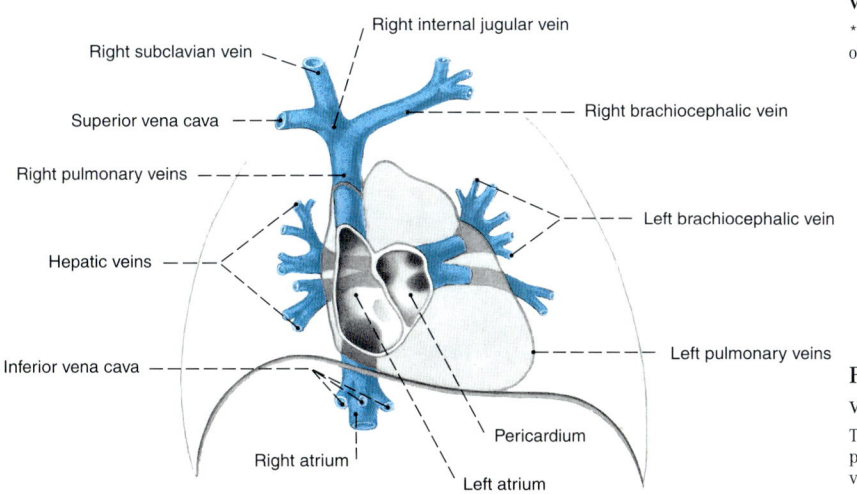

Fig. 870 Pericardium; anterior parts of pericardium as well as heart and great blood vessels removed; ventral aspect.

* Reflection of visceral layer [epicardium] into parietal layer of serous pericardium.

Fig. 871 Great veins draining into the heart; ventral aspect.

The so-called "venous cross" is formed by the horizontal pulmonary veins and the vertical superior and inferior venae cavae.

92 Thoracic viscera

Right main bronchus

Right superior lobar bronchus
 1 = apical segmental bronchus [B I]
 2 = posterior segmental bronchus [B II]
 3 = anterior segmental bronchus [B III]

Middle lobar bronchus
 4 = lateral segmental bronchus [B IV]
 5 = medial segmental bronchus [B V]

Right inferior lobar bronchus
 6 = superior segmental bronchus [B VI]
 7 = medial basal segmental bronchus [B VII]
 8 = anterior basal segmental bronchus [B VIII]
 9 = lateral basal segmental bronchus [B IX]
 10 = posterior basal segmental bronchus [B X]

Left main bronchus

Left superior lobar bronchus
 1, 2 = apicoposterior segmental bronchus [B I+II]
 3 = anterior segmental bronchus [B III]
 4 = superior lingular segmental bronchus [B IV]
 5 = inferior lingular segmental bronchus [B V]

Left inferior lobar bronchus
 6 = superior segmental bronchus [B VI]
 7 = medial basal segmental bronchus [B VII]
 8 = anterior basal segmental bronchus [B VIII]
 9 = lateral basal segmental bronchus [B IX]
 10 = posterior basal segmental bronchus [B X]

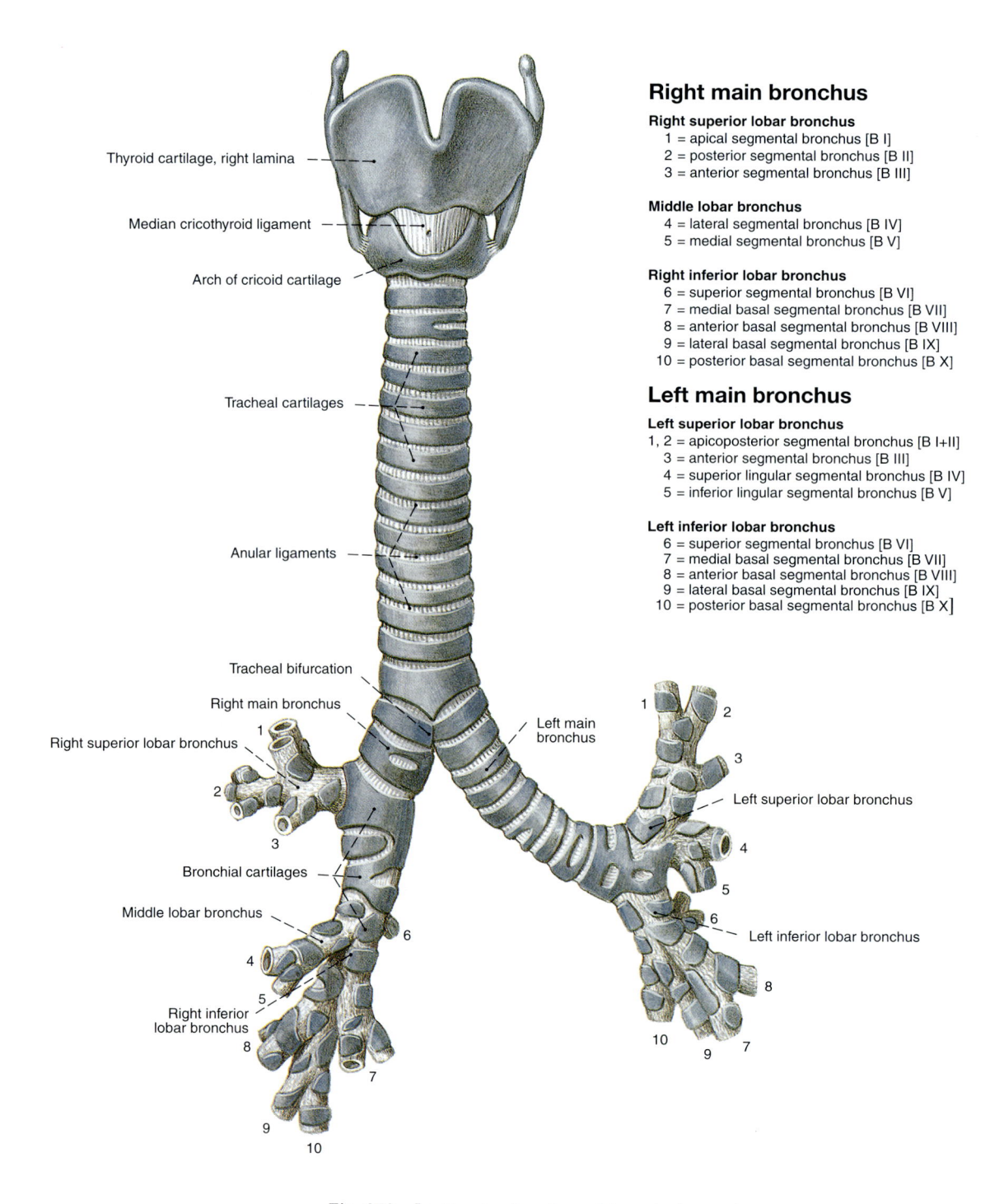

Labels: Thyroid cartilage, right lamina — Median cricothyroid ligament — Arch of cricoid cartilage — Tracheal cartilages — Anular ligaments — Tracheal bifurcation — Right main bronchus — Right superior lobar bronchus — Bronchial cartilages — Middle lobar bronchus — Right inferior lobar bronchus — Left main bronchus — Left superior lobar bronchus — Left inferior lobar bronchus

Fig. 872 Larynx; trachea; bronchi; ventral aspect. On the left side the medial basal segmental bronchus [B VII] is frequently missing.

Bronchi and trachea 93

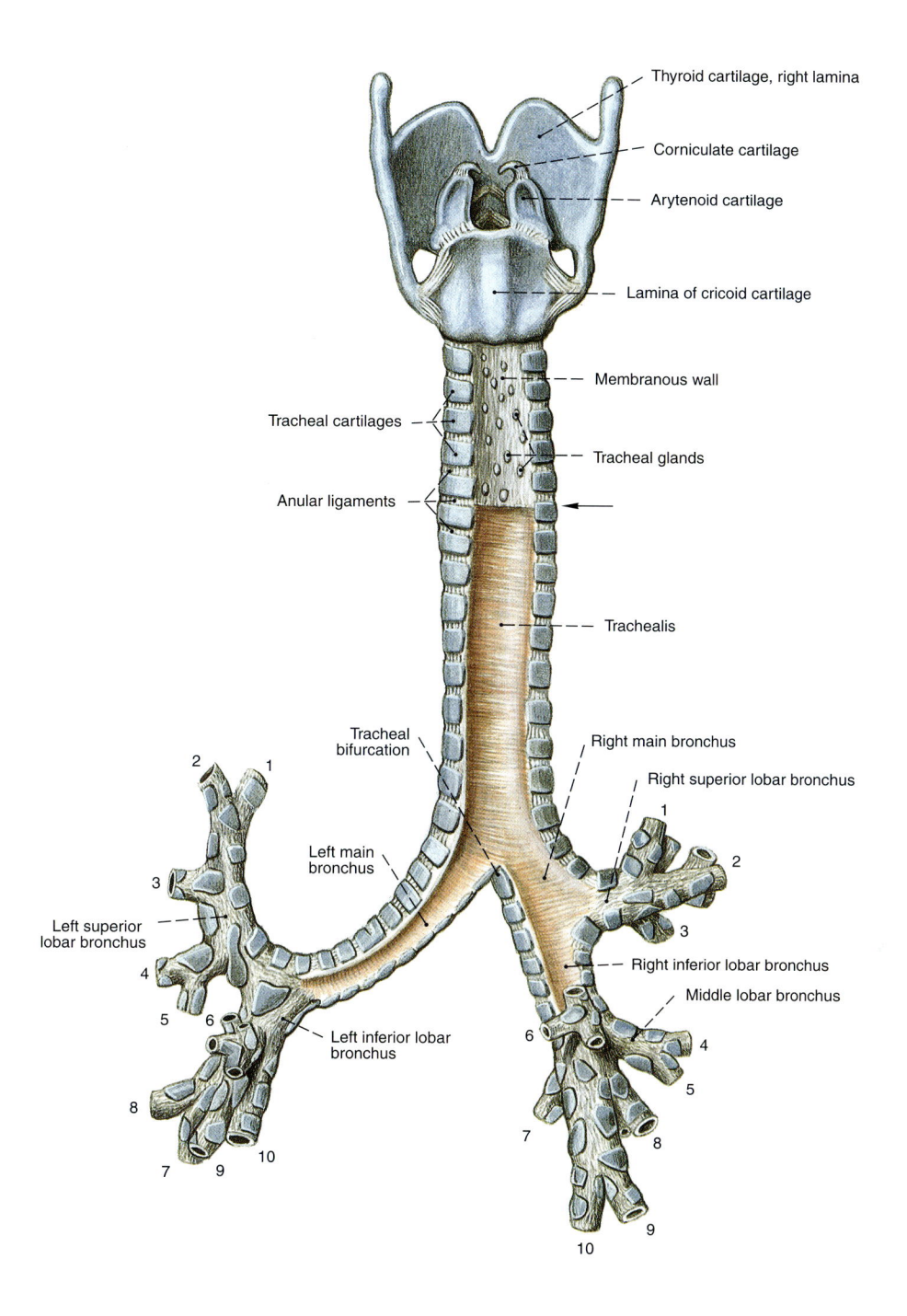

Fig. 873 Larynx; trachea; bronchi; below the arrow the superficial layer of the membranous wall is removed to expose the trachealis muscle; dorsal aspect.
Numbers refer to segmental bronchi (compare page 92).

94 *Thoracic viscera*

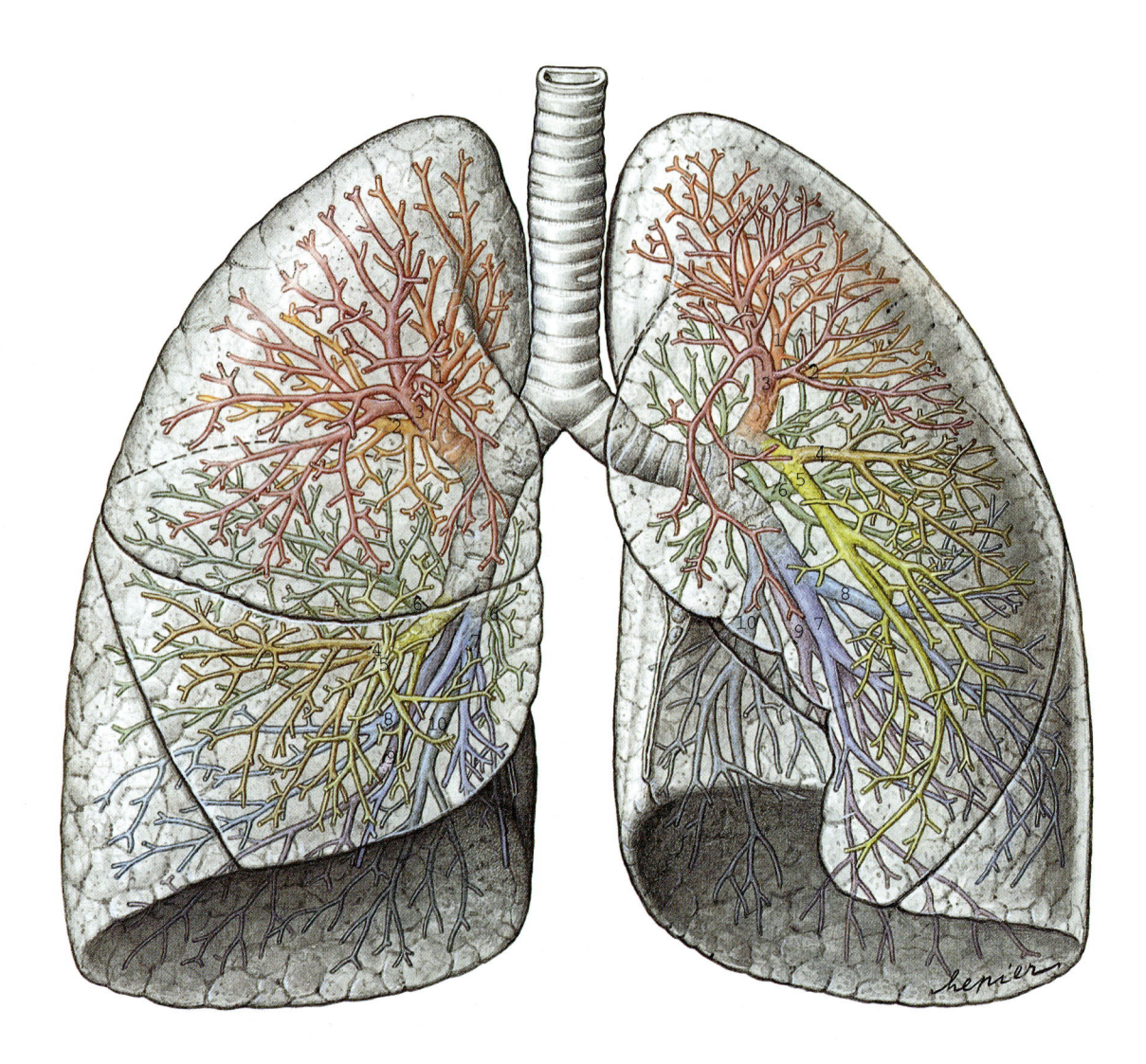

Fig. 874 Lungs, bronchi; lobar and segmental bronchi projected onto the lung in different colors; ventral aspect. Numbers refer to segmental bronchi (compare page 92). In the left lung the segments S I and S II frequently arise from a common bronchus; the medial basal segment S VII is frequently missing.

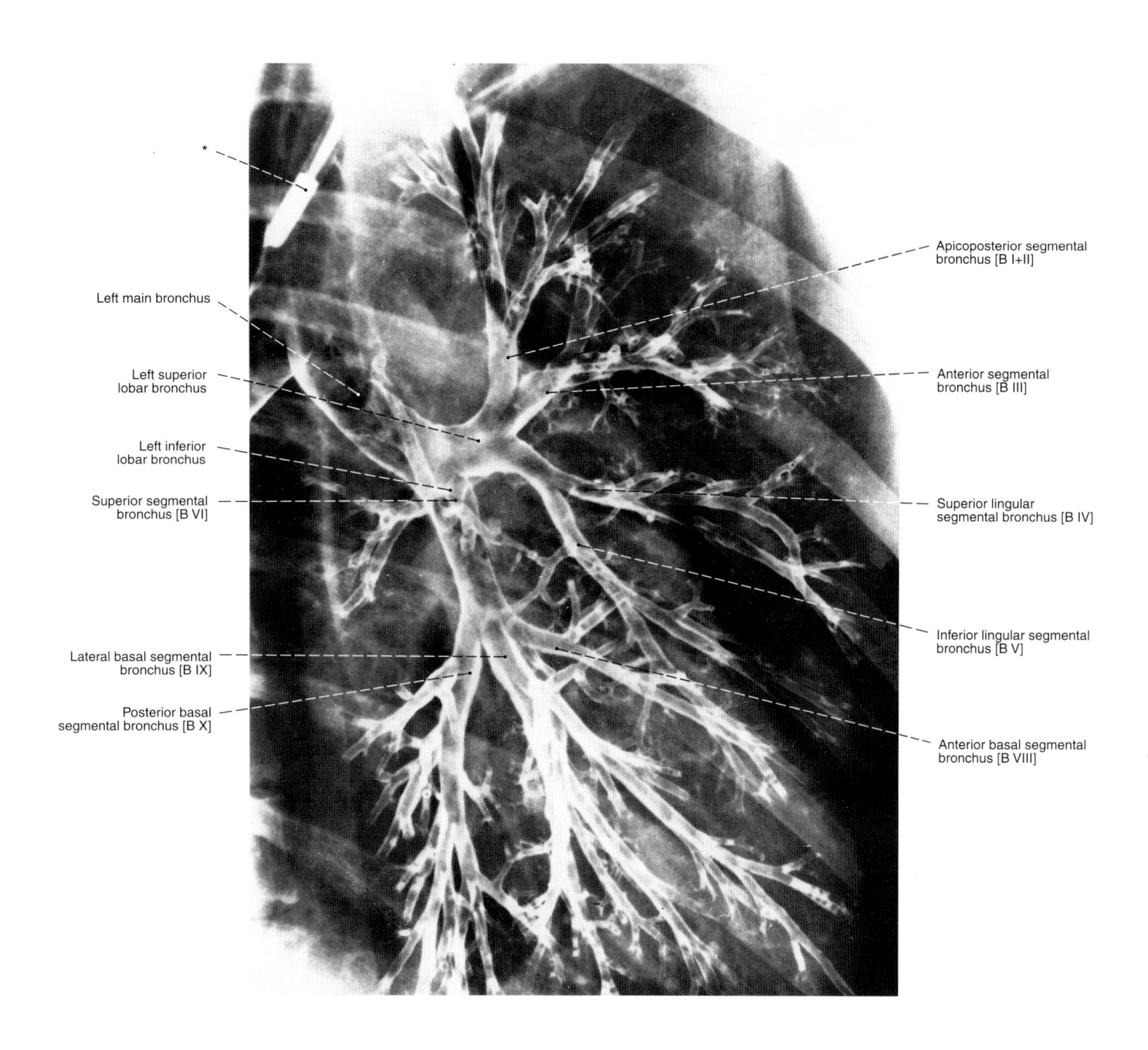

Fig. 875 Left bronchi; AP bronchogram (bronchial tree is visualized by administration of contrast medium powder); ventral aspect.

* Bronchography catheter in trachea.

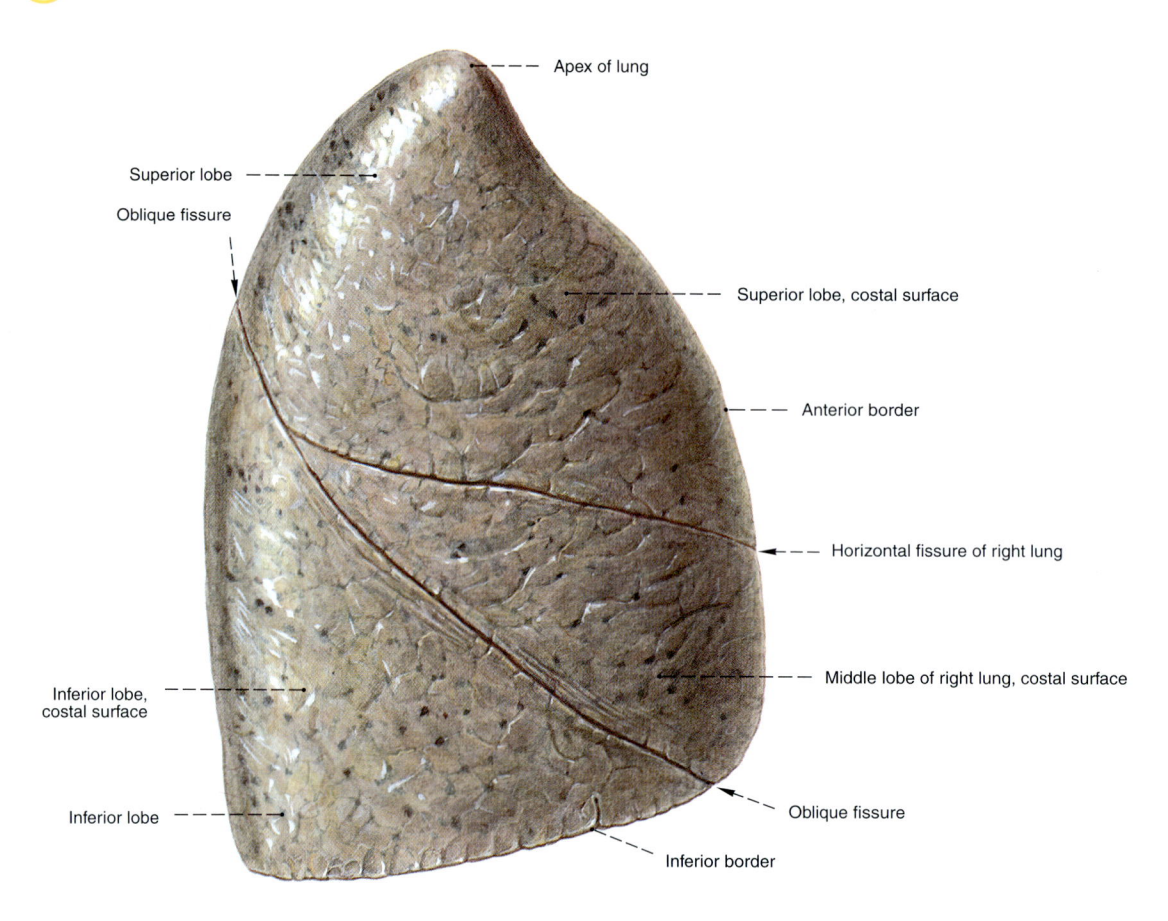

96 Thoracic viscera

Fig. 876 Right lung; lateral aspect.
Note the grey-black spots of the lung, that are caused by deposits of inhaled dust particles ("anthracotic pigment") under the visceral pleura.

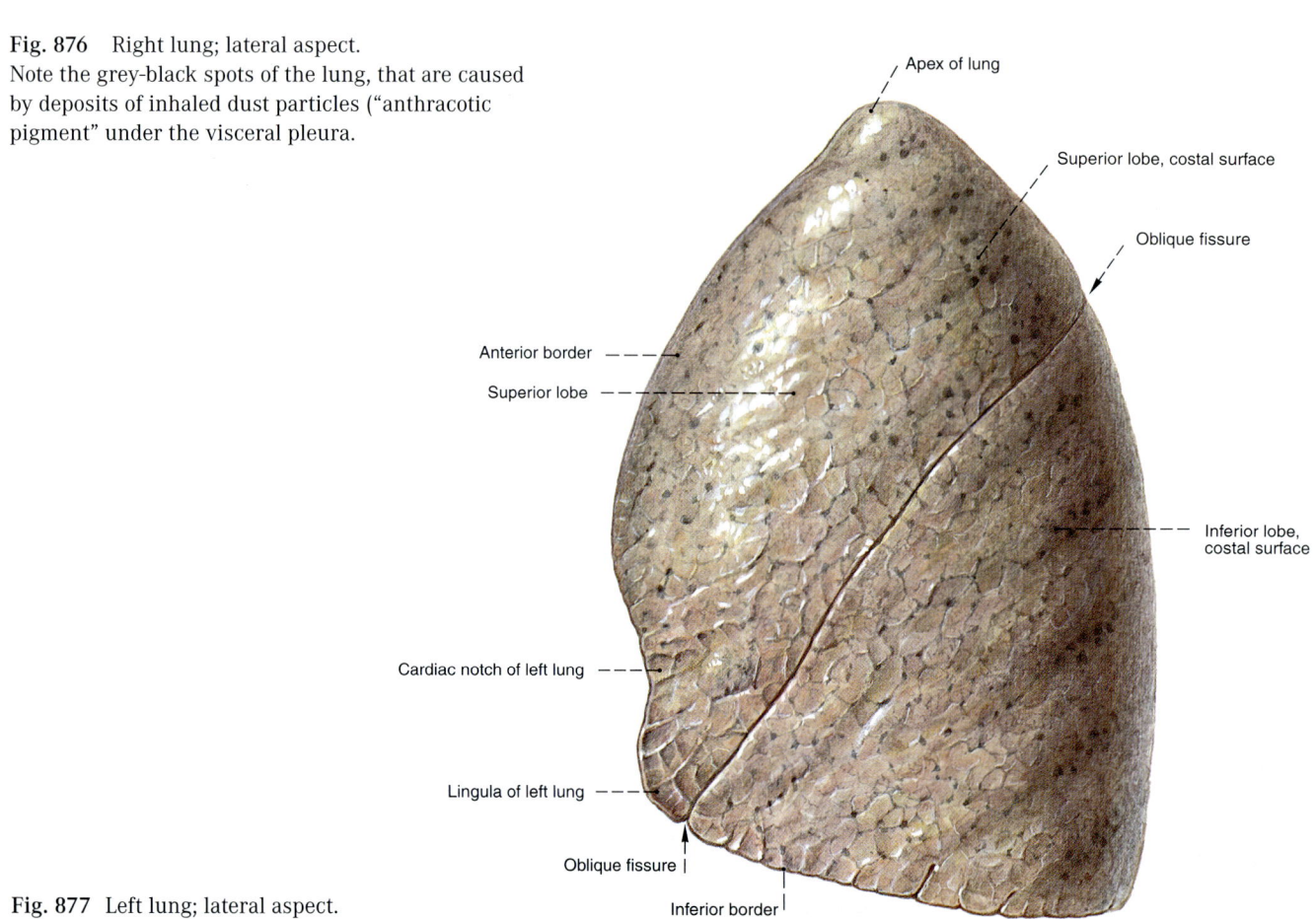

Fig. 877 Left lung; lateral aspect.

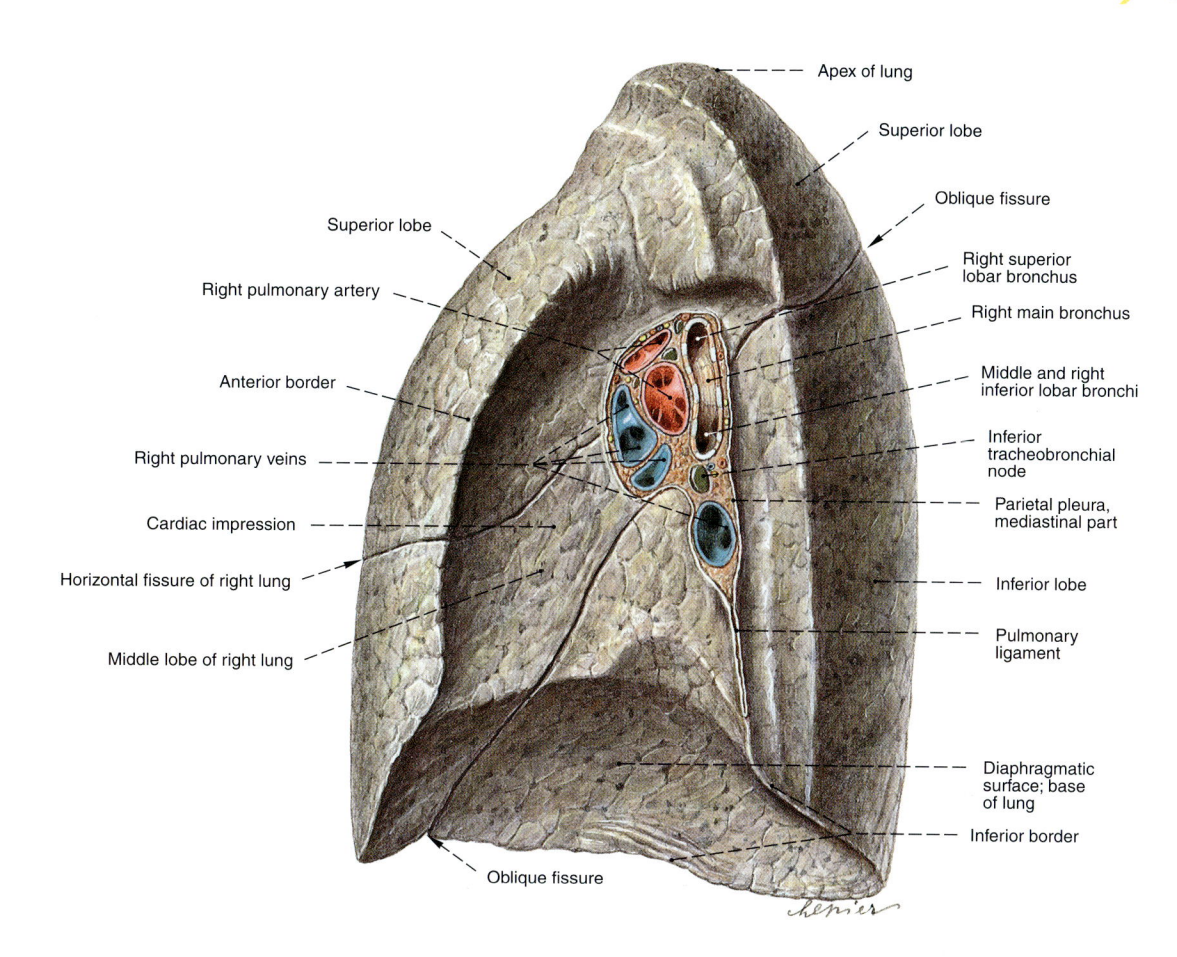

Lung 97

Fig. 878 Right lung; medial aspect.
In older people or in persons heavily exposed to dust in the workplace the hilar lymph nodes are blackened by deposits of inhaled soot or other particles ("anthracotic nodes").

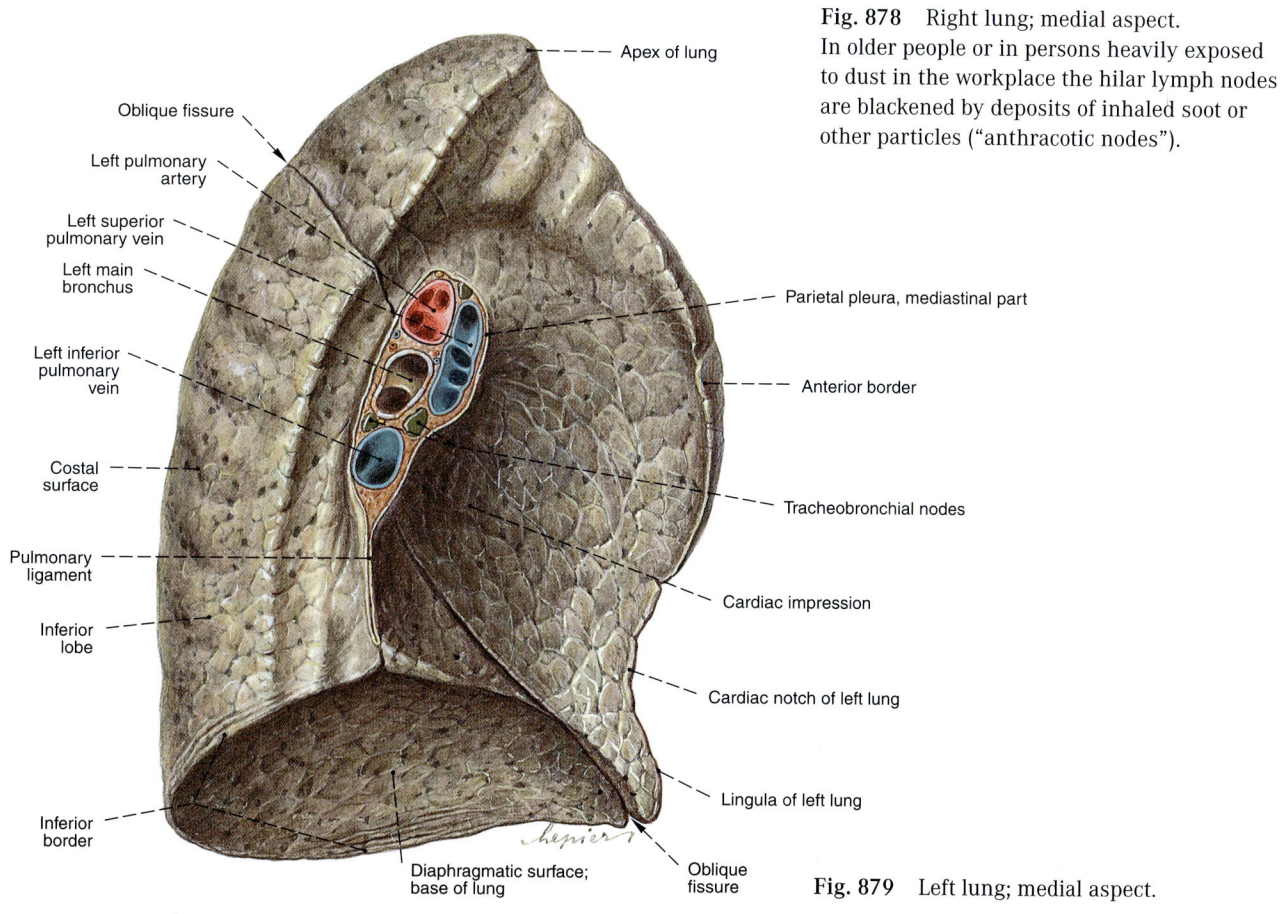

Fig. 879 Left lung; medial aspect.

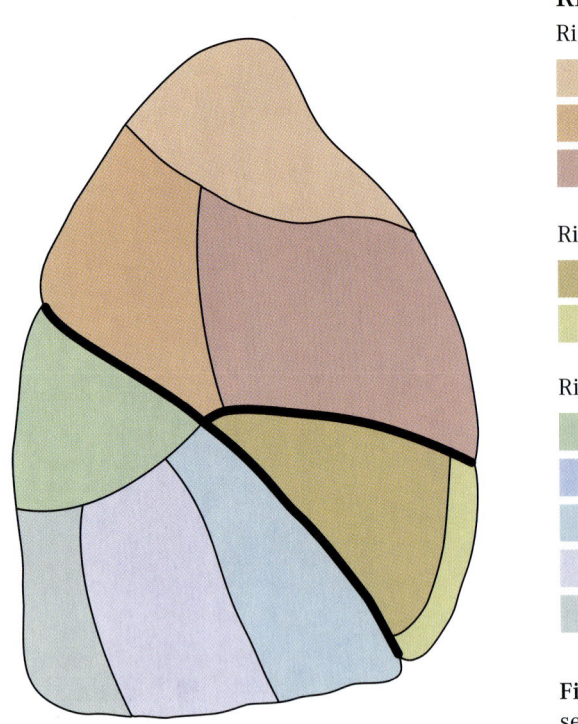

98 *Thoracic viscera*

Right lung
Right lung, superior lobe
- Apical segment [S I]
- Posterior segment [S II]
- Anterior segment [S III]

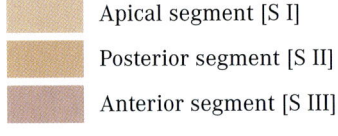

Right lung, middle lobe
- Lateral segment [S IV]
- Medial segment [S V]

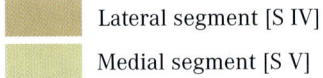

Right lung, inferior lobe
- Superior segment [S VI]
- Medial basal segment [S VII]
- Anterior basal segment [S VIII]
- Lateral basal segment [S IX]
- Posterior basal segment [S X]

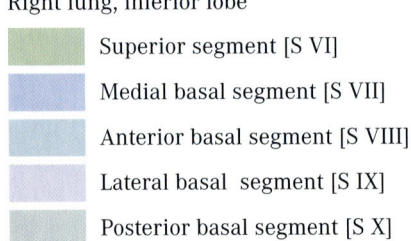

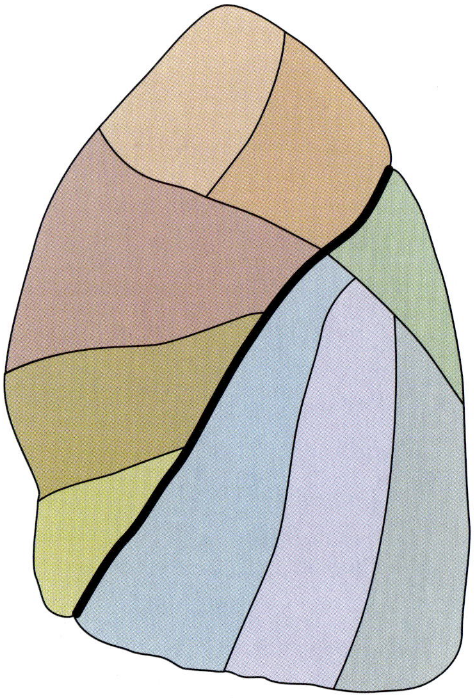

Fig. 880 Right lung; bronchopulmonary segments; lateral aspect.

Left lung
Left lung, superior lobe
- Apicoposterior segment [S I+II]
- Anterior segment [S III]
- Superior lingular segment [S IV]
- Inferior lingular segment [S V]

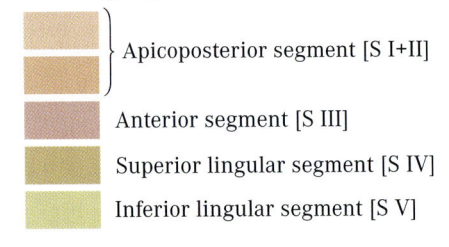

Left lung, inferior lobe
- Superior segment [S VI]
- Medial basal segment [S VII] *
- Anterior basal segment [S VIII]
- Lateral basal segment [S IX]
- **Posterior basal segment [S X]**

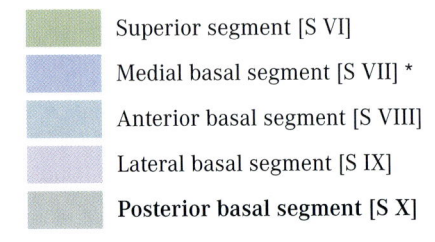

Fig. 881 Left lung; bronchopulmonary segments; lateral aspect.
*Generally this segment is not a separate unit, but fused with the anterior basal segment.

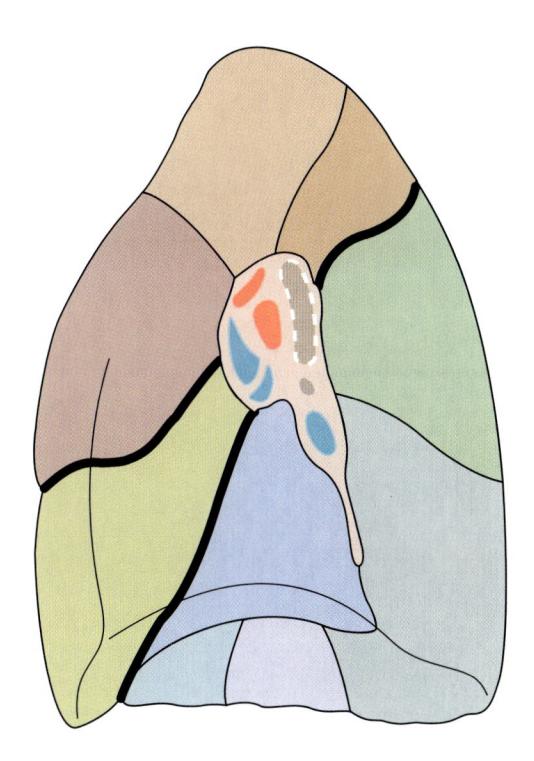

Lungs 99

Fig. 882 Right lung; bronchopulmonary segments; medial aspect.
For color code and names of segments see page 98.

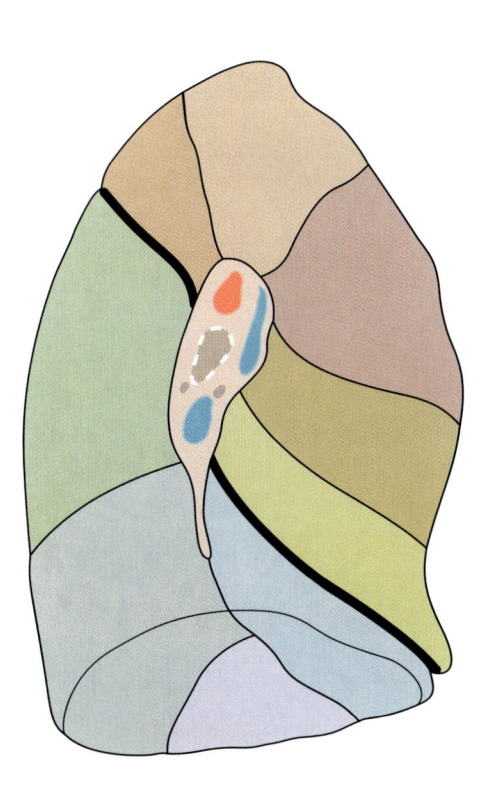

Fig. 883 Left lung; bronchopulmonary segments; medial aspect.
For color code and names of segments see page 98.

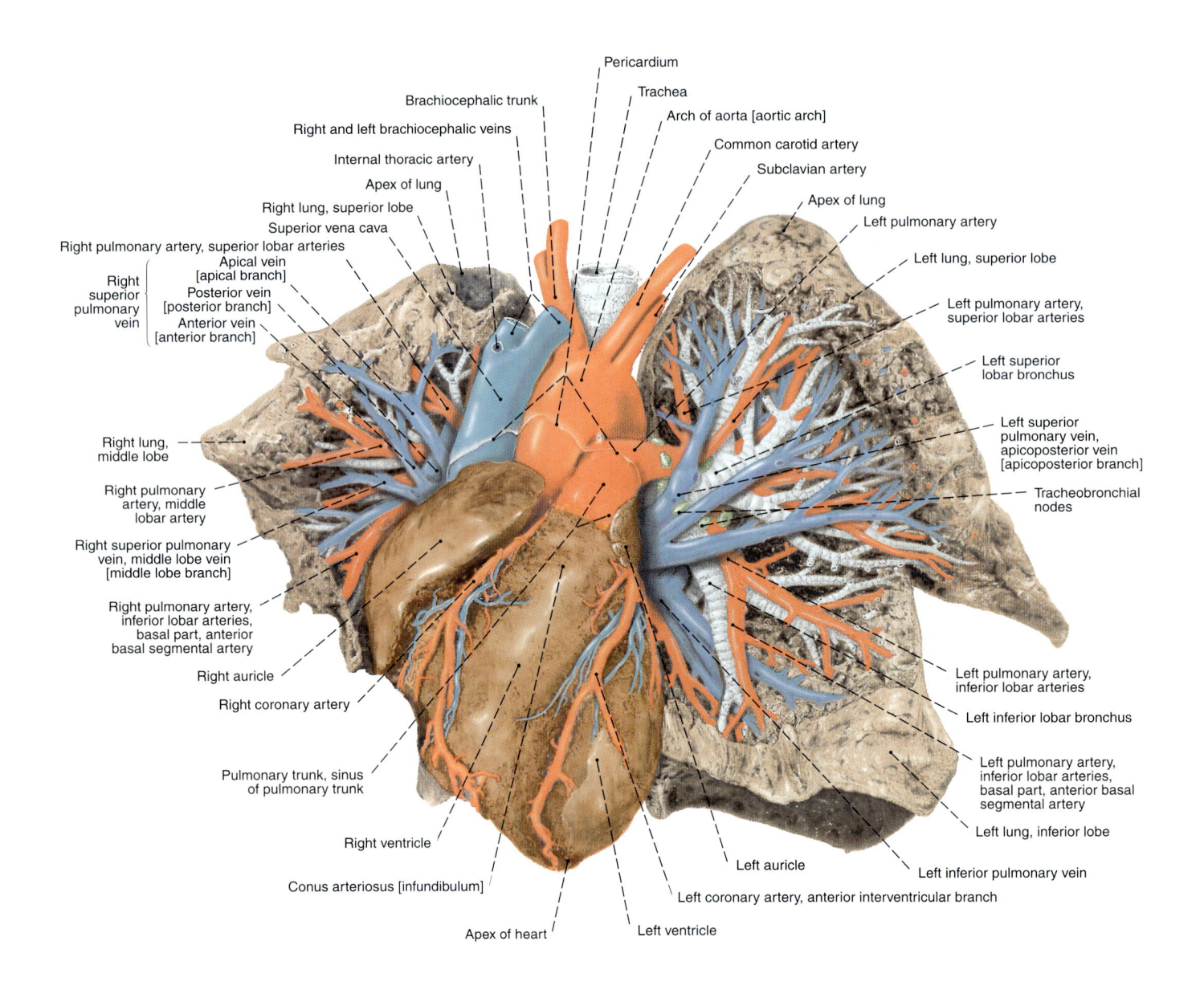

Fig. 884 Heart and lungs; arteries, veins, and bronchi of lungs dissected up to the surface of the lungs; apex of heart retracted to the right for better exposure of the structures of the left lung; ventral aspect.

Lungs **101**

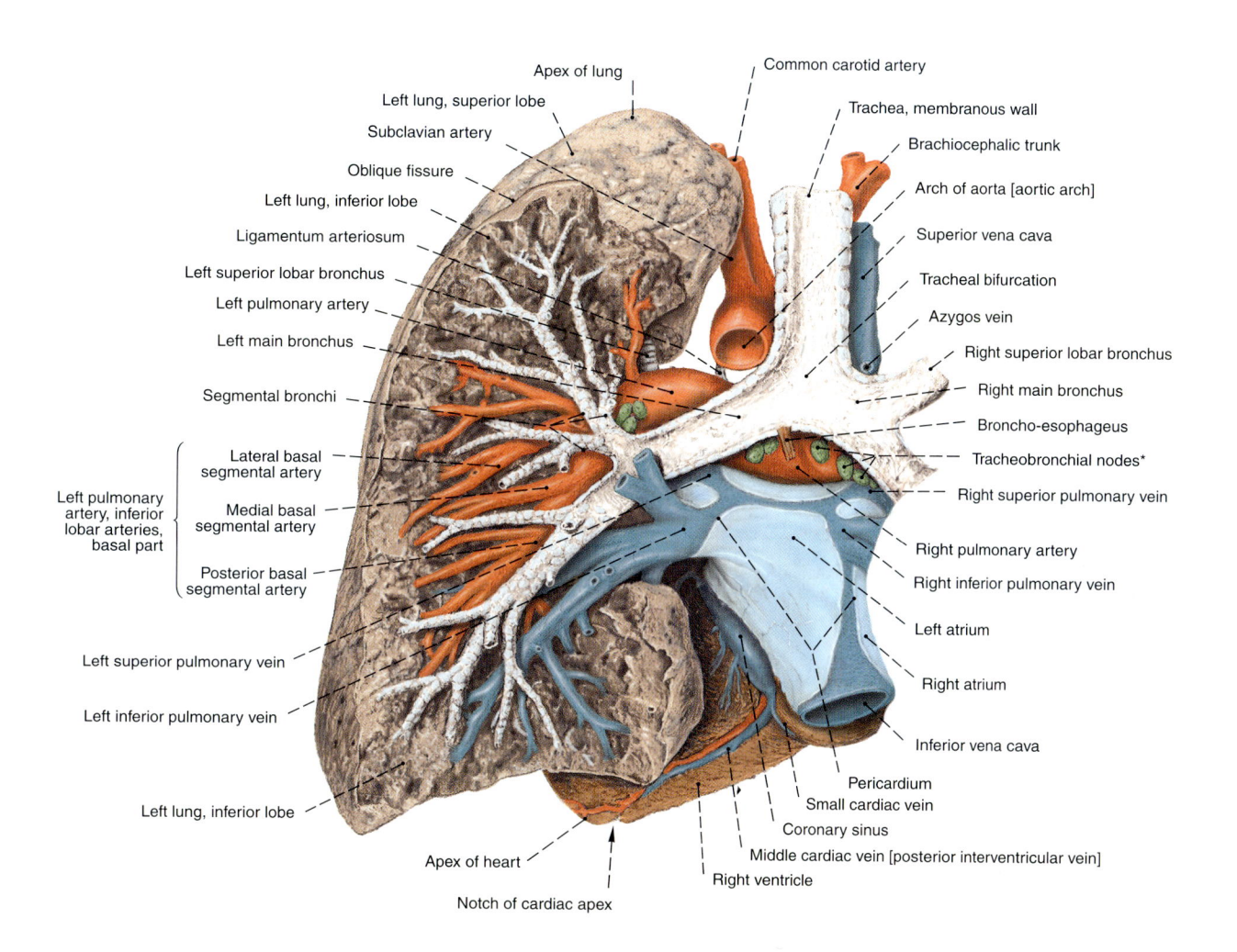

Fig. 885 Left lung; large bronchi, pulmonary veins and arteries as well as hilar lymph nodes dissected; dorsal aspect.
* Clinically: hilar lymph nodes.

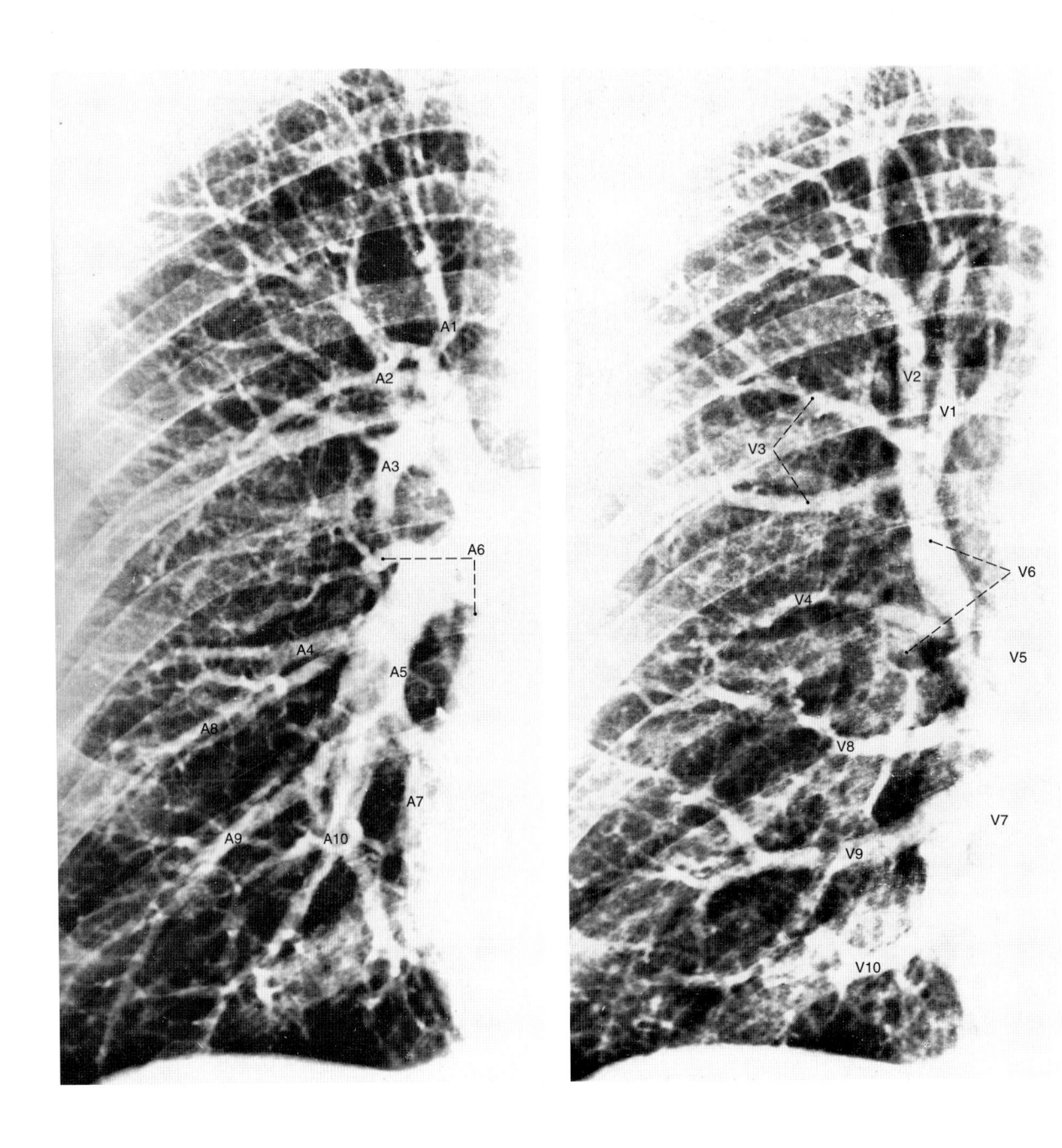

Fig. 886 Arteries of right lung; right pulmonary arteries; AP radiograph (pulmonary angiogram); injection of contrast medium into the right ventricle; ventral aspect.
Note the similar course of arteries and bronchi (Figs. 874, 875). Numbers refer to respective segmental arteries.

Fig. 887 Veins of right lung; right pulmonary veins; AP radiograph (reflux of contrast medium from the lung after injection into the right ventricle); ventral aspect.
Note the different course of the veins compared to the pulmonary arteries (Fig. 886).

Thoracic cage

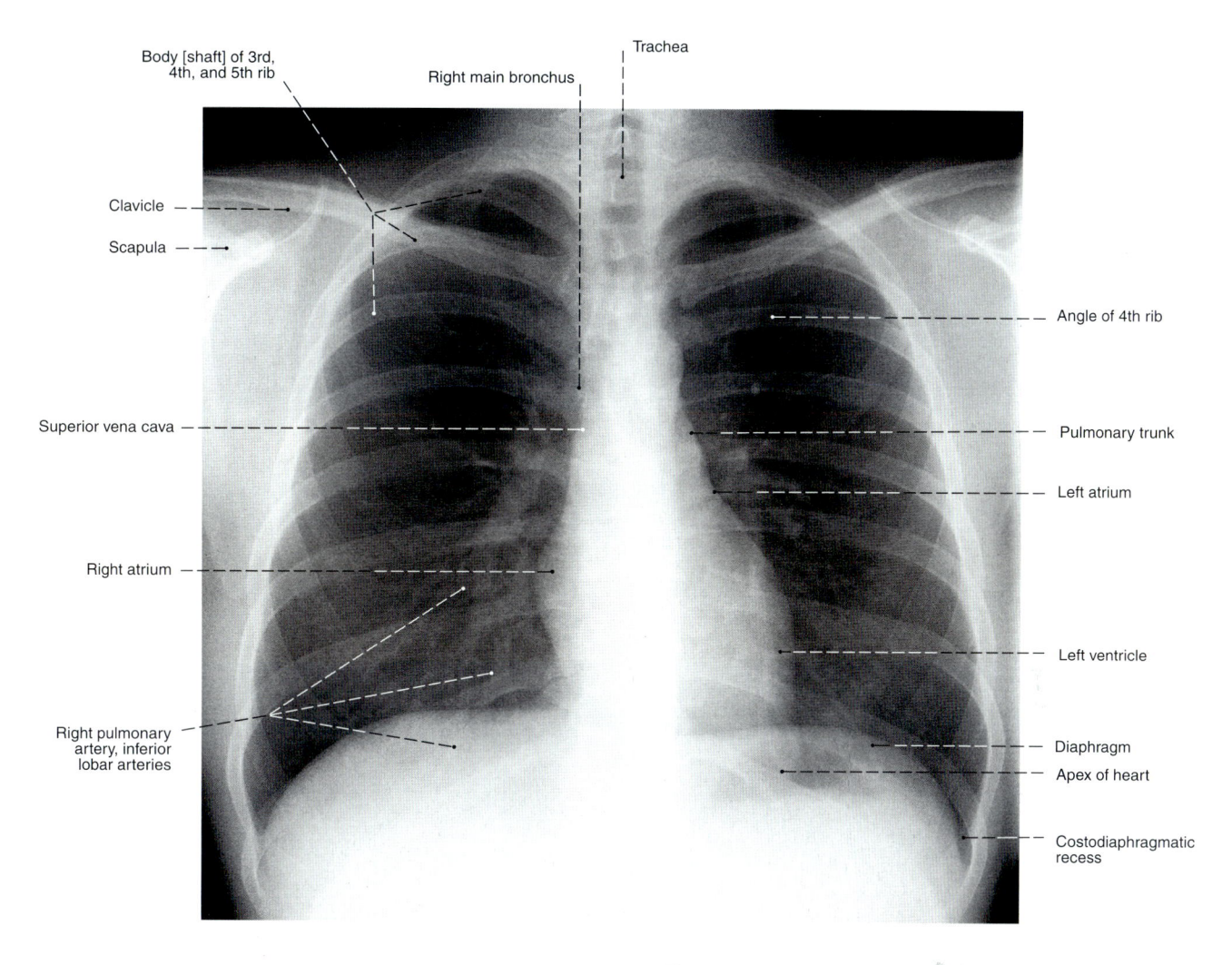

Fig. 888 Thoracic cage and viscera; PA radiograph of a 27-years-old male; beam directed sagittally onto the center of the sternum.
Position and size of the heart, the lung, and the bony structures of the thoracic cage as well as the vertebral column can be viewed.

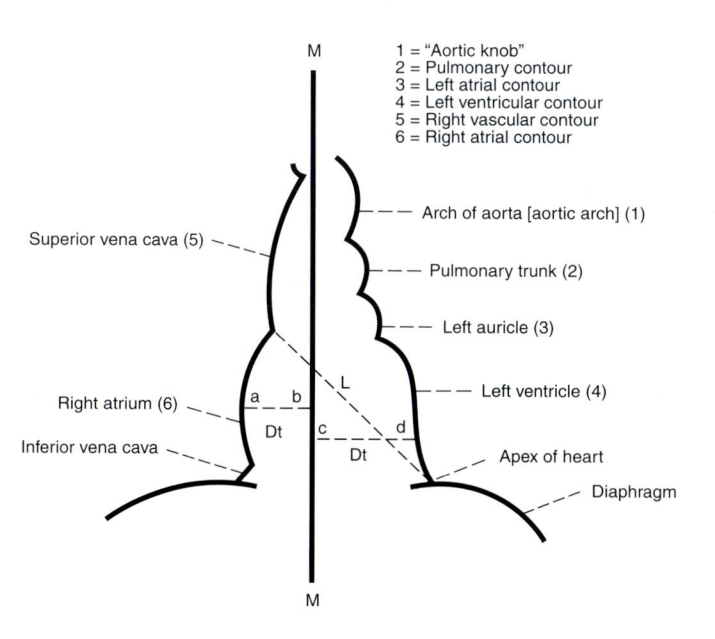

1 = "Aortic knob"
2 = Pulmonary contour
3 = Left atrial contour
4 = Left ventricular contour
5 = Right vascular contour
6 = Right atrial contour

Fig. 889 Diagram of silhouette of heart in the radiograph,
Dt = Transverse diameter, ab + cd = 13-14 cm
L = Longitudinal axis of heart (from superior end of right atrial contour to apex of heart) = 15-16 cm
M = Median plane of body

104 Thoracic viscera

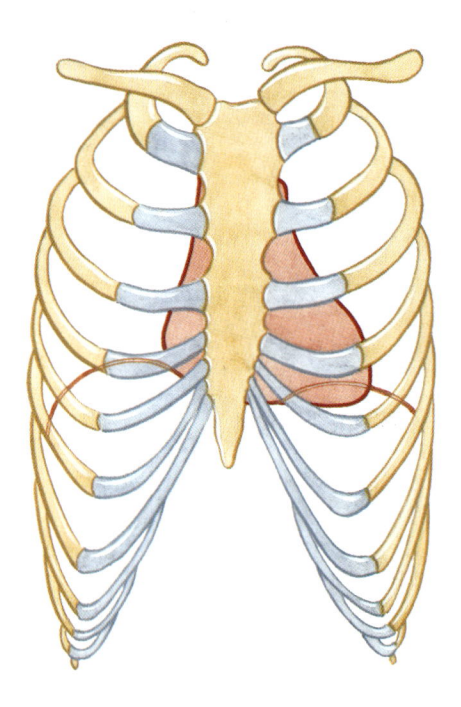

Fig. 890 Position of heart in the thorax during expiration; ventral aspect.

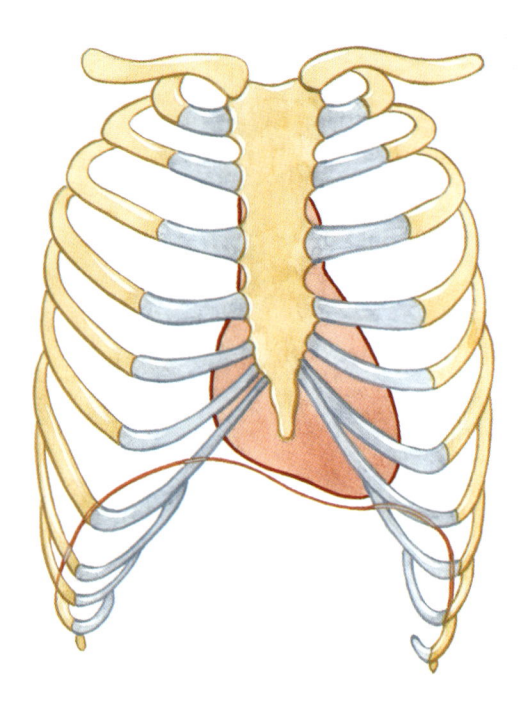

Fig. 891 Position of heart in the thorax during inspiration; ventral aspect.
The heart is positioned more vertical; the apex of heart is directed medially and caudally.

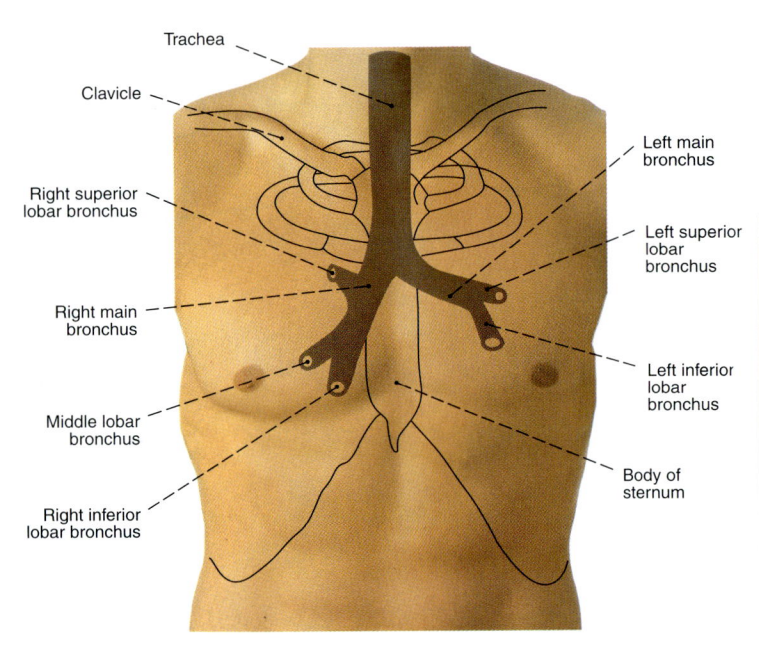

Fig. 892 Trachea and bronchi in a living person; projection onto the anterior thoracic wall.

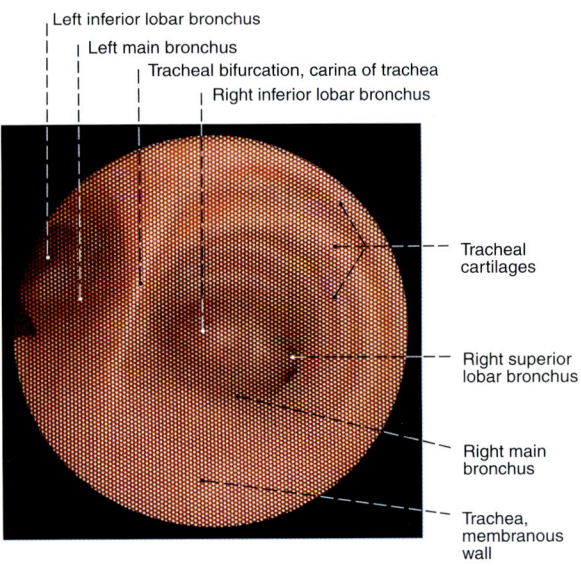

Fig. 893 Tracheal bifurcation; endoscopic view (bronchoscopy).

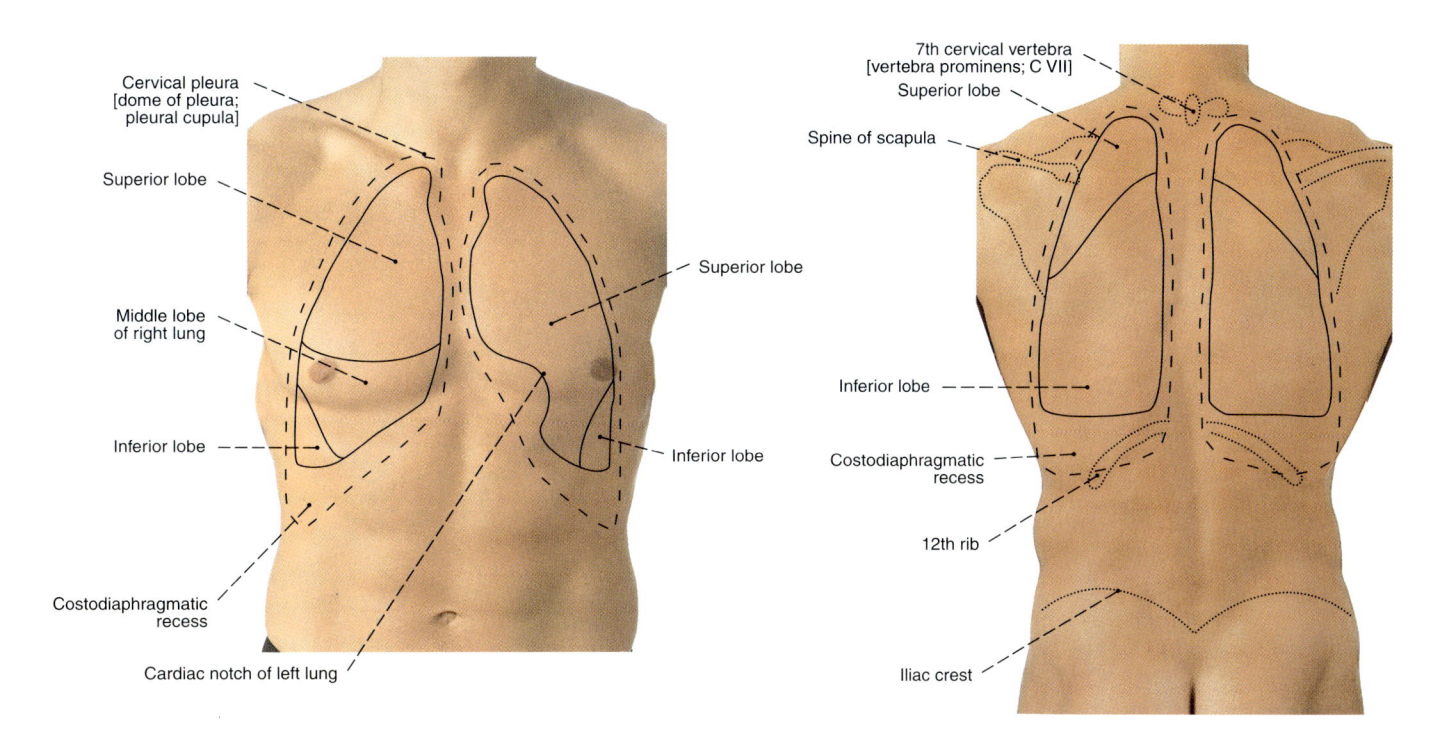

Pulmonary and pleural boundaries

Fig. 894 Projection of pulmonary and pleural boundaries onto the anterior thoracic wall; ventral aspect.
Pulmonary boundaries are solid lines; pleural boundaries are broken lines.

Fig. 895 Projection of pulmonary and pleural boundaries onto the anterior thoracic wall; dorsal aspect.
Pulmonary boundaries are solid lines; pleural boundaries are broken lines.

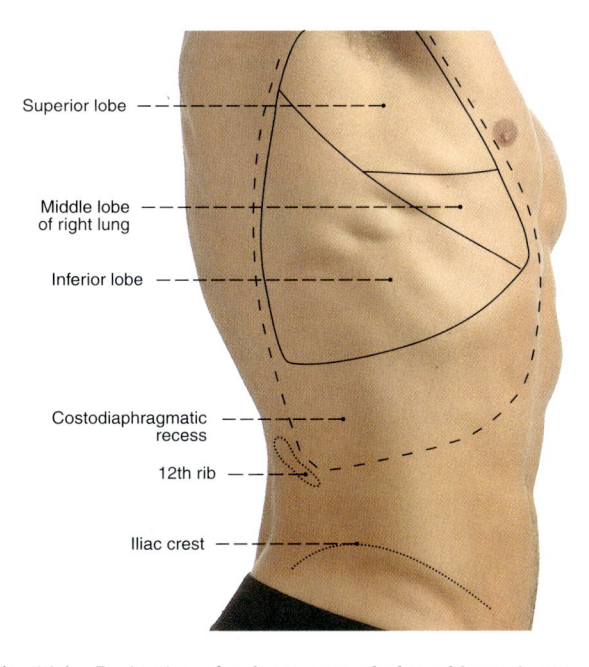

Fig. 896 Projection of pulmonary and pleural boundaries onto the anterior thoracic wall; right lateral aspect.
Pulmonary boundaries are solid lines; pleural boundaries are broken lines.

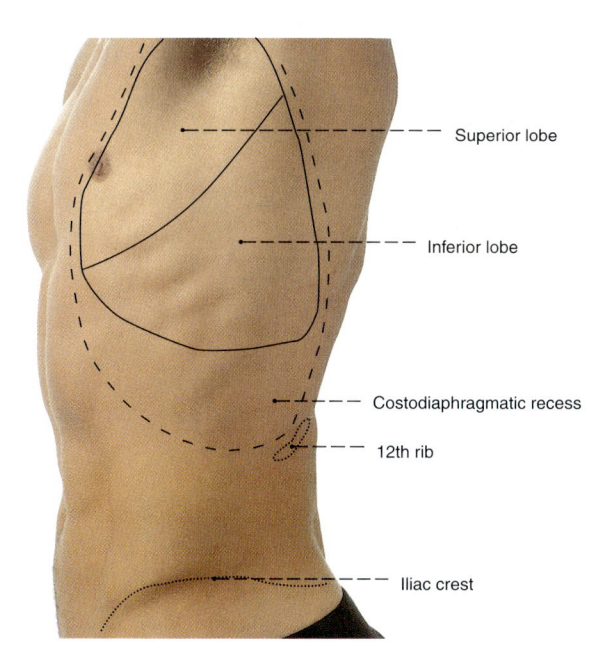

Fig. 897 Projection of pulmonary and pleural boundaries onto the anterior thoracic wall; left lateral aspect.
Pulmonary boundaries are solid lines; pleural boundaries are broken lines.

106 *Thoracic viscera*

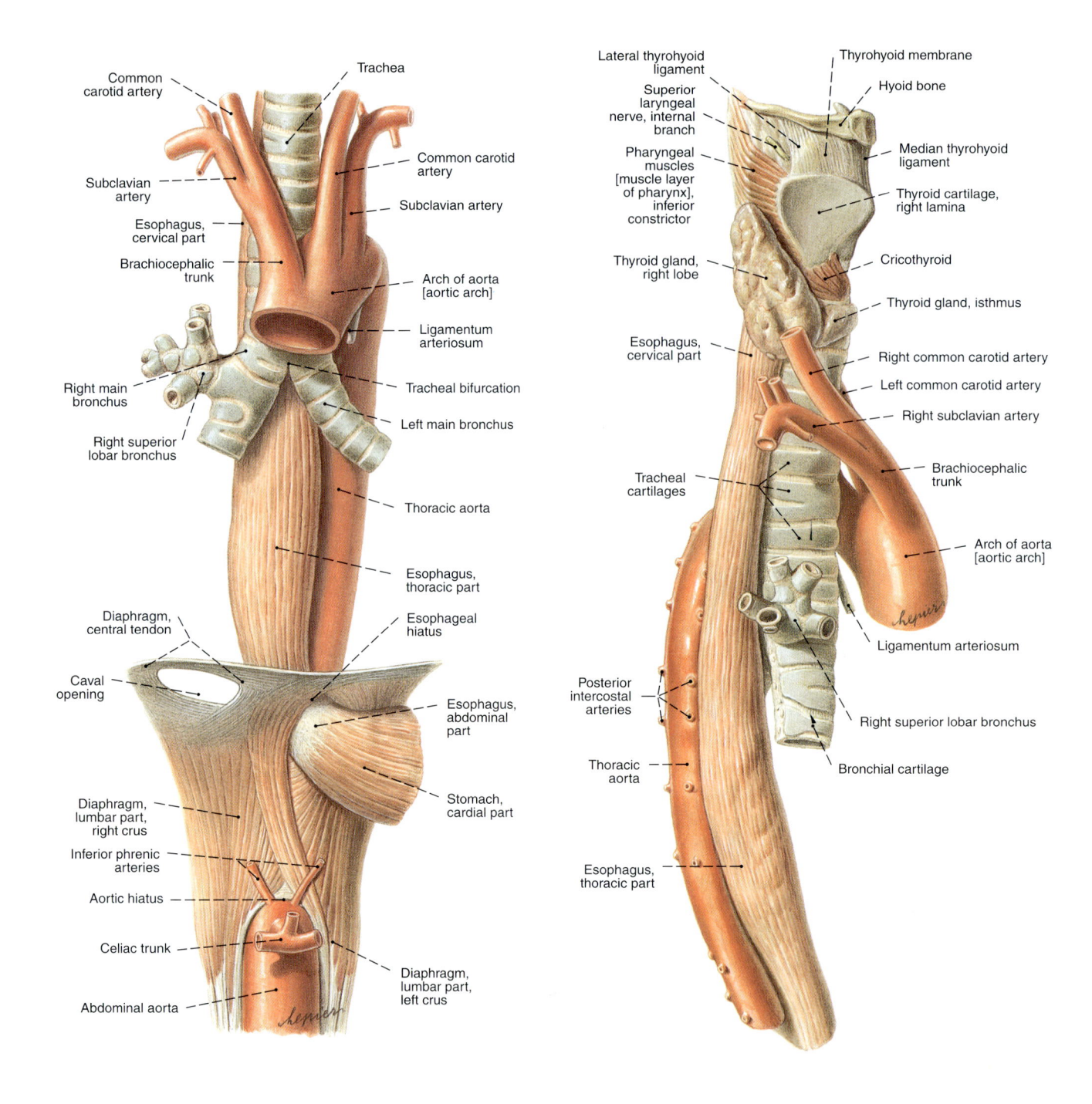

Fig. 898   Esophagus, trachea; thoracic aorta; parts of diaphragm retained to show openings for aorta, inferior vena cava, and esophagus; ventral aspect.

Fig. 899   Esophagus, trachea; thoracic aorta; right lateral aspect.

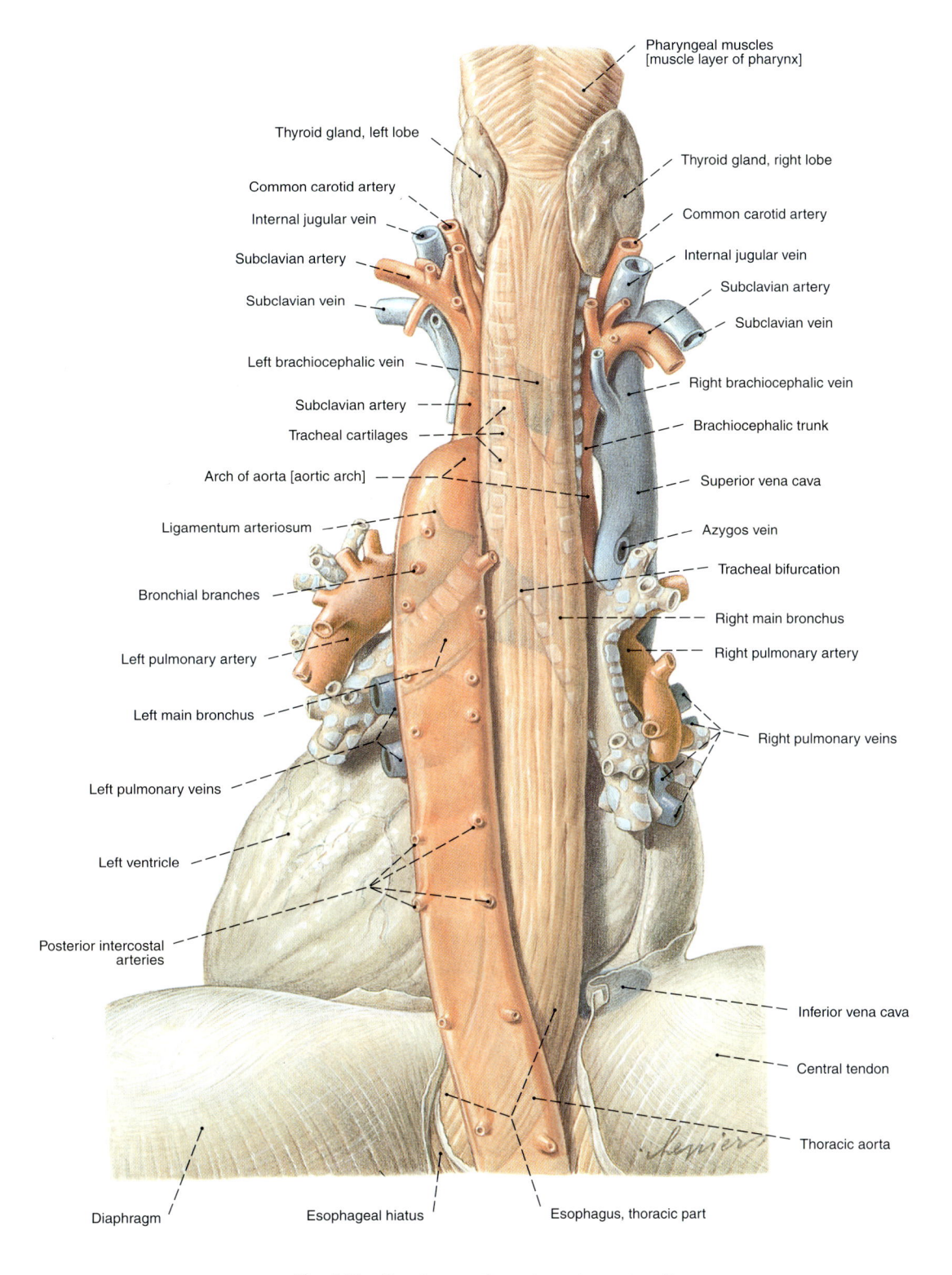

Esophagus and aorta

Fig. 900 Esophagus, thoracic aorta; pericardium; dorsal aspect.

Thoracic viscera

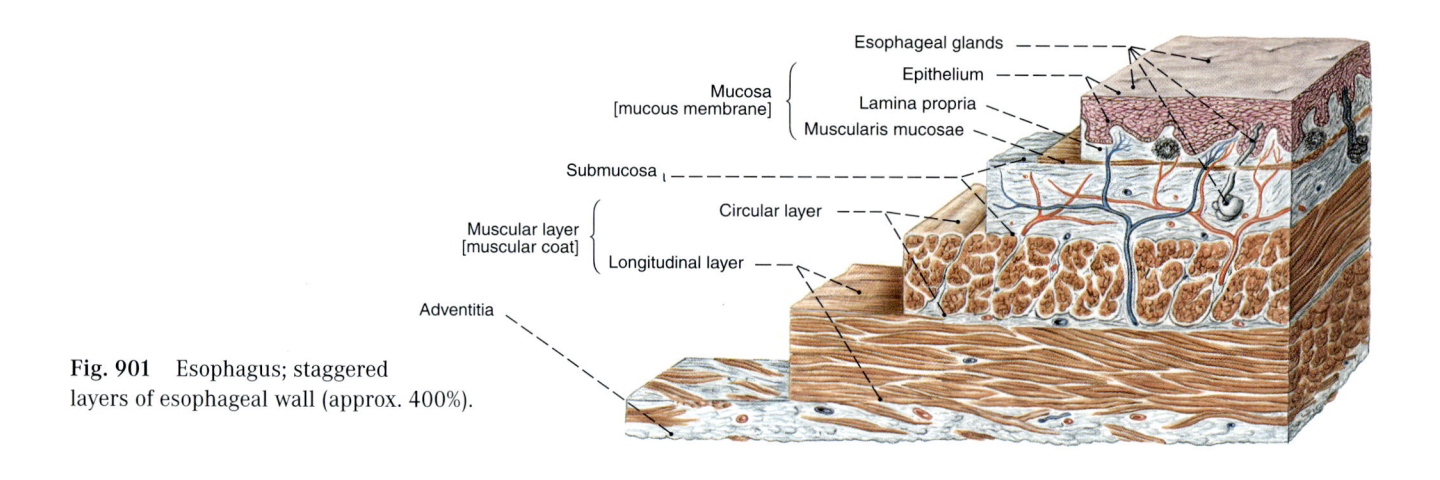

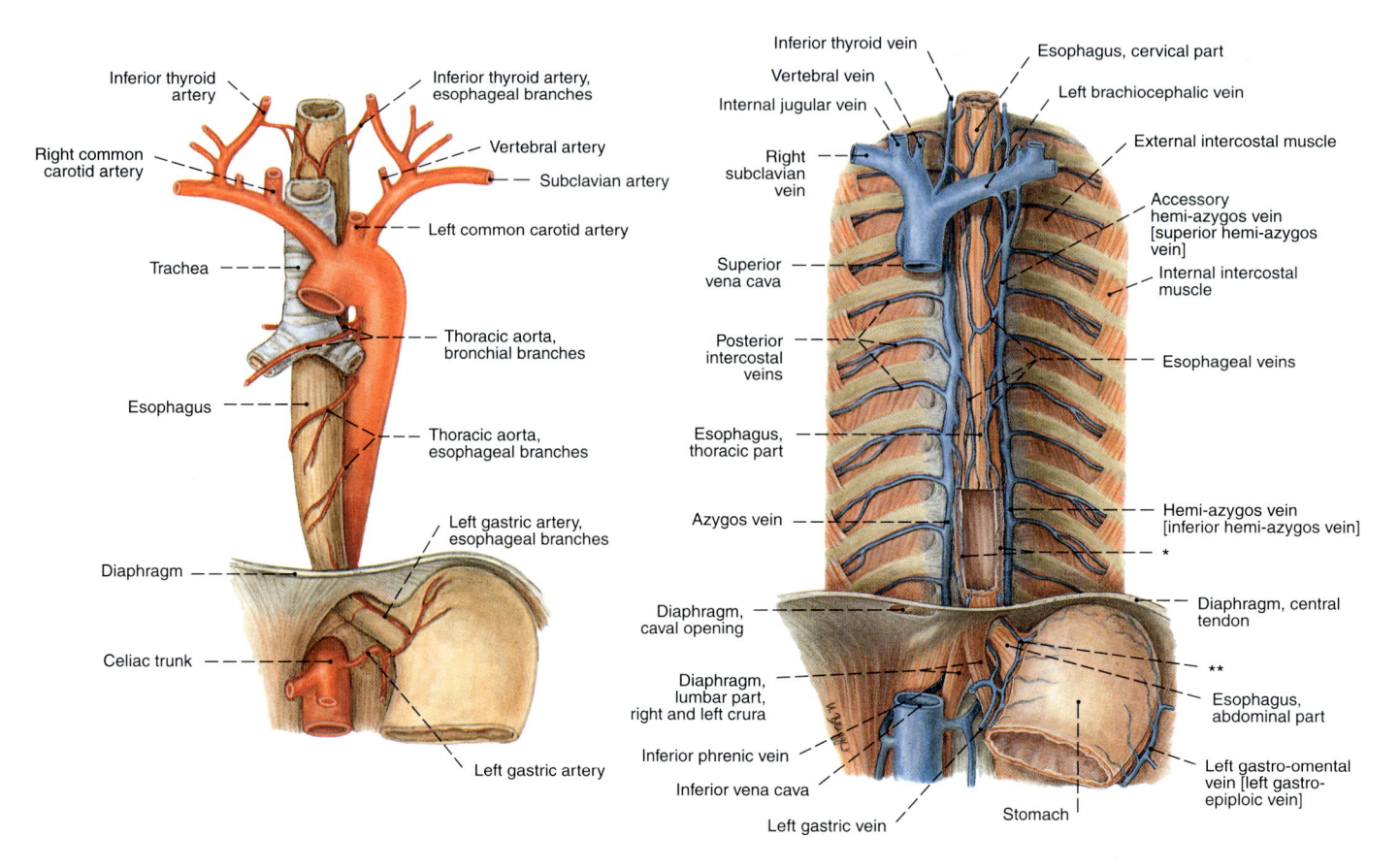

Fig. 901 Esophagus; staggered layers of esophageal wall (approx. 400%).

Fig. 902 Esophagus and its arterial supply; ventral aspect.

Fig. 903 Esophageal veins; parts of diaphragm and stomach removed; in the lower thoracic part anterior wall of esophagus removed.

* Veins of esophageal mucosa.
** Connecting branch between veins of stomach and esophagus.

Thoracic lymph nodes 109

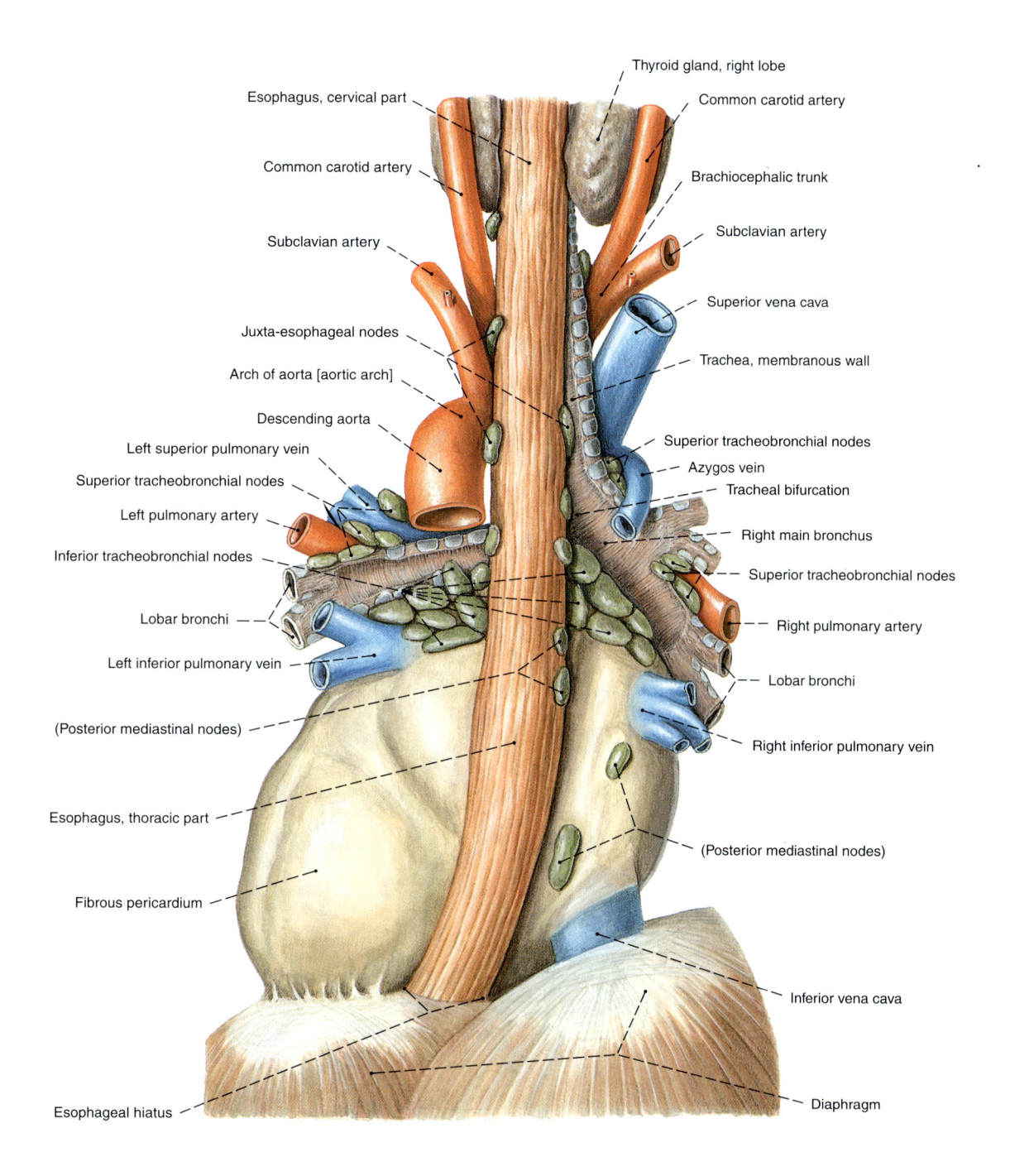

Fig. 904 Thoracic lymph nodes; bronchi sectioned after division into lobar bronchi; great blood vessels retained in mediastinum; dorsal aspect. Lymph nodes in the healthy adult are usually smaller than shown here.

Thoracic viscera

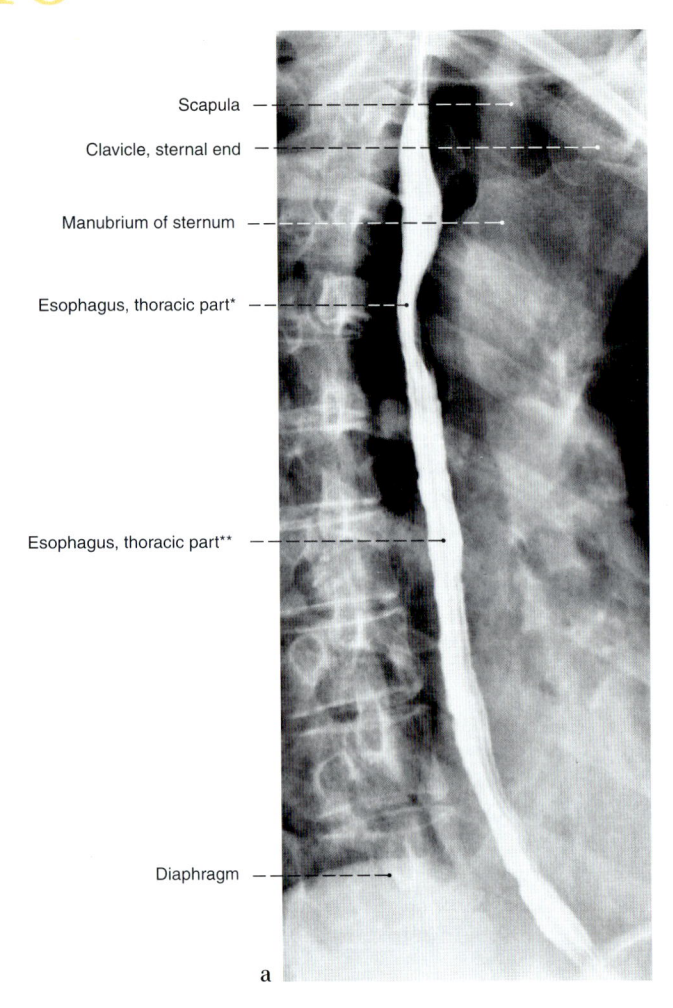

Fig. 905 a, b Esophagus; radiograph (after swallowing contrast medium);
a Right anterior oblique (RAO) position (beam from left anterior to right posterior)
b Left anterior oblique (LAO) position (beam from right anterior to left posterior)

* Thoracic constriction [broncho-aortic constriction].
** Retrocardial part.
*** Constriction at beginning of esophagus.

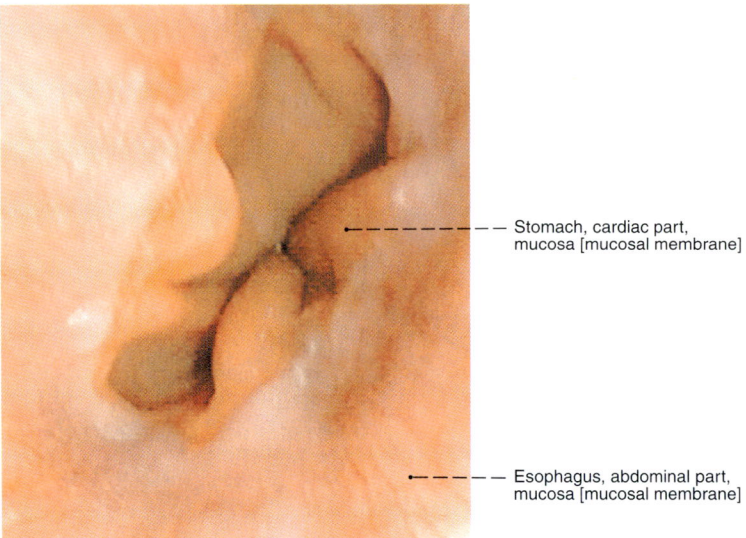

Fig. 906 Esophagus; mucosa viewed by endoscope (esophagoscopy); superior aspect.

Thymus 111

Fig. 907 Thymus of a 2-year-old child; ventral aspect.

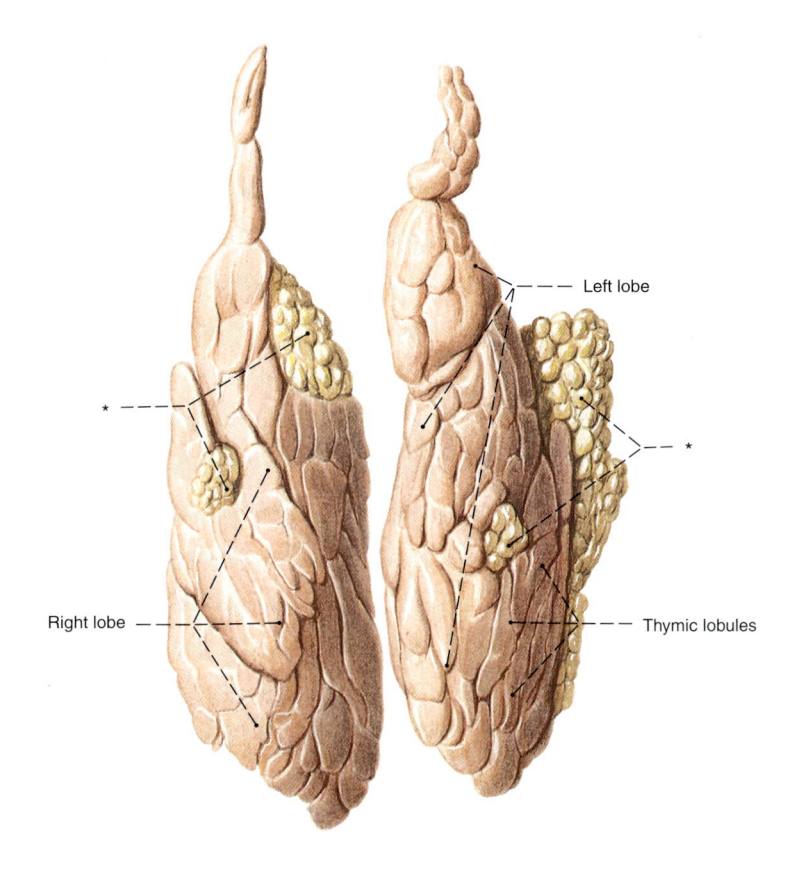

Fig. 908 Thymus of a 42-year-old; fatty tissue extensively removed; ventral aspect.

* Parathymic fat.

In this specimen shape and size of the thymus were unusually preserved.

112 *Thoracic viscera*

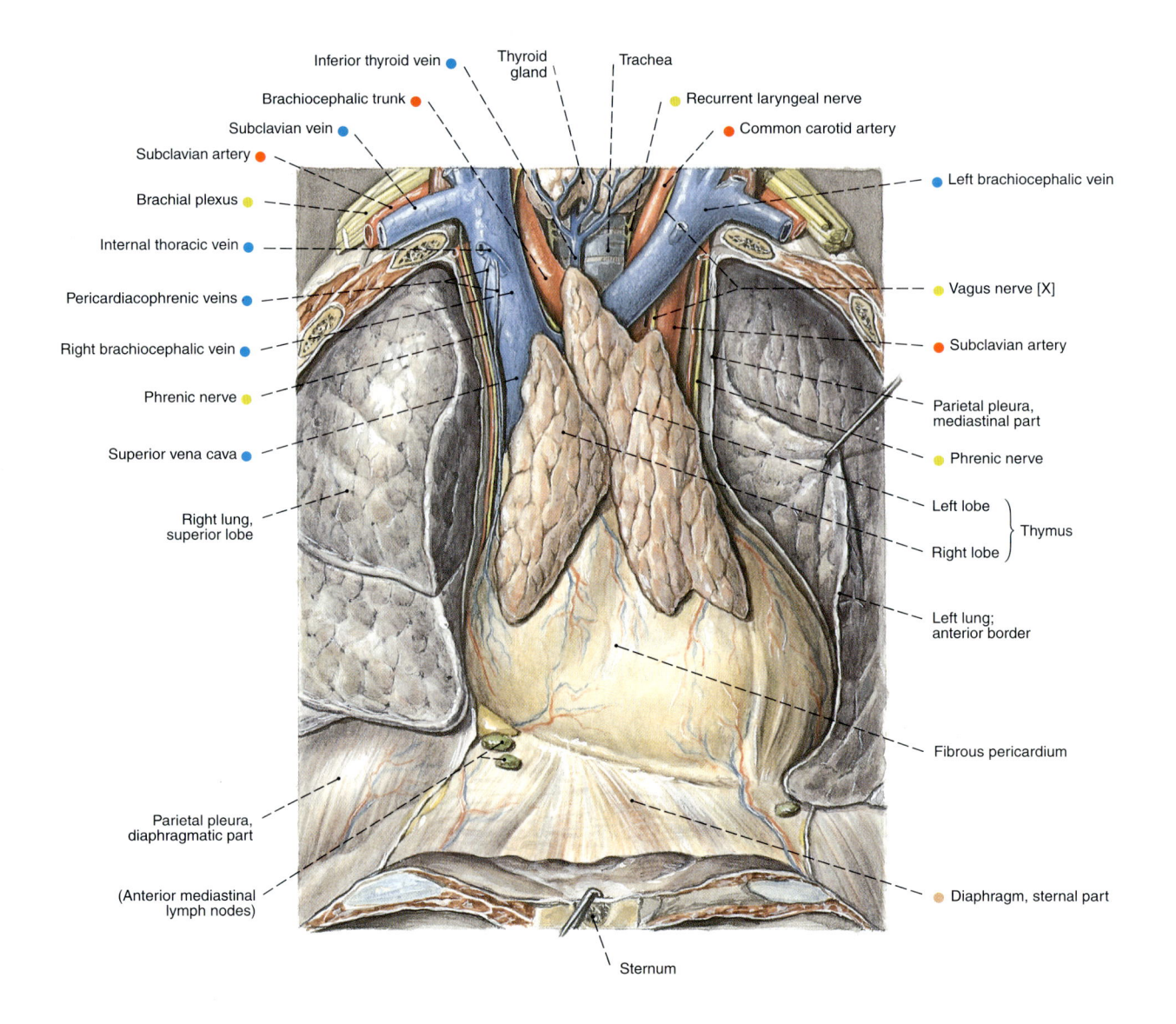

Fig. 909 Thymus in the adolescent; anterior thoracic wall removed, pleural cavity opened and left lung retracted laterally; ventral aspect. Compare size of thymus of newborn (Fig. 999) and 2-year-old child (Fig. 907).

Thoracic viscera 113

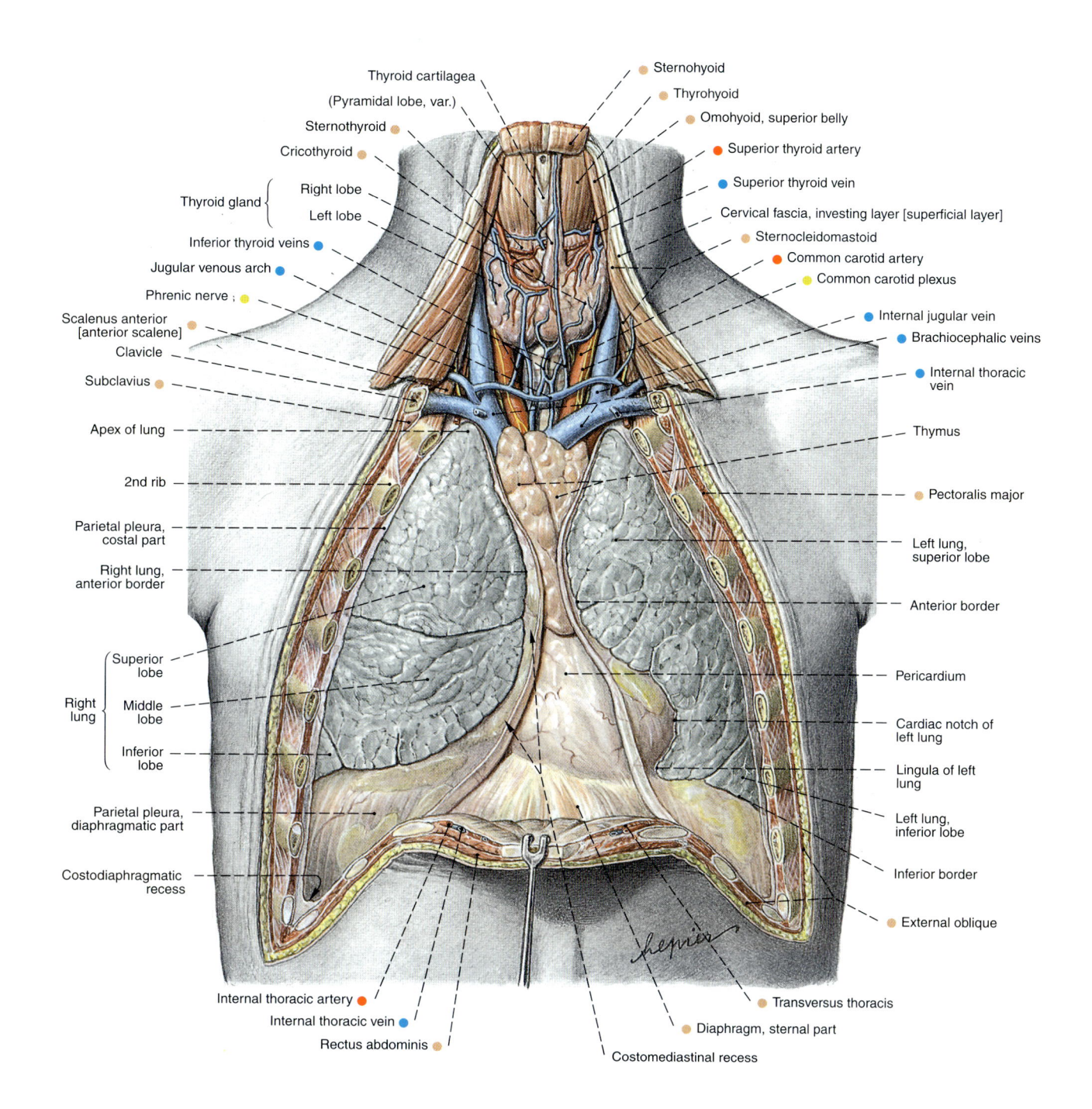

Fig. 910 Thymus; pericardium; lungs; anterior thoracic wall removed, pleural cavity opened; ventral aspect. Note the size of thymus in the young adult. In the older individuals thymic tissue is almost entirely replaced by fat.

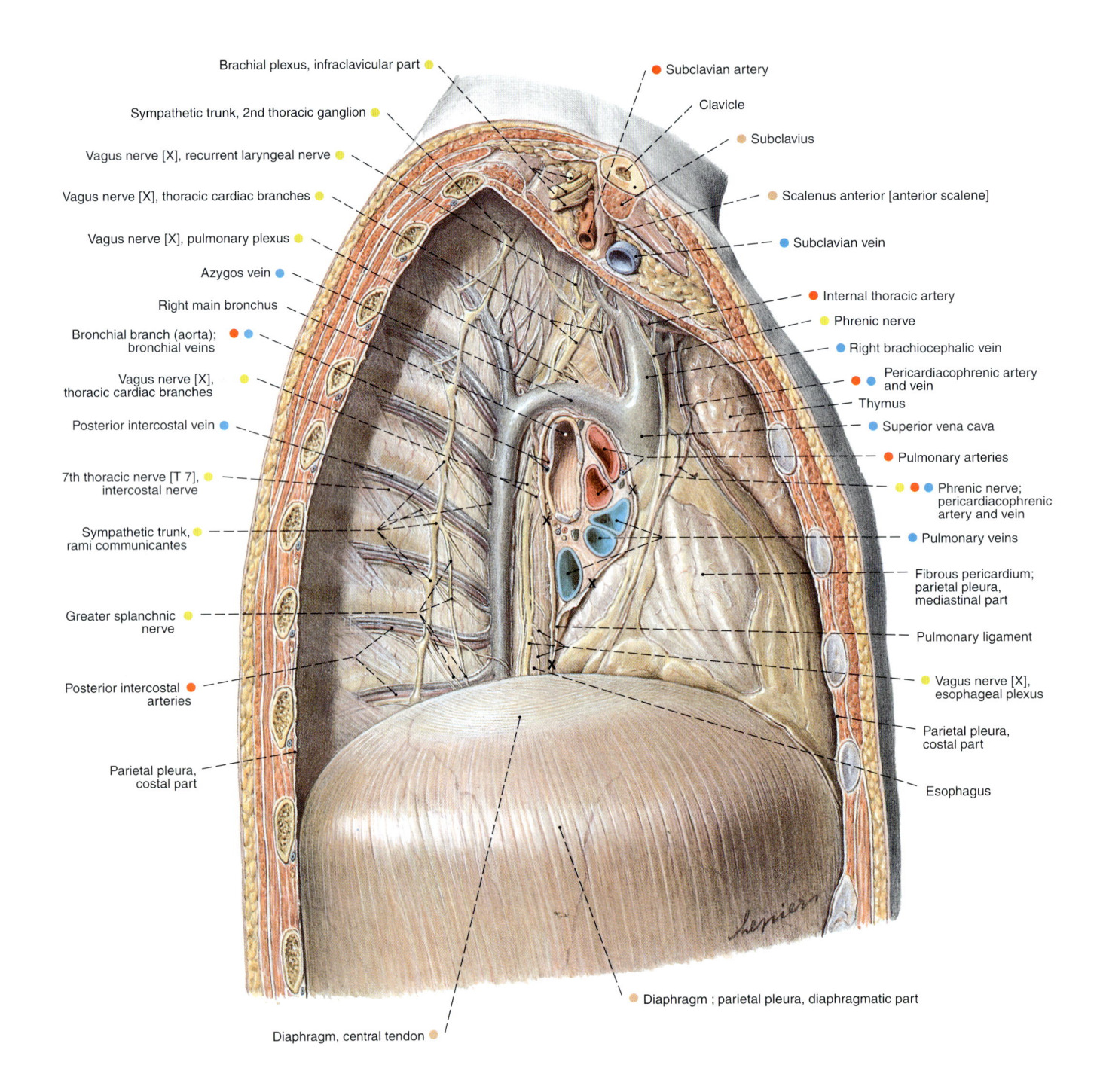

Fig. 911 Pleural cavity; mediastinum; lateral thoracic wall and right lung removed; parts of mediastinal and costal pleura resected to expose the blood vessels and nerves; right lateral aspect.
Areas marked with an "x" indicate reflection of the visceral pleura into the parietal pleura surrounding the root of lung and the pulmonary ligament.

Pleural cavity and mediastinum

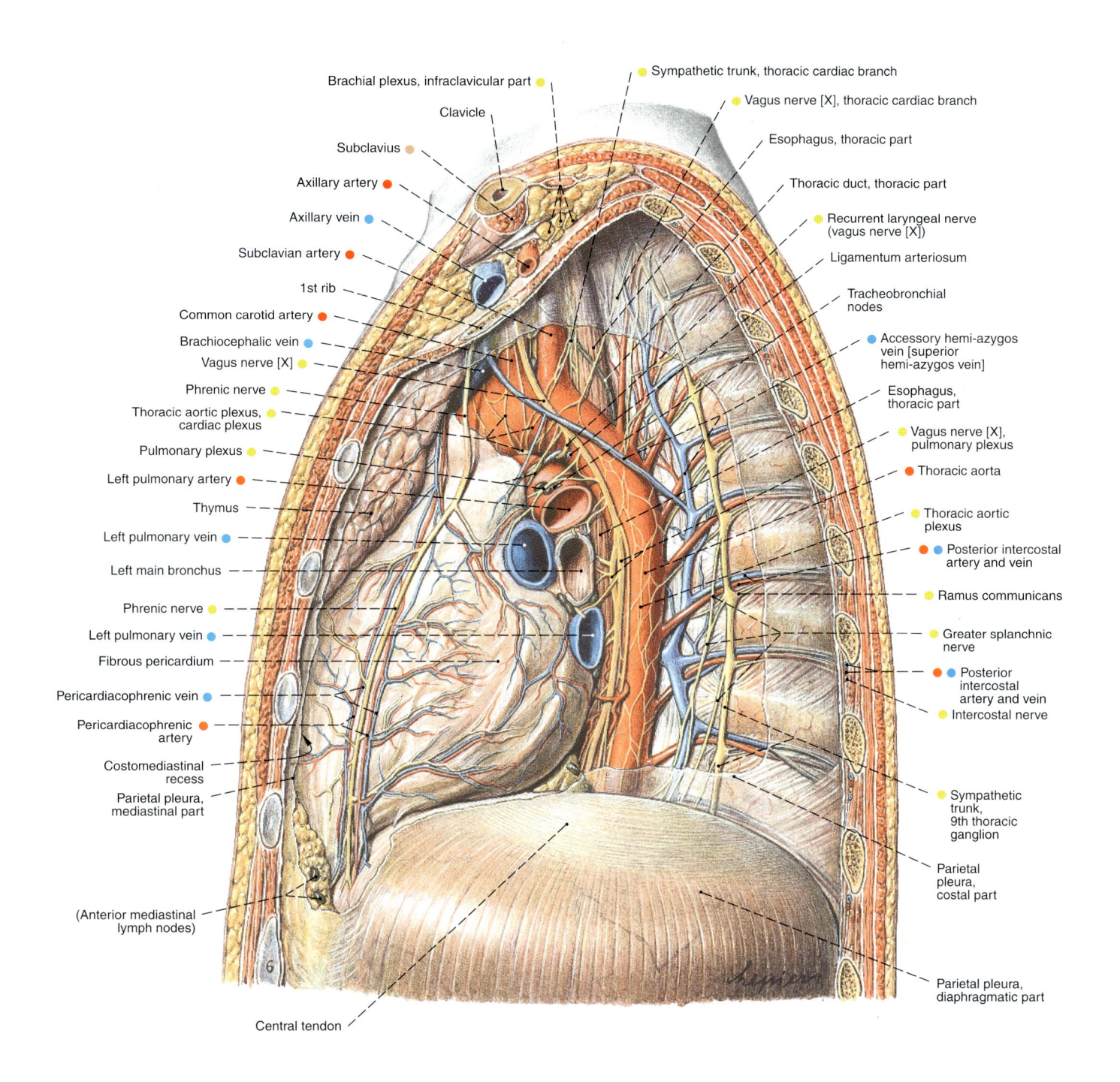

Fig. 912 Pleural cavity; mediastinum; lateral thoracic wall and left lung removed; parts of mediastinal and costal pleura resected to expose the blood vessels and nerves; left lateral aspect.

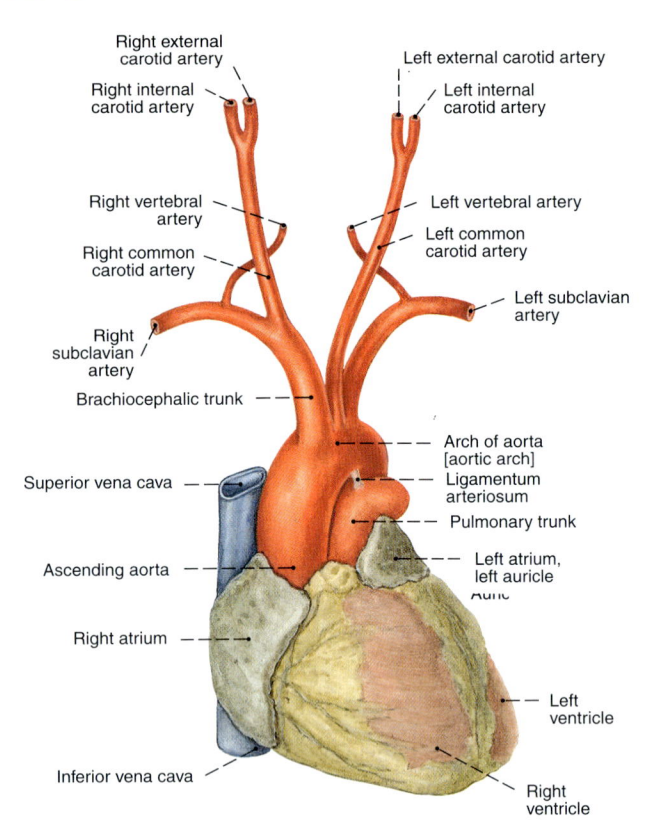

Pleural cavity and mediastinum

Fig. 913 Heart; arch of aorta [aortic arch] with origins of large arteries; ventral aspect.

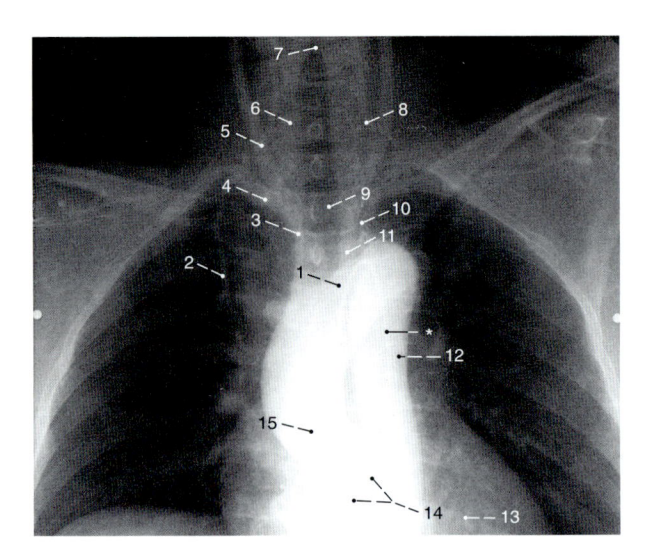

Fig. 914 Arch of aorta [aortic arch] and branches; AP radiograph (after injection of contrast medium into the aortic bulb [infundibulum]; ventral aspect.
* Catheter.

1 Arch of aorta [aortic arch]
2 Internal thoracic artery
3 Brachiocephalic trunk
4 Right subclavian artery
5 Right common carotid artery
6 Right vertebral artery
7 Rima glottidis
8 Left vertebral artery
9 Trachea
10 Left subclavian artery
11 Left common carotid artery
12 Descending aorta
13 Heart
14 Aortic valve
15 Ascending aorta

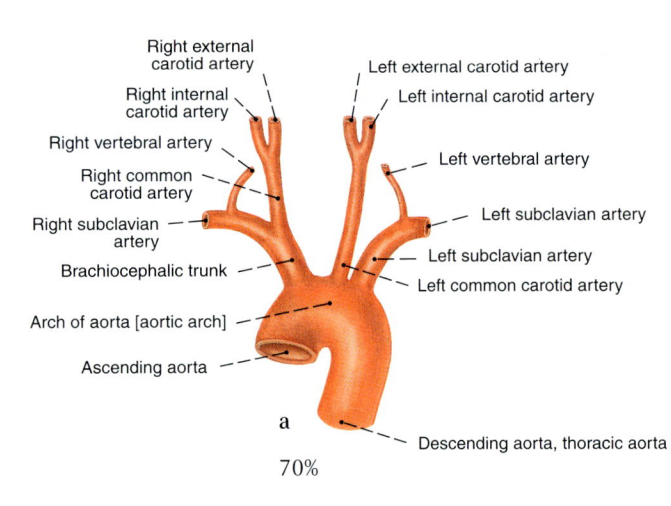

Fig. 915 a–e Variations of origins of large arteries from arch of aorta [aortic arch].
a "Normal case"
b Common origin of brachiocephalic trunk and left common carotid artery
c Common stem of brachiocephalic trunk and left common carotid artery
d Independent origin of left vertebral artery from arch of aorta [aortic arch]
e Right subclavian artery as the last branch of arch of aorta [aortic arch]

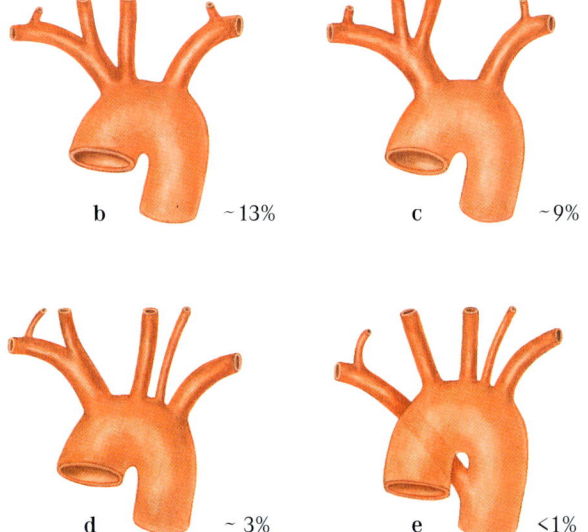

This abnormal artery usually crosses to the right behind the esophoagus, causing difficulties in swallowing (dysphagia lusoria).

Thoracic and abdominal aorta, mediastinum

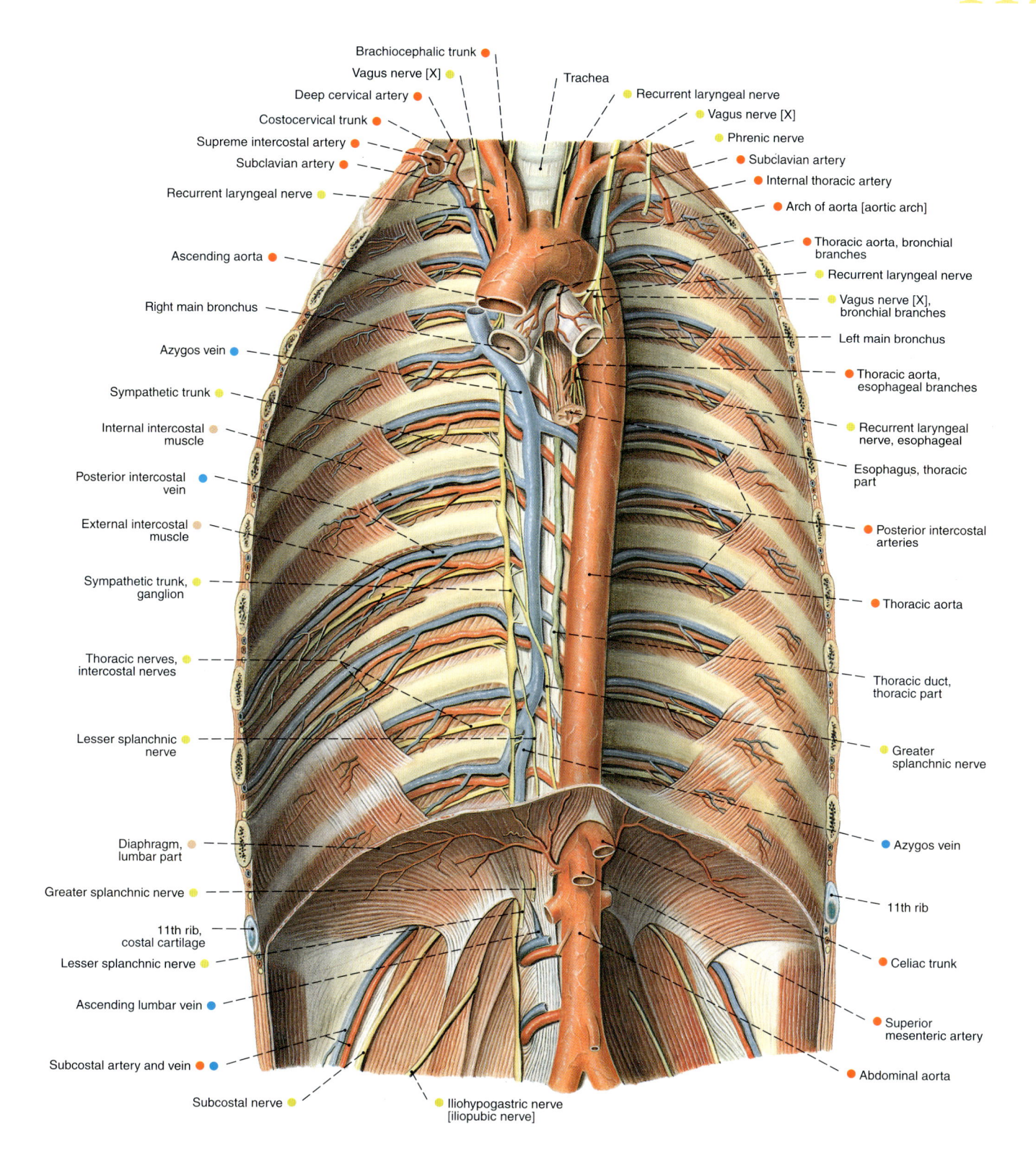

Fig. 916 Thoracic and abdominal aorta; posterior mediastinum; pleura removed to expose intercostal nerves and sympathetic trunk; ventral aspect.

118 *Thoracic viscera*

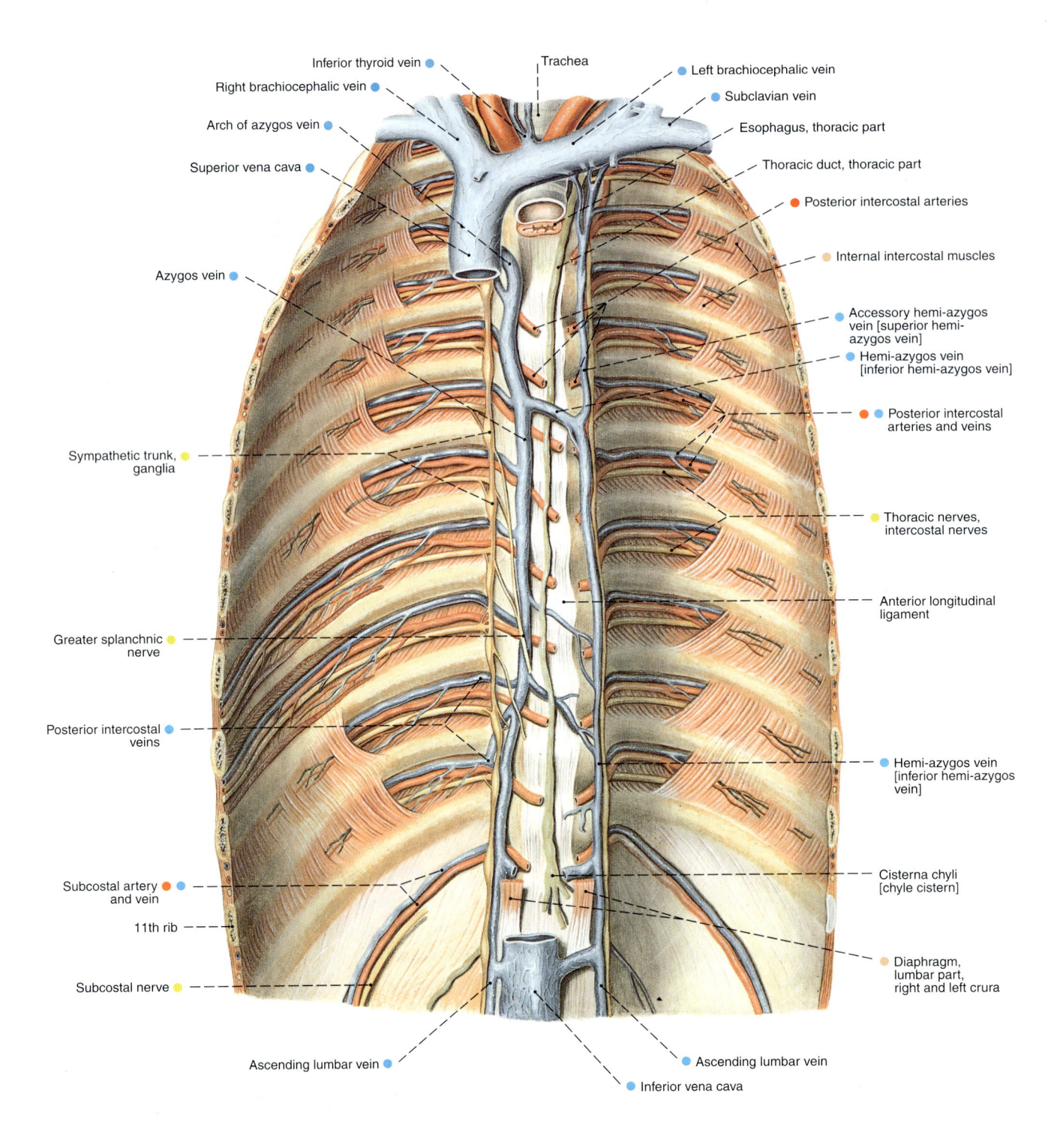

Fig. 917 Blood vessels and nerves of posterior mediastinum; pleura, aorta, and esophagus removed to expose thoracic duct, azygos vein, and intercostal blood vessels and nerves; ventral aspect.

Esophagus and mediastinum 119

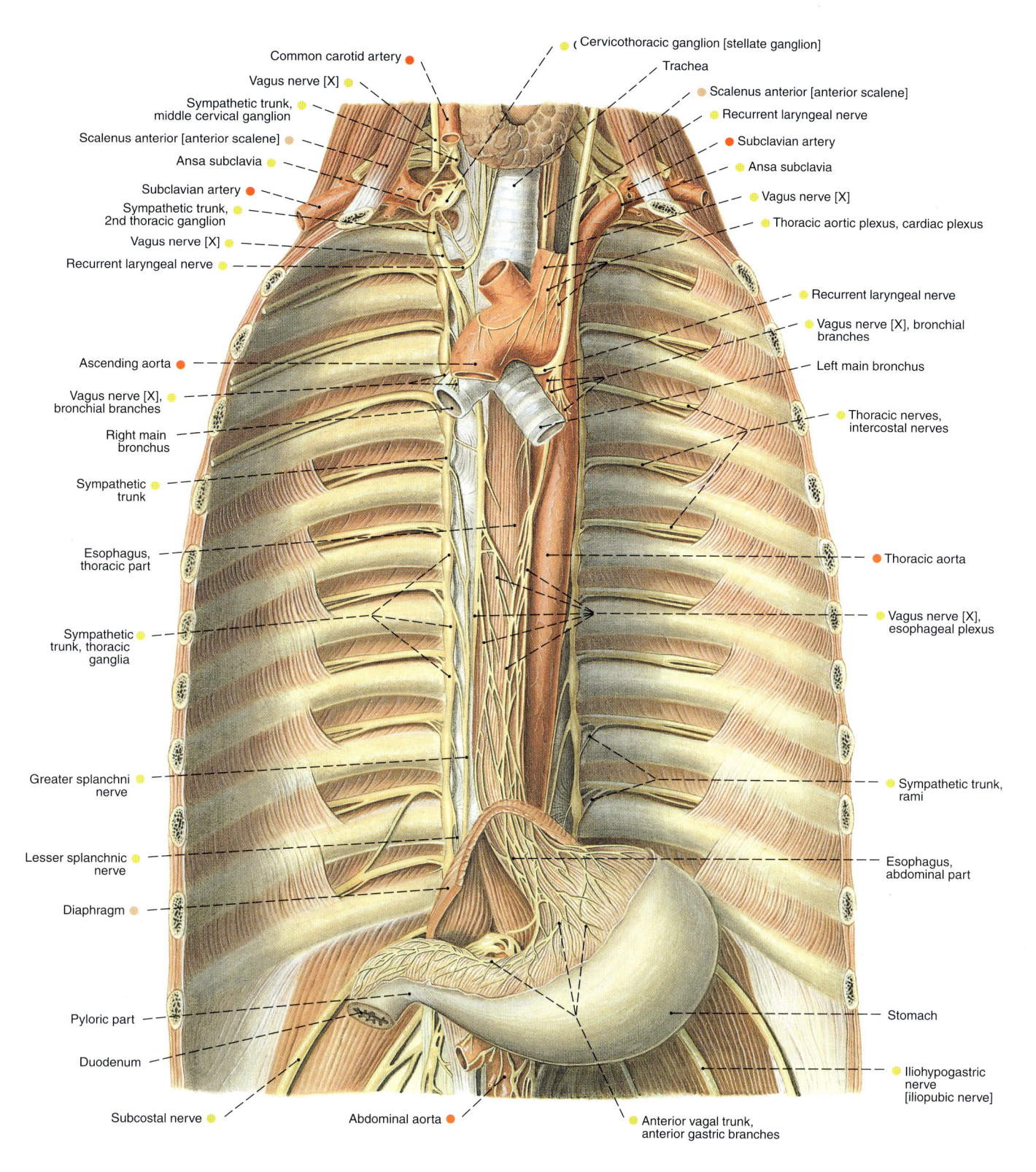

Fig. 918 Esophagus; aorta; autonomic division [part] of peripheral nervous system; stomach.
Only dorsal parts of diaphragm retained; pleura removed to expose sympathetic trunk and its connections to intercostal nerves; ventral aspect.

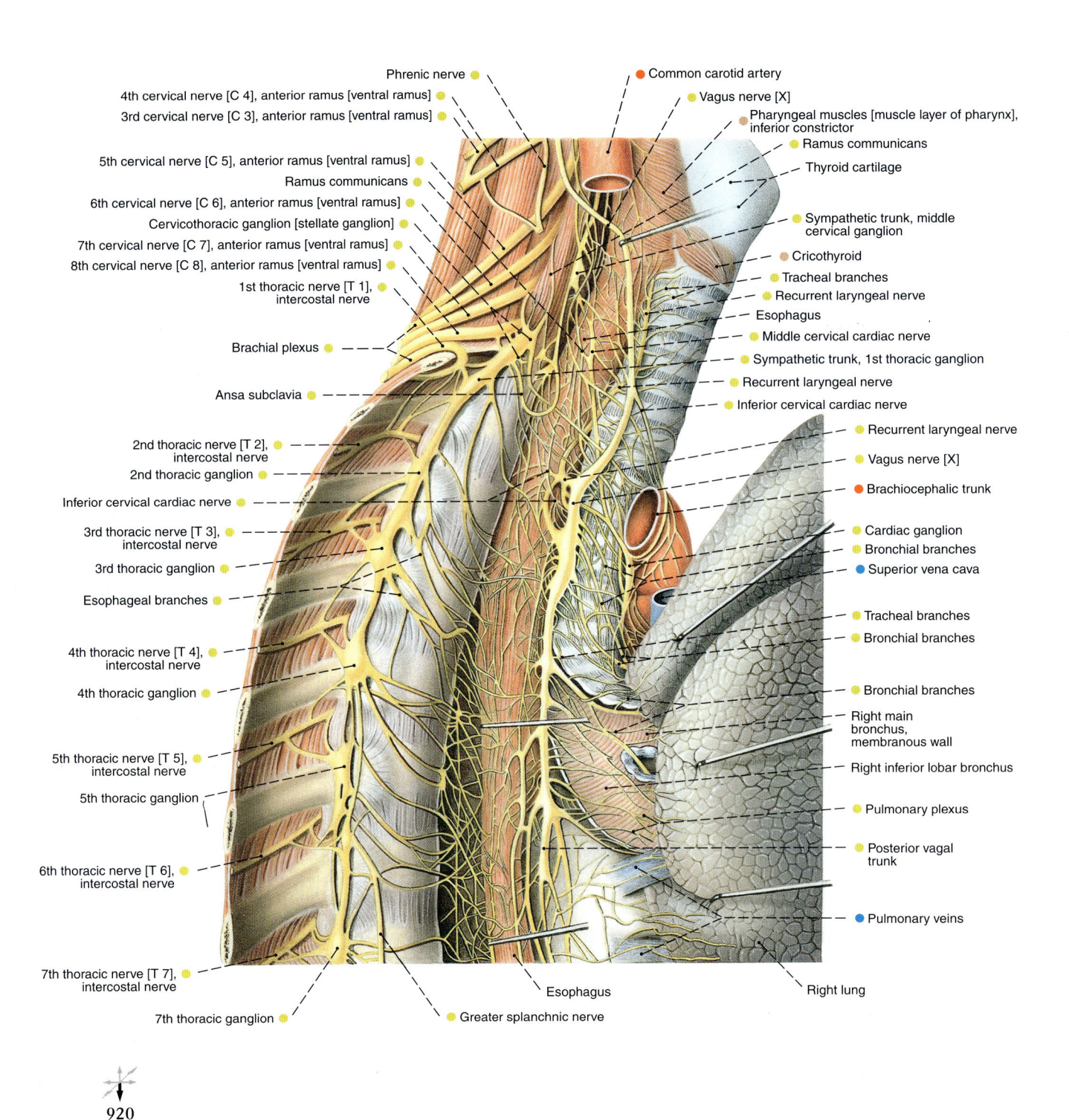

Fig. 919 Lower cervical and upper thoracic part of autonomic division of peripheral nervous system; vagus nerve and right lung retracted anteriorly to expose esophagus; right lateral aspect.

Mediastinum, autonomic division [part] of peripheral nervous system

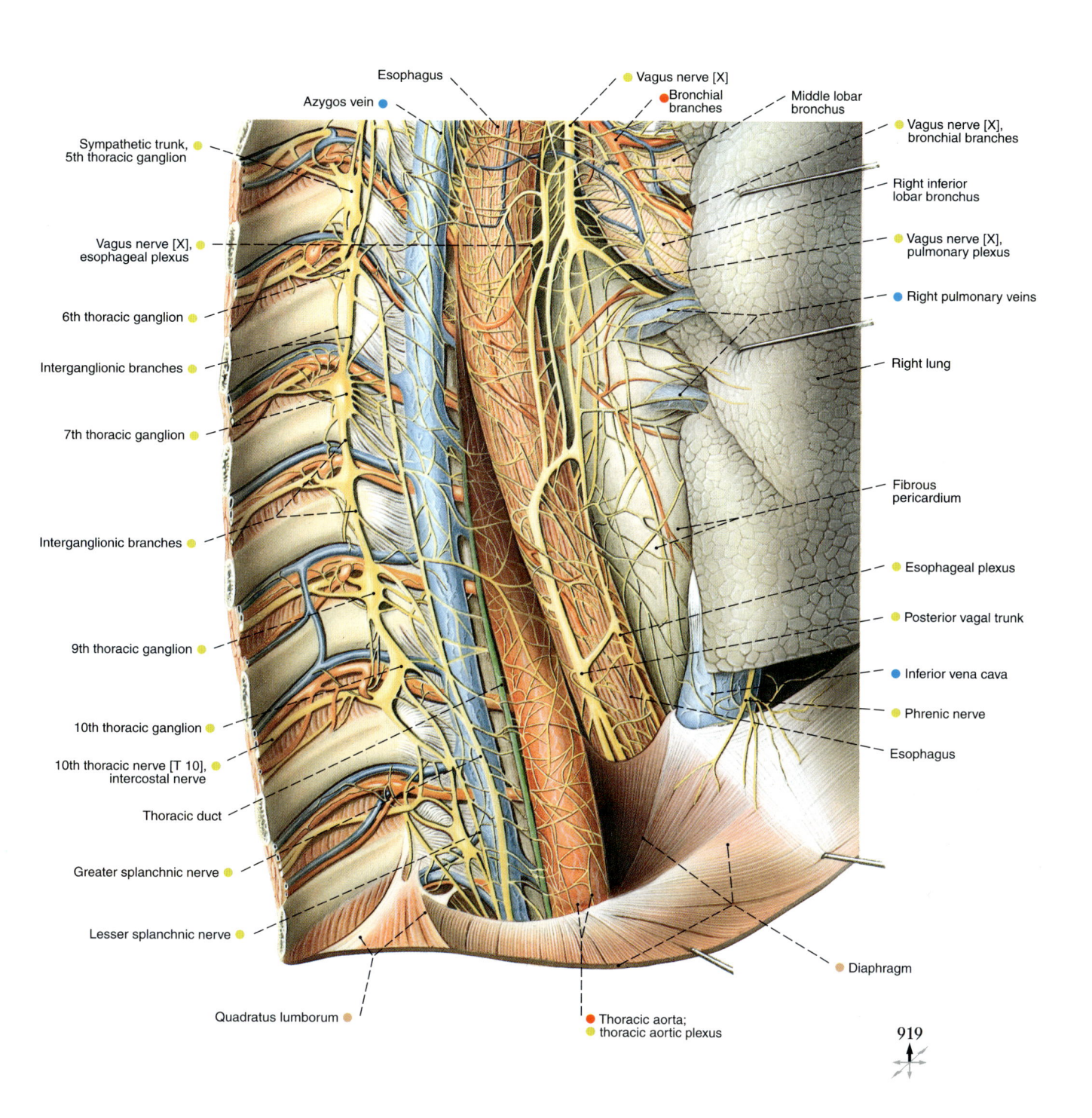

Fig. 920 Lower thoracic part of autonomic division of peripheral nervous system; dissection similar to Fig. 919; aorta, thoracic duct, and azygos vein, however, retained; right lateral aspect.

122 Thoracic viscera

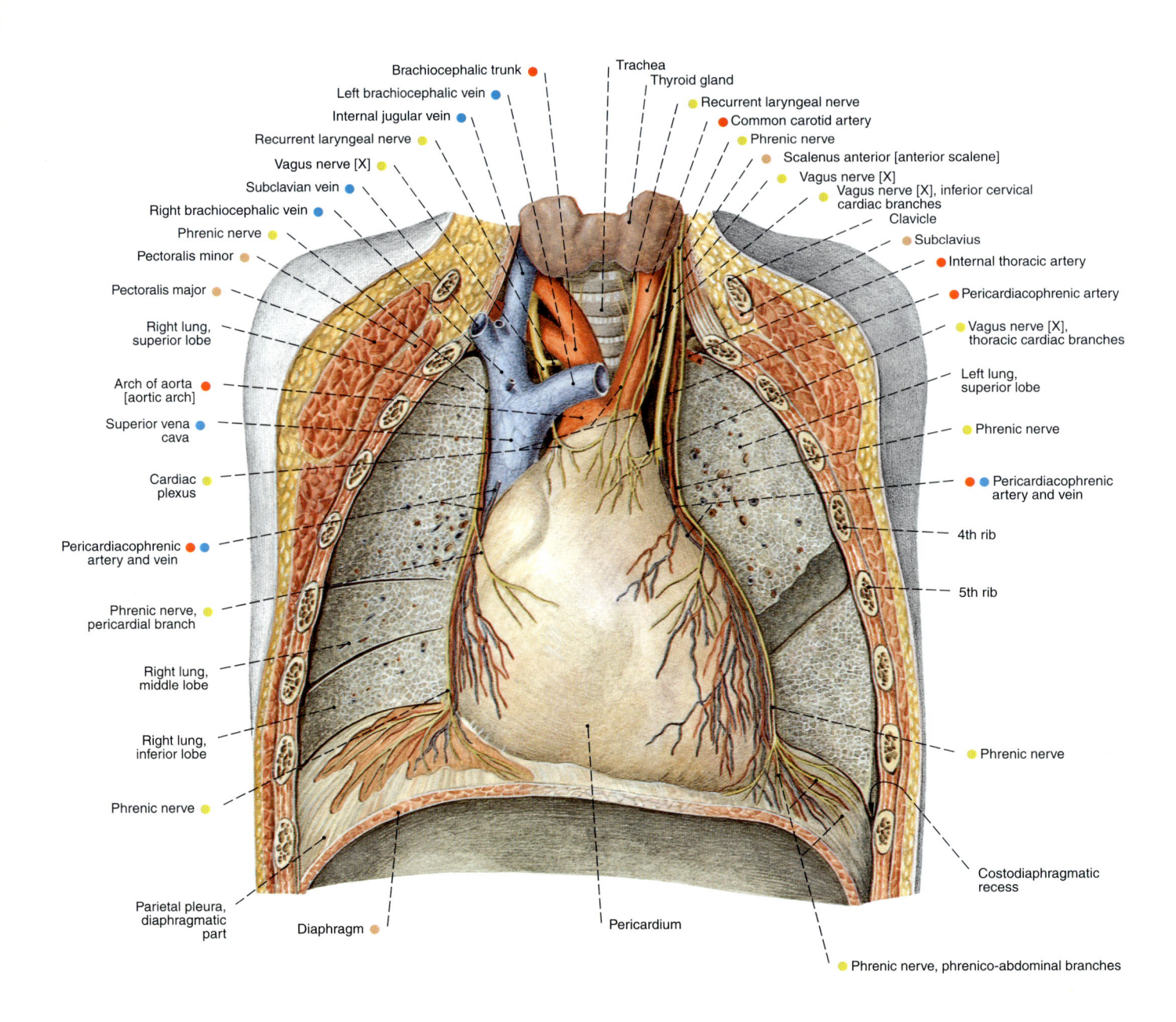

Fig. 921 Thoracic cavity in an adult; anterior thoracic wall removed; right and left lung sectioned in the frontal plane; mediastinal and diaphragmatic pleura removed to expose pericardiacophrenic artery and branches of phrenic nerve; ventral aspect.

Thoracic viscera 123

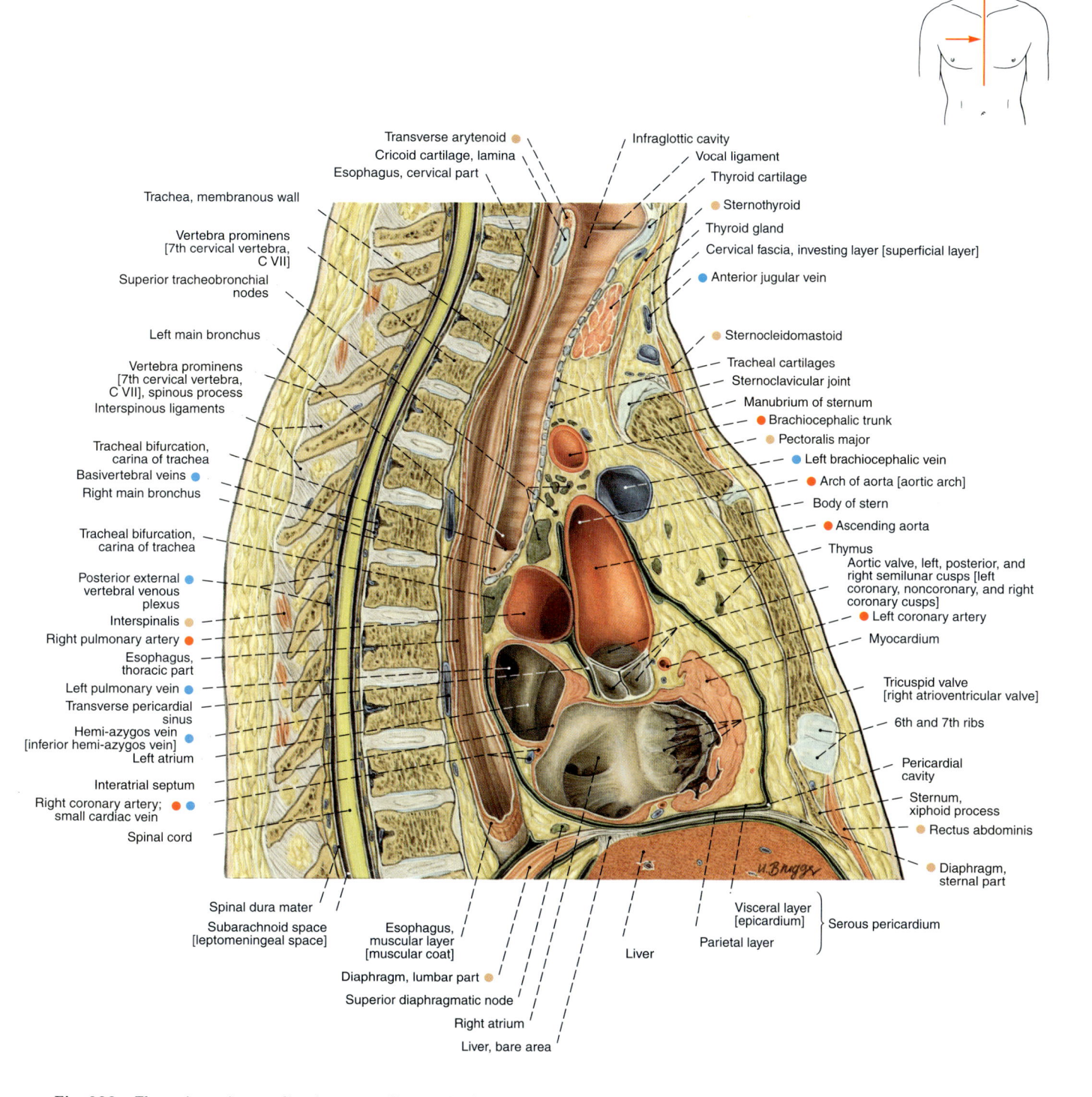

Fig. 922 Thoracic cavity; mediastinum; median sagittal section through neck and thorax. Due to a slight asymmetry of the thorax the sternoclavicular joint is sectioned above the manubrium of sternum; right lateral aspect.
Due to the proximity of the left atrium to the esophagus, an enlargement of the left atrium can be recognized by displacement of the esophagus in the radiograph. The heart may be examined with ultrasound through the esophagus (transesophageal ultrasonography).

124 Thoracic viscera

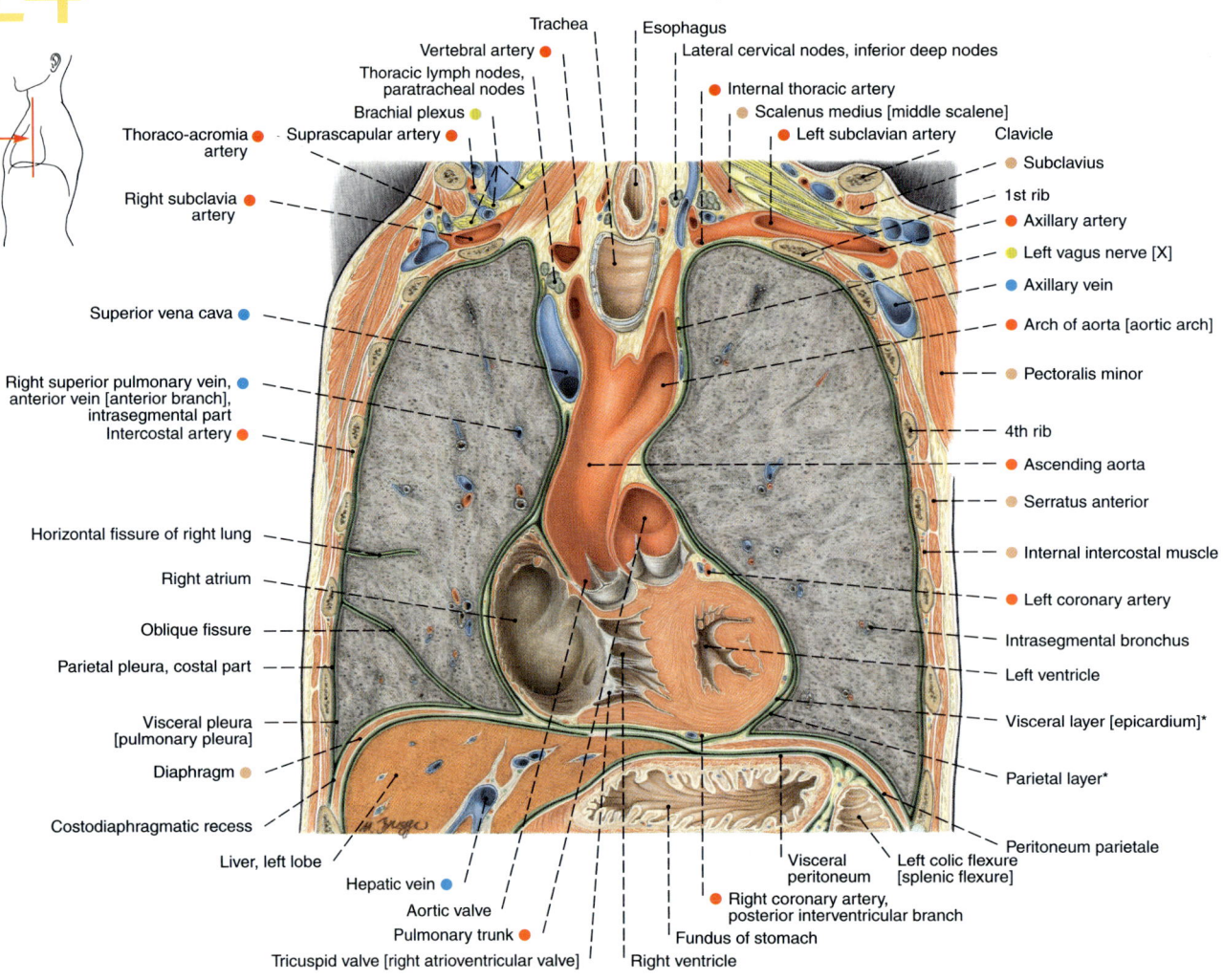

Fig. 923 Thoracic cavity; frontal section; ventral aspect.

* Serous pericardium.

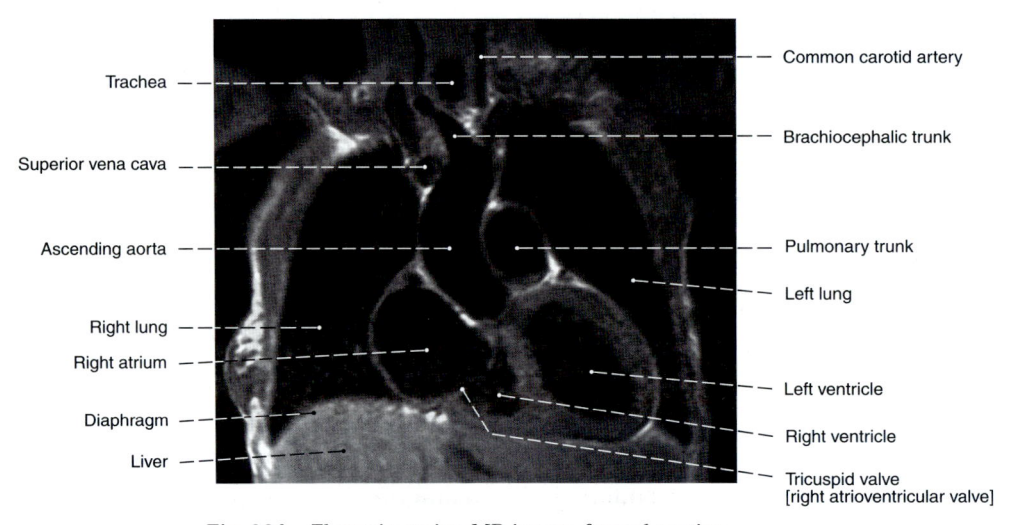

Fig. 924 Thoracic cavity; MR image; frontal section at level of superior vena cava; ventral aspect. Compare Fig. 913.

Frontal sections through thorax

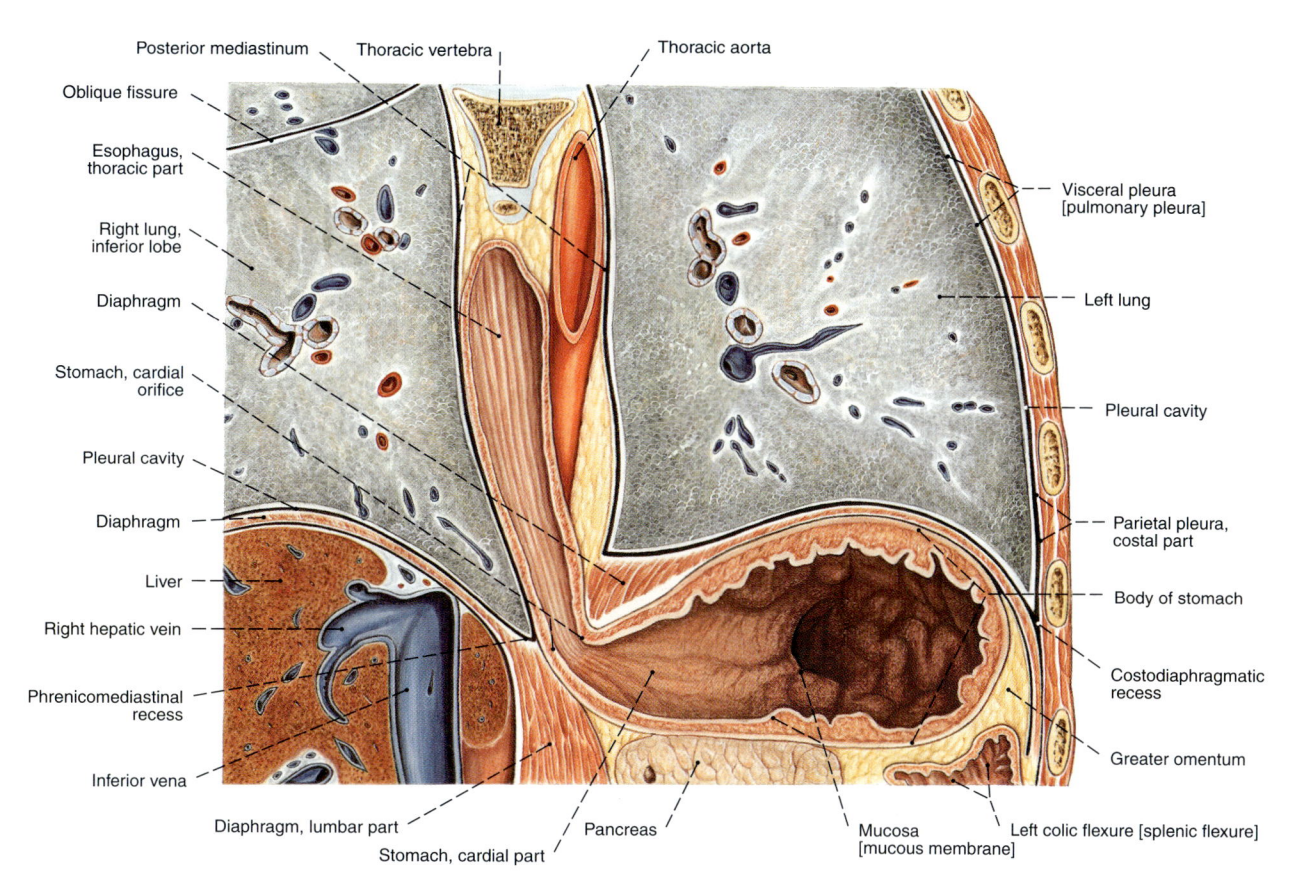

Fig. 925 Diaphragm; esophagus and junction to stomach; frontal section through lower part of thoracic and upper part of abdominal cavities; ventral aspect.

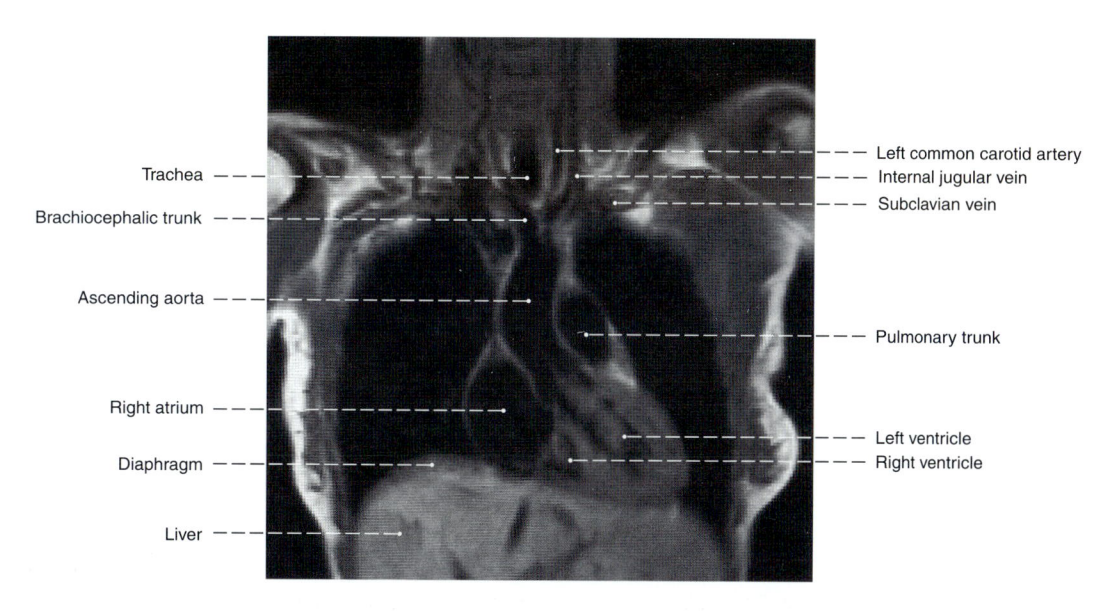

Fig. 926 Thoracic cavity; MR image; frontal section at level of aortic valve; ventral aspect. Compare Figs. 913 and 923.

Thoracic viscera

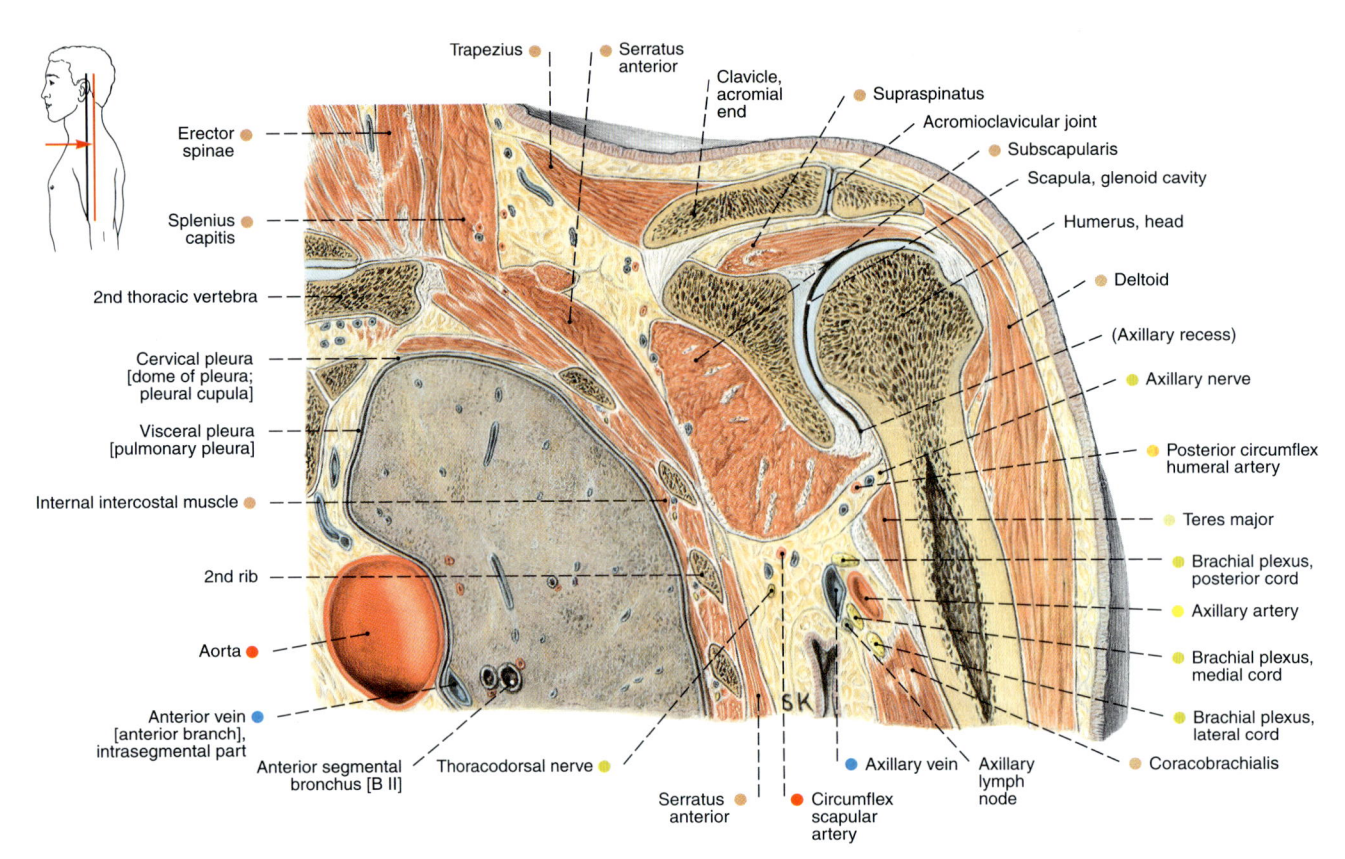

Fig. 927 Neck; axillary fossa; thoracic cavity; frontal section of left side; ventral aspect.

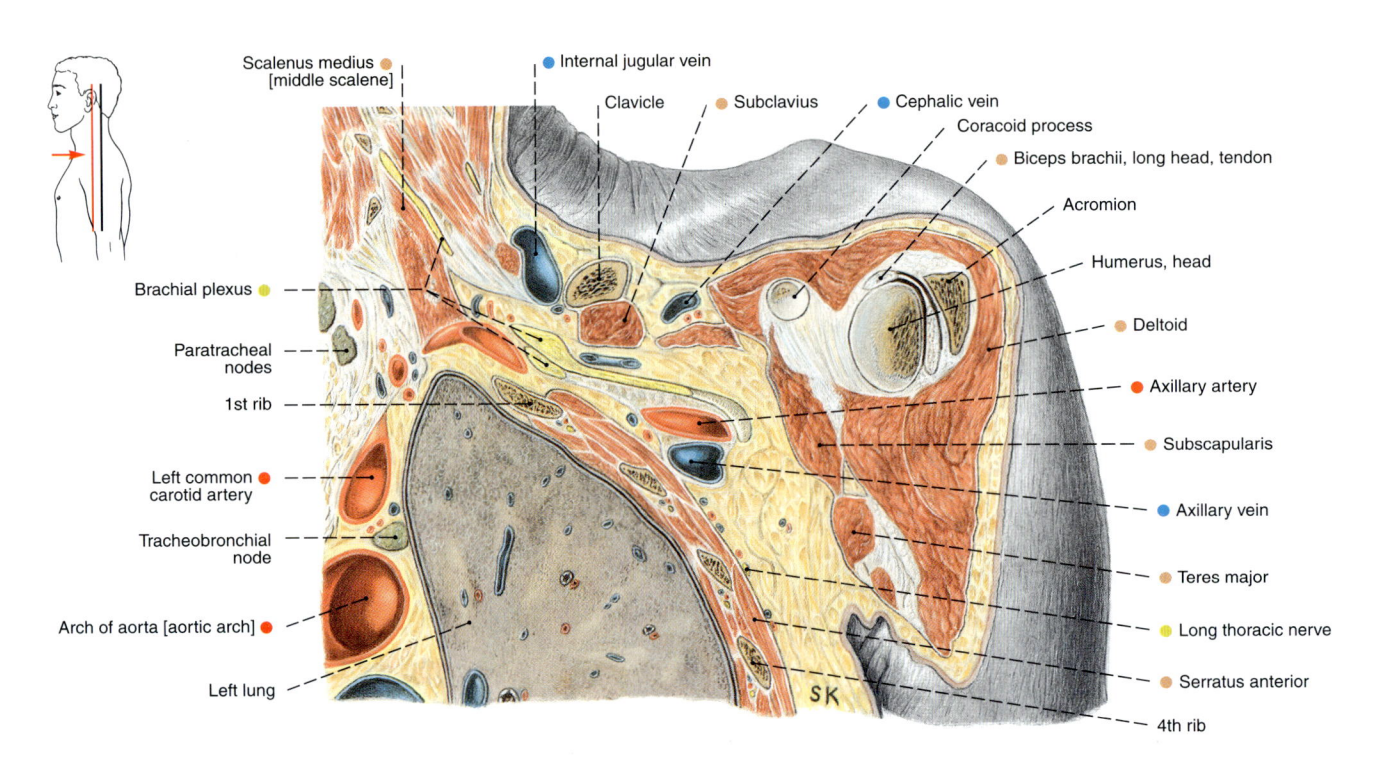

Fig. 928 Neck; axillary fossa; thoracic cavity; frontal section of left side; ventral aspect.

Horizontal section through thorax **127**

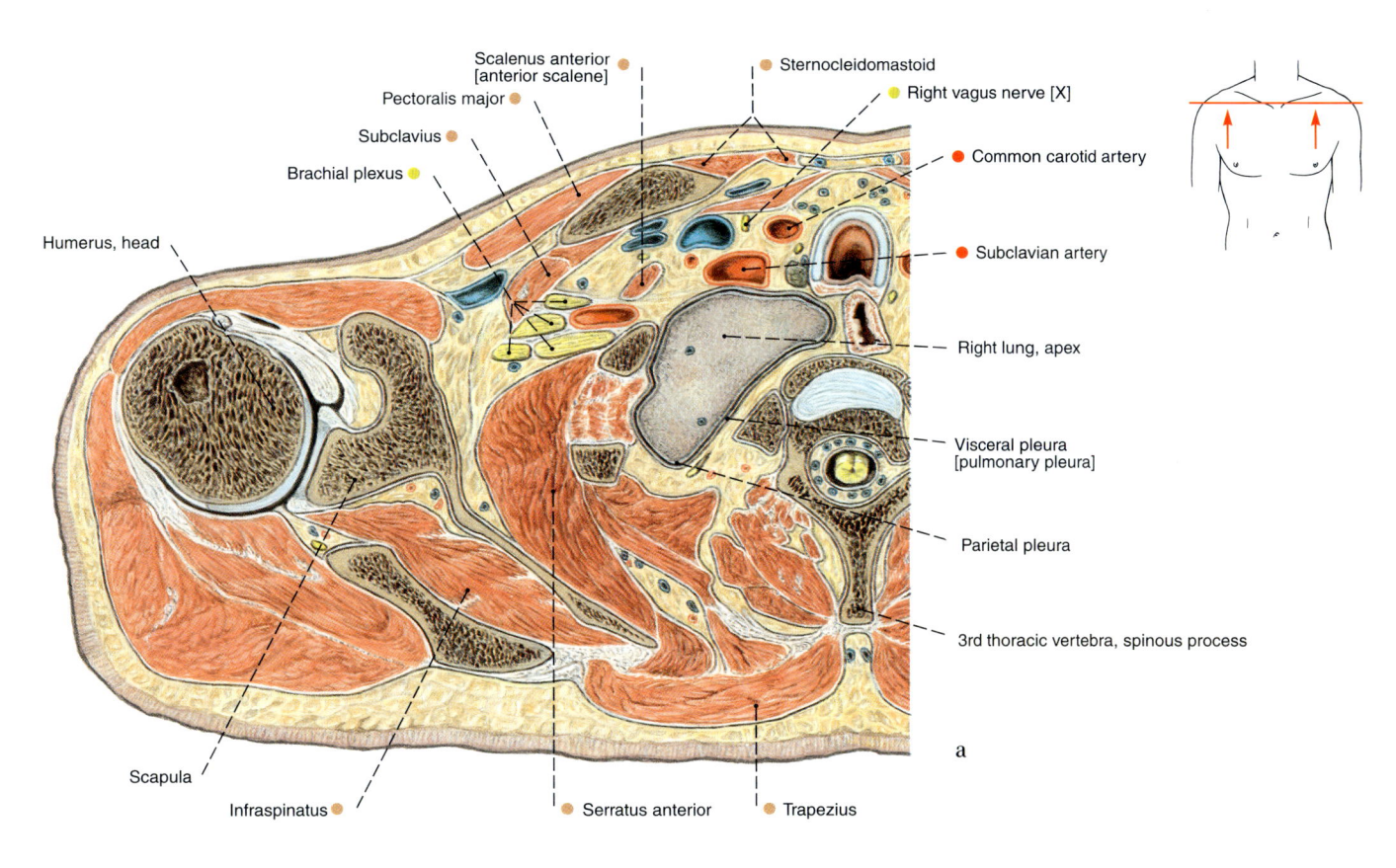

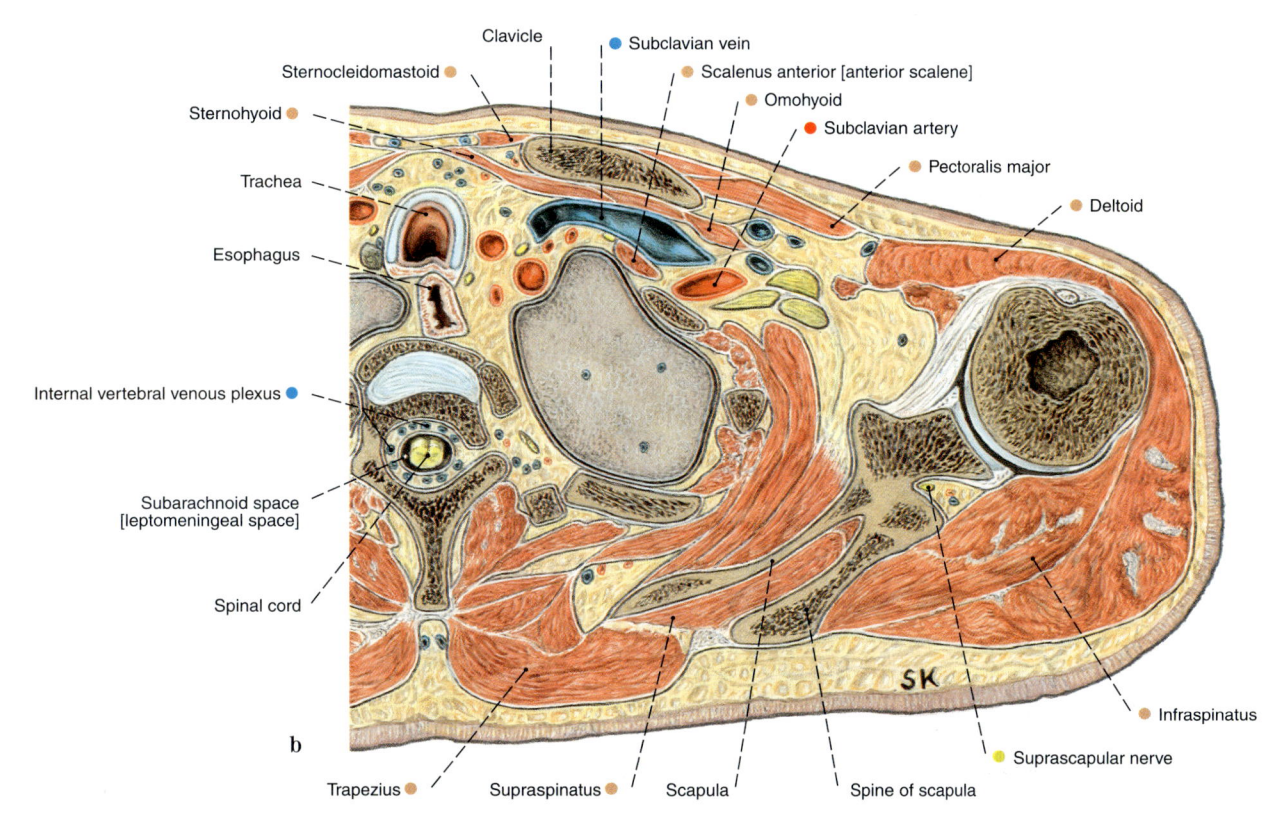

Fig. 929 a, b Thoracic cavity; horizontal section to expose cervical pleura [dome of pleura; pleural cupula] and apices of lungs; caudal aspect.

a Right side of body
b Left side of body

128 Thoracic viscera

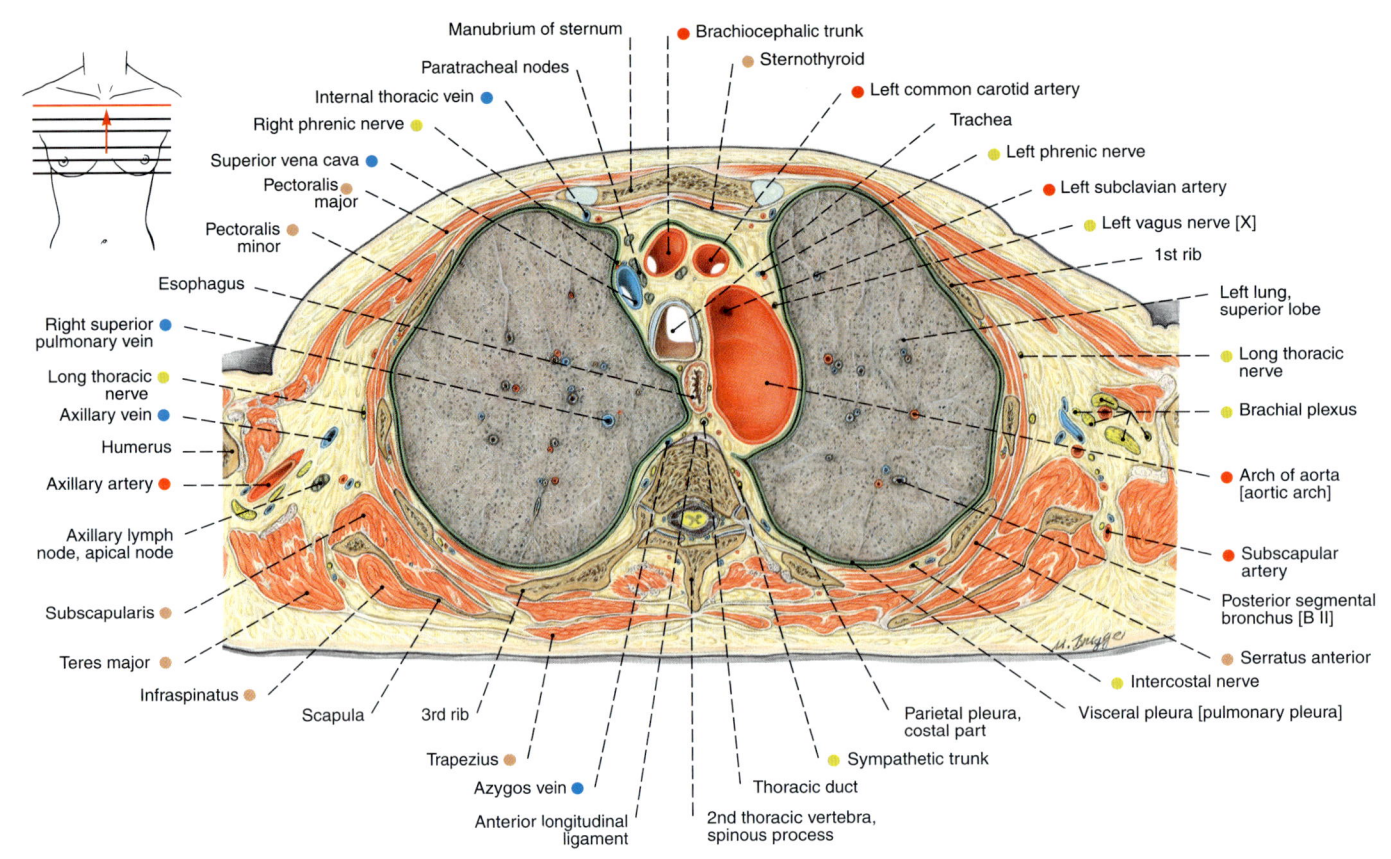

Fig. 930 Thoracic cavity; horizontal section at level of arch of aorta [aortic arch]; caudal aspect.

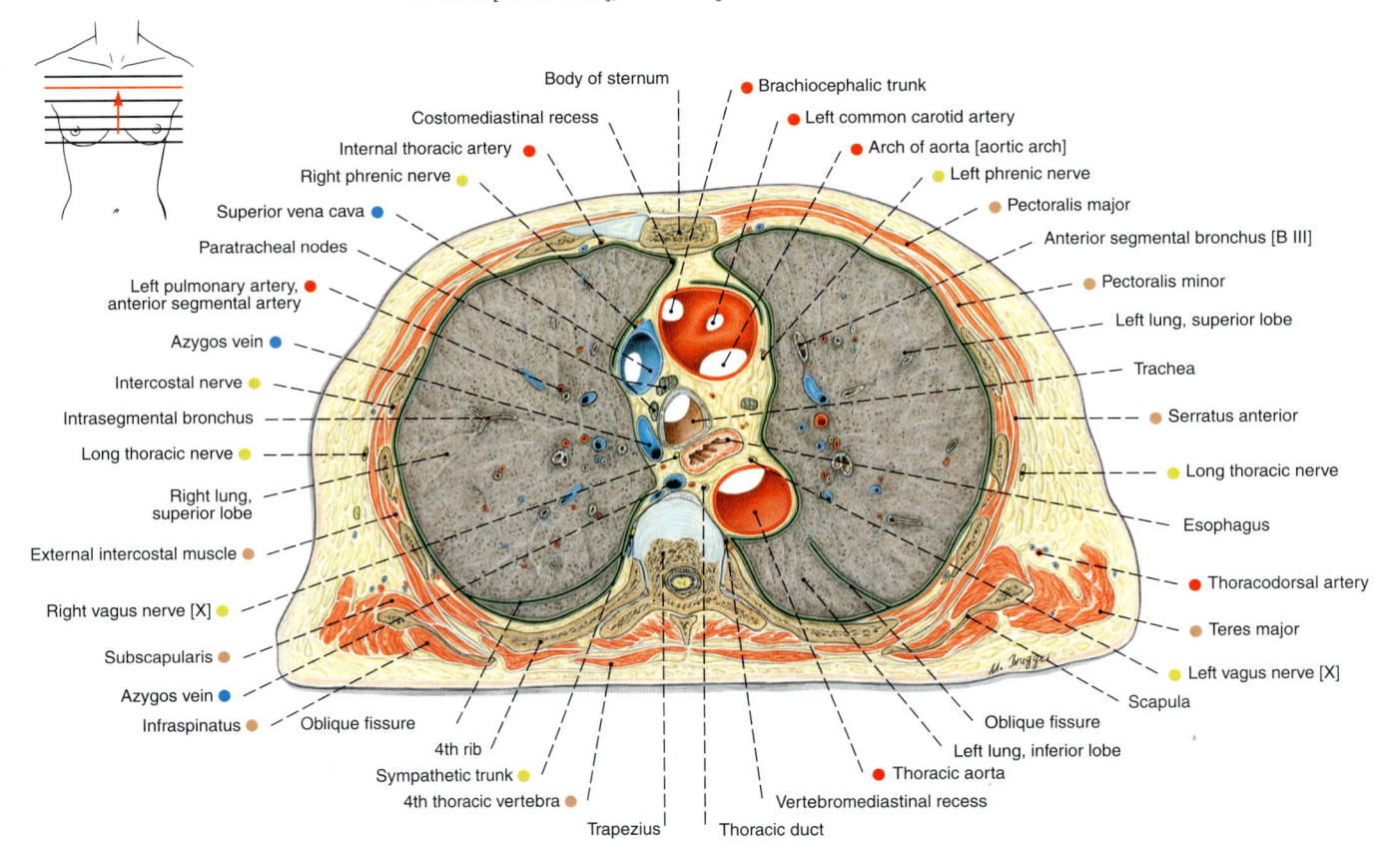

Fig. 931 Thoracic cavity; horizontal section at level of 4th thoracic vertebra; caudal aspect.

Horizontal sections through thorax

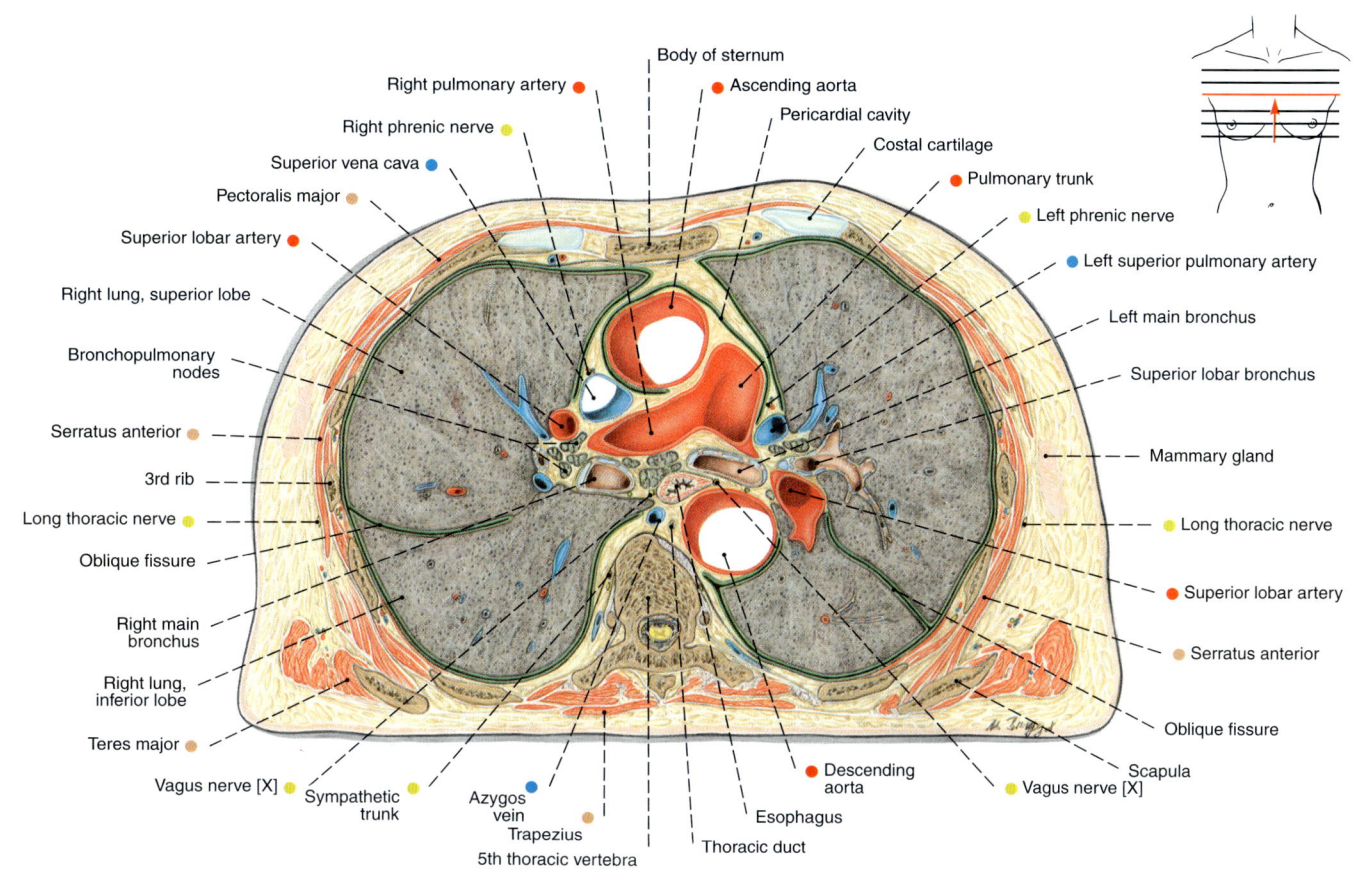

Fig. 932 Thoracic cavity; horizontal section at level of bifurcation of pulmonary trunk; caudal aspect.

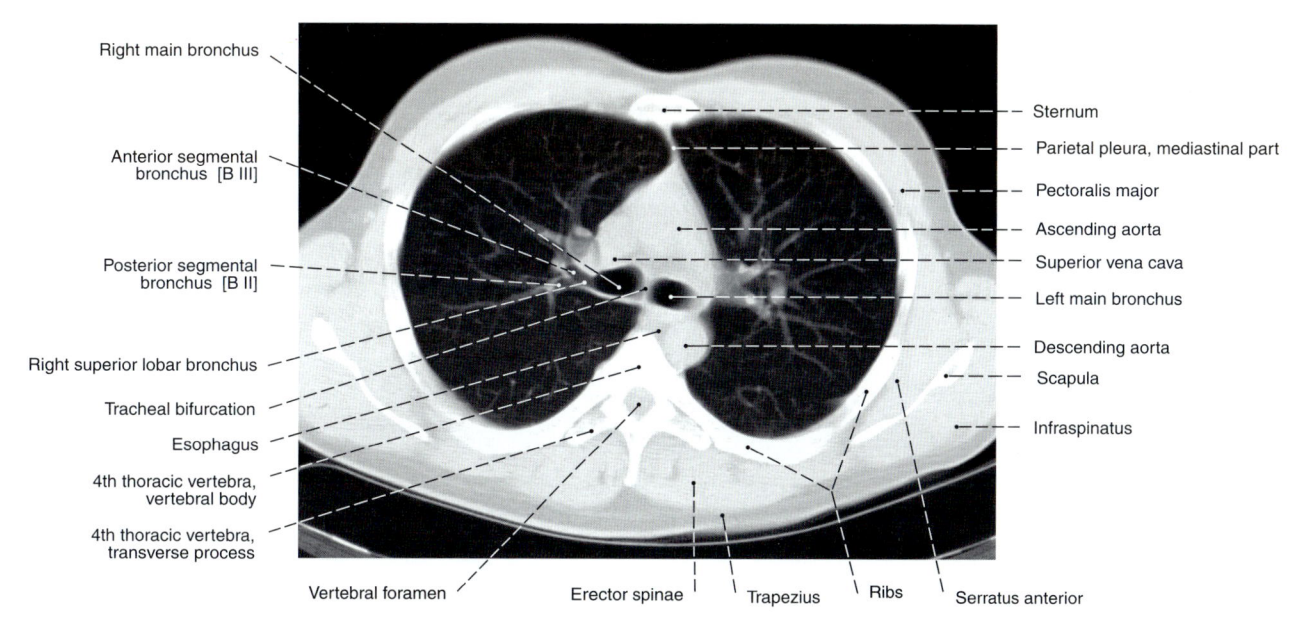

Fig. 933 Thoracic cavity; computer tomographic horizontal section at level of tracheal bifurcation; caudal aspect. Depending on electronic processing, either the lung or the skeletal system can be visualized.

130 Thoracic viscera

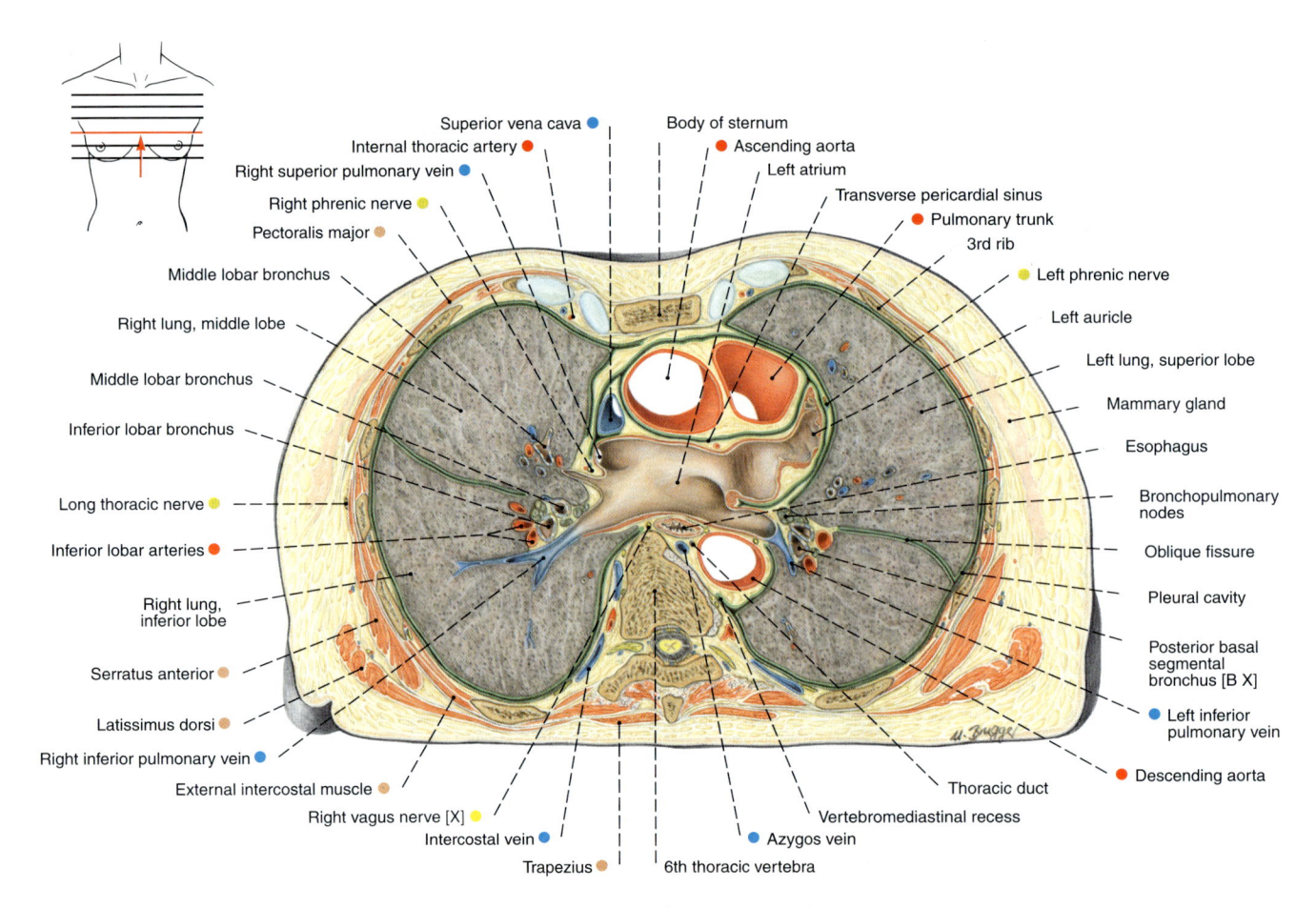

Fig. 934 Thoracic cavity; horizontal section at level of left atrium; caudal aspect.

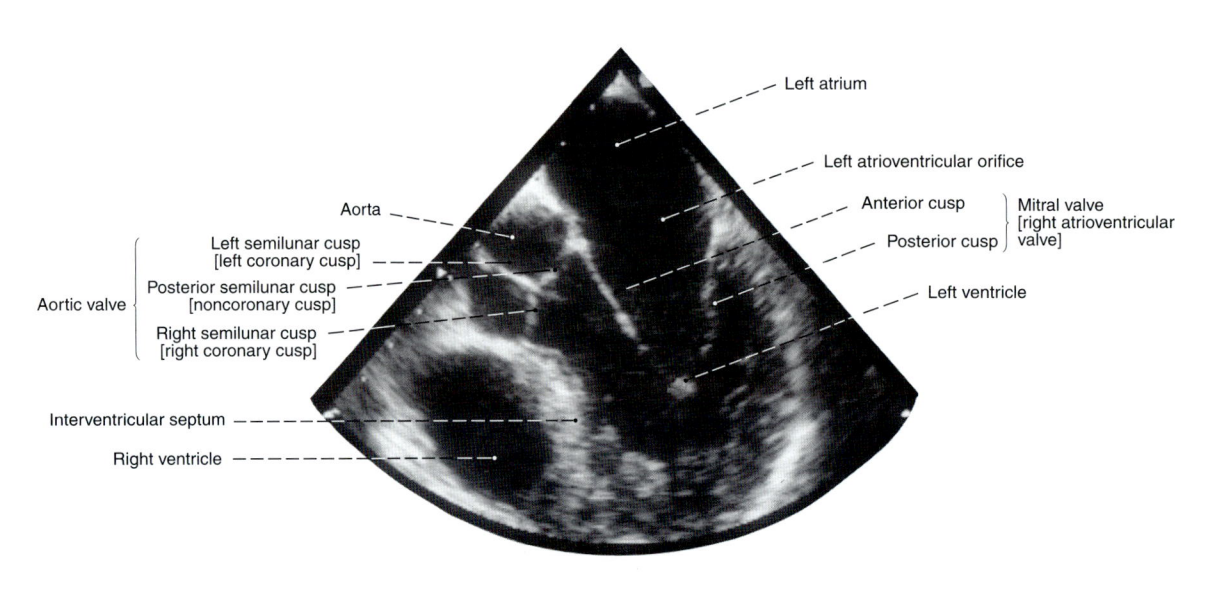

Fig. 935 Thoracic cavity; ultrasound image; transducer in the esophagus via endoscope to visualize the left heart and its valves; transducer at top of triangle; superior left aspect.

Horizontal sections through thorax

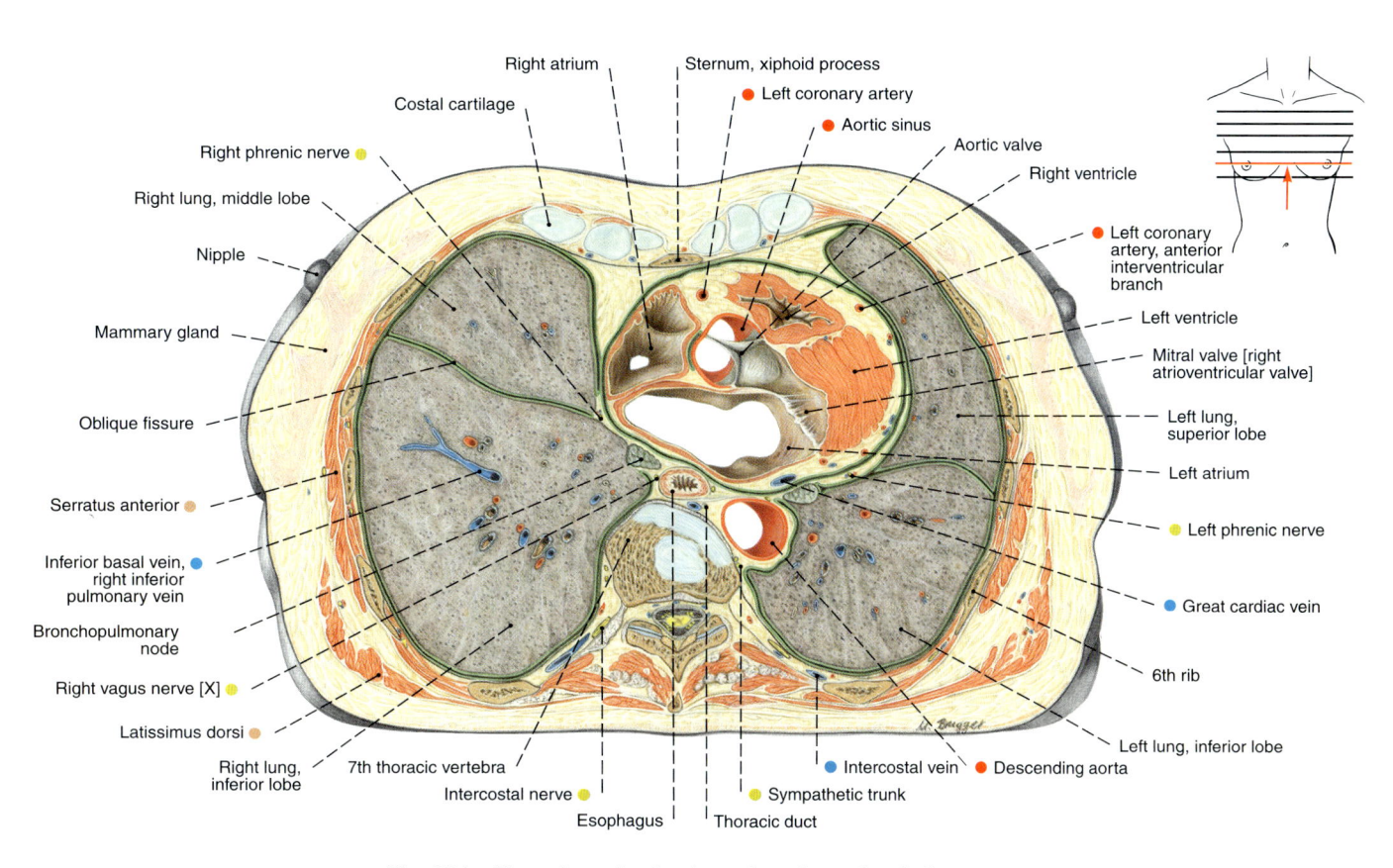

Fig. 936 Thoracic cavity; horizontal section at level of 7th thoracic vertebra; caudal aspect.

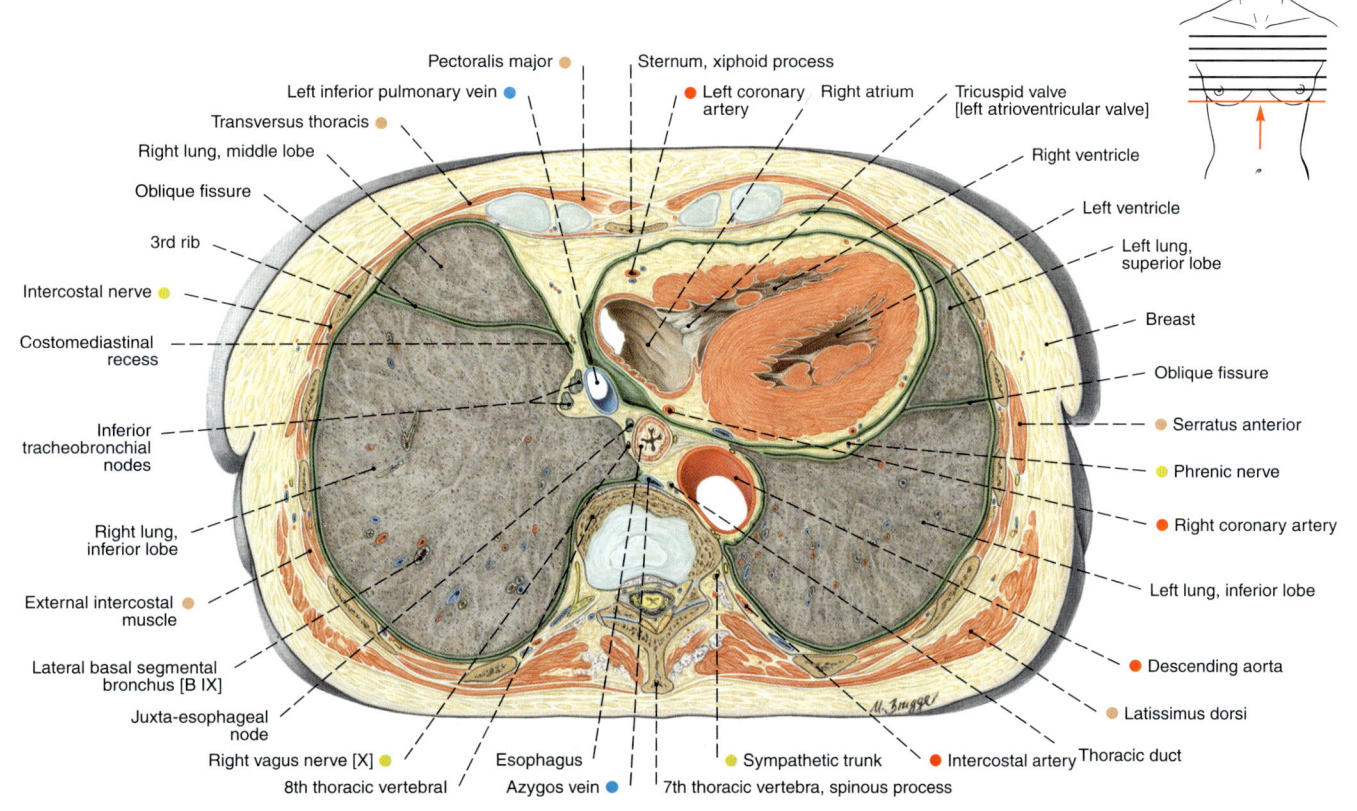

Fig. 937 Thoracic cavity; horizontal section at level of 8th thoracic vertebra; caudal aspect.

Abdominal viscera

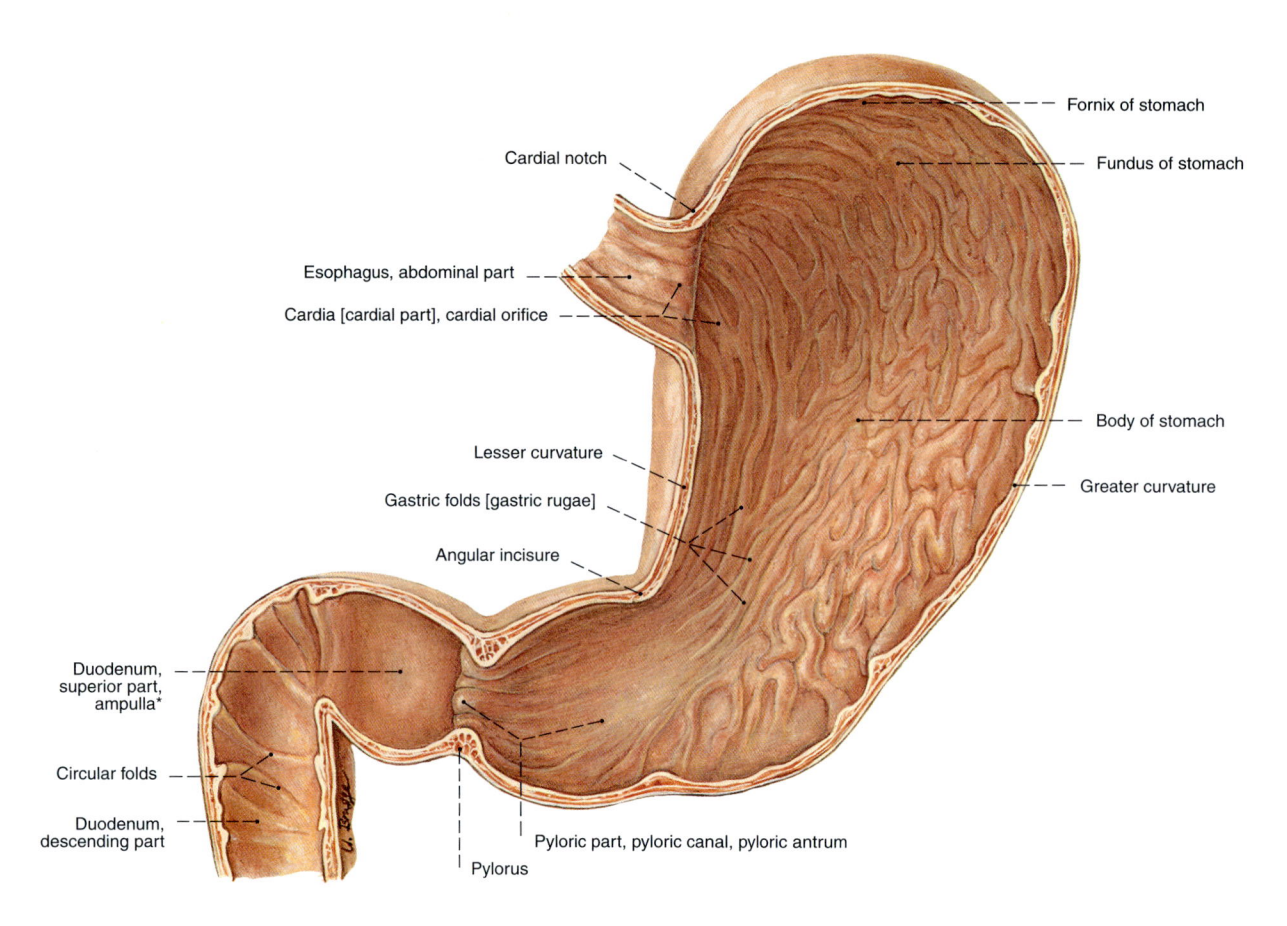

Fig. 938 Stomach; duodenum; anterior wall removed to expose folds of gastric and intestinal mucosa [mucous membrane]; ventral aspect.
The circular muscular layer is especially pronounced at the pylorus.
*Clinically: duodenal cap [duodenal bulb].

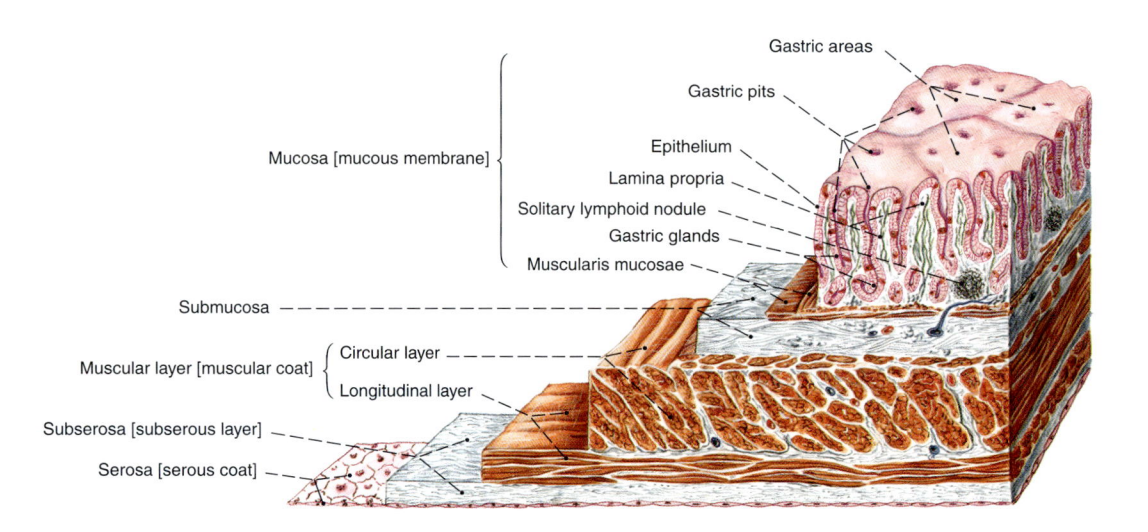

Fig. 939 Diagram of staggered wall of stomach; low power magnification.

Stomach 133

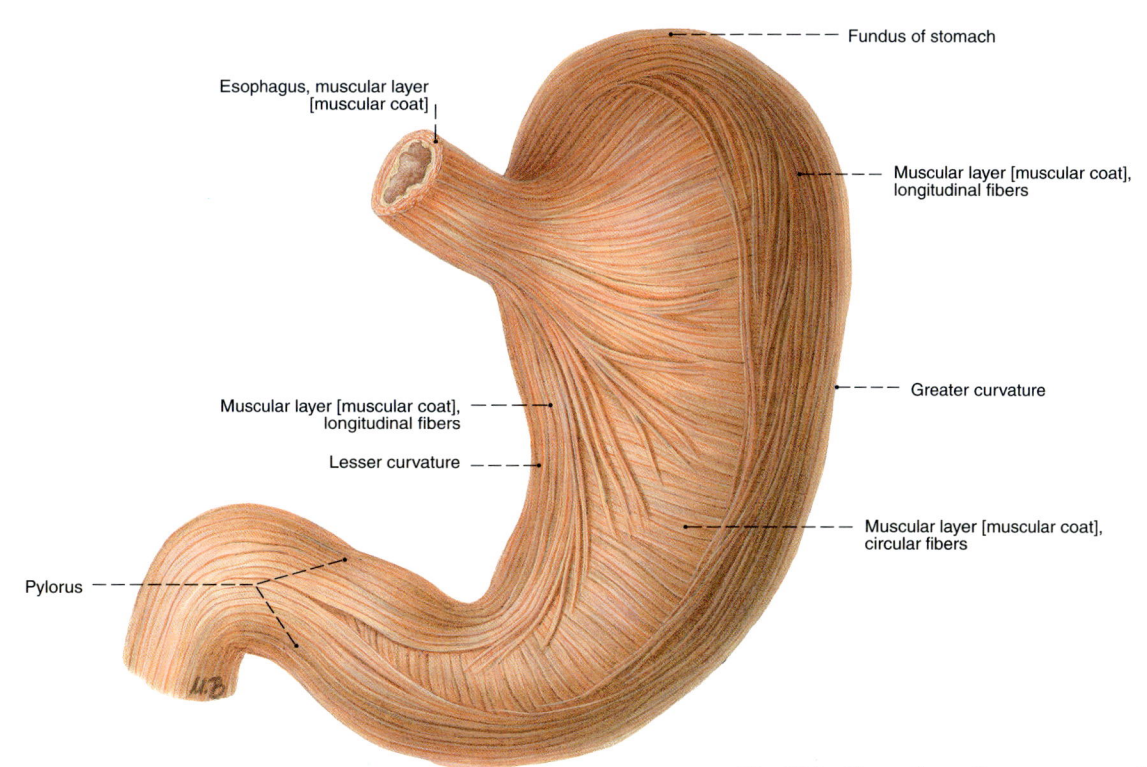

Fig. 940 Stomach; peritoneum removed to expose external muscular layers of anterior wall of stomach; ventral aspect.

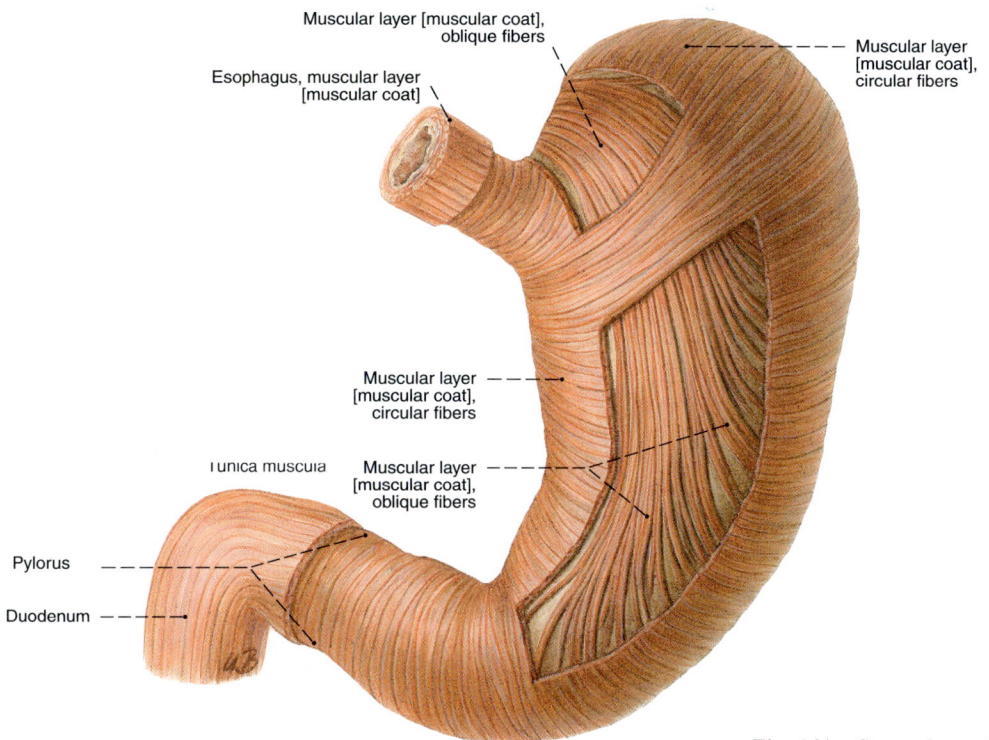

Fig. 941 Stomach; peritoneum removed; external muscular layer partially resected to expose oblique fibers internally; ventral aspect.

134 Abdominal viscera

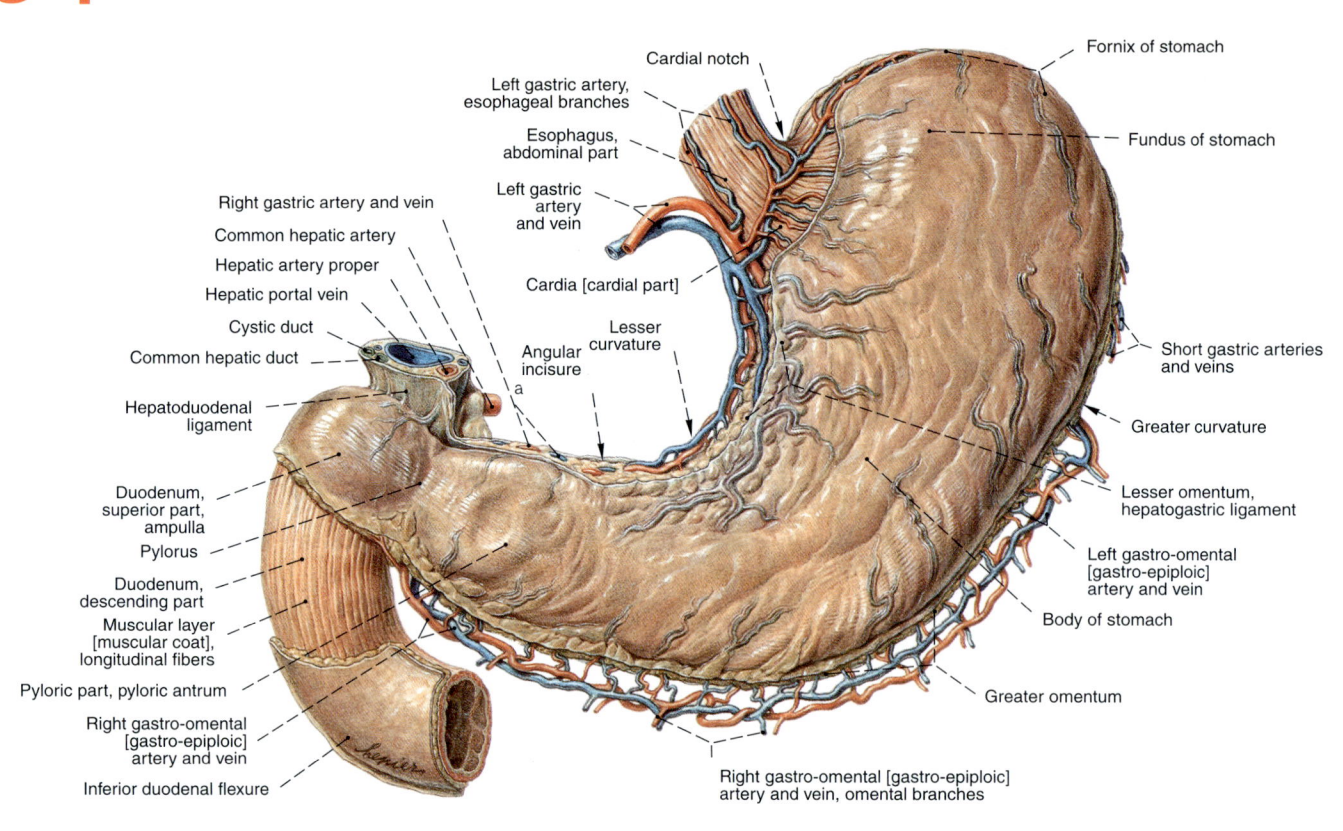

Fig. 942 Stomach; duodenum; peritoneum partially removed; ventral aspect.

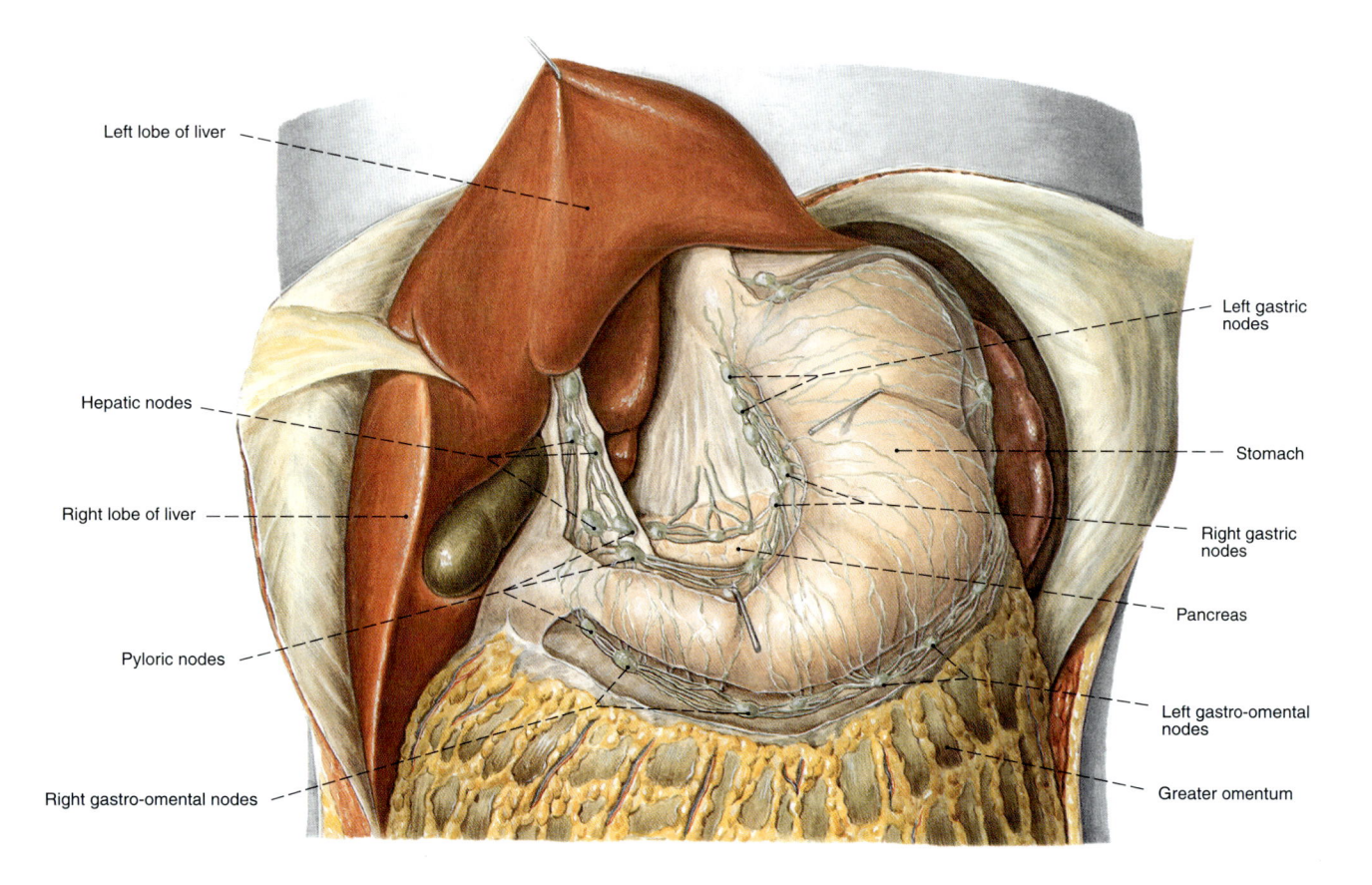

Fig. 943 Stomach and liver, with lymph nodes; left lobe of liver retracted superiorly; peritoneum removed from the lesser and the greater curvatures to expose the lymph nodes; ventral aspect.
Number and size of gastric lymph nodes vary considerable.

Stomach 135

1 = Esophagus with contrast medium. In the passage (1a) to the fundus of the stomach the grooves between the folds are visible as dark stripes.
2 = Fundus of stomach with air bubble
3 = Body of stomach
3a = Lesser curvature
3b = Greater curvature.
At the boundary between 3a and 3b notches according to the relief of the mucosa are visible.
4 = Peristaltic contraction at angular incisure
5 = Pyloric part just before progression of a portion of the contents of the stomach.
6 = Duodenum, superior part, ampulla
7 = Duodenum, descending part with circular folds
8 = Jejunum
9 = Left dome of diaphragm
10 = Left colic flexure [splenic flexure] (with air)

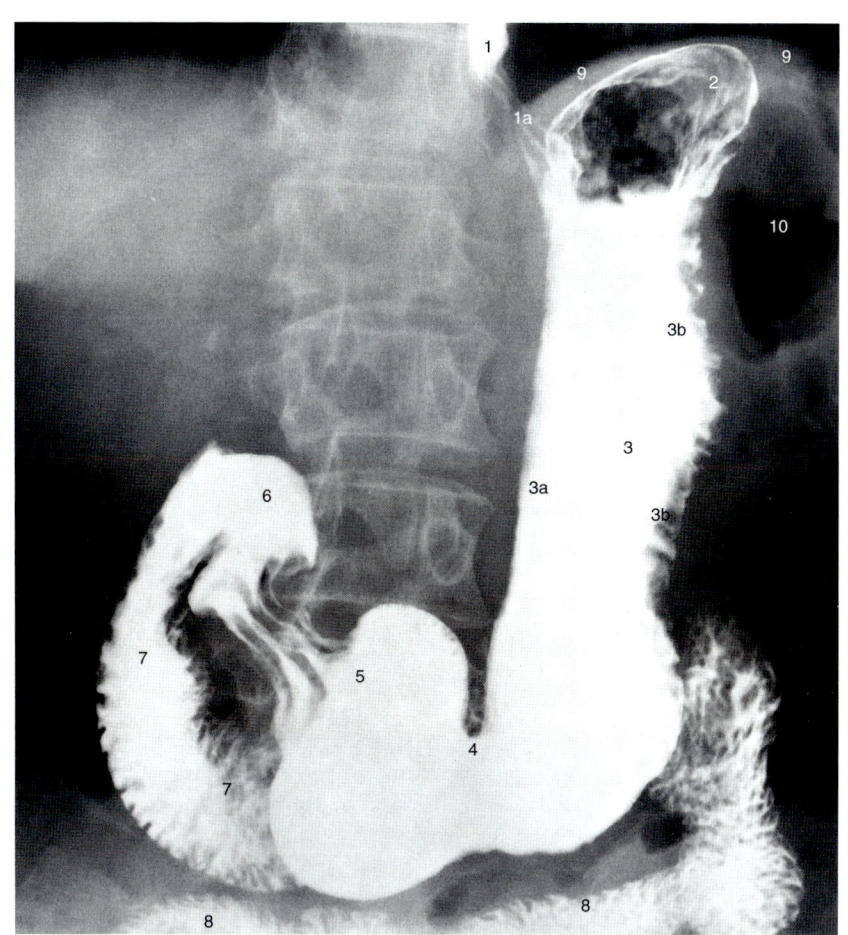

Fig. 944 Stomach; duodenum; AP radiograph after oral intake of contrast medium in upright position; ventral aspect.
In the radiograph of an upright patient an air bubble can be seen in the fundus of stomach, which is bordered by a fluid balance inferiorly.

The stripes in the junction between the esophagus and the stomach and in the pylorus are caused by longitudinal folds of the mucosa.

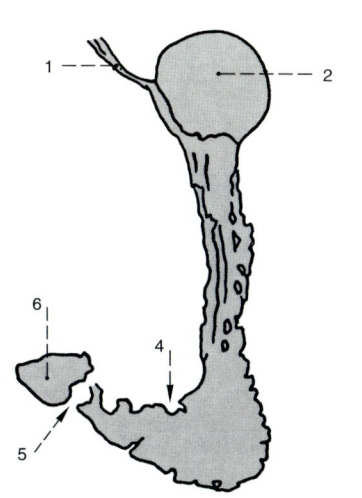

Fig. 945 Stomach; line drawing of relief of mucosa from an AP radiograph in an upright patient; ventral aspect. The pyloric part is constricted; the wall of the pyloric antrum is relaxed.

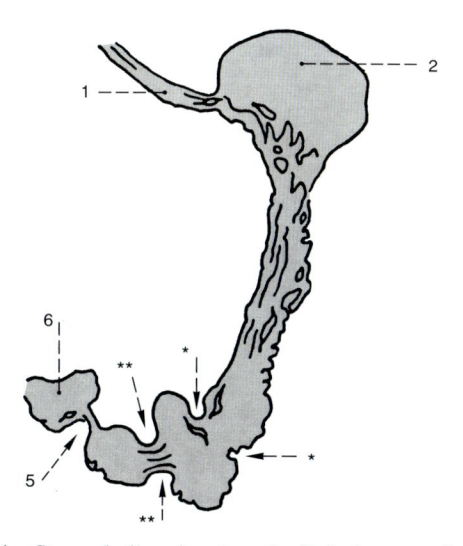

Fig. 946 Stomach; line drawing of relief of mucosa from an AP radiograph in an upright patient; ventral aspect. The two constrictions at the angular incisure (*) and in the area of the pyloric antrum (**) indicate a peristaltic wave.

Abdominal viscera

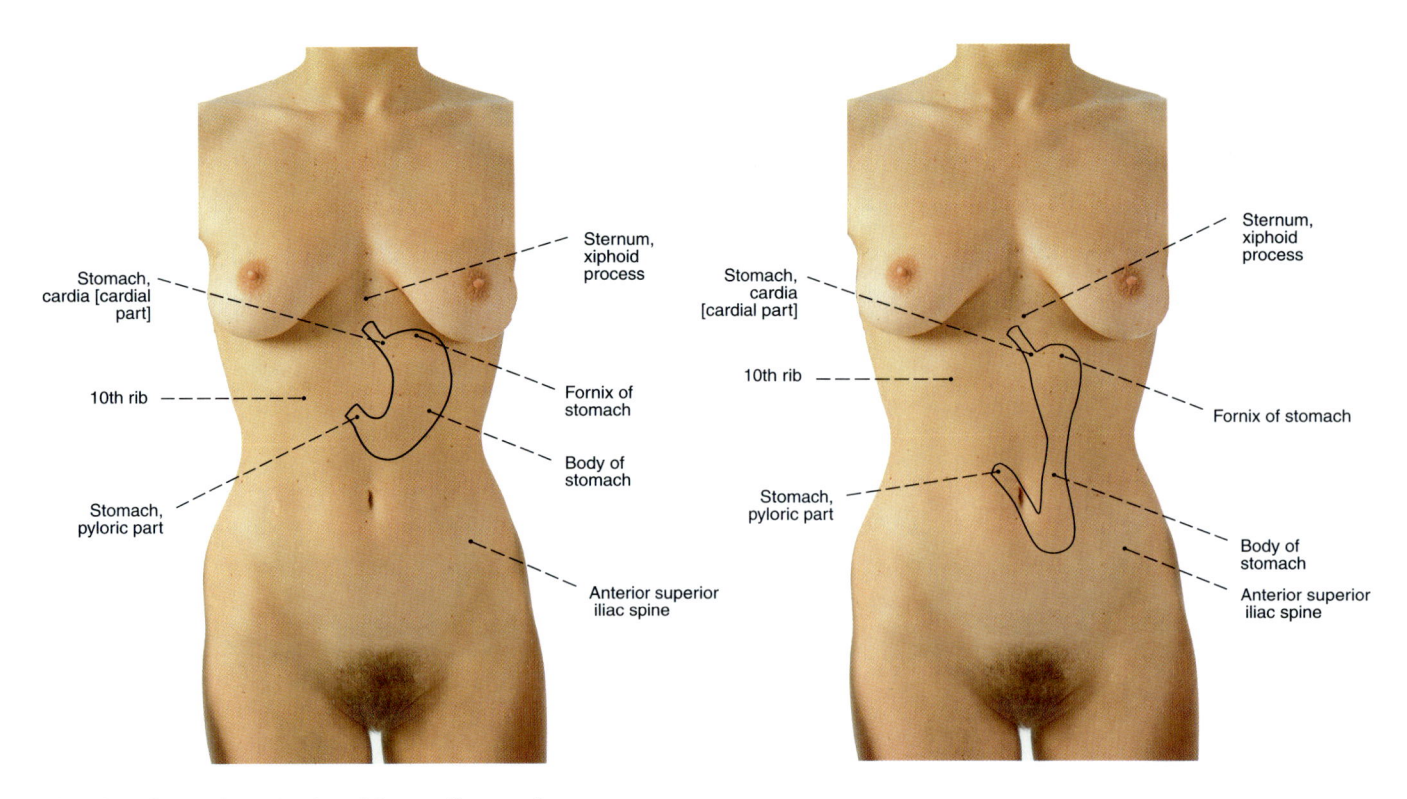

Fig. 947 Stomach; projection of "normal" stomach onto the anterior abdominal wall in the upright position.

Fig. 948 Stomach; projection of "long" stomach onto the anterior abdominal wall in the upright position. The stomach is fixed at its inlet and its outlet. Size and position of the other parts of the stomach largely depend on filling status and body position. Moreover, there are many variations among individuals.

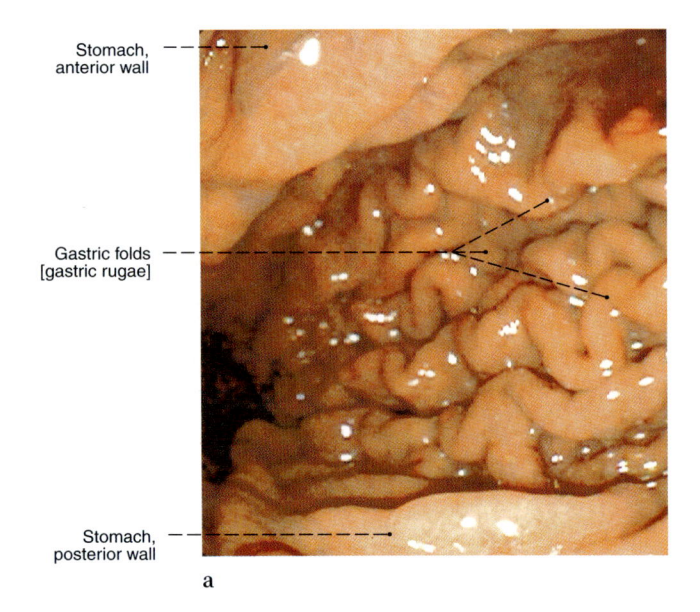

Fig. 949a, b Stomach; endoscopic view of stomach (gastroscopy); superior aspect.

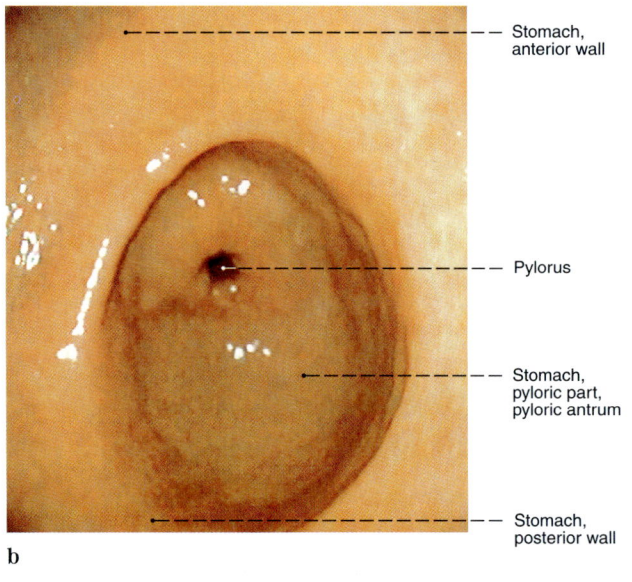

a Body of stomach with well-developed longitudinal folds of mucosa (gastric folds [gastric rugae]).
b Pyloric antrum with mainly smooth mucosa.

Small intestine

Fig. 950 Small intestine; cross-section through upper small intestine.

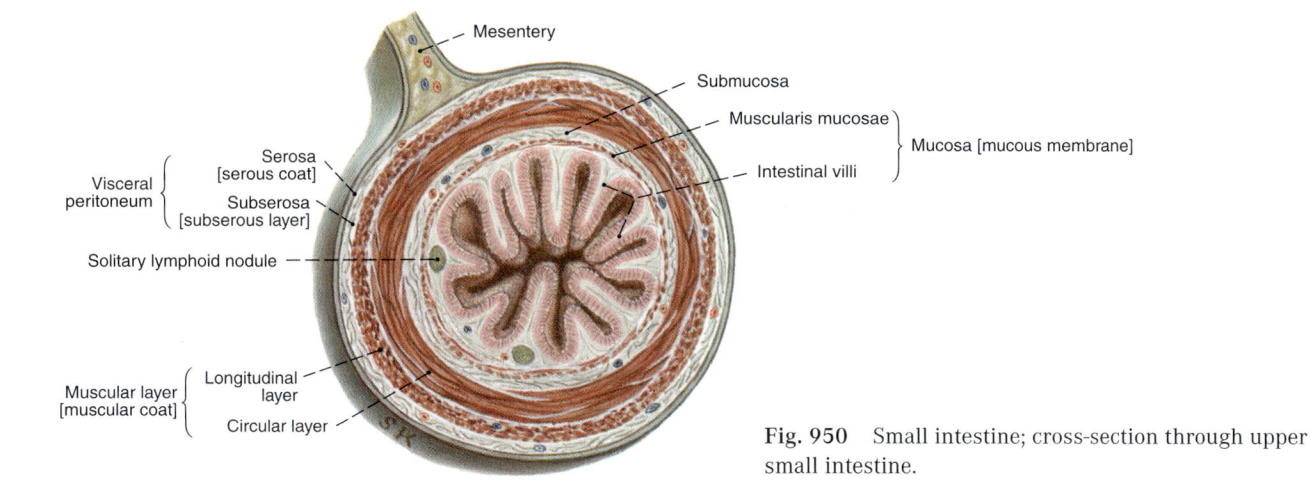

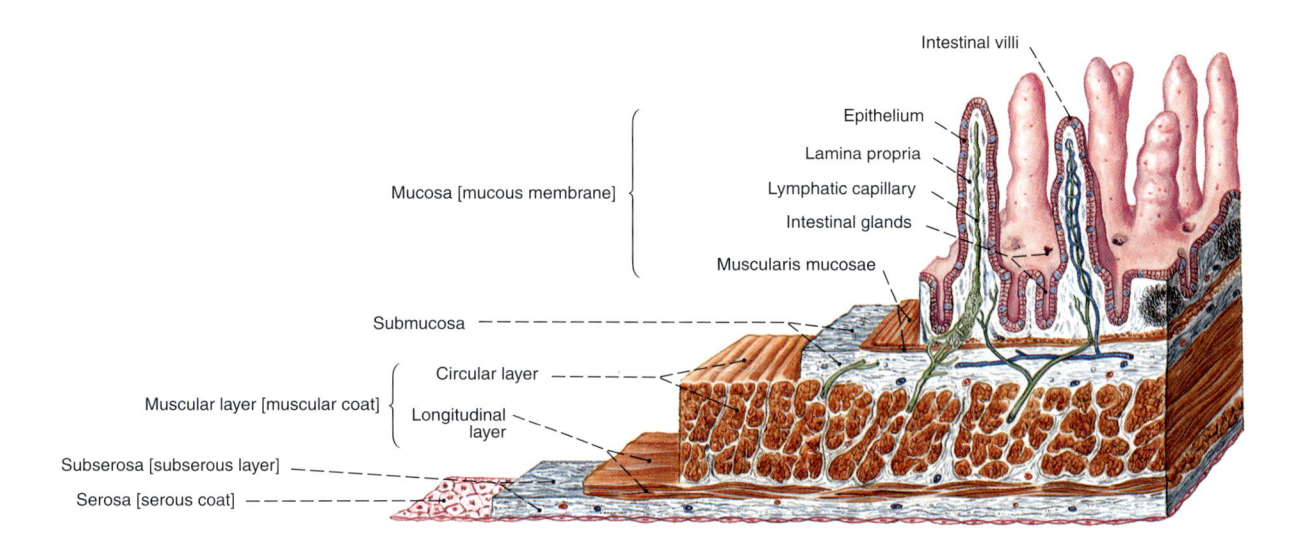

Fig. 951 Small intestine; staggered layers of wall; low-power magnification.

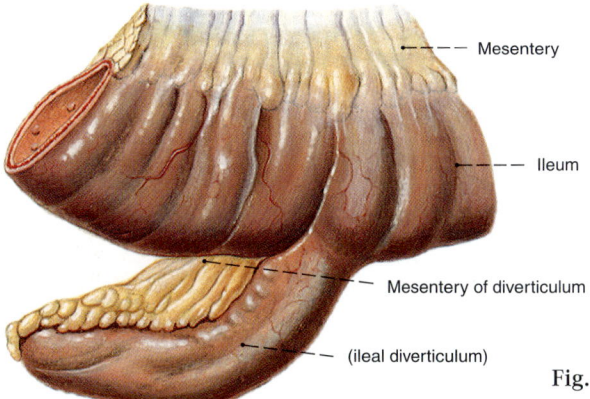

Fig. 952 MECKEL's diverticulum (ileal diverticulum). In 1-3% of people, such a diverticulum is present as a residuum of the vitelline duct (yolk stalk).

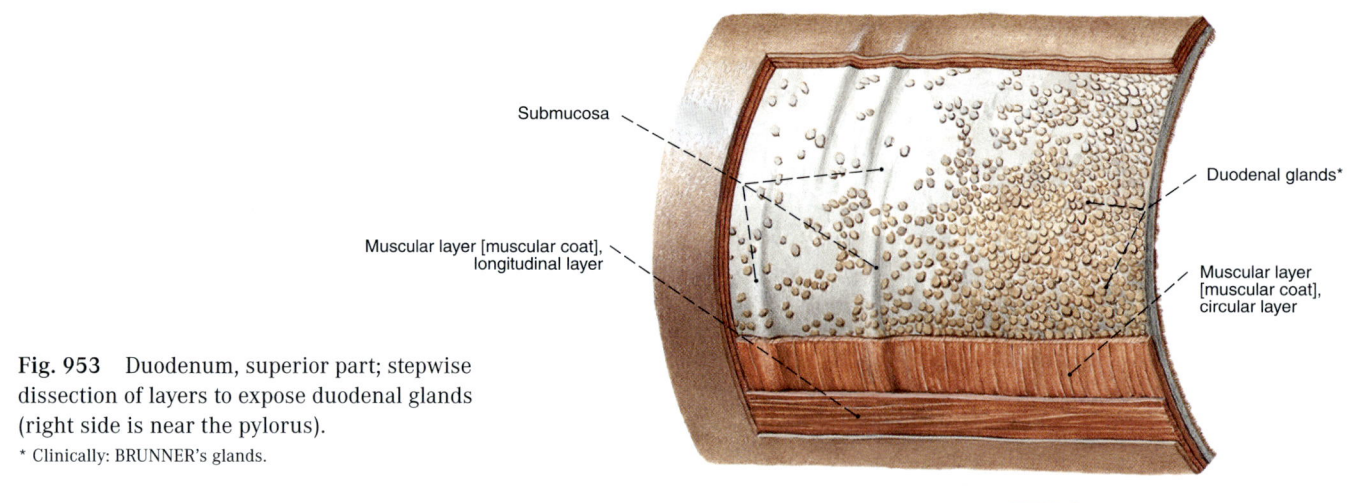

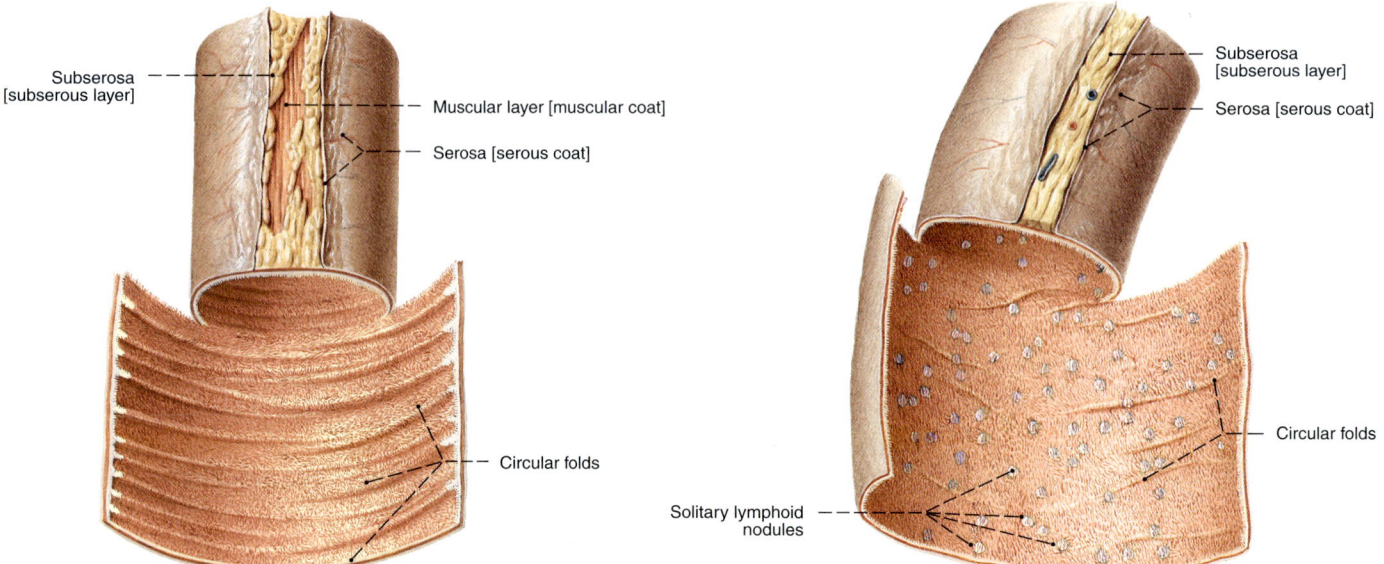

Fig. 953 Duodenum, superior part; stepwise dissection of layers to expose duodenal glands (right side is near the pylorus).
* Clinically: BRUNNER's glands.

Fig. 954 Upper small intestine: jejunum; wall partially opened along the attachment of the mesentery to expose the mucosa [mucous membrane]. Compare number of folds in Fig. 955.

Fig. 955 Lower small intestine: ileum; wall partially opened along the attachment of the mesentery to expose the mucosa [mucous membrane]. Compare with Fig. 954.

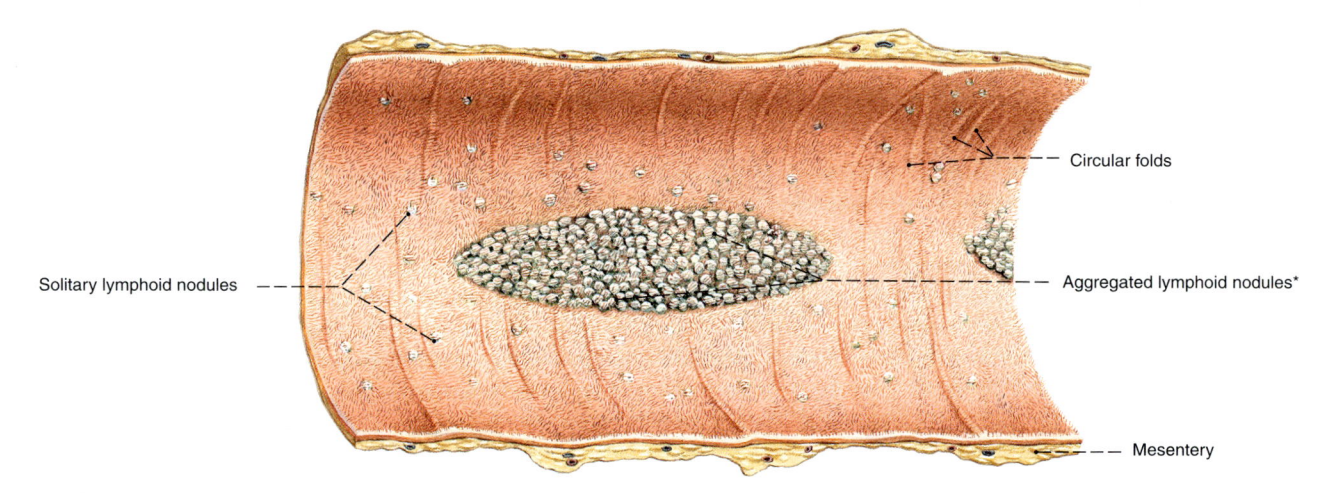

Fig. 956 Lowest small intestine: terminal ileum; wall opened along the attachment of the mesentery. PEYER'S patches are also found in the duodenum and the jejunum and are not characteristic of the ileum.
* Clinically: PEYER'S patches.

Duodenum

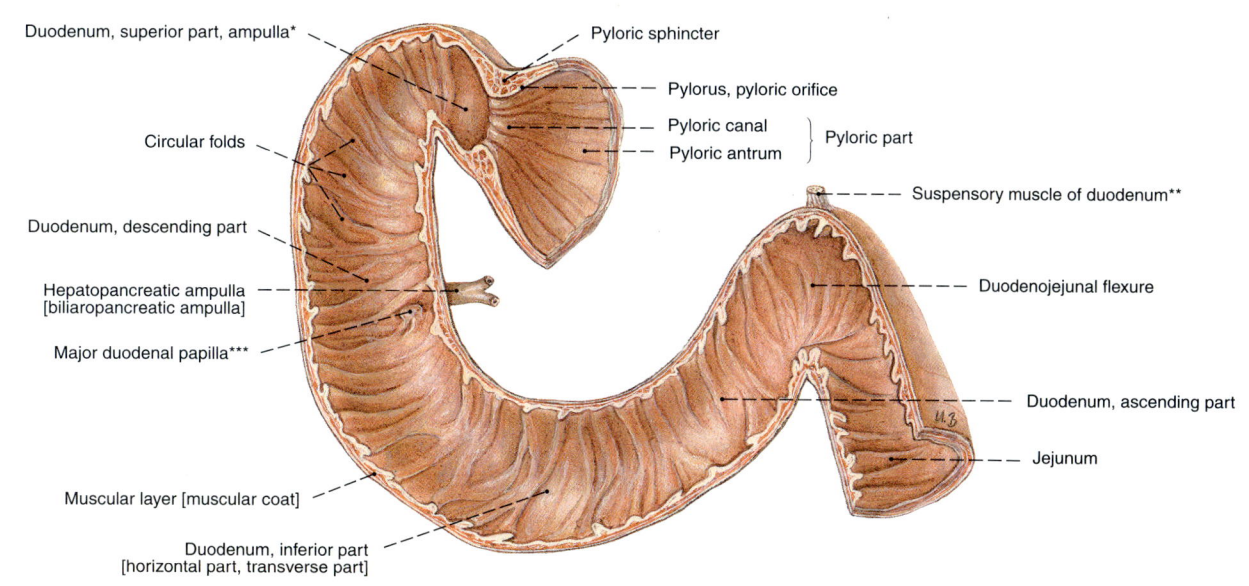

Fig. 957 Duodenum; anterior wall removed to expose the mucosa [mucous membrane]; ventral aspect.
The superior part courses from the stomach dorsocranially to the right; ND at the duodenojejunal flexure the duodenum swings ventrocaudally.

* Clinically: Duodenal cap [bulb].
** Clinically: muscle of TREITZ.
*** Clinically: tubercle of VATER.

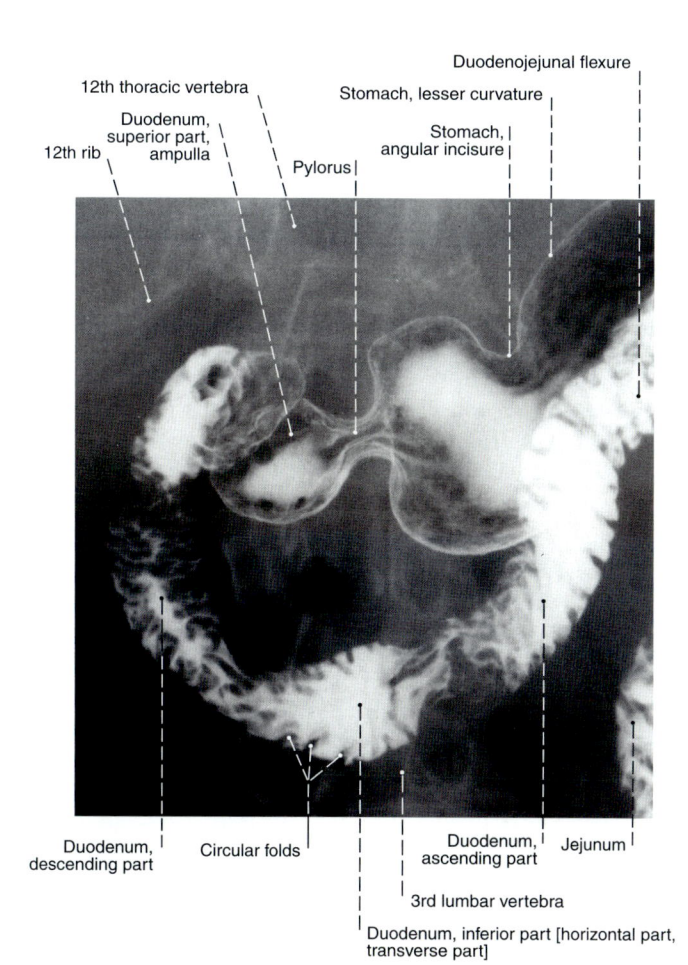

Fig. 958 Duodenum; AP radiograph after oral application of contrast medium; upright position; ventral aspect.

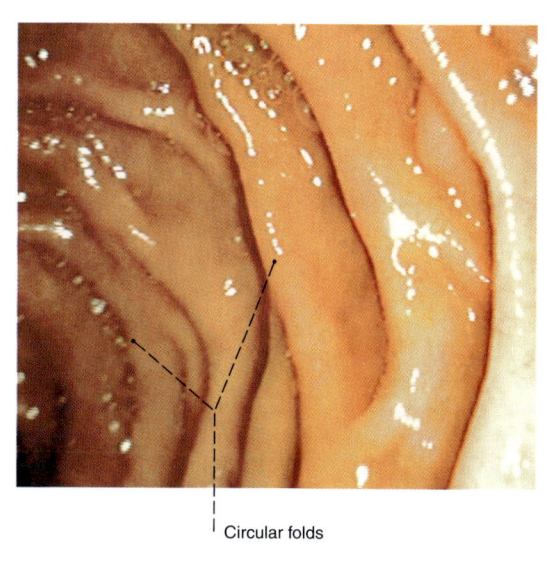

Fig. 959 Duodenum; endoscopic view of the mucosa [mucous membrane] with circular folds; superior aspect.

Abdominal viscera

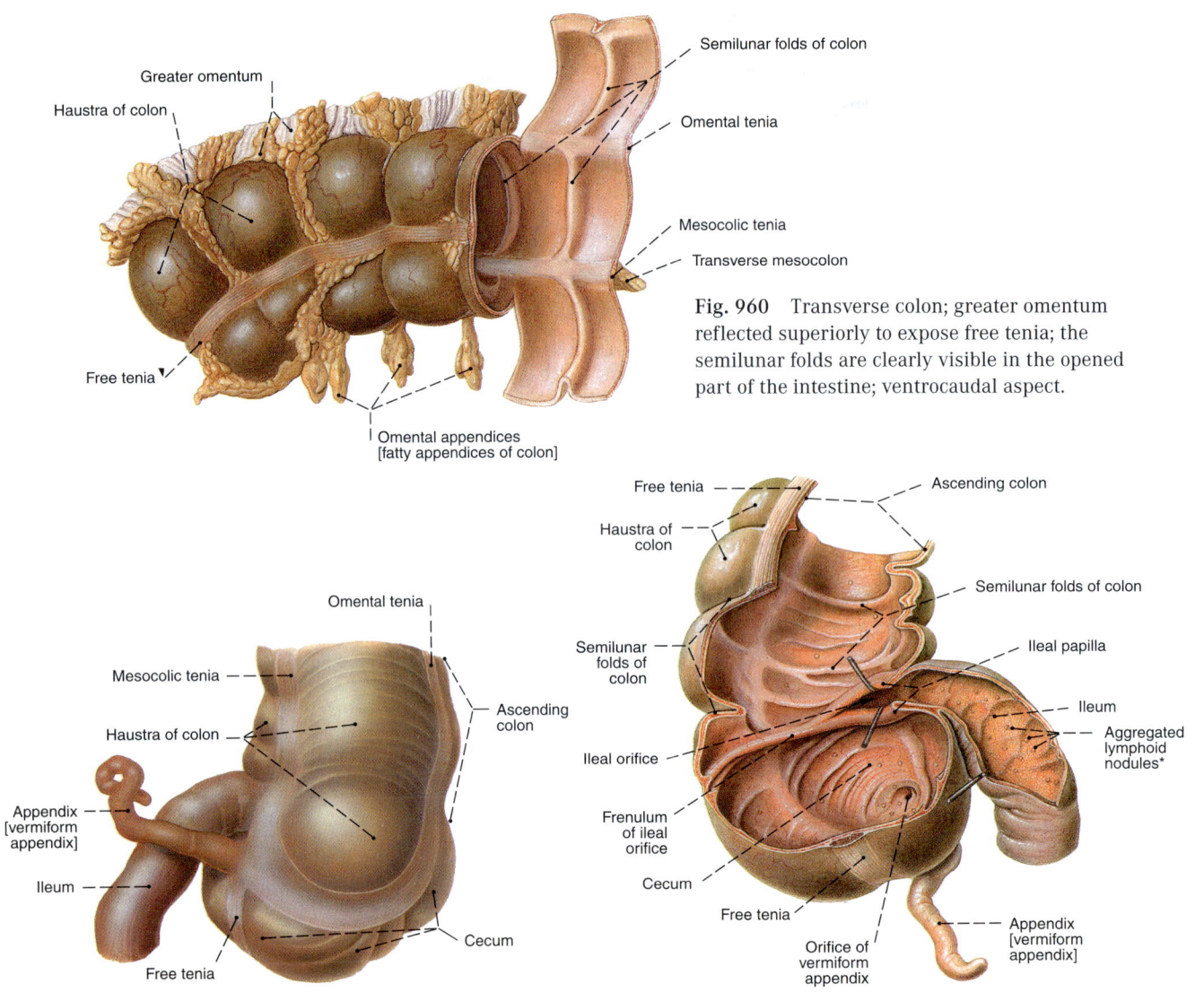

Fig. 960 Transverse colon; greater omentum reflected superiorly to expose free tenia; the semilunar folds are clearly visible in the opened part of the intestine; ventrocaudal aspect.

Fig. 961 Cecum; appendix [vermiform appendix]; terminal ileum; dorsal aspect.

Fig. 962 Ascending colon; cecum; appendix [vermiform appendix]; intestine opened by a frontal section to expose ileal orifice [orifice of ileal papilla; BAUHIN's valve]; orifice is held open with hooks; ventral aspect.
*PEYER's patches.

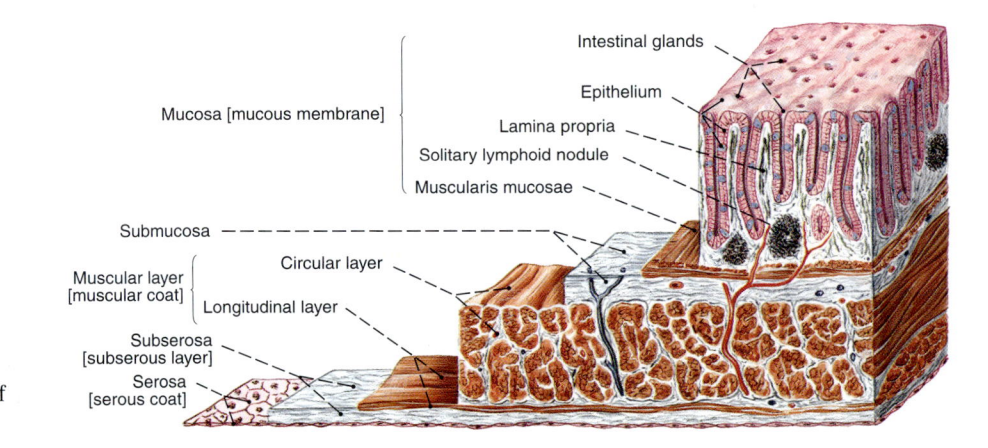

Fig. 963 Colon; staggered layers of wall; low-power magnification.

Colon

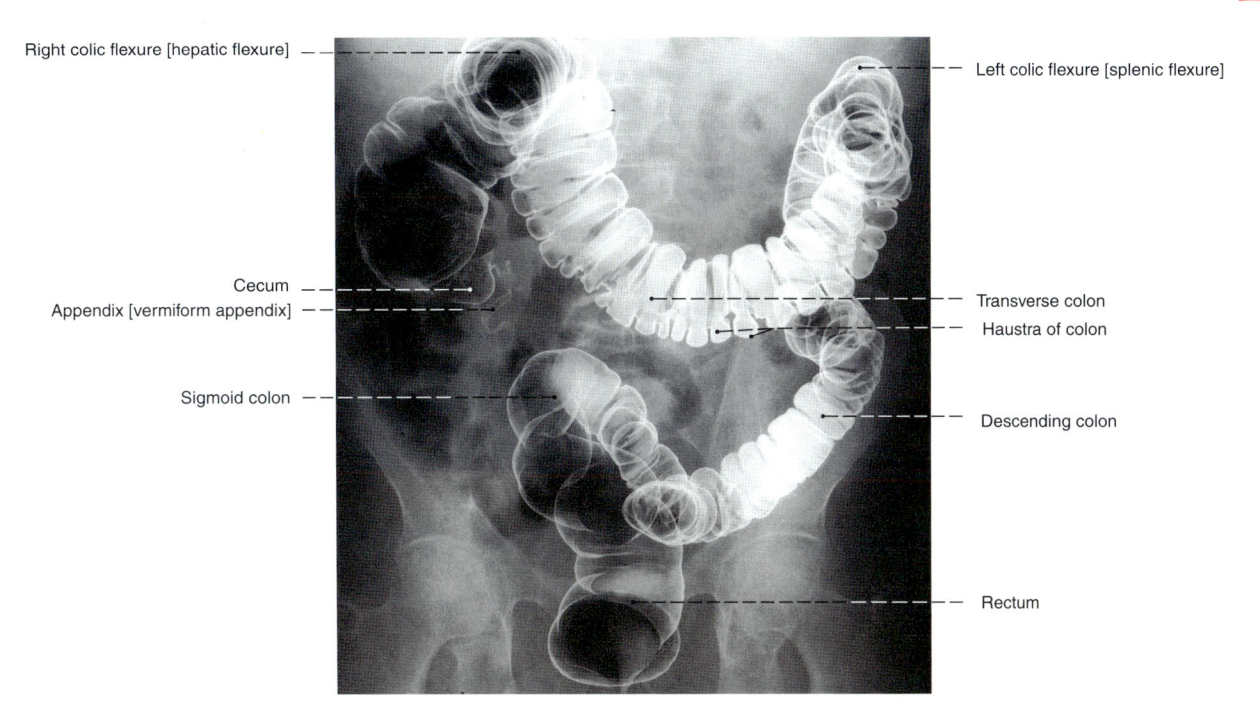

Fig. 964 Colon; rectum; AP radiograph after filling with contrast agent and air (double-contrast method). Compare the topography of colon in Figs. 1005 and 1008.

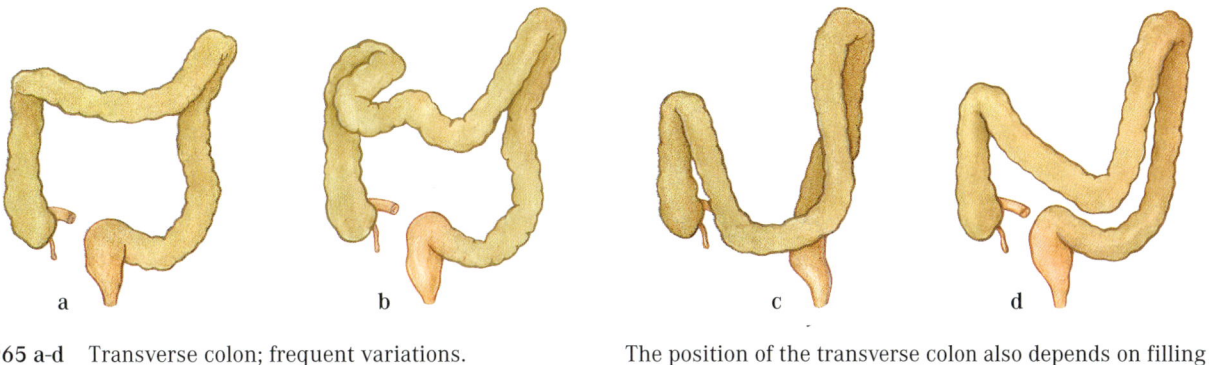

Fig. 965 a-d Transverse colon; frequent variations.
a normal position; **b** twisted; **c** U-shaped; **d** V-shaped. The position of the transverse colon also depends on filling status and on body position; ventral aspect.

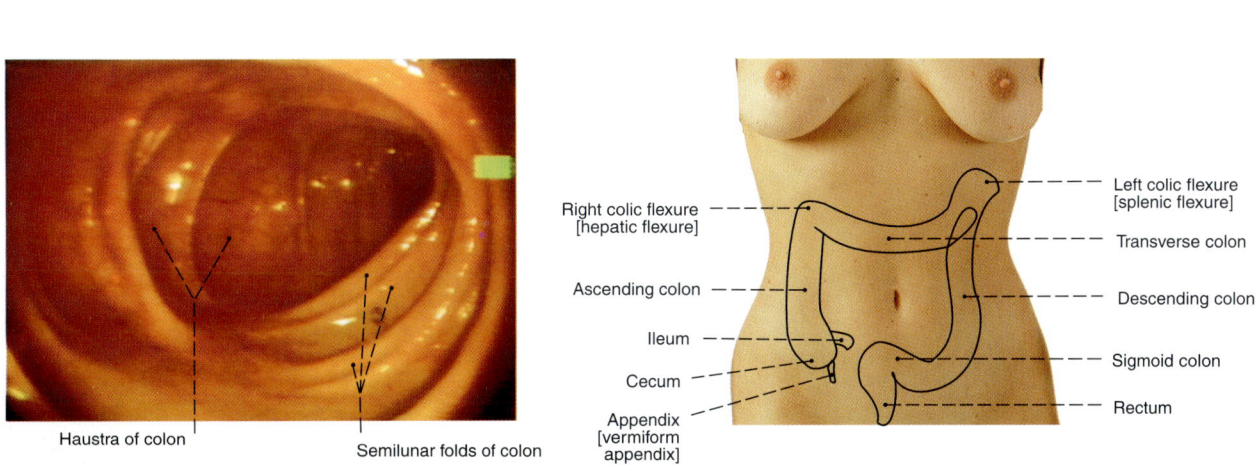

Fig. 966 Ascending colon; endoscopic (colonoscopic) view; endoscope inserted via rectum, sigmoid, and descending colon.

Fig. 967 Colon; projection onto anterior abdominal wall. Position of transverse and sigmoid colon vary considerably (compare Fig. 965).

142 Abdominal viscera

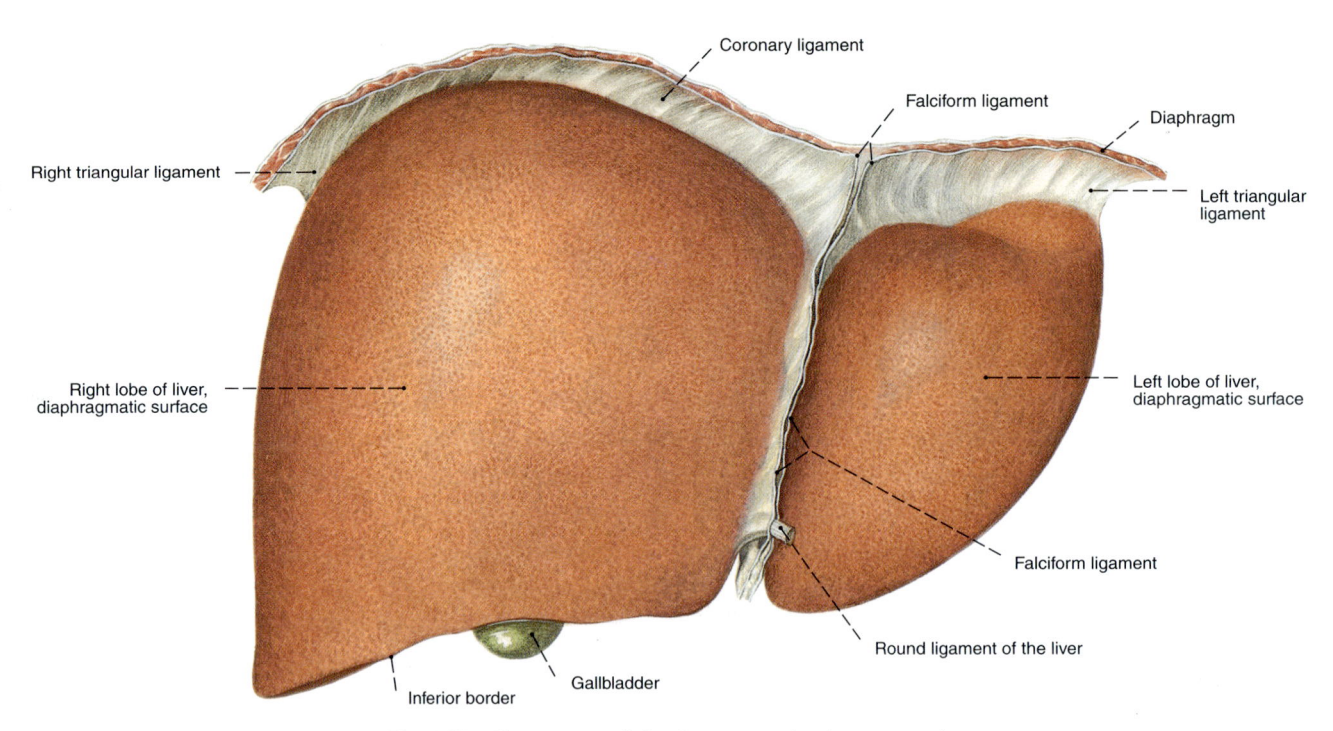

Fig. 968 Liver; parts of diaphragm retained to expose its attachment to the liver; the falciform ligament and the round ligament of the liver severed; ventral aspect.

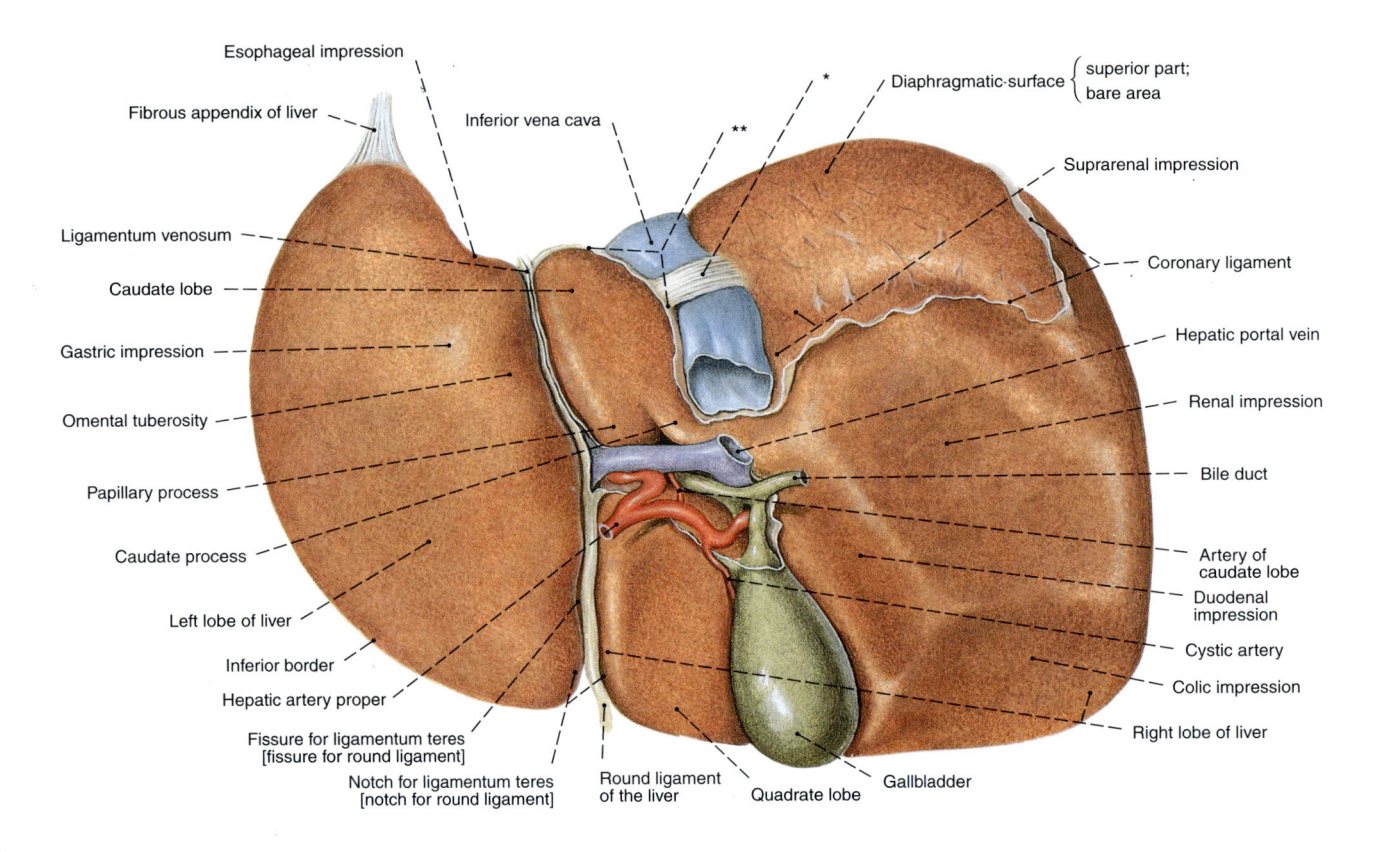

Fig. 969 Liver; porta hepatis; ligaments of the liver and blood vessels severed; dorsal aspect.

* Also: ligament of vena cava.
** Boundary of superior recess of omental bursa [lesser sac].

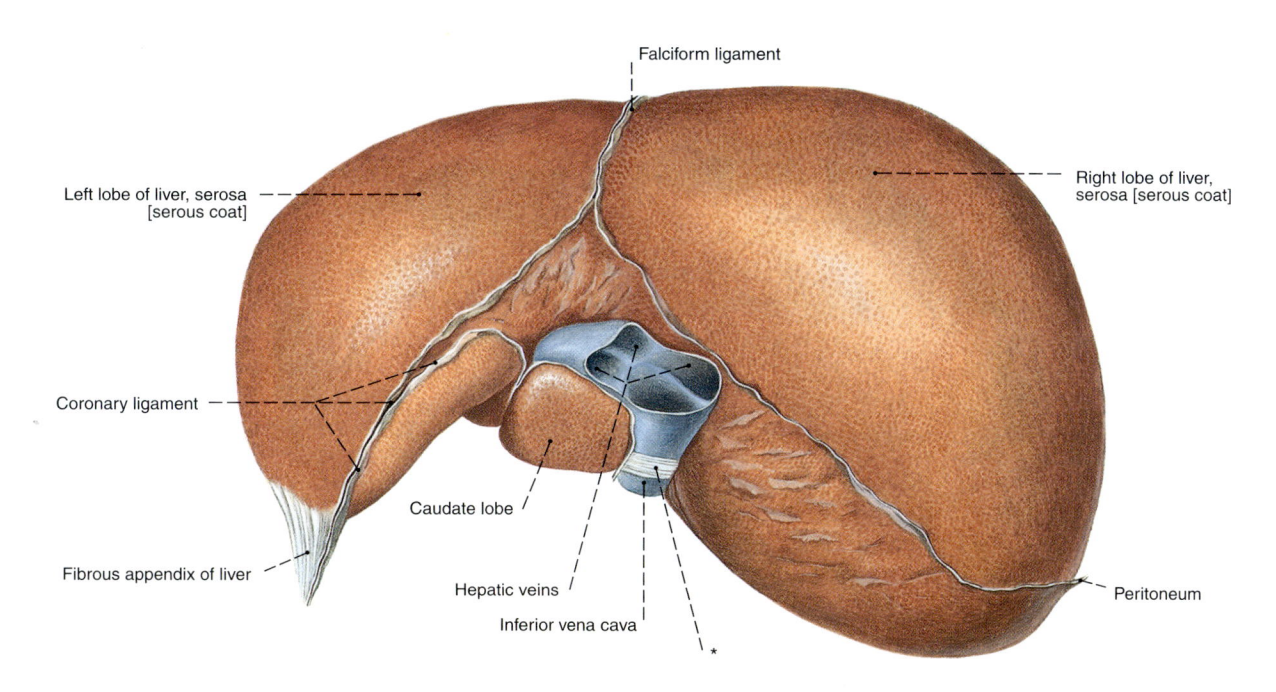

Liver 143

Fig. 970 Liver; reflections of peritoneum sectioned; cranial aspect.

The bare area without peritoneum can be recognized by its roughened surface.

* Also: ligament of vena cava.

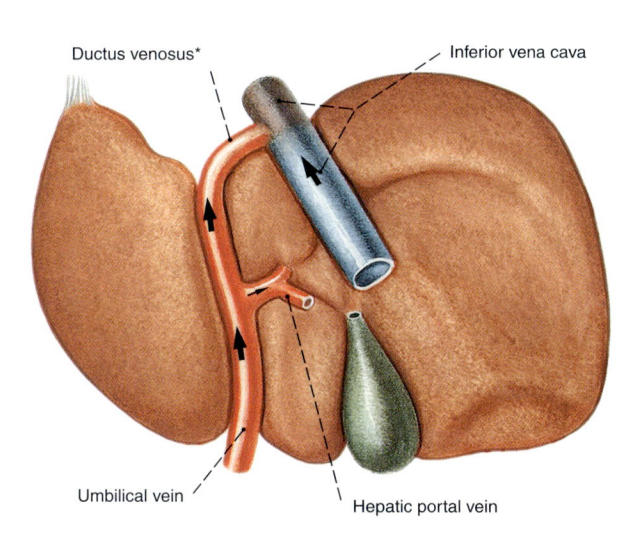

Fig. 971 Liver of a fetus; colors indicate oxygen content of blood, arrows indicate direction of blood flow; dorsal aspect. The liver parenchyma is bypassed by the ductus venosus, that carries oxygen-rich blood from the placenta to the inferior vena cava.

* Also: ARTANTIUS' duct.

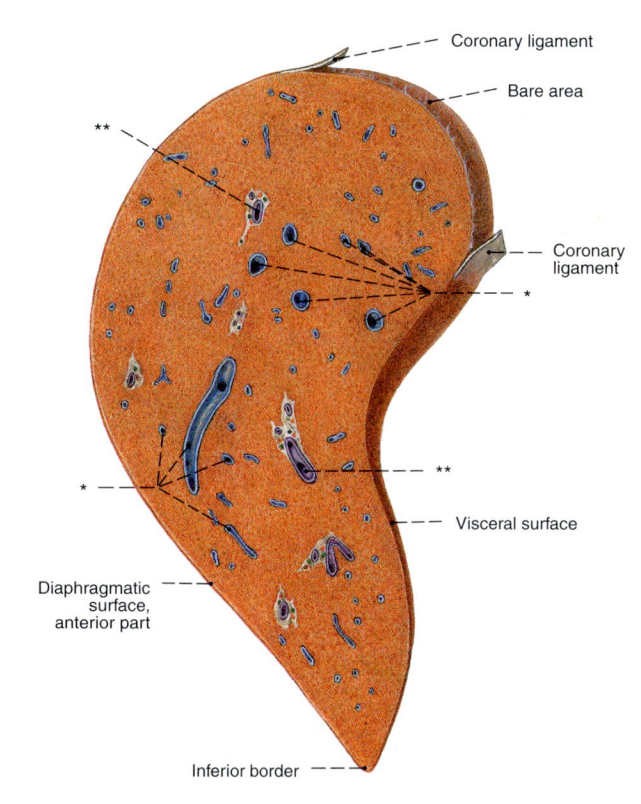

Fig. 972 Liver of a fetus; sagittal section through right lobe of liver to expose branches of both hepatic and portal veins.

* Intrahepatic branches of hepatic veins.
** Intrahepatic branches of hepatic portal vein and hepatic artery.

Abdominal viscera

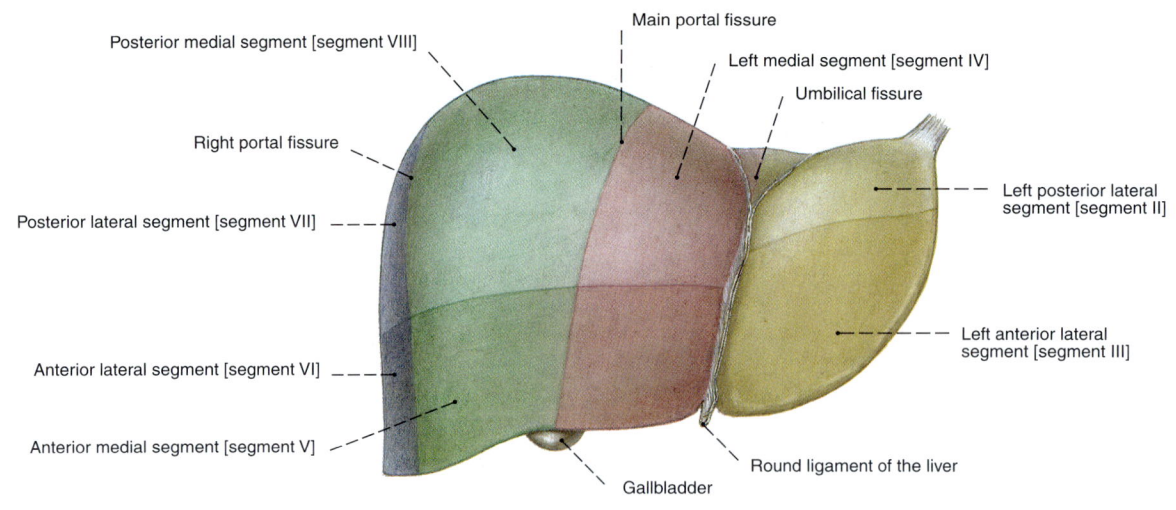

Fig. 973 Liver; colors indicate different liver segments; ventral aspect.

Surgically, the 4th segment is divided into an upper (IV a) and lower (IV b) subsegment.

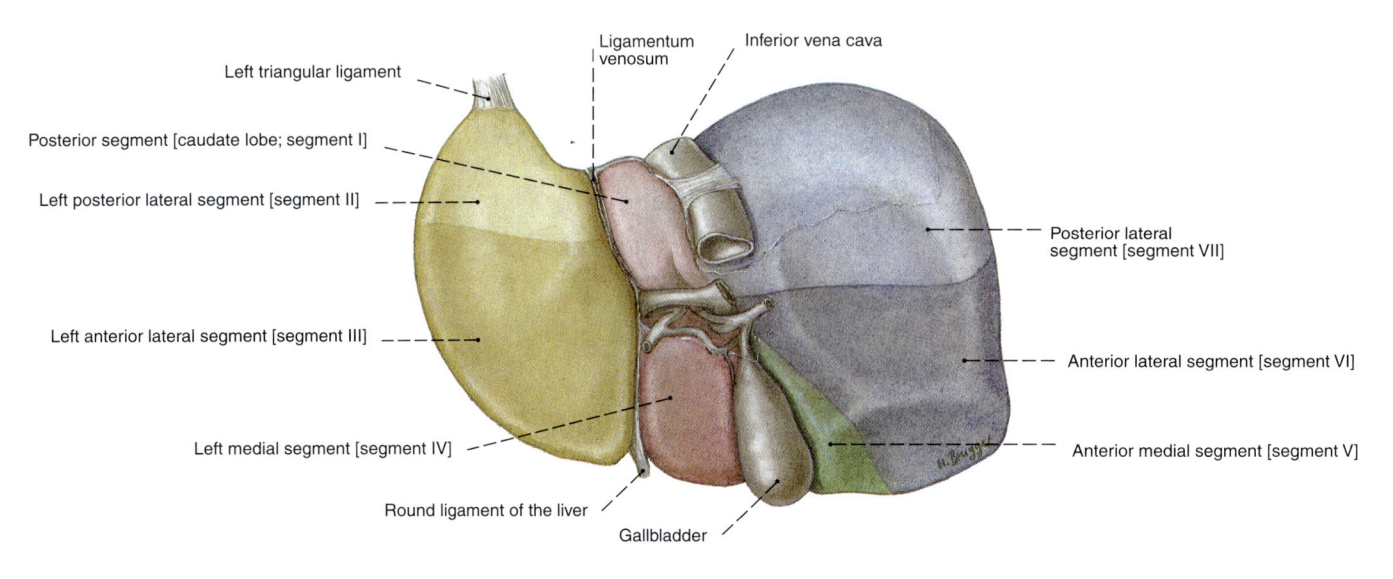

Fig. 974 Liver; colors indicate same liver segments as in Fig. 973; dorsal aspect.

Hepatic segmentation

Left liver [left part of liver]	Posterior liver [posterior part of liver, caudate lobe]	Posterior segment [caudate lobe; segment I]
	Left lateral division	Left posterior lateral segment [segment II]
		Left anterior lateral segment [segment III]
	Left medial division	Left medial segment [segment IV]
Right liver [right part of liver]	Right medial division	Anterior medial segment [segment V]
		Posterior medial segment [segment VIII]
	Right lateral division	Anterior lateral segment [segment VI]
		Posterior lateral segment [segment VII]

Traditionally, the liver is divided into a right and a left lobe with regard to the falciform ligament. The classification in parts and divisions, however, based on the branching pattern of hepatic artery, hepatic portal vein, and hepatic duct, are based on practical aspects, e.g. the requirements for surgical resection of parts of the liver. Moreover, in this classification also developmental aspects are taken into account.
The separate parts are divided by fissures, which do not correspond to superficially visible clefts.

Liver 145

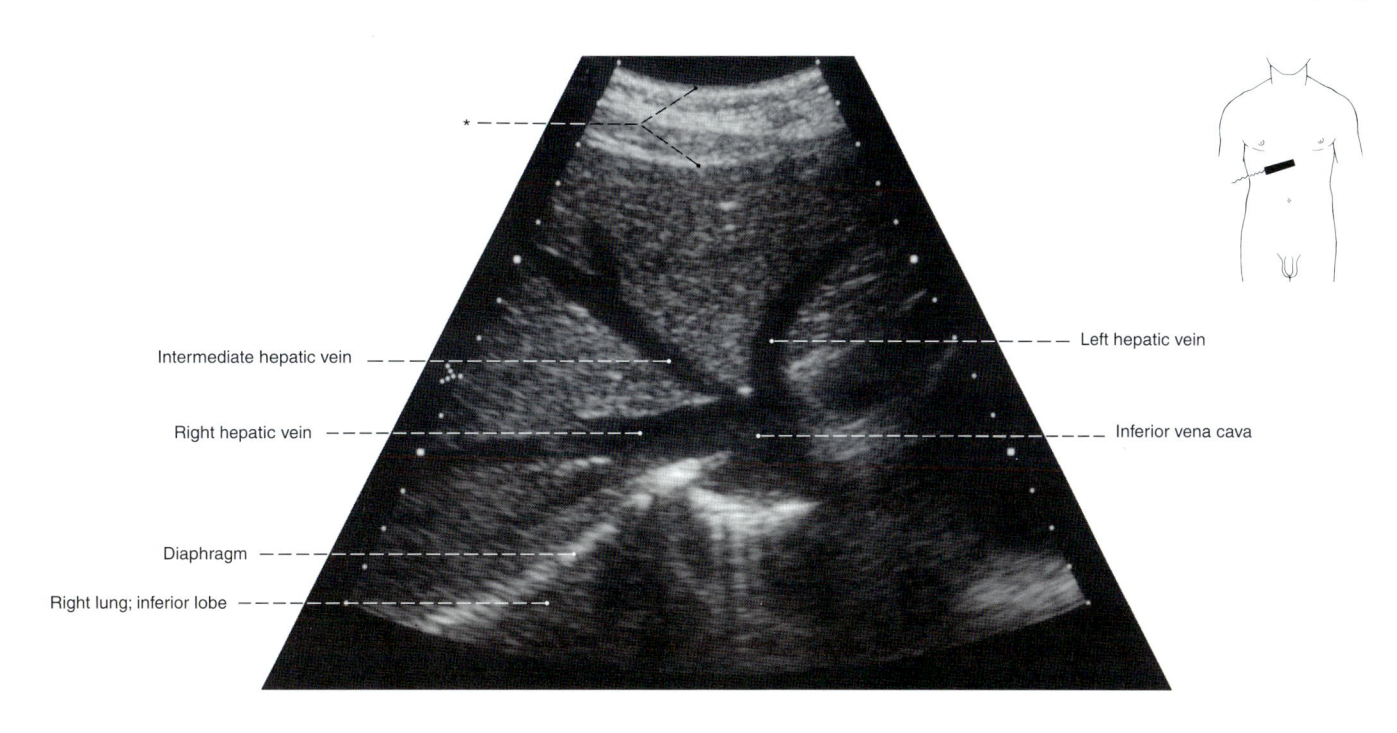

Fig. 975 Hepatic veins; ultrasound scan of openings of hepatic veins into inferior vena cava; inferior aspect.
* Abdominal wall.

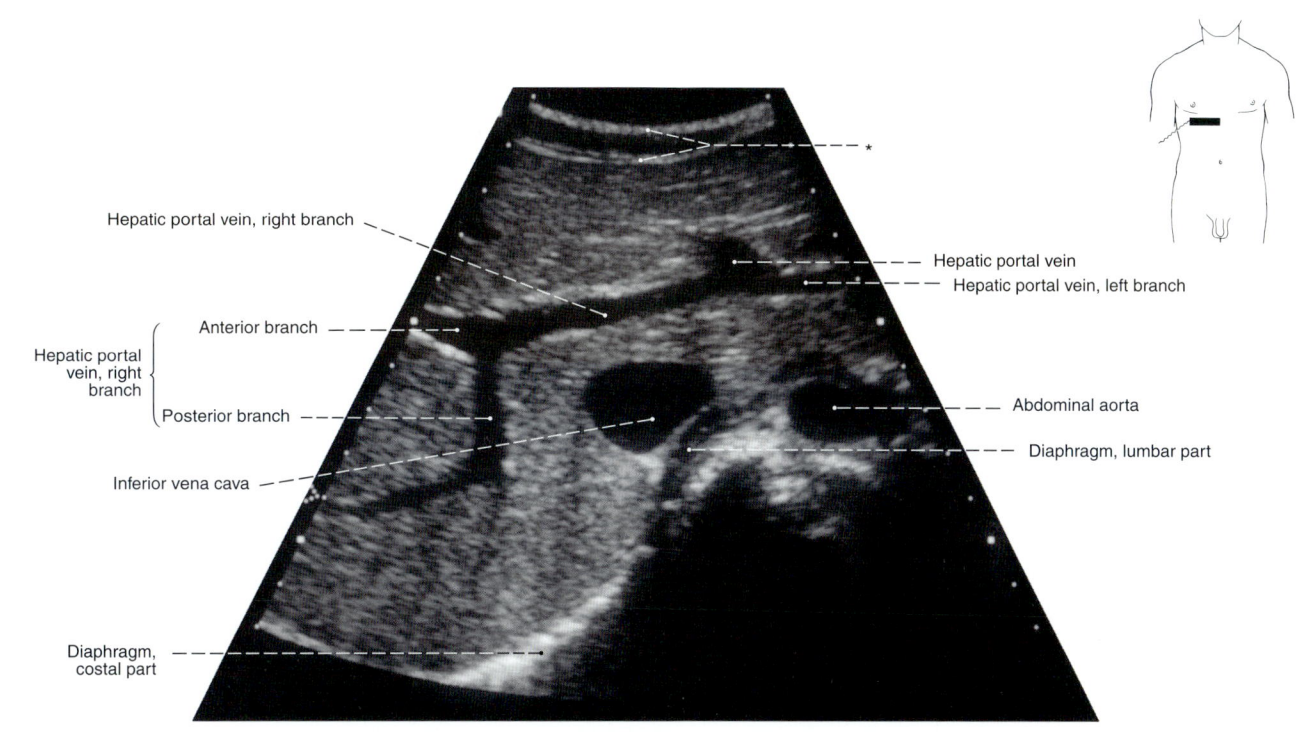

Fig. 976 Hepatic portal vein; ultrasound scan of division of hepatic portal vein into main branches; inferior aspect.
Compare Fig. 982.
* Abdominal wall.

Abdominal viscera

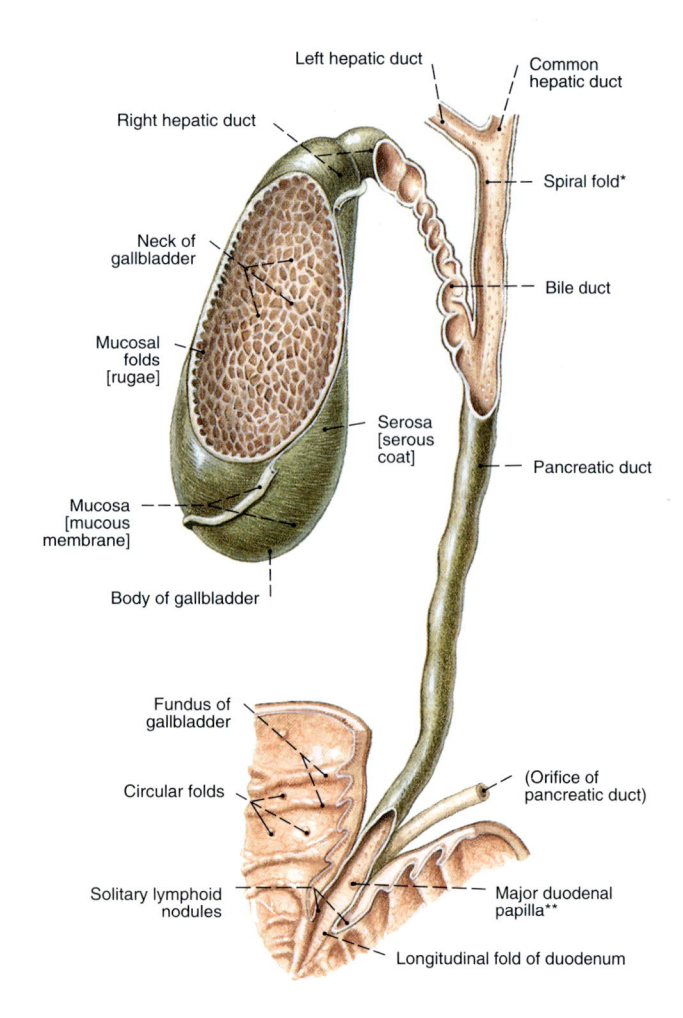

Fig. 977 Gallbladder; biliary duct system; parts of anterior wall of gallbladder, biliary duct system, and duodenum removed to expose mucosa [mucous membrane]; ventral aspect.
* Clinically: HEISTER's valve.
** Clinically: Tubercle of VATER.

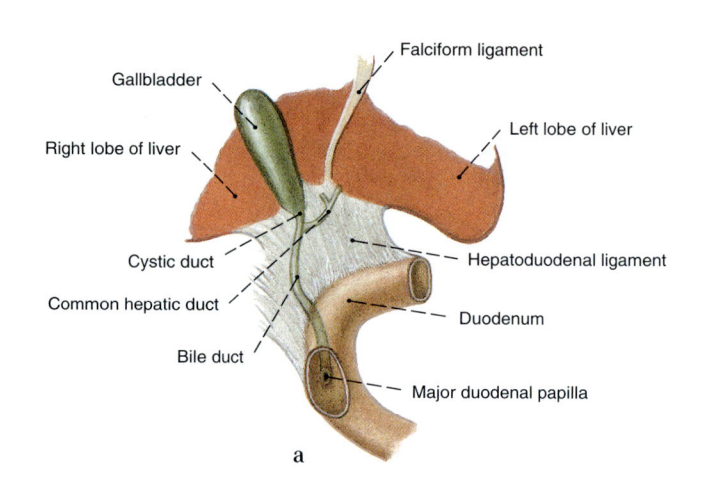

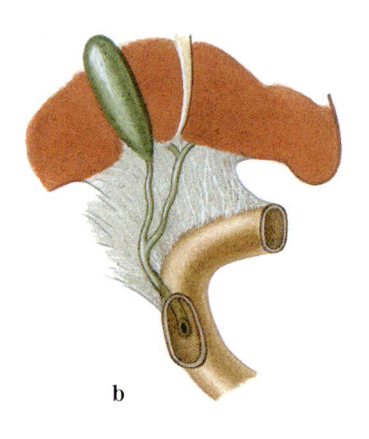

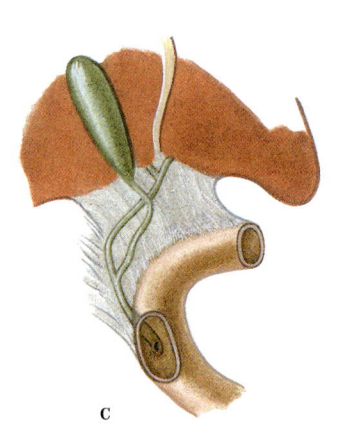

Fig. 978 a–c Variability of biliary duct system, common hepatic duct, bile duct.
a High union of common hepatic duct and cystic duct
b Low union of common hepatic duct and cystic duct
c Low union after cystic duct crossing over common hepatic duct

Gallbladder 147

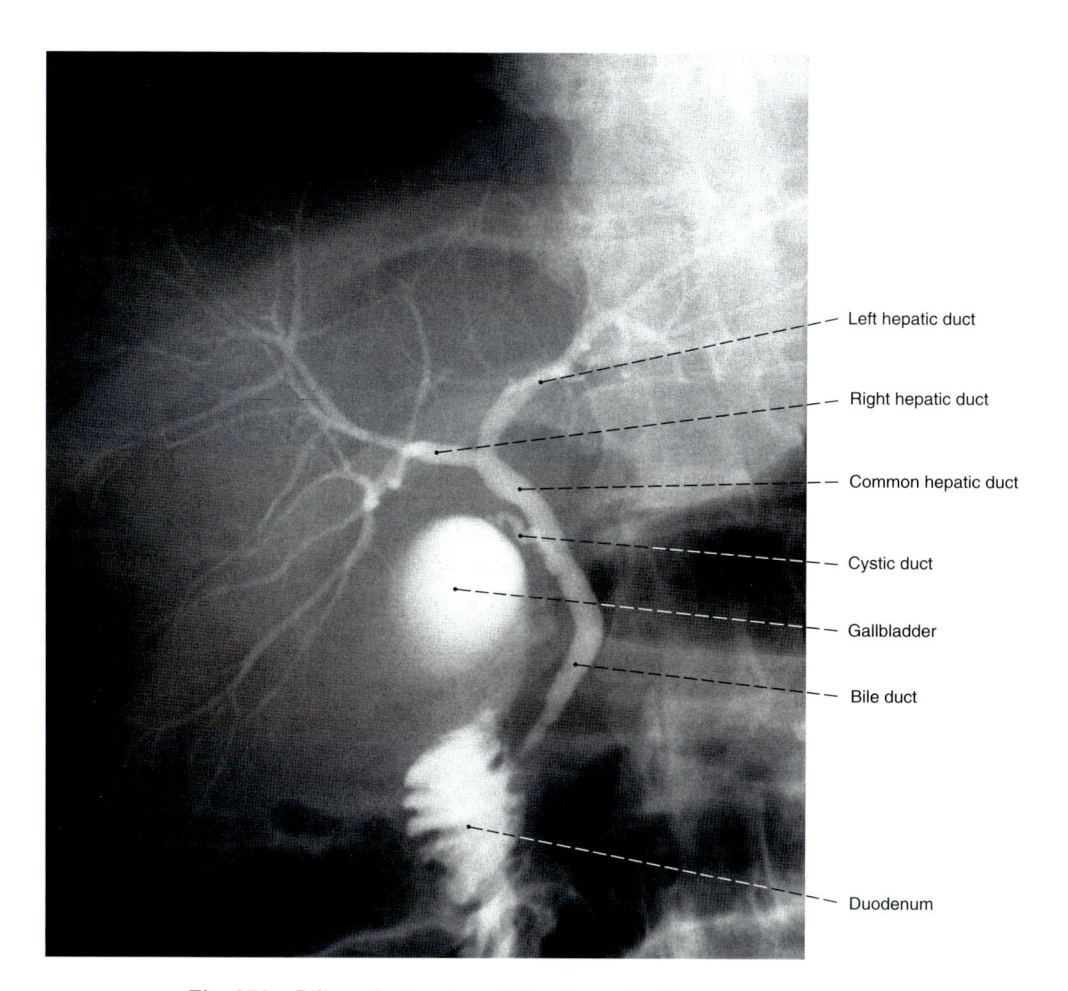

Fig. 979 Biliary duct system; AP radiograph after administration of contrast medium; upright position; ventral aspect.

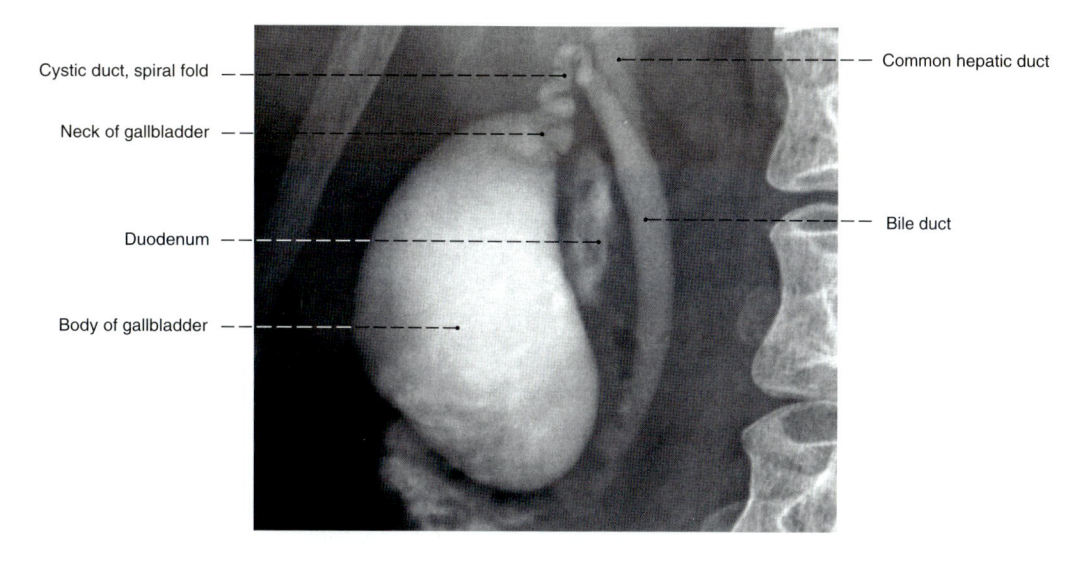

Fig. 980 Gallbladder and biliary duct system; AP radiograph after administration of contrast medium; upright position; ventral aspect.

148　Abdominal viscera

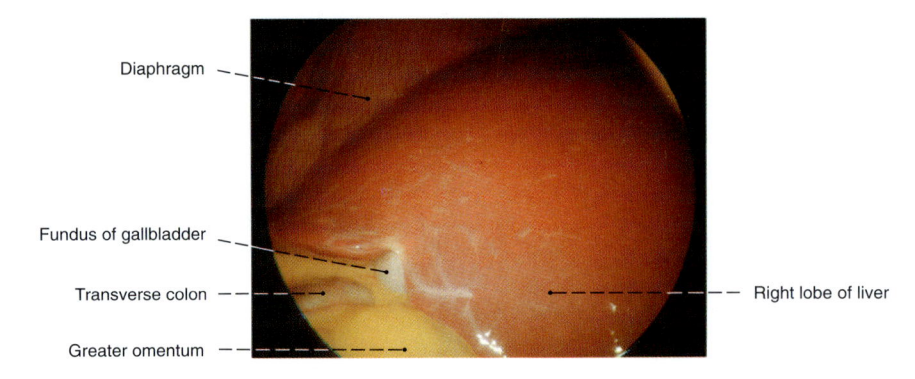

Fig. 981 Liver; gallbladder; endoscopy (laparoscopy) allows visualization of color, surface, and shape of the liver; ventral, left inferior aspect. Insufflation of gas into the peritoneal cavity causes a space between the diaphragm and the liver, thus, allowing a comprehensive exploration of liver and gallbladder.

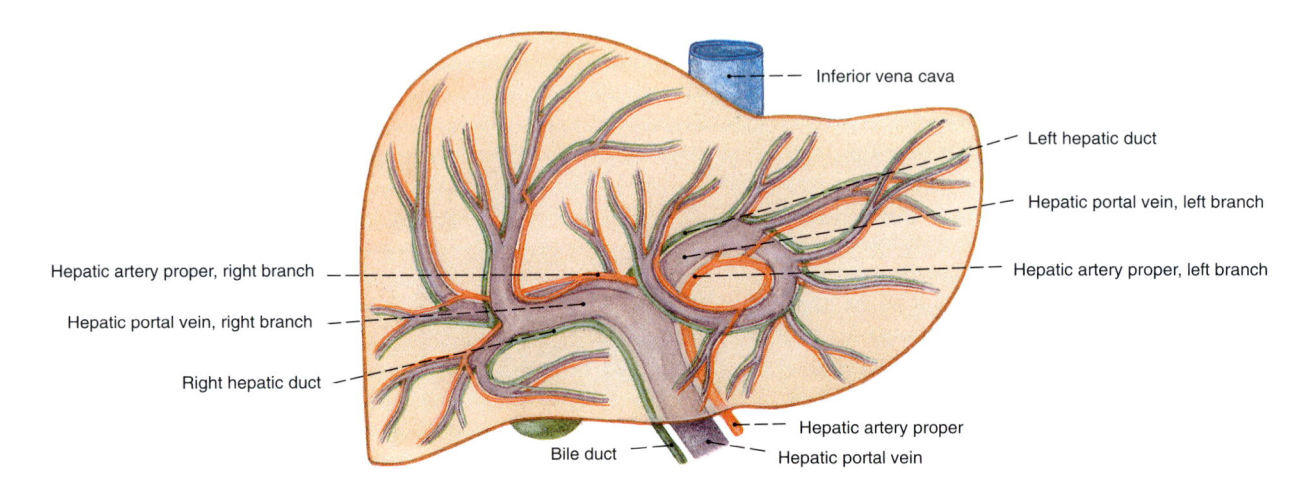

Fig. 982 Liver; hepatic portal vein; diagram of branching pattern of hepatic portal vein projected onto the surface of the liver; ventral aspect.

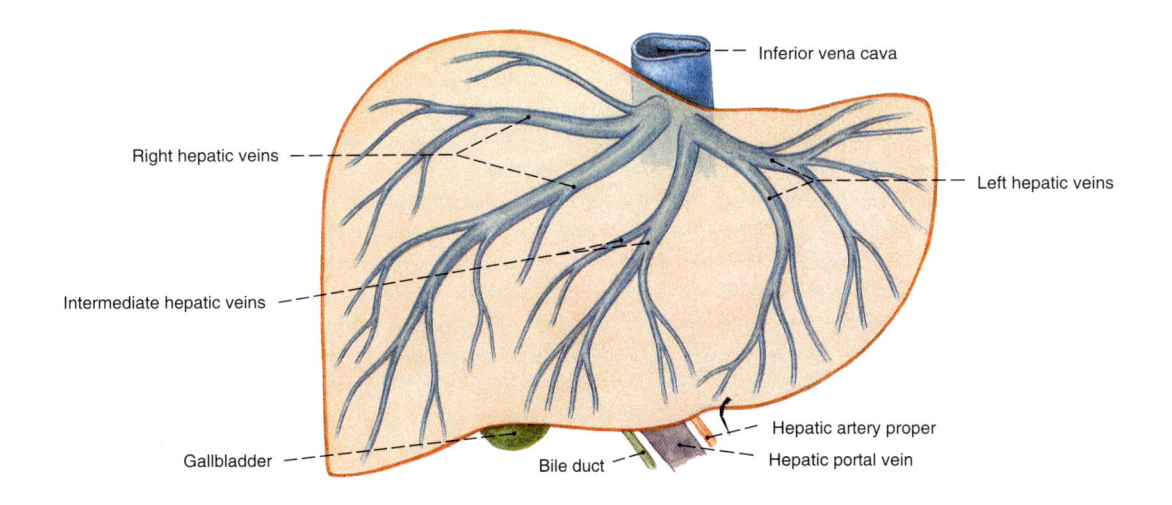

Fig. 983 Liver; hepatic veins; diagram of branching pattern of hepatic veins projected onto the surface of the liver; ventral aspect.

Position of upper viscera **149**

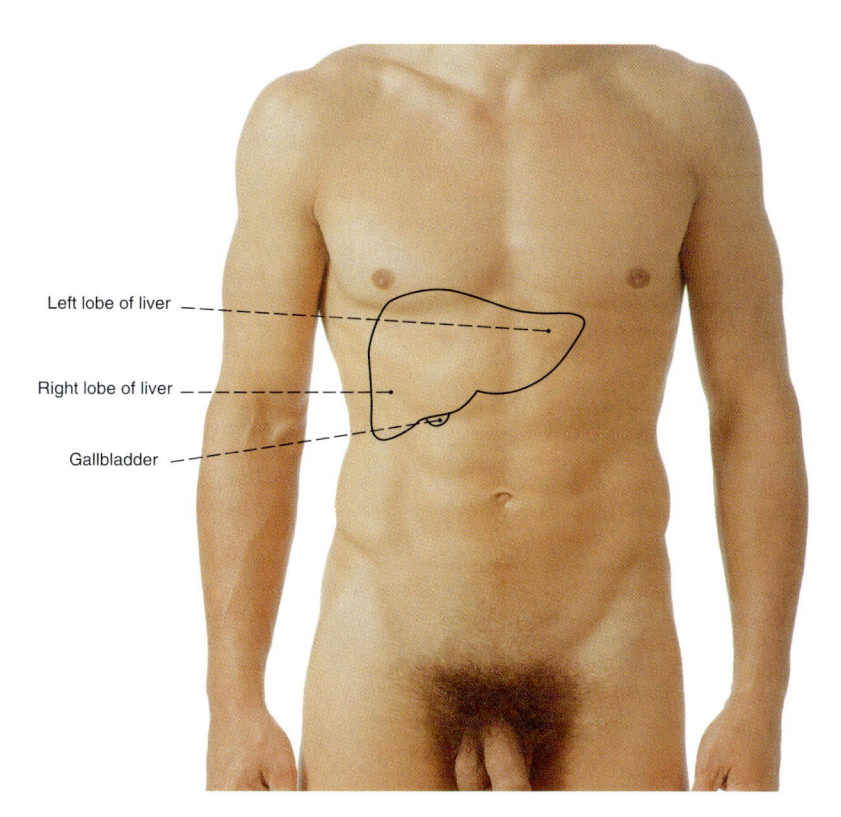

Fig. 984 Liver; projection onto the anterior abdominal wall; in midrespiratory position. Position of the liver highly depends on the respiratory cycle. In inspiration the diaphragm flattens and the diaphragmatic dome descends caudally. This pushes the healthy liver caudally to the costal margin [costal arch], and the inferior border becomes palpable.

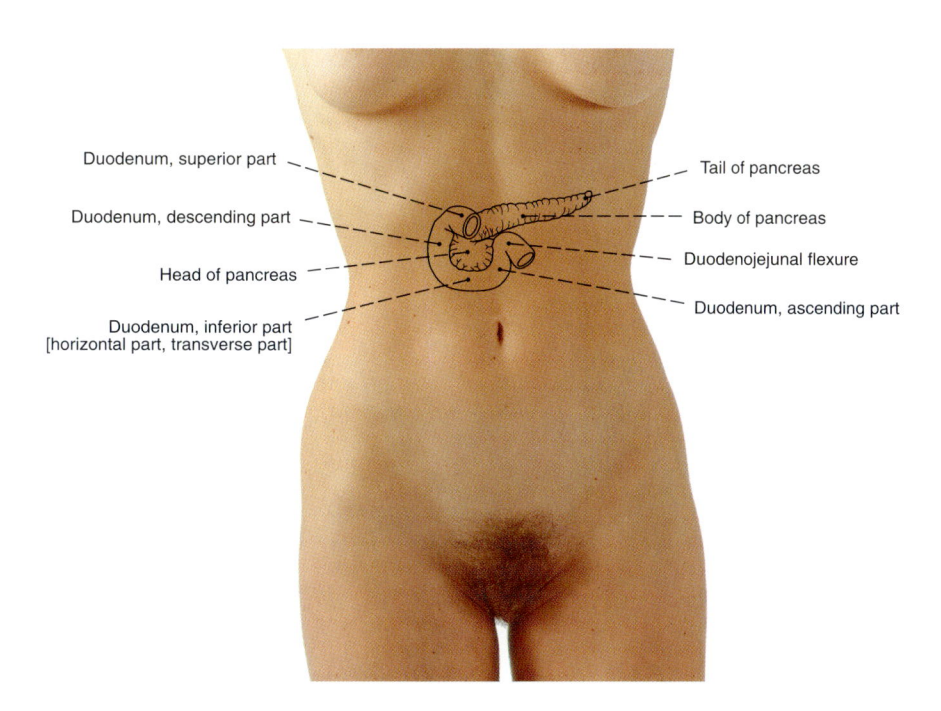

Fig. 985 Duodenum; pancreas; projection onto the anterior abdominal wall.

150 Abdominal viscera

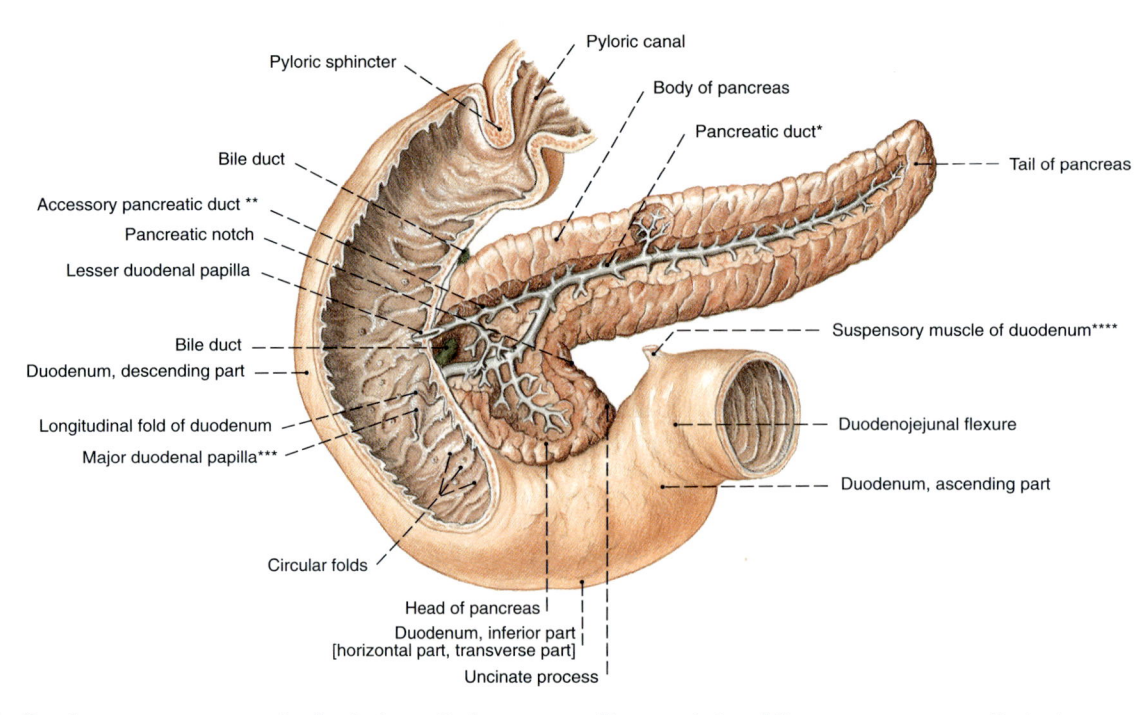

Fig. 986 Duodenum; pancreas; parts of anterior wall of duodenum removed to expose the opening of the pancreatic duct; pancreatic duct dissected; ventral aspect.

Shape and size of the accessory pancreatic duct vary considerably (in ~30% adjacent branch, in less than 10% main excretory duct).

* Clinically: duct of WIRSUNG.
** Clinically: SANTORINI's duct.
*** Clinically: muscle of TREITZ.
**** Clinically: tubercle of VATER.

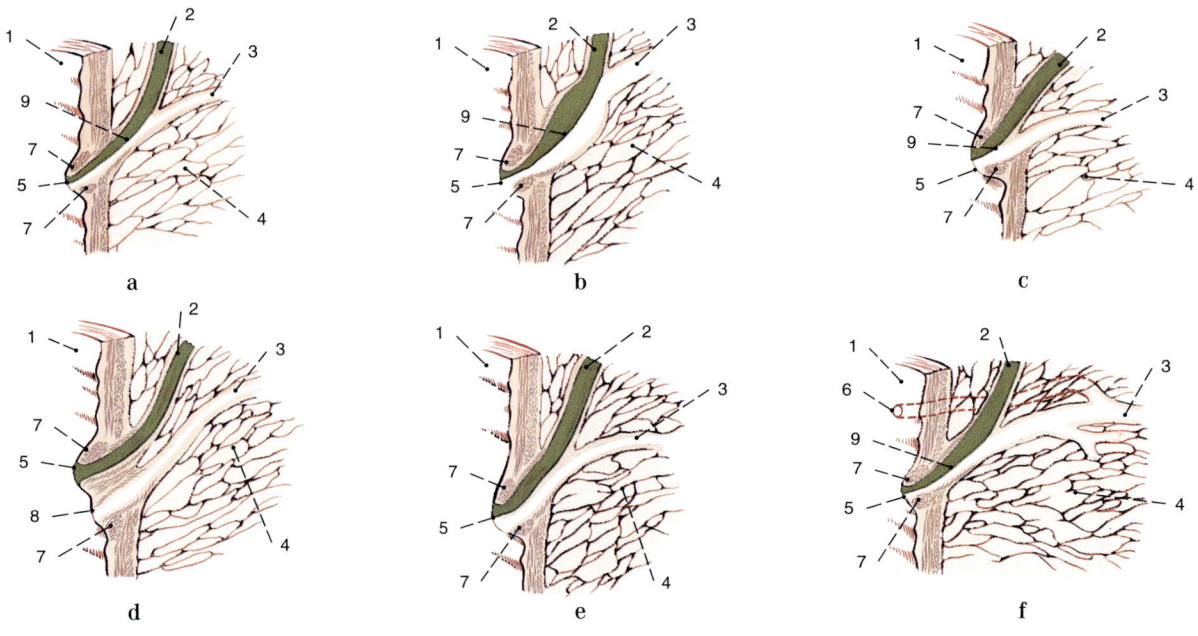

Fig. 987 a-f Variability of opening of bile duct and pancreatic duct.
- a Long common section
- b Ampullar enlargement of terminal part
- c Short common section
- d Separate openings
- e Common opening with septum in the common section
- f Additional duct, accessory pancreatic duct

1 = Duodenum
2 = Bile duct
3 = Pancreatic duct
4 = Pancreas
5 = Major duodenal papilla
6 = Minor duodenal papilla, accessory pancreatic duct
7 = Sphincter of ampulla
8 = Pancreatic duct (in bipartite papilla)
9 = Hepatopancreatic ampulla [biliaropancreatic ampulla]

Pancreas 151

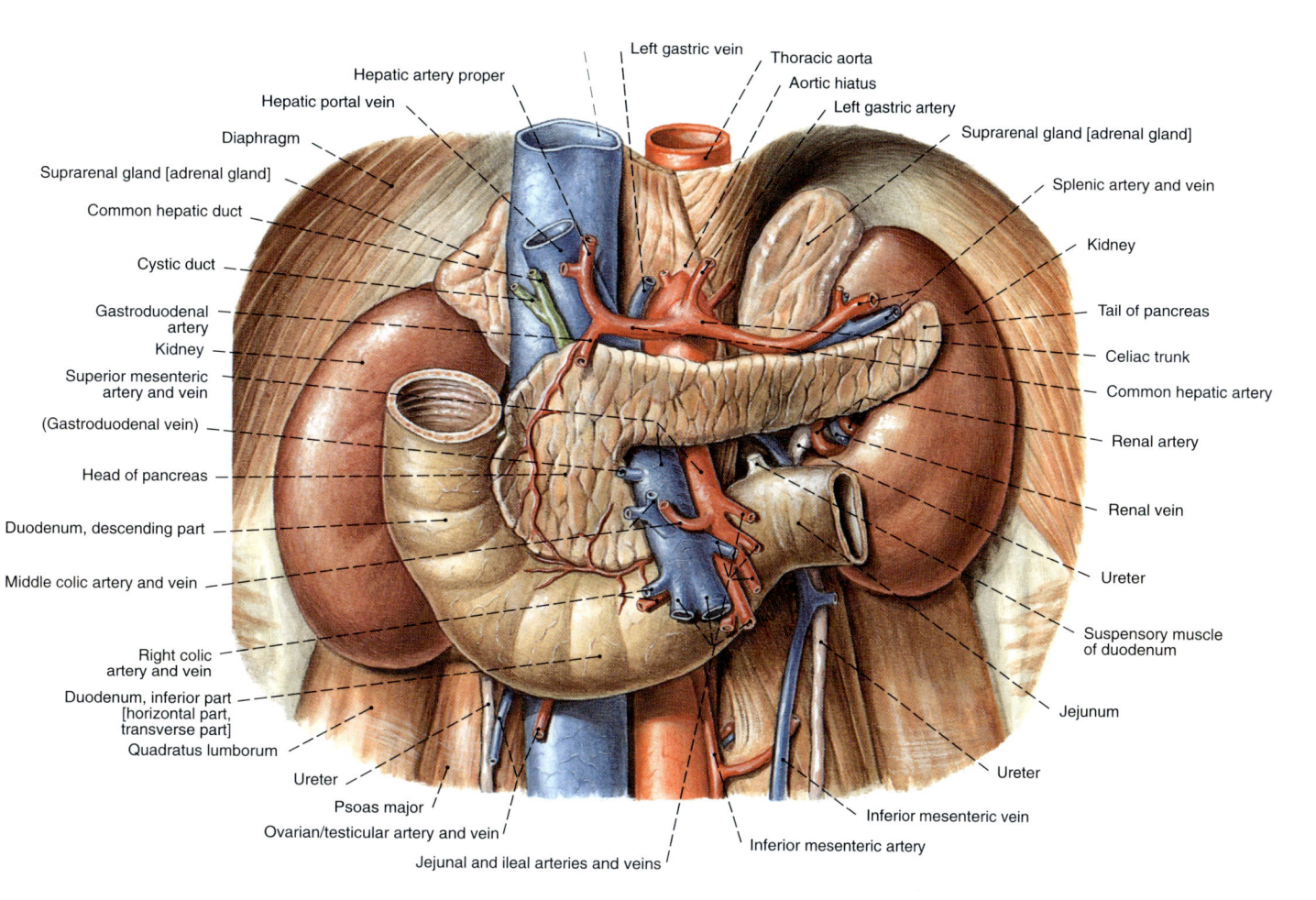

Fig. 988 Retroperitoneal organs and blood vessels of upper abdomen; ventral aspect. Lymph nodes are not shown.

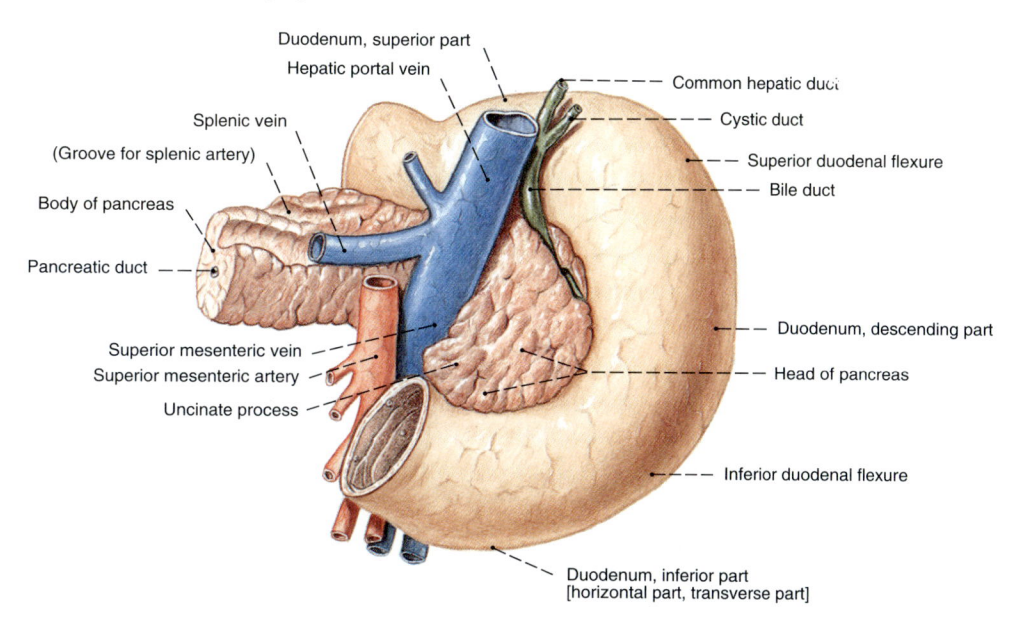

Fig. 989 Duodenum; pancreas; body of pancreas severed to expose pancreatic duct; dorsal aspect. The bile duct courses through the pancreas; the head of pancreas embraces the superior mesenteric vein.

Abdominal viscera

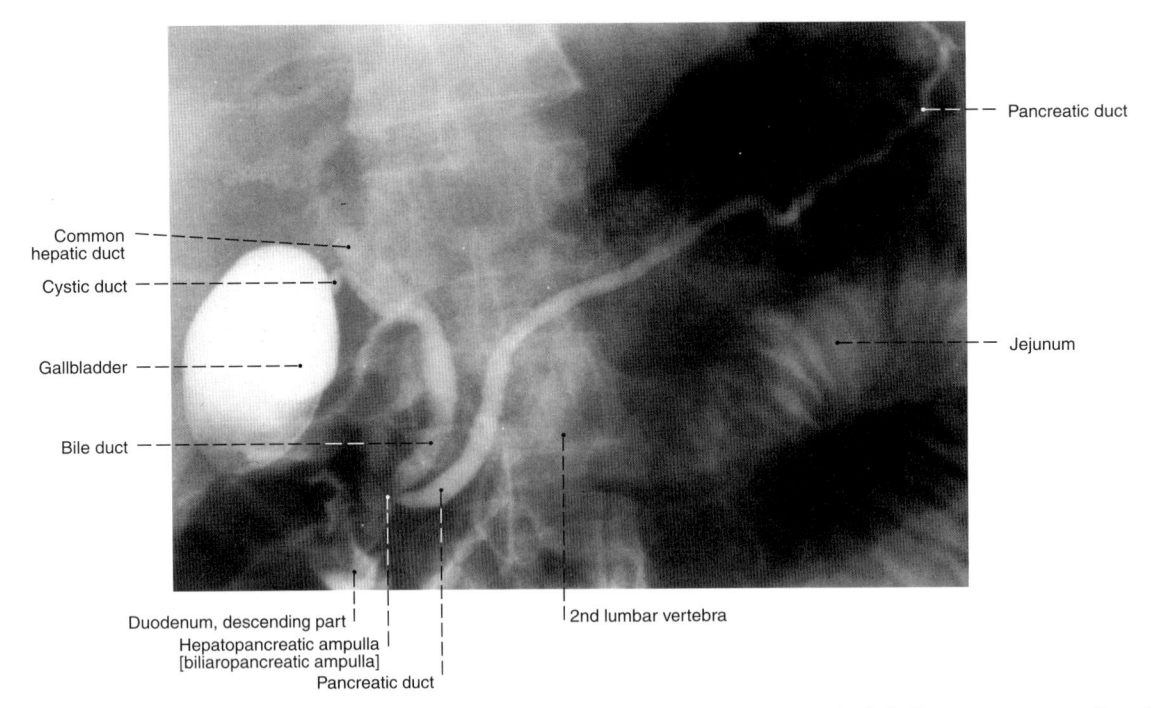

Fig. 990 Pancreatic duct; bile duct; gallbladder; AP radiograph; supine position; after endoscopic cannulation of the common excretory duct of pancreas and liver and injection of contrast medium; ventral aspect.

Clinically: ERCP (endoscopic retrograde cholangiopancreatography). The pancreatic duct is visible throughout its entire length up to the splenic hilum and shows a typical oblique course superiorly toward the left. Some contrast medium has flowed into the small intestine; thus, parts of duodenum and jejunum are also visible. When the contrast medium is injected with higher pressure also, the side branches of the pancreatic duct are visible (compare Fig. 986). This, however, may lead to damage of the pancreas.

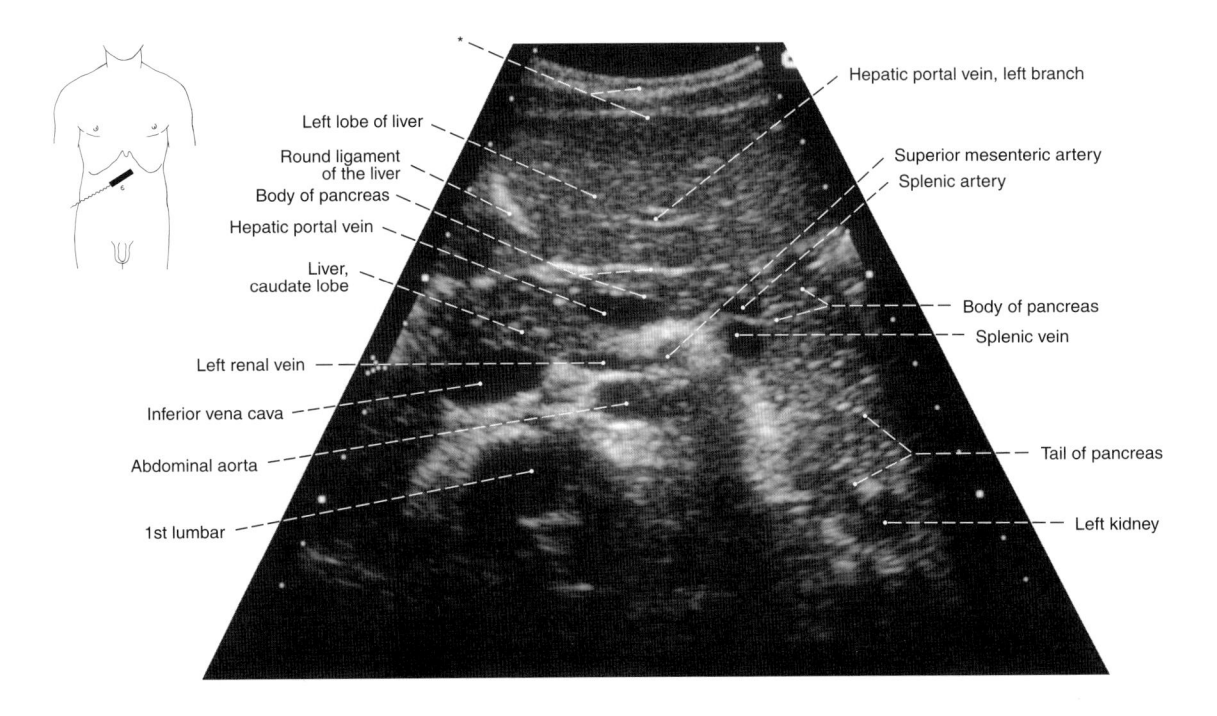

Fig. 991 Pancreas; ultrasound scan visualizing pancreas and neighboring blood vessels in deep inspiration; the tail of pancreas extends far dorsally; inferior aspect.
* Abdominal wall.

Spleen 153

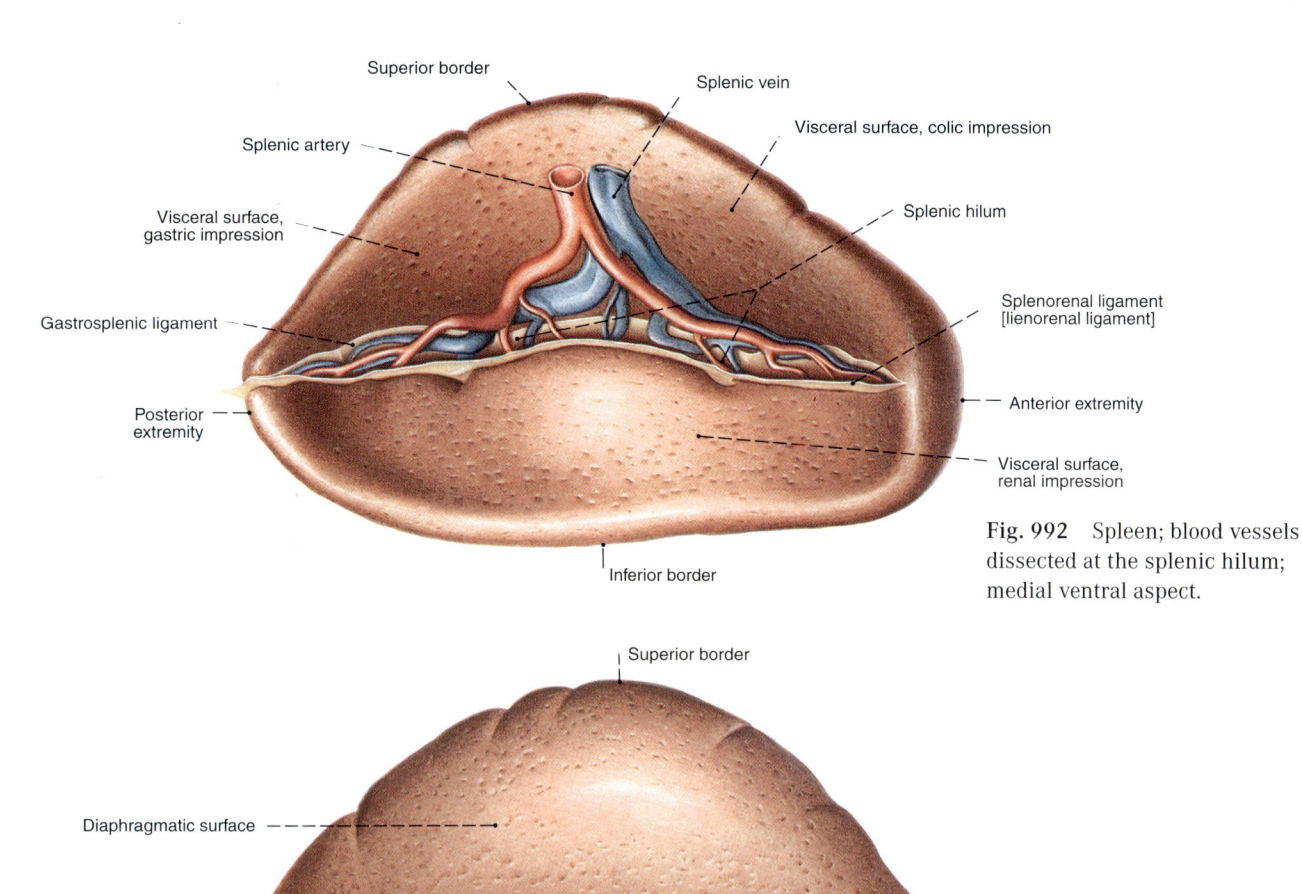

Fig. 992 Spleen; blood vessels dissected at the splenic hilum; medial ventral aspect.

Fig. 993 Spleen; lateral cranial aspect.

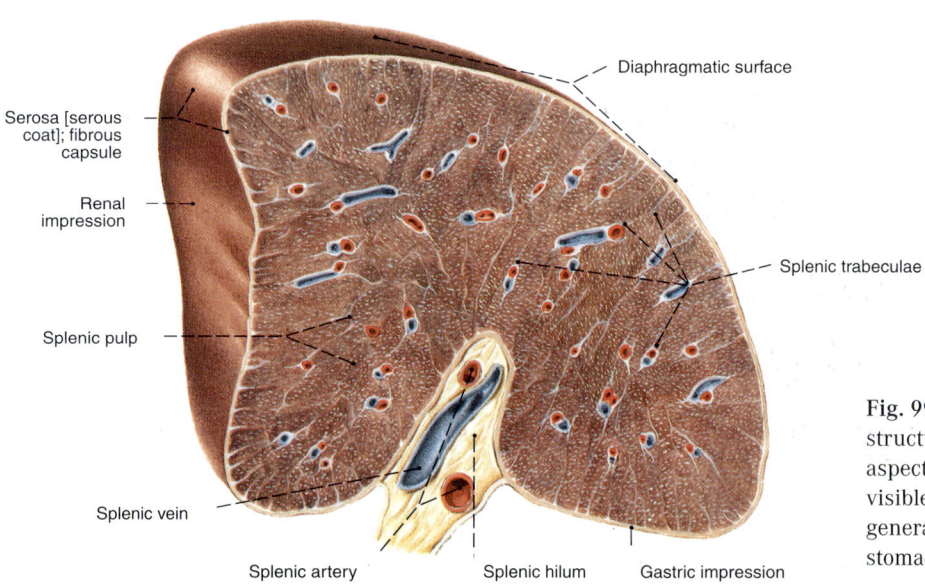

Fig. 994 Spleen; cross-section exposing the structure and the splenic hilum; medial cranial aspect. In this section no lymph nodes are visible at the splenic hilum, although they are generally present at the hilum, draining the stomach and the tail of pancreas.

154 *Abdominal viscera*

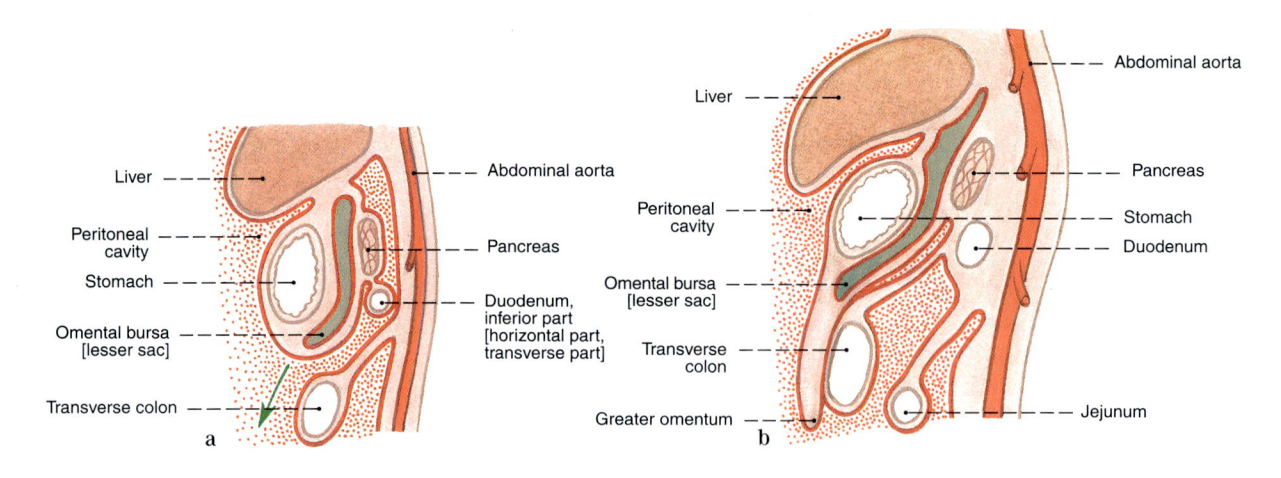

Fig. 995 a, b Development of peritoneal cavity and relationship of peritoneum; schematic median section; lateral aspect.
a Early development
b During formation of greater omentum

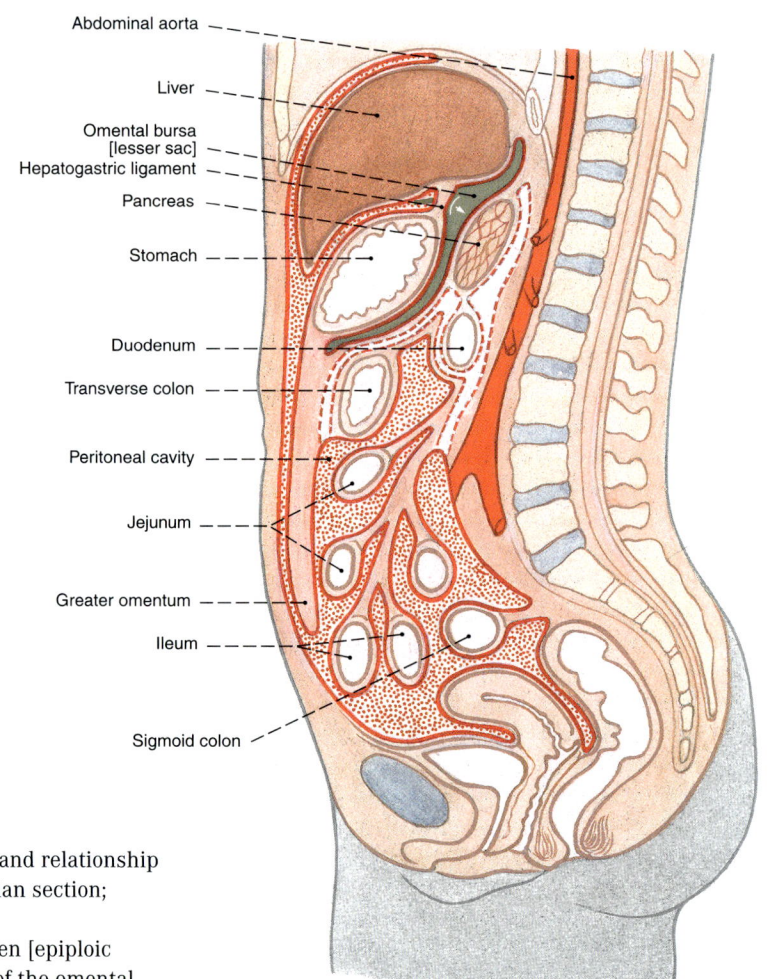

Fig. 996 Development of peritoneal cavity and relationship of peritoneum in the female; schematic median section; lateral aspect.
  The arrow indicates the omental foramen [epiploic foramen]; the arrowhead is in the vestibule of the omental bursa [lesser sac].

Peritoneal cavity 155

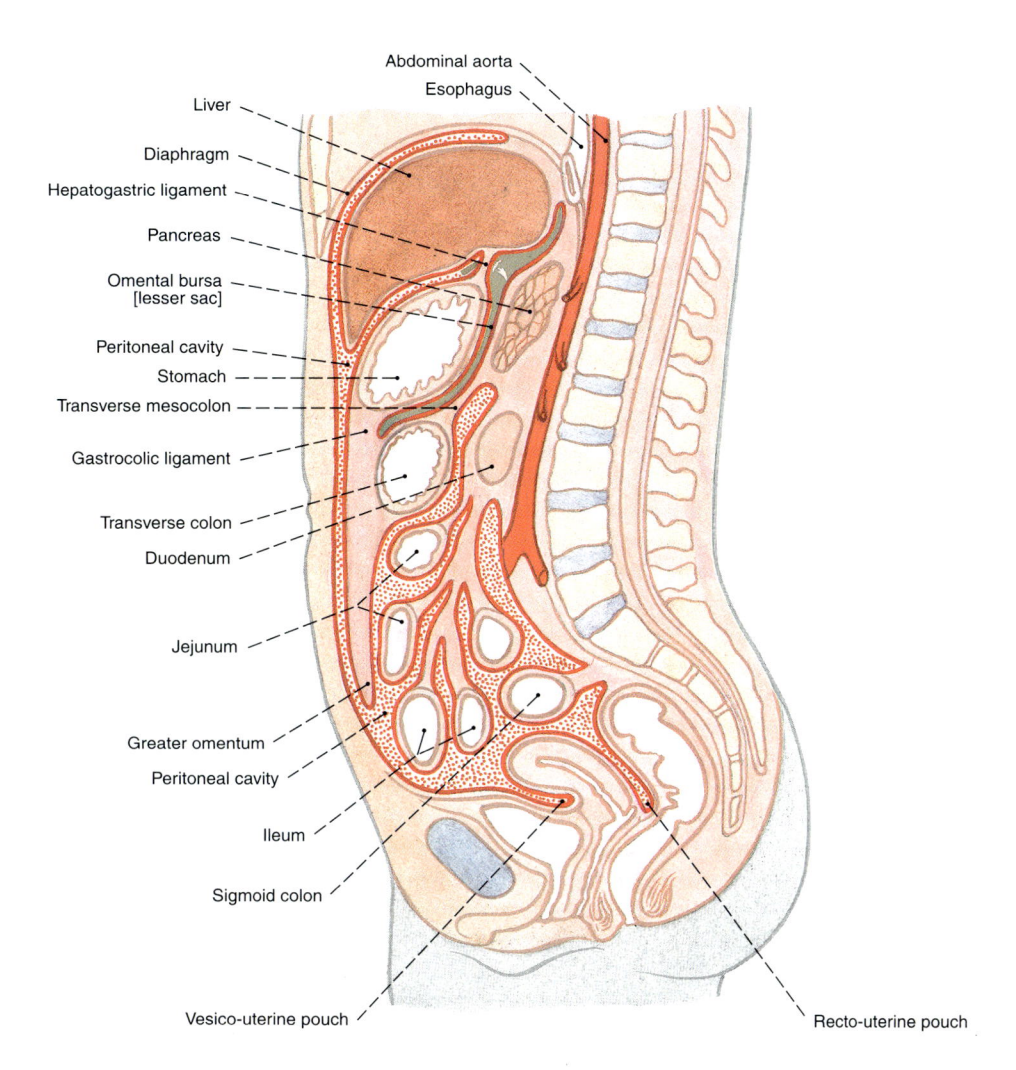

Fig. 997 Development of peritoneal cavity and relationship of peritoneum in the female; final state of peritoneal cavity with fixation of the transverse colon to the greater omentum; schematic median section; lateral aspect.
* Clinically: pouch of DOUGLAS.

Figs. 995-997 The development of the intestines is presented highly schematically; in fact, several developmental steps take place at the same time. The peritoneal cavity is enlarged for didactic reasons. In reality, the organs lie tightly adjacent to each other, separated only by a small capillary space. The volume of the peritoneal fluid is only a few milliliters.

Peritoneal cavity: dotted red; omental bursa [lesser sac]: olive; red dotted line: original arrangement of peritoneum. Arrow in omental foramen [epiploic foramen].

156 Abdominal viscera

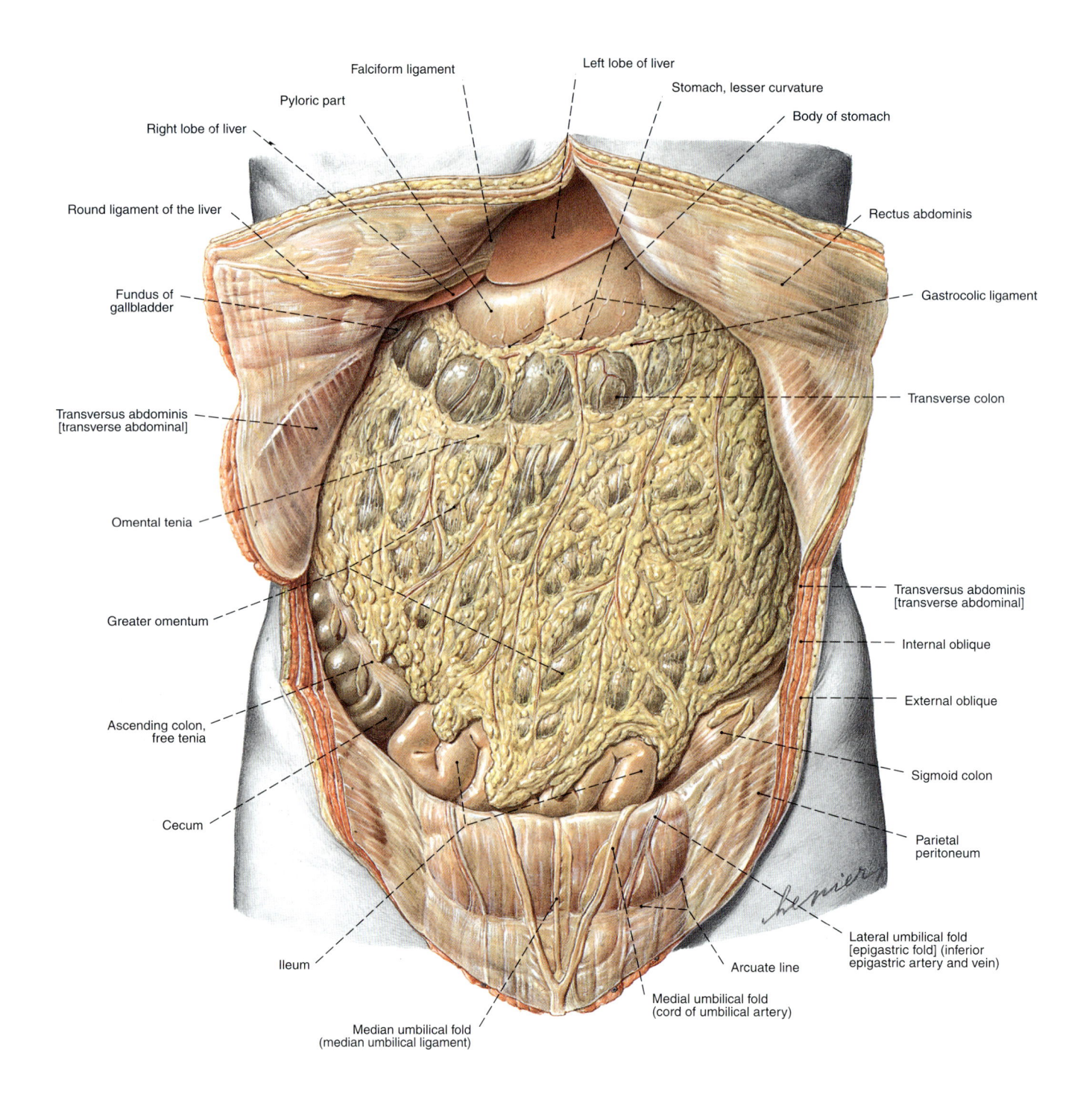

Fig. 998 Position of abdominal viscera; greater omentum; ventral aspect.
The lower part of the peritoneal cavity is also called "intestinal abdomen."

Thoracic and abdominal viscera in the newborn

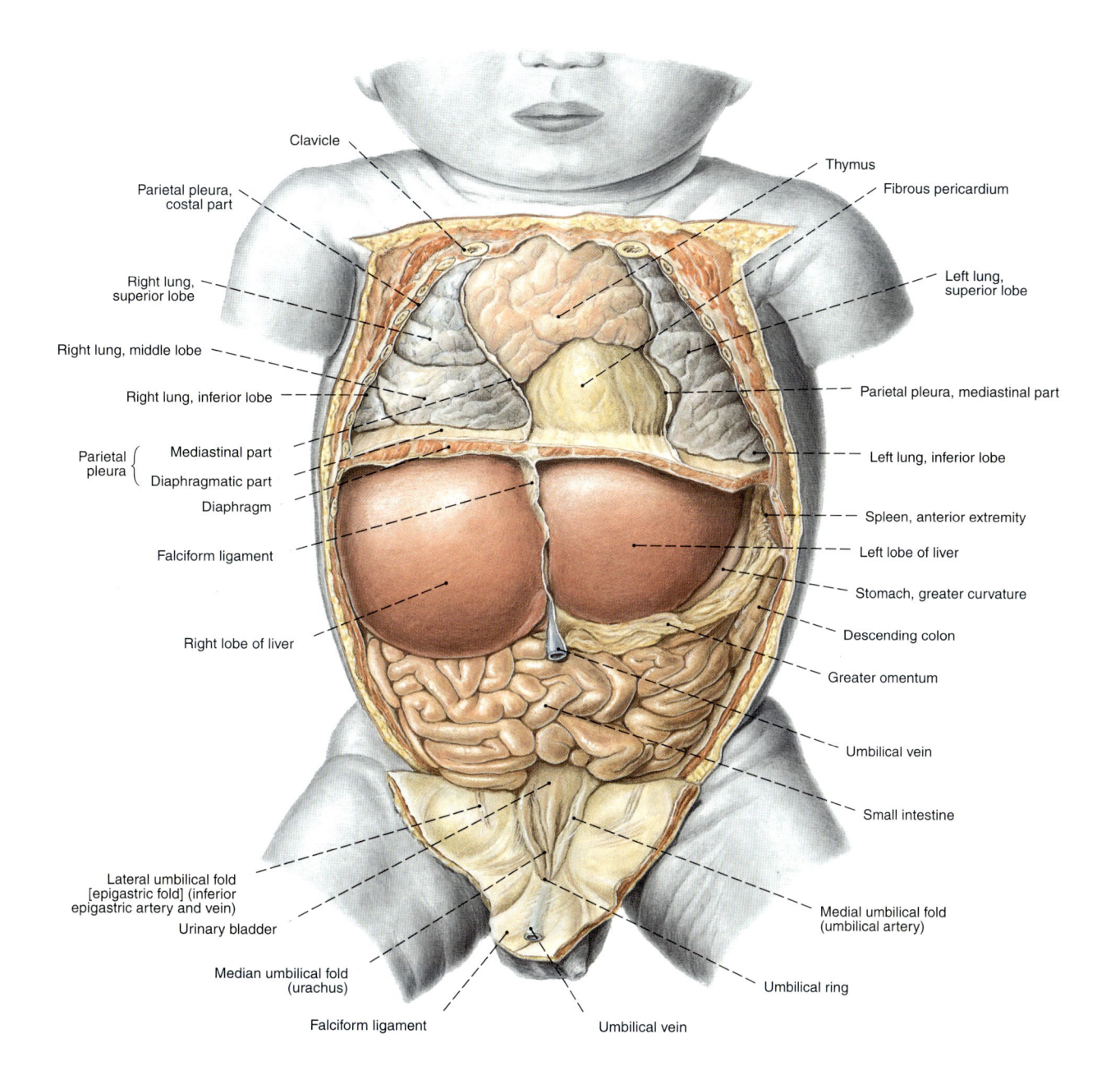

Fig. 999 Position of viscera in the newborn; anterior thoracic and abdominal walls, as well as parts of diaphragm, removed; ventral aspect.
Note the relative size of the liver, the limited extension of the greater omentum, and the size of the medial umbilical folds and the umbilical vein compared to that of the adult (Fig. 998).

158 Abdominal viscera

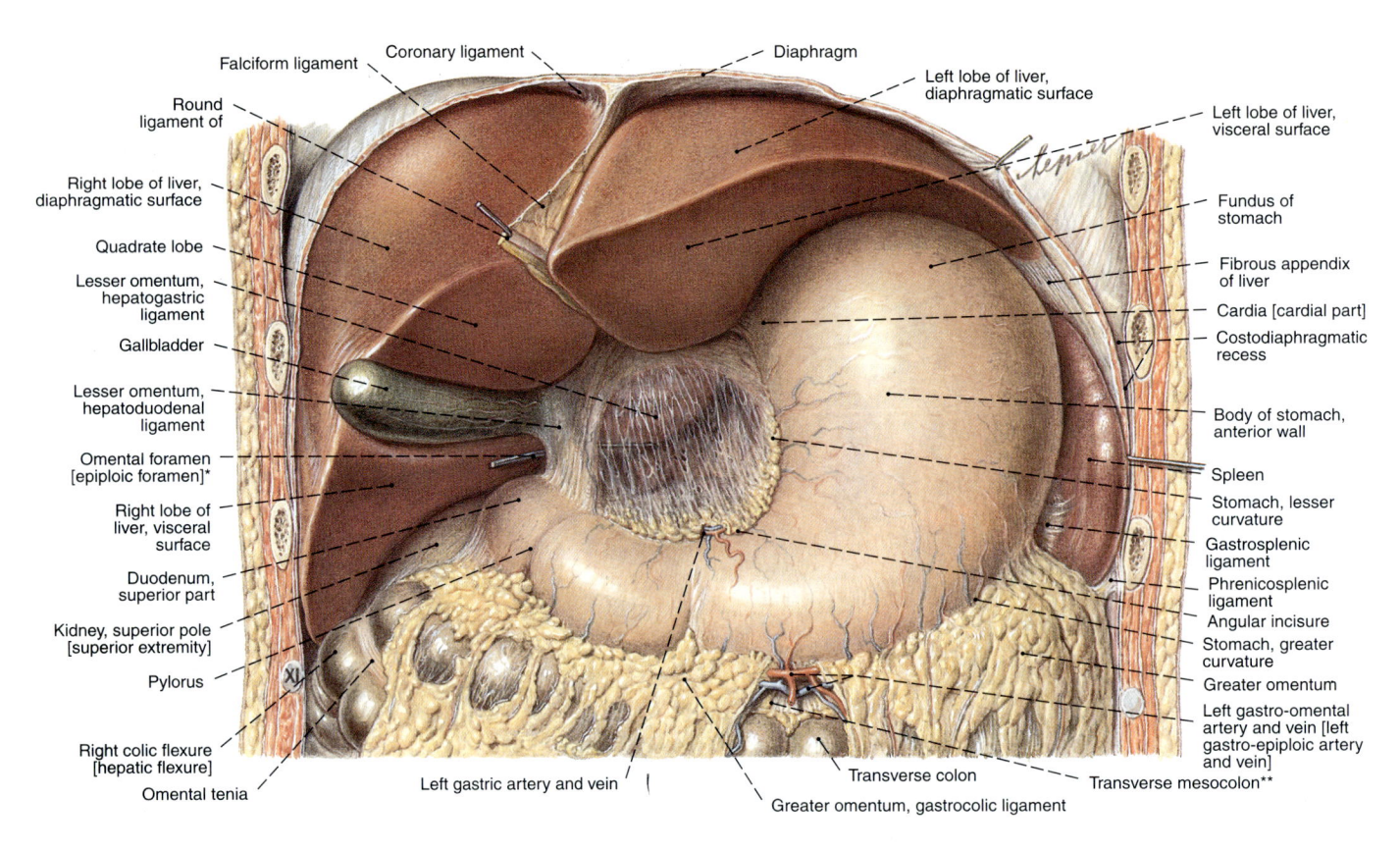

Fig. 1000 Position of viscera in the upper abdomen; anterior thoracic and abdominal walls, as well as parts of diaphragm, removed; ventral aspect.

This part of the peritoneal cavity is also called "glandular abdomen."

* Also: foramen of WINSLOW.

** Omental bursa [lesser sac] partially opened.

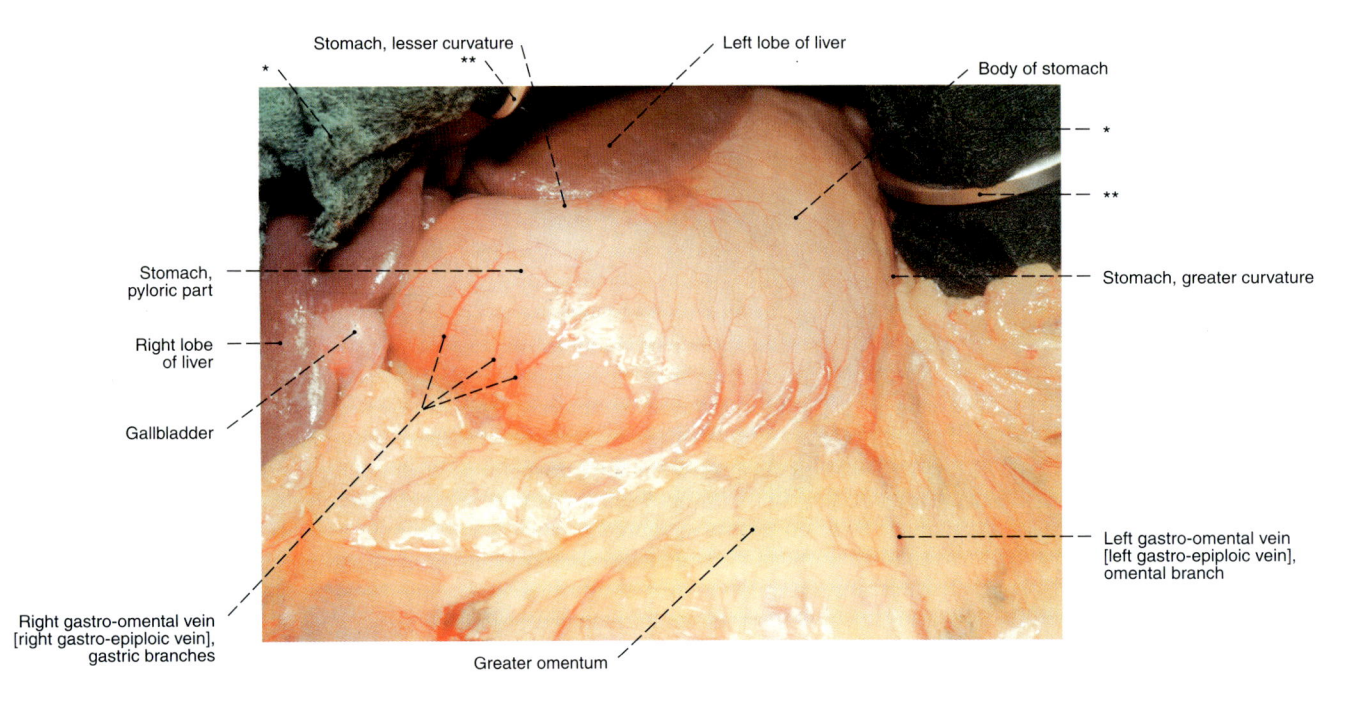

Fig. 1001 Stomach; greater omentum; intra-operative photograph; organs in natural positions; ventral aspect.

* Surgical drape.

** Surgical hook.

Upper abdominal viscera 159

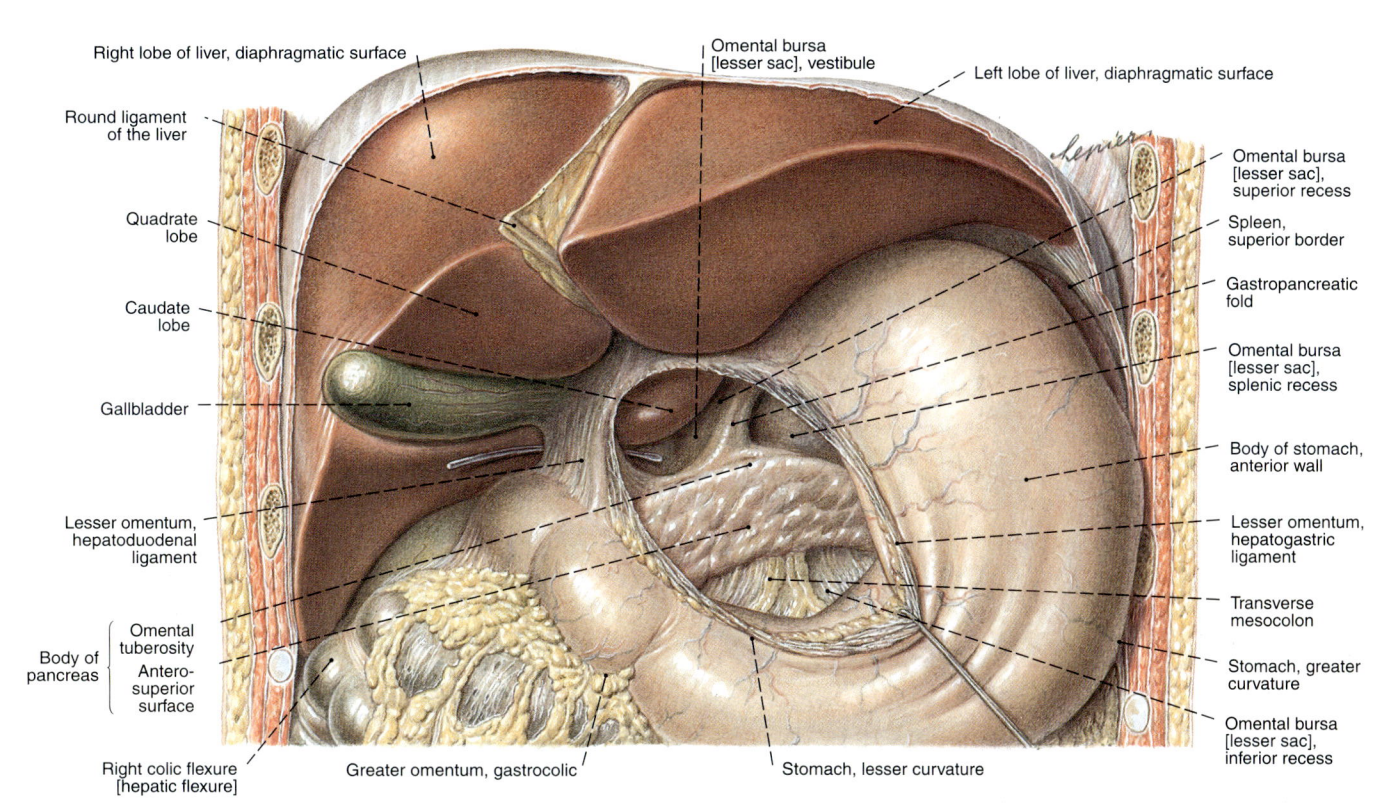

Fig. 1002 Upper abdominal viscera; parts of lesser omentum (hepatogastric ligament) removed to expose omental bursa [lesser sac] and body of pancreas; smaller curvature of stomach retracted inferiorly to the right; ventral aspect.

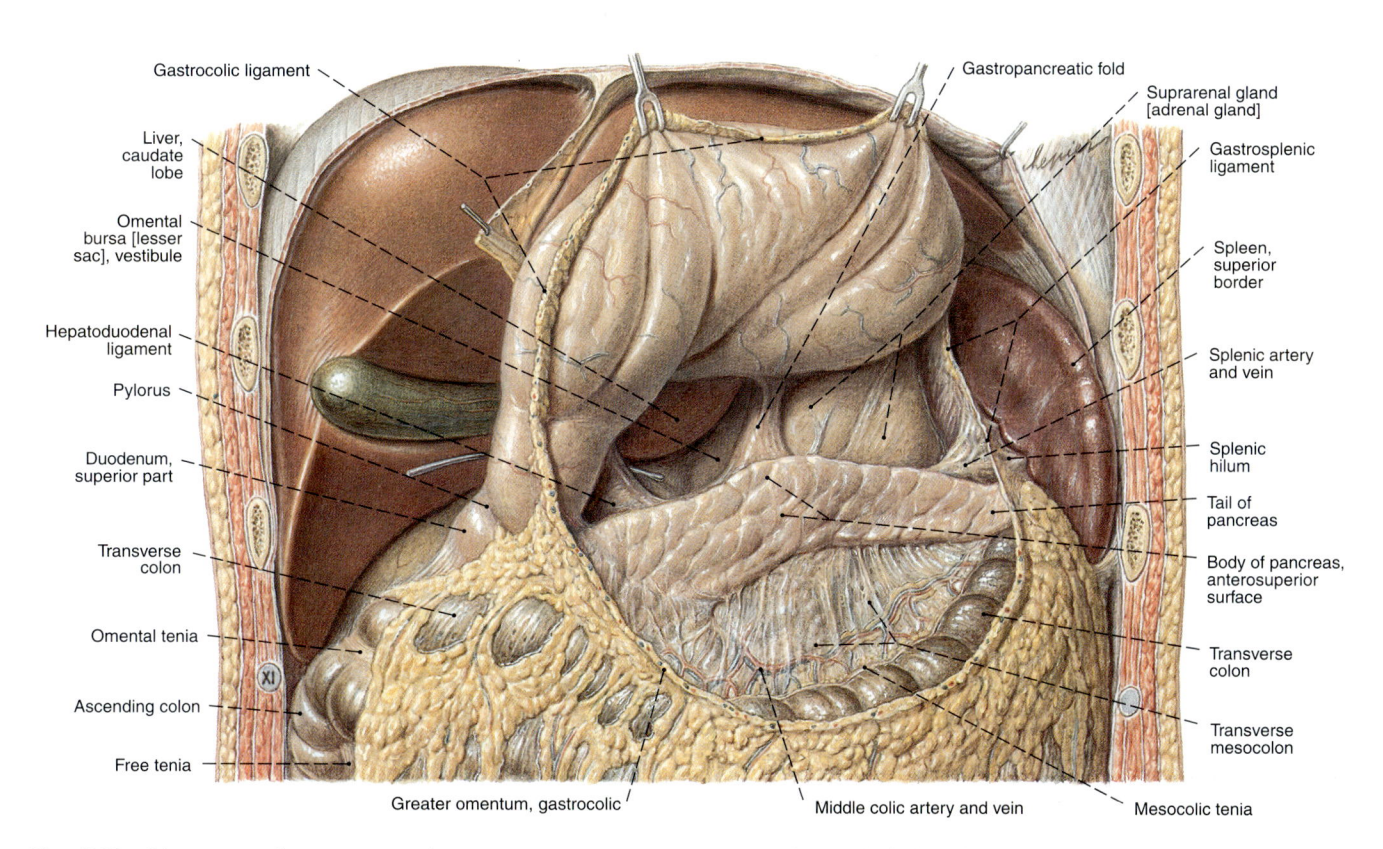

Fig. 1003 Liver; stomach; pancreas; spleen; greater omentum severed in the gastrocolic ligament; greater curvature of stomach retracted superiorly by a hook to expose omental bursa [lesser sac]; ventral aspect.

160 Abdominal viscera

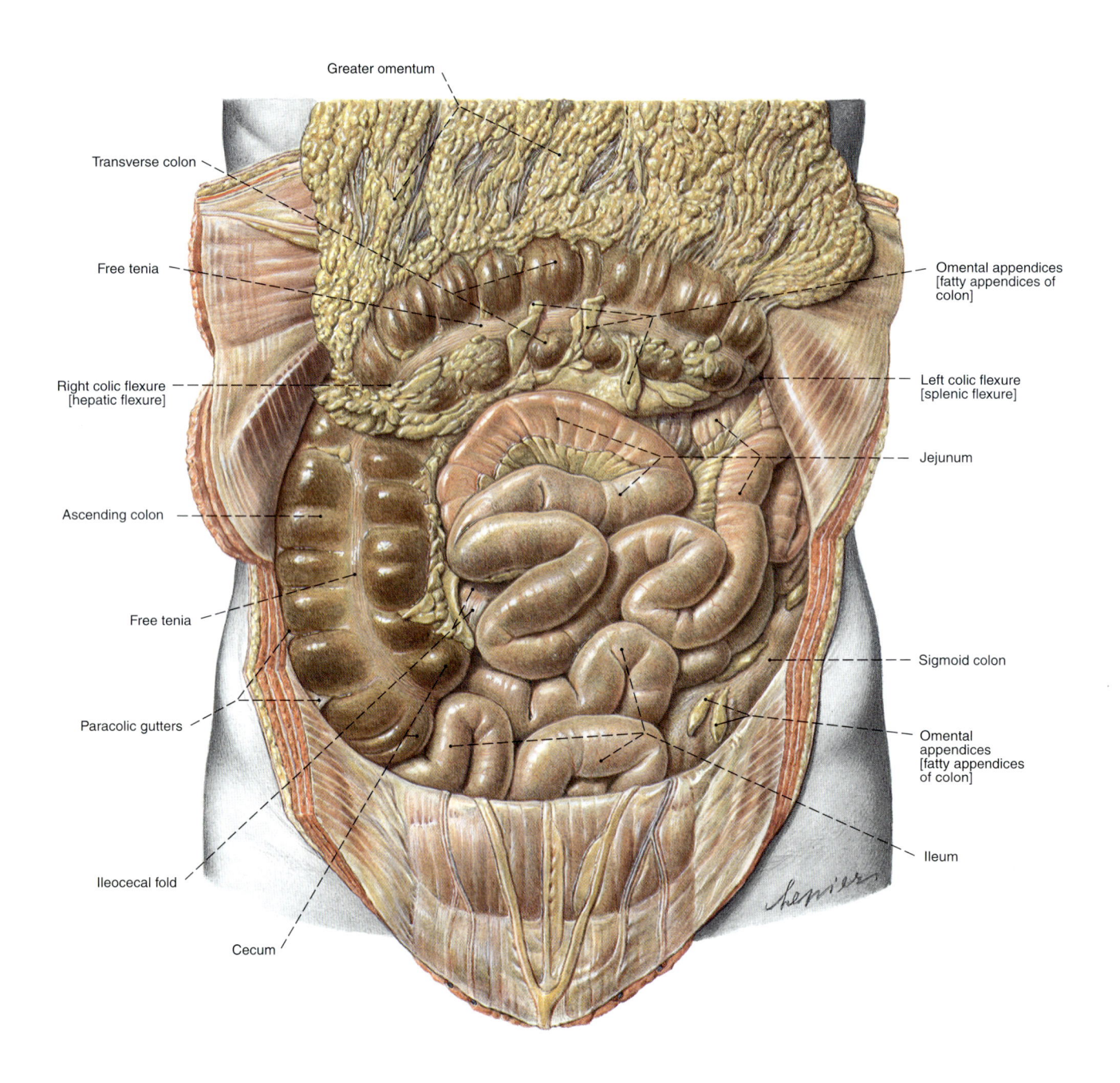

Fig. 1004   Position of abdominal viscera; greater omentum and transverse colon retracted cranially; ventral aspect.

Position of abdominal viscera **161**

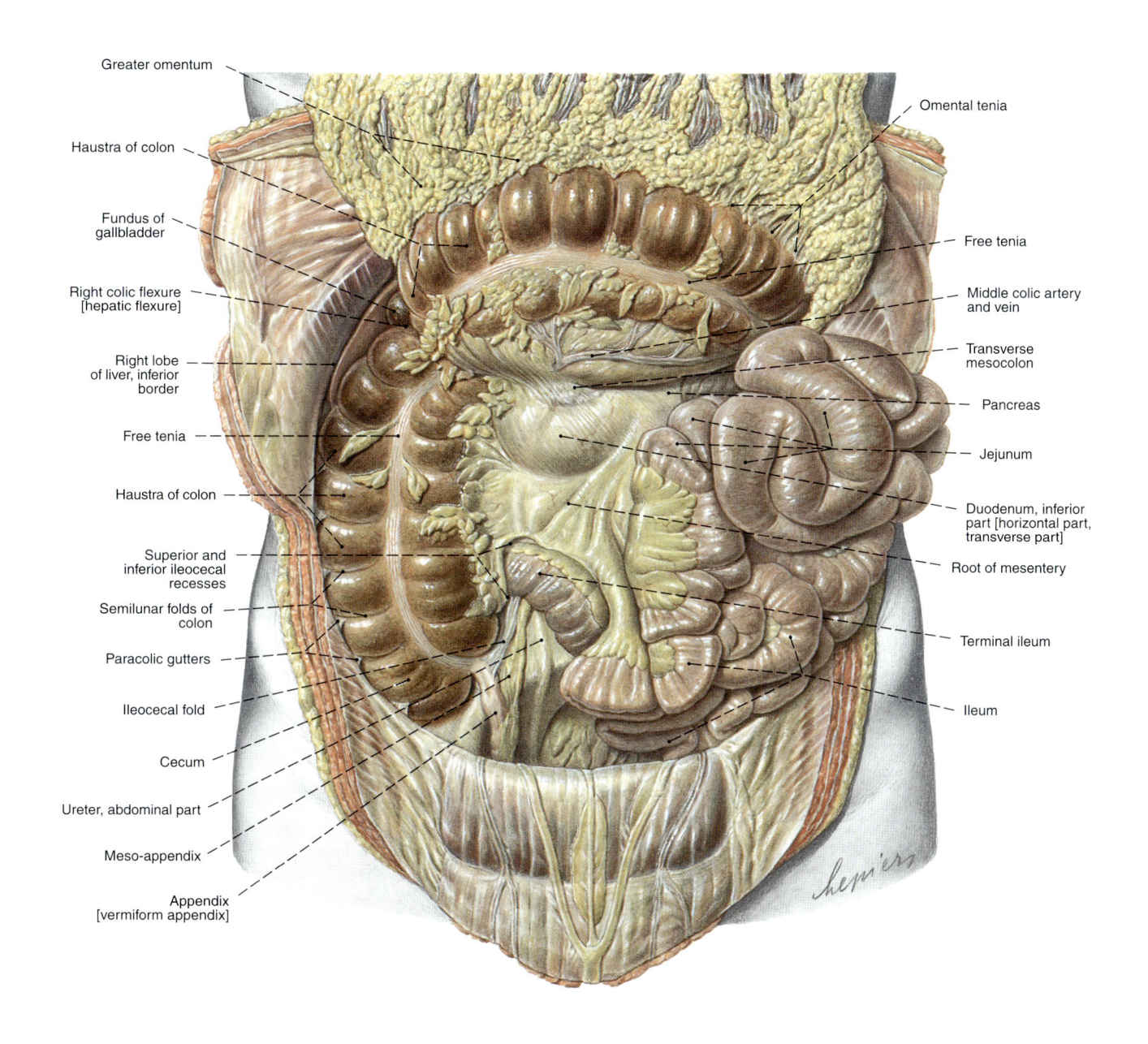

Fig. 1005 Small and large intestines; greater omentum and transverse colon reflected cranially, small intestine retracted laterally to the left to expose cecum and appendix [vermiform appendix]; ventral aspect.

Note the thin subcutaneous tissue layer and the respective thin fatty deposits in the mesentery.

Abdominal viscera

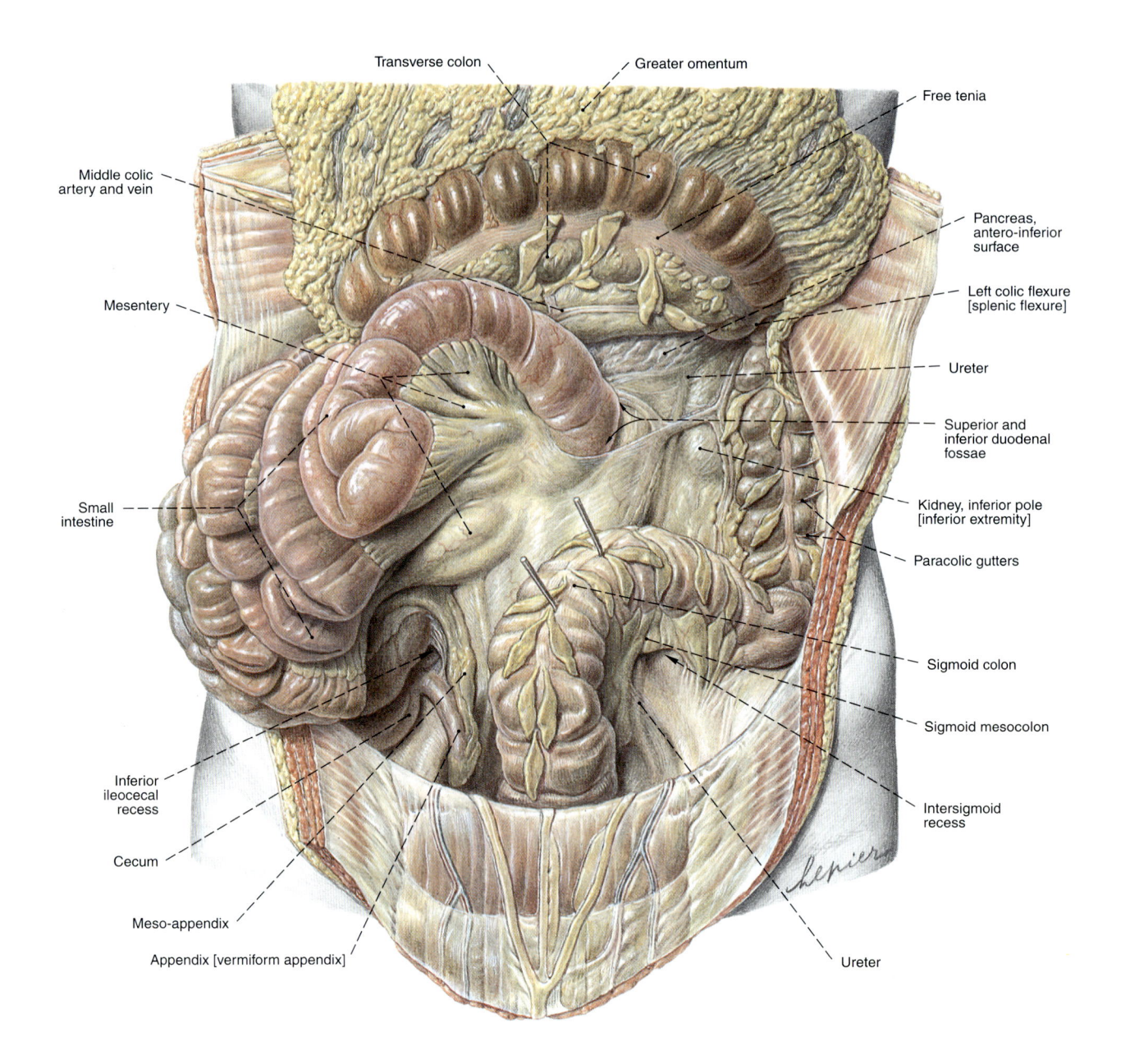

Fig. 1006 Small and large intestines; greater omentum and transverse colon reflected cranially, small intestine retracted laterally to the right; sigmoid colon retracted to the right by a hook; ventral aspect.

The recesses/ fossae/ spaces at the changes between retroperitoneal and intraperitoneal parts of the intestine vary considerably.

Position of abdominal viscera

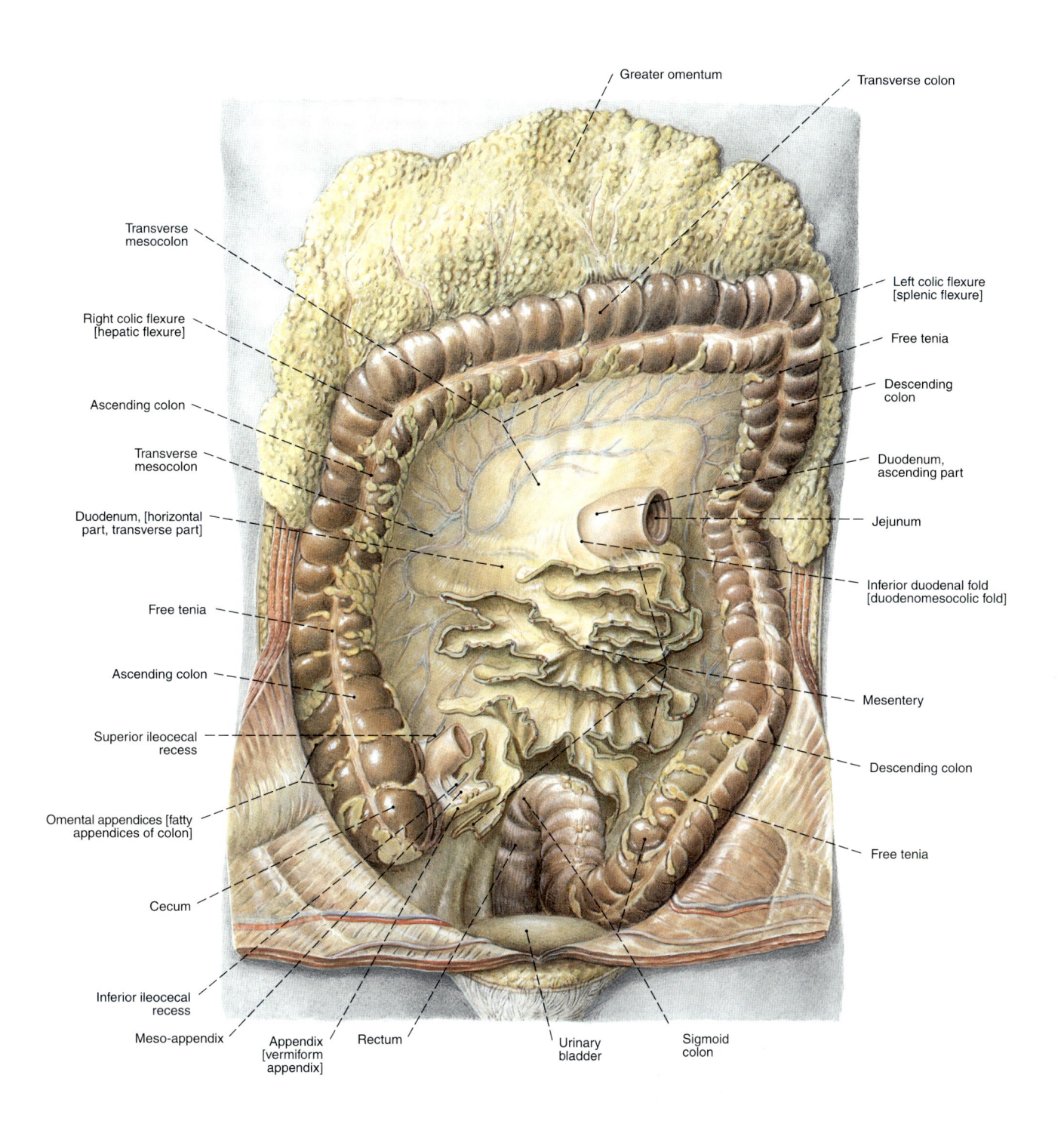

Fig. 1007 Mesentery; large intestine; greater omentum and transverse colon reflected cranially, small intestine severed next to the duodenojejunal flexure, at the terminal ileum and at the mesentery, and then removed; ventral aspect.

164 Abdominal viscera

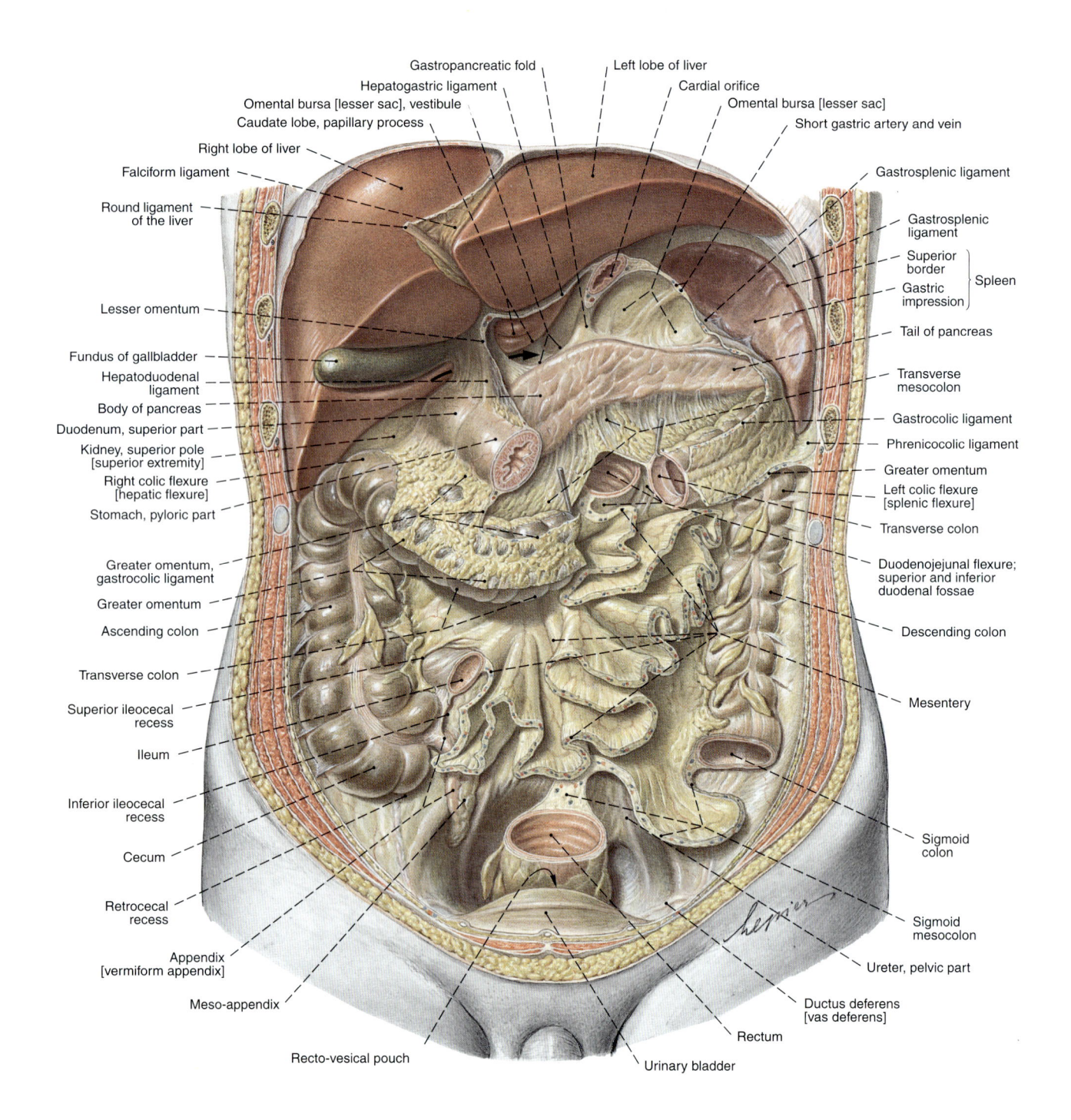

Fig. 1008 Position of abdominal viscera; stomach between cardia and pylorus, small intestine between duodenojejunal flexure and terminal ileum, and parts of transverse and sigmoid colon removed; omental bursa [lesser sac] visible with all recesses/fossae/spaces; ventral aspect.

Position of abdominal viscera 165

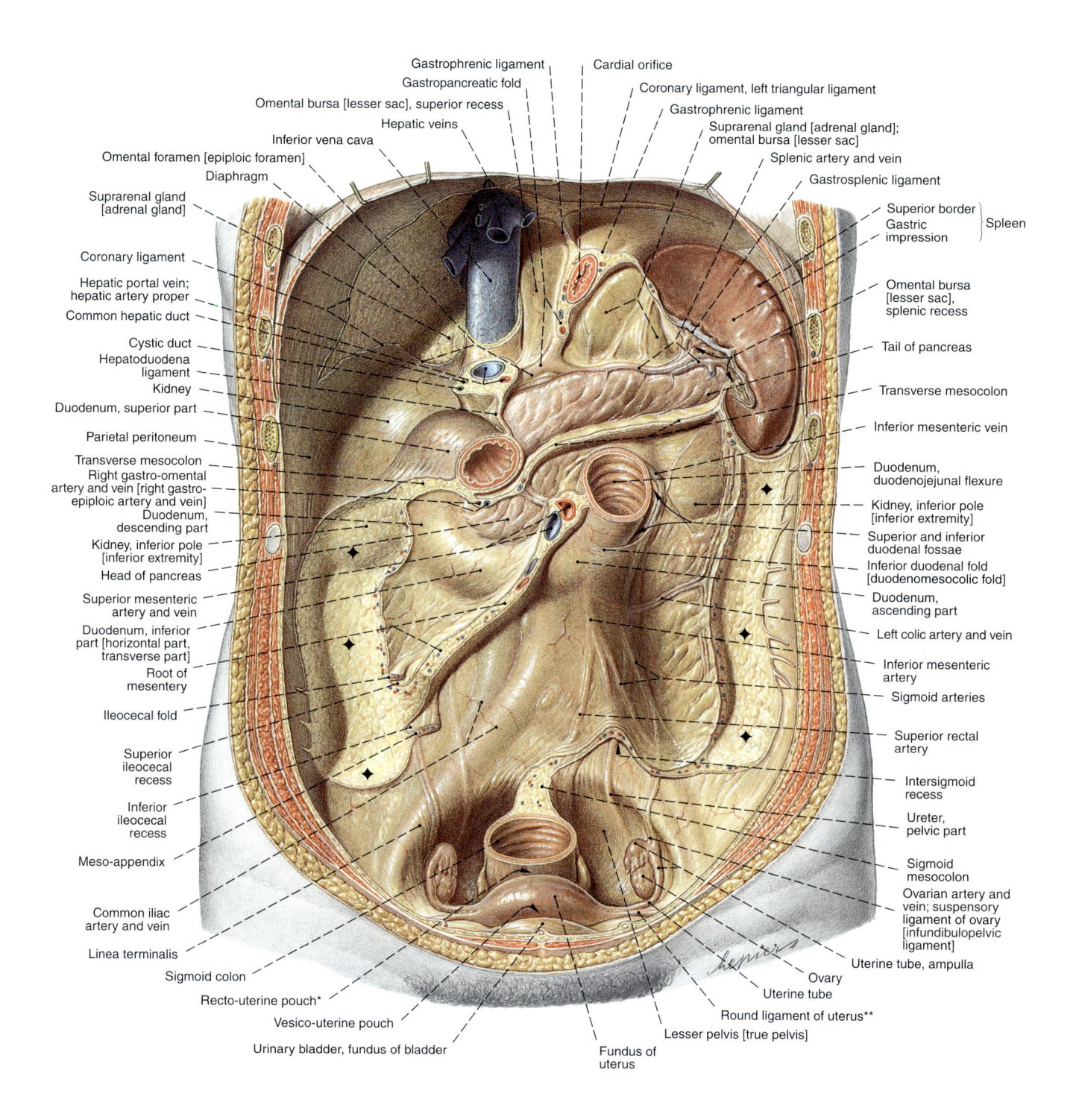

Fig. 1009   Dorsal wall of peritoneal cavity and spleen in the female after removal of liver and stomach; small intestine, except duodenum and colon, removed to expose pancreas, root of mesentery, and areas of attachment of ascending and descending colon; ventral aspect.

The areas of attachment of ascending and descending colon are marked (_).

* Clinically: pouch of DOUGLAS.
** Clinically: HUNTER's ligament.

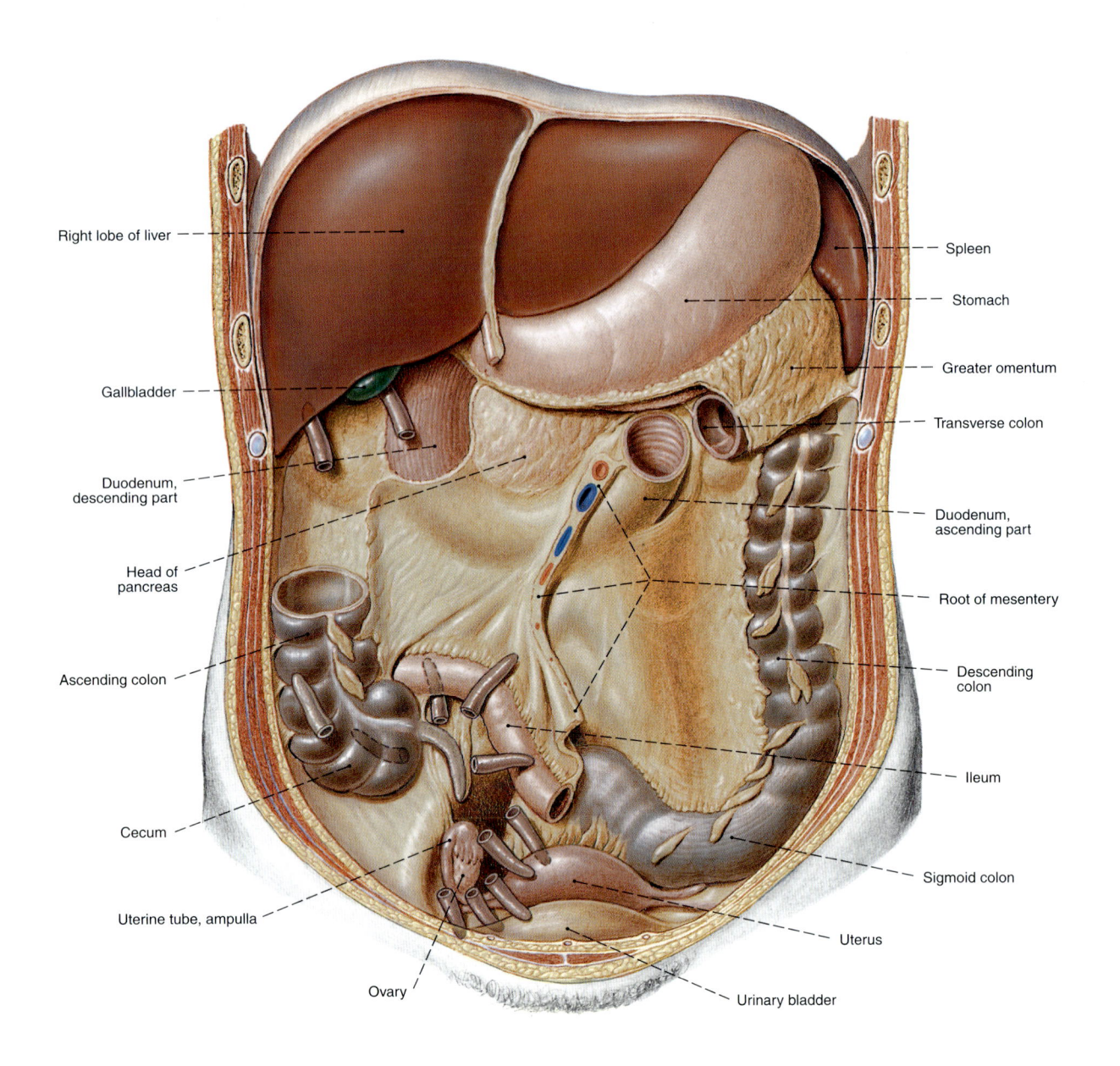

Fig. 1010 Appendix [vermiform appendix]; variations of position; ventral aspect.

Larger deviations from the normal position are frequently caused either by atypical position of the cecum (e.g.: high cecum) or by lack of peritoneal fixation of the cecum (e.g. mobile cecum).

Appendix [veriform appendix] 167

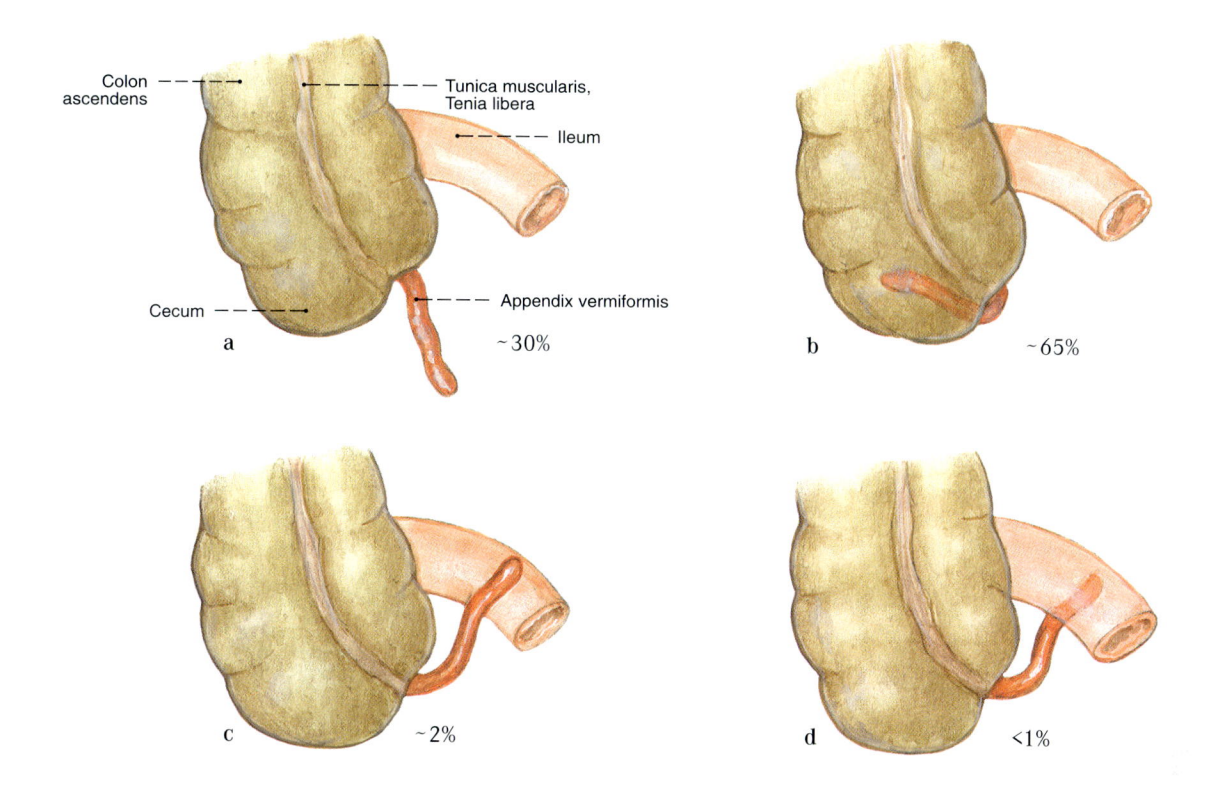

Fig. 1011 a-d Appendix [vermiform appendix]; variations of position.
    a   Descending into lesser pelvis [true pelvis]
    b   Retrocecal
    c   Pre-ileal
    d   Retro-ileal

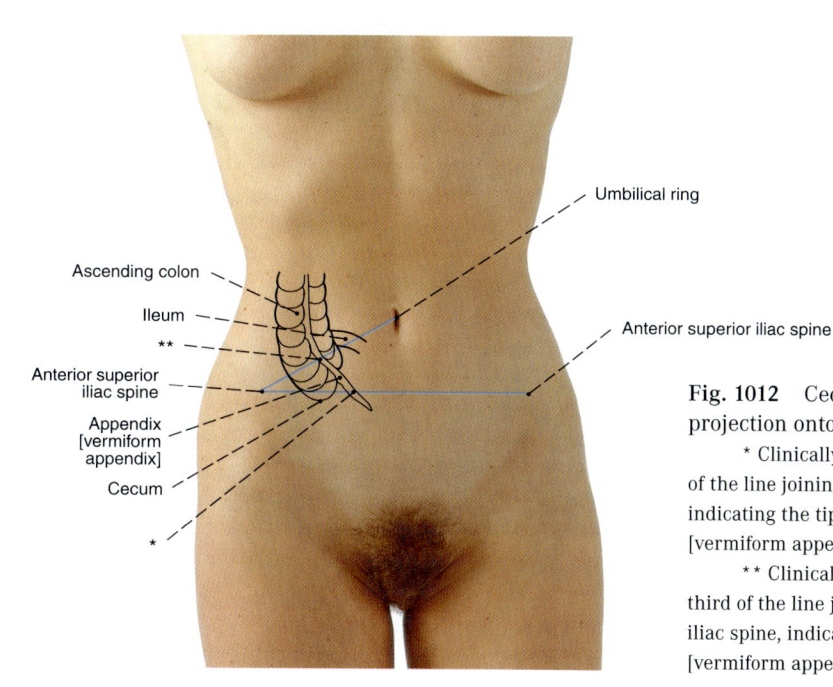

Fig. 1012 Cecum and appendix [vermiform appendix]; projection onto anterior abdominal wall.
    * Clinically: v. LANZ's point, point at the right third of the line joining the anterior superior iliac spines, indicating the tip of the descending appendix [vermiform appendix].
    ** Clinically: McBURNEY's point, point at the lateral third of the line joining umbilicus and right anterior superior iliac spine, indicating the base of the appendix [vermiform appendix].

168 Abdominal viscera

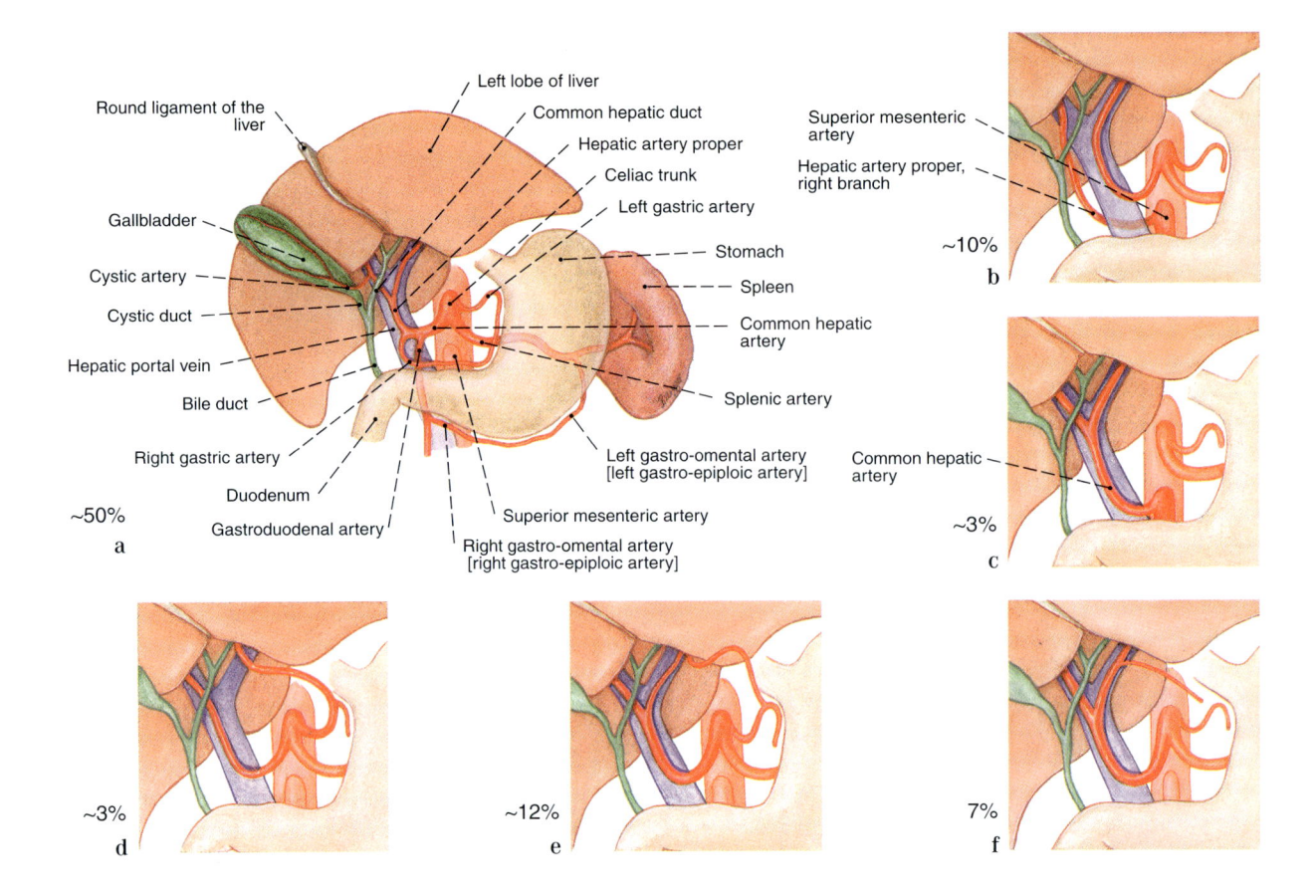

Fig. 1013 a–d Variations in the blood supply of the liver.

    a "Normal textbook case"
    b Superior mesenteric artery, participating in the supply of the right lobe of liver
    c Common hepatic artery, originating from the superior mesenteric artery
    d Left gastric artery, supplying the left lobe of liver
    e Branch of left gastric artery, participating in the supply of the left lobe of liver, in addition to left branch of hepatic artery proper
    f Accessory branch of hepatic artery proper, supplying the lesser curvature of the stomach

In 25% the superior mesenteric artery participates in the arterial blood supply of the liver.

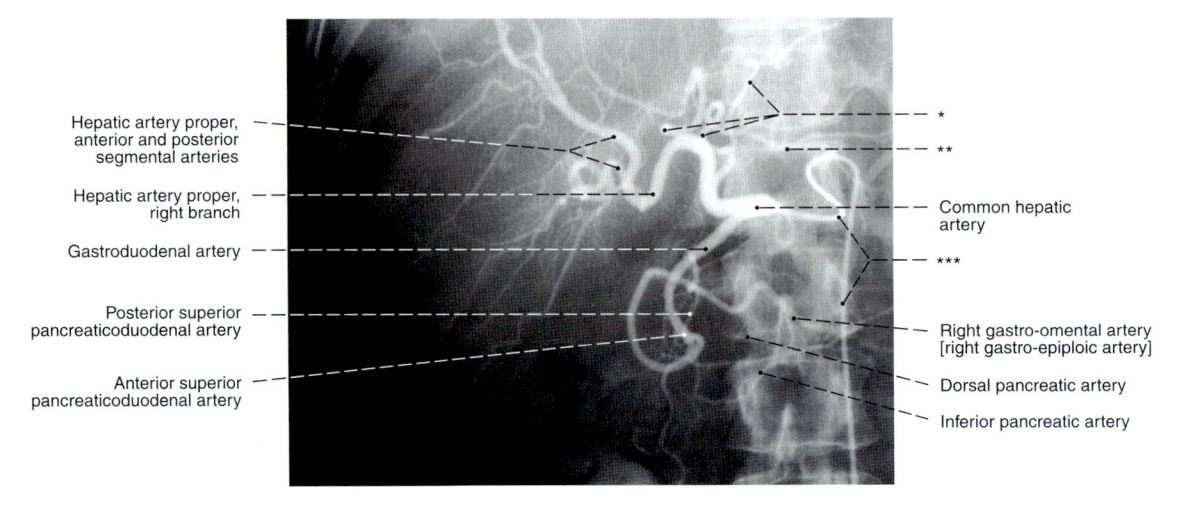

Fig. 1014 Common hepatic artery; AP radiograph after selective injection of contrast medium into the common hepatic artery; ventral aspect.

    * Branches to the left lobe of liver, replacing the left branch of hepatic artery proper.
    ** Accessory branch from the hepatic artery to the lesser curvature of the stomach.
    *** Catheter in aorta.

Position of abdominal viscera

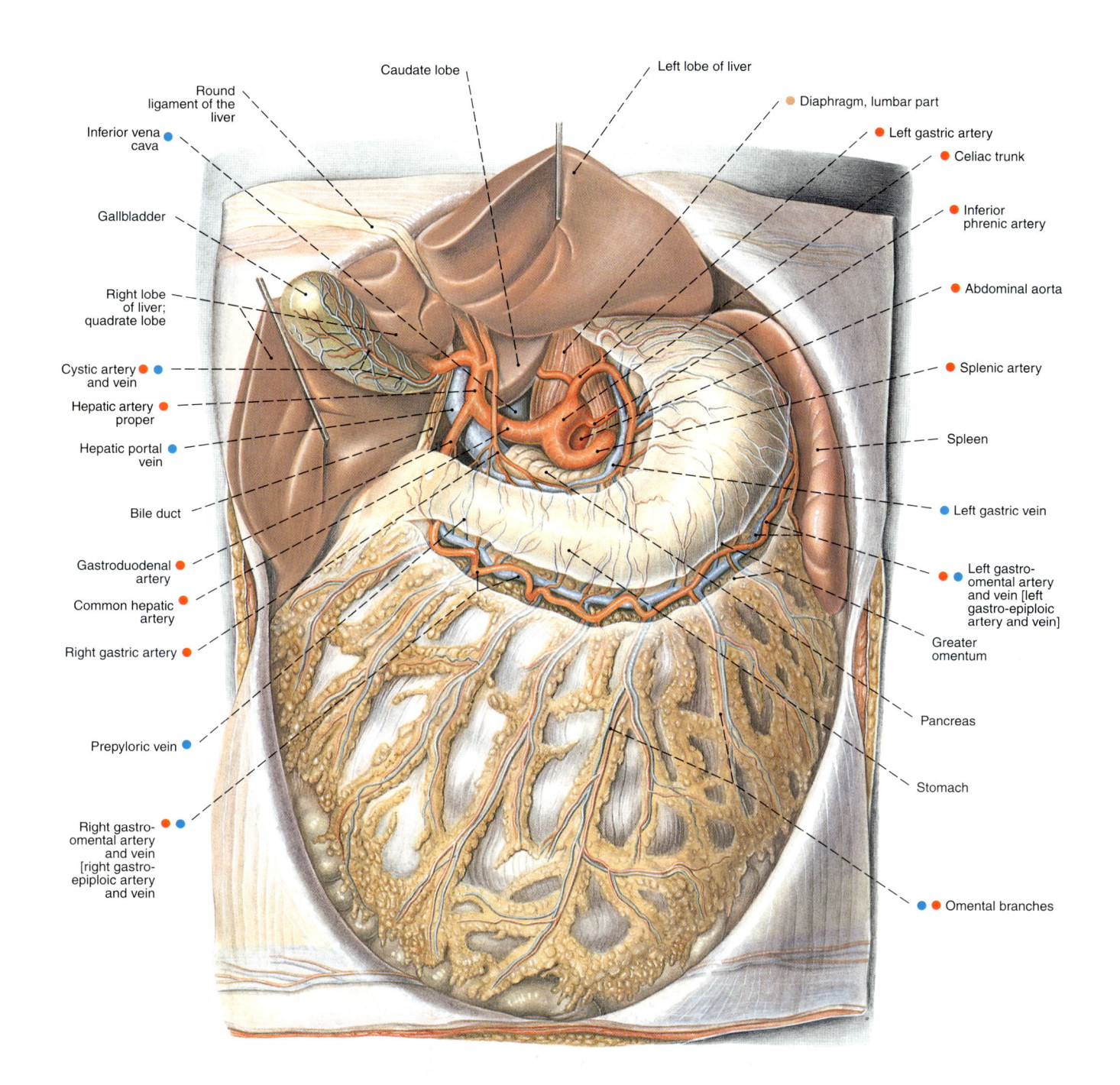

Fig. 1015 Blood vessels of the upper abdomen; lesser omentum removed to expose celiac trunk and its branches; the gastrocolic ligament and the gastro-omental [gastro-epiploic] arteries and veins dissected at the greater curvature of the stomach; the vestibule of the omental bursa [lesser sac] opened; ventral aspect.

The distance of the arteries from the lesser and greater curvature is variable.

170 Abdominal viscera

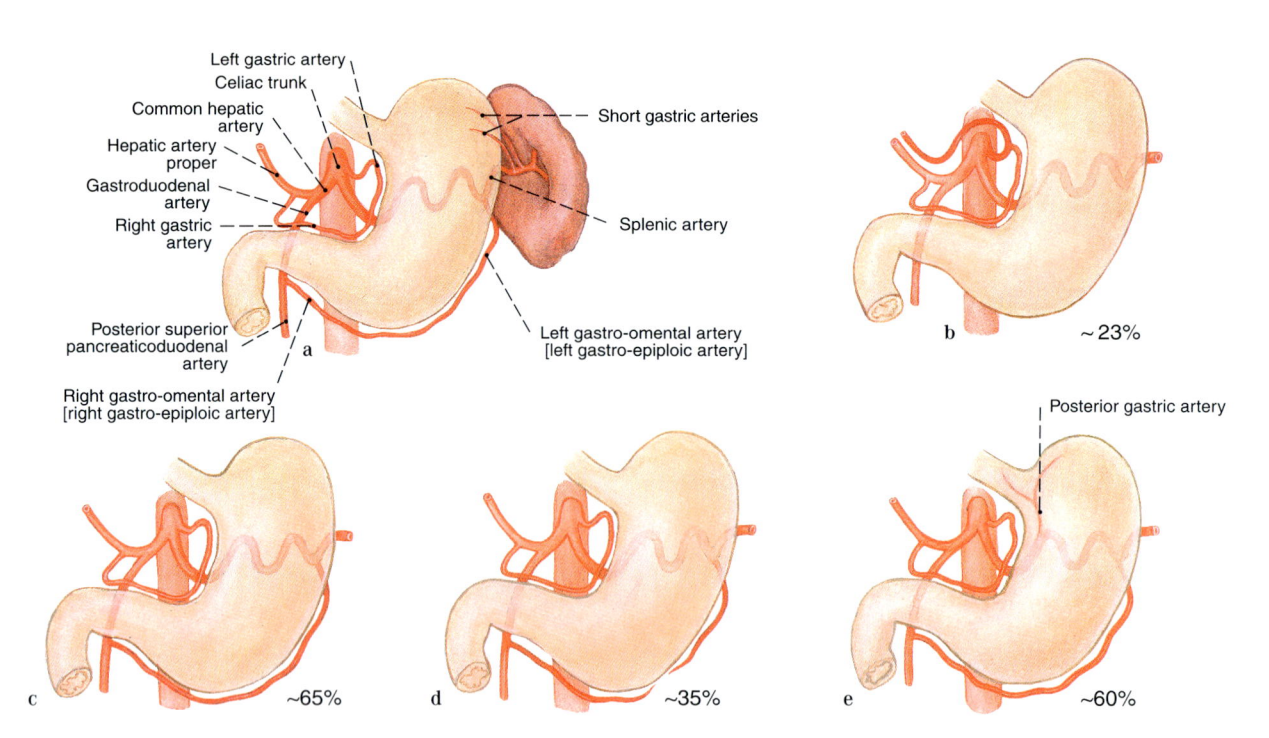

Fig. 1016 a-d Variations in the arterial blood supply of the stomach.
 a "Normal textbook case," closed arcade at the lesser and greater curvature
 b Left gastric artery participating in the supply of the left lobe of liver
 c Anastomosis between right and left gastro-omental arteries [left gastro-epiploic arteries] at greater curvature (closed arcade)
 d No anastomosis between right and left gastro-omental arteries [left gastro-epiploic arteries] at greater curvature (not closed arcade)
 e Accessory posterior gastric artery branching off the splenic artery and supplying the posterior wall of stomach

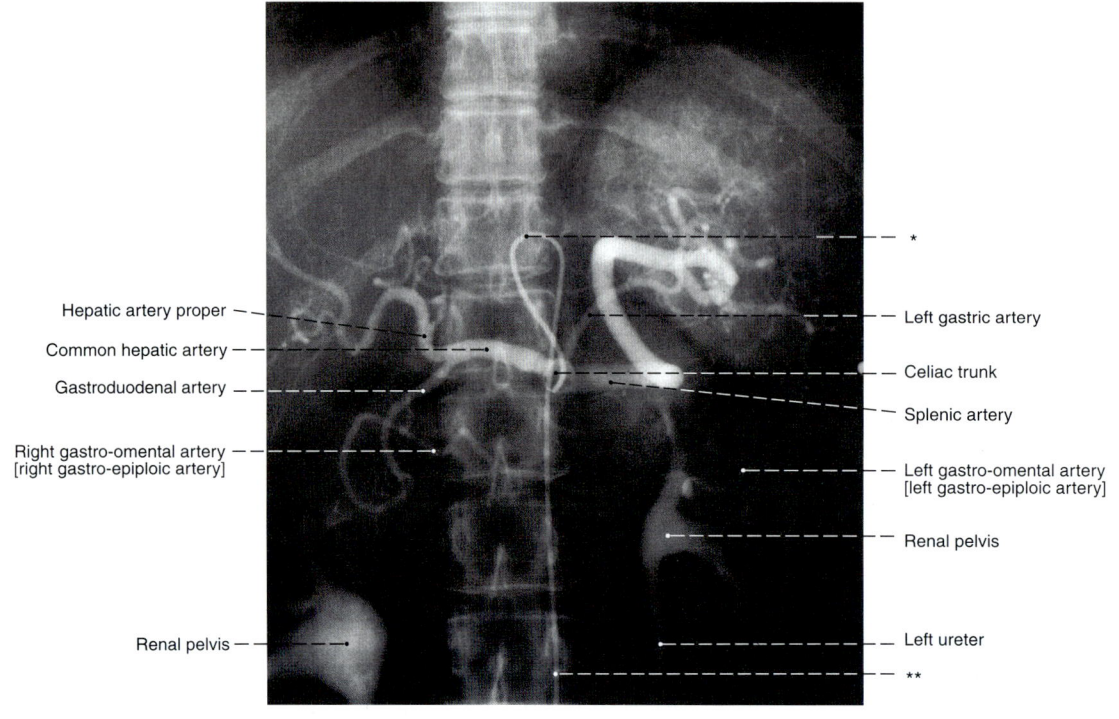

Fig. 1017 Arteries of stomach, spleen, and liver; AP radiograph after selective injection of contrast medium into the celiac trunk (celiac arteriography) and simultaneous visualization of the renal pelvis after intravenous injection of a renal-excreted contrast medium; ventral aspect.
 * Loop of catheter in aorta.
 ** Catheter in aorta.

Position of abdominal viscera 171

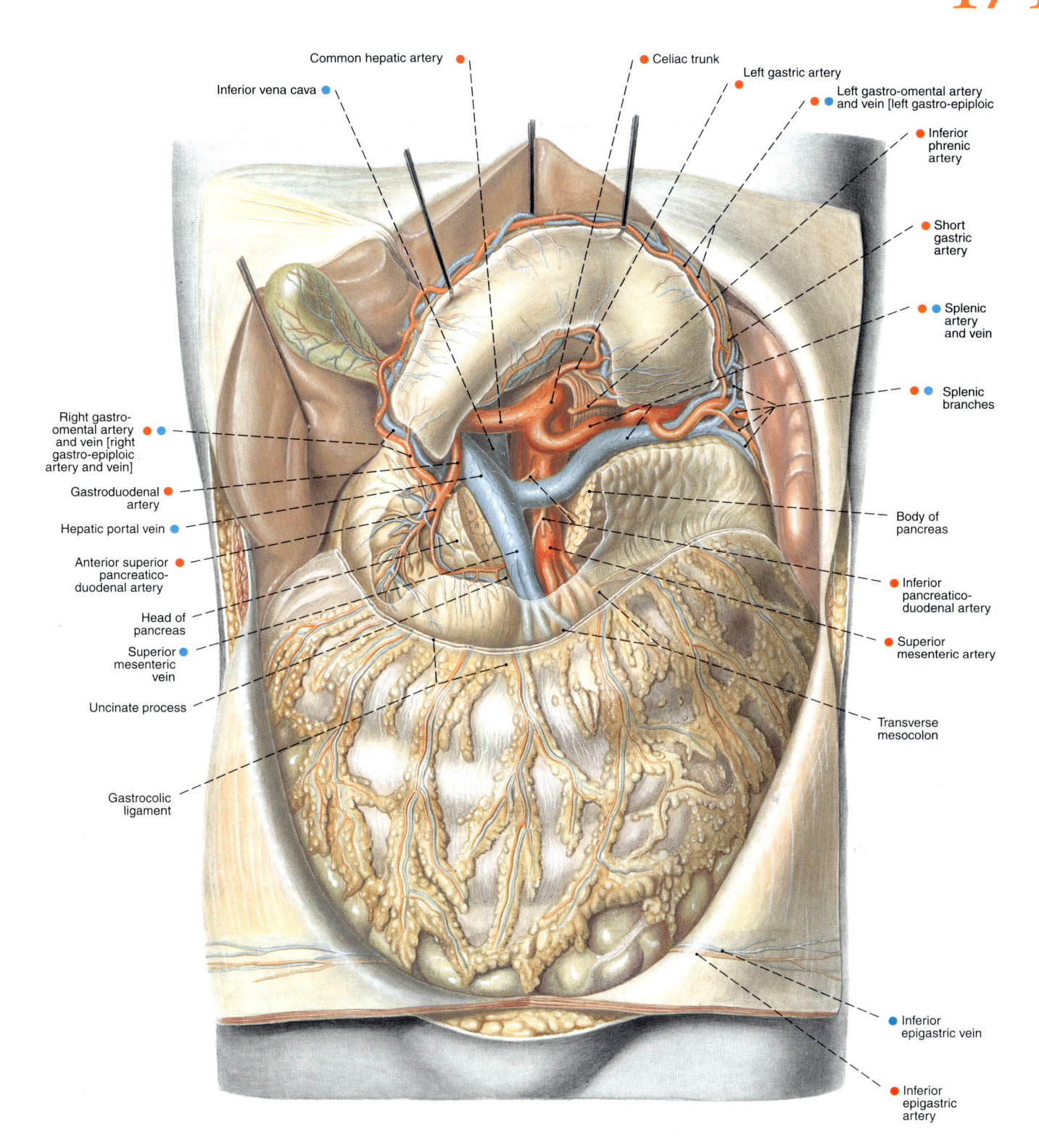

Fig. 1018 Blood vessels of the upper abdomen; gastrocolic ligament severed; stomach retracted cranially by a hook to expose celiac trunk; body of pancreas partially removed to expose the junction of the splenic and superior mesenteric veins; omental bursa [lesser sac] opened; ventral aspect.

The uncinate process of pancreas frequently pushes far behind the mesenteric blood vessels.

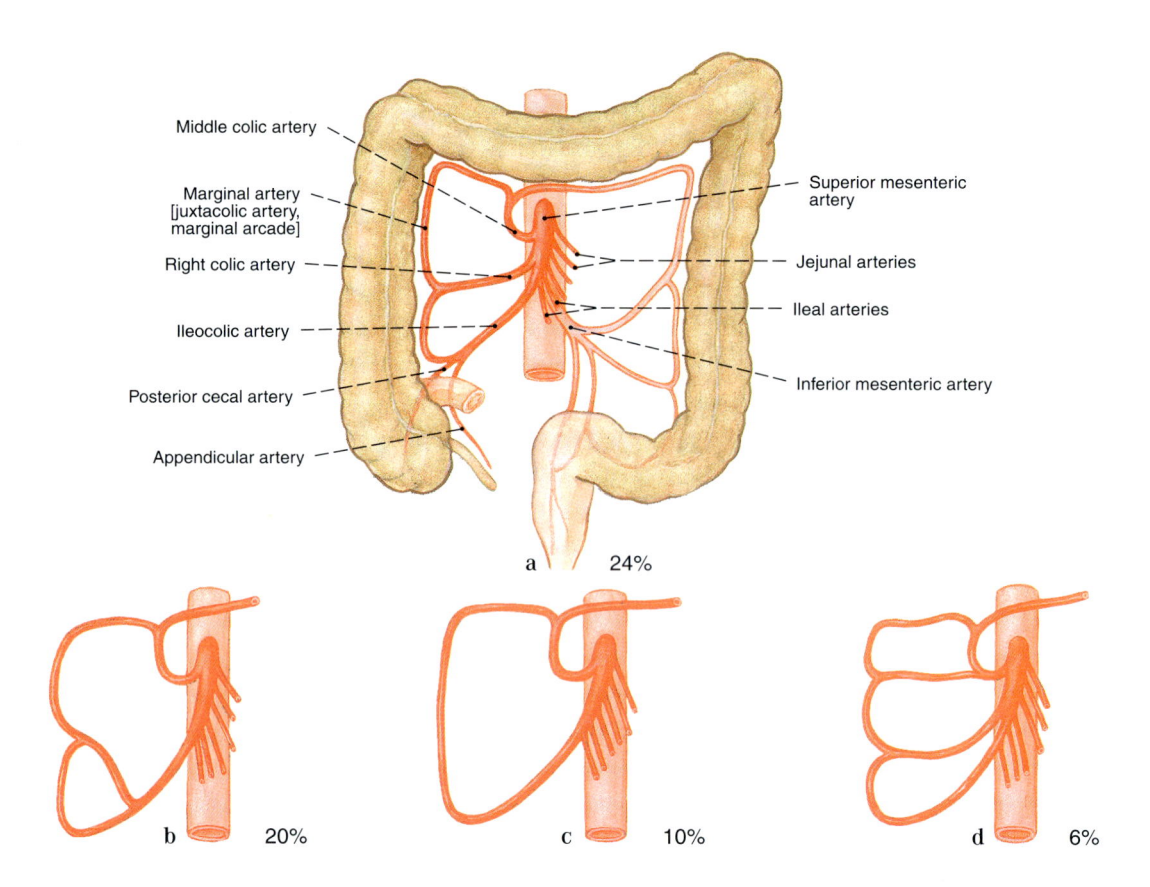

172 Abdominal viscera

Fig. 1019 a–d Variations in the branches of the superior mesenteric artery to the large intestine.

    a   "Normal textbook case," ascending and transverse colon supplied by three branches

b   Trunk-formation of ileocolic and right colic arteries
c   Two branches only with right colic artery absent
d   Double right colic artery

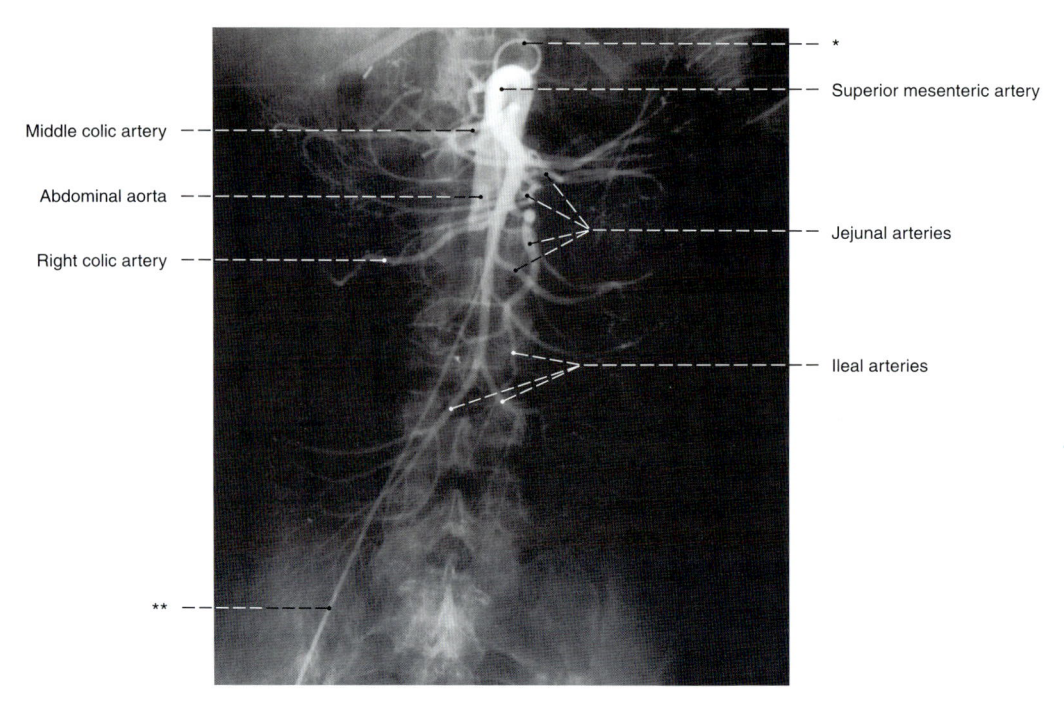

Fig. 1020 Superior mesenteric artery; AP radiograph after selective injection of contrast medium into the beginning of the superior mesenteric artery; ventral aspect.

* Catheter in aorta.
** Catheter in the common iliac artery.

Superior mesenteric artery and vein

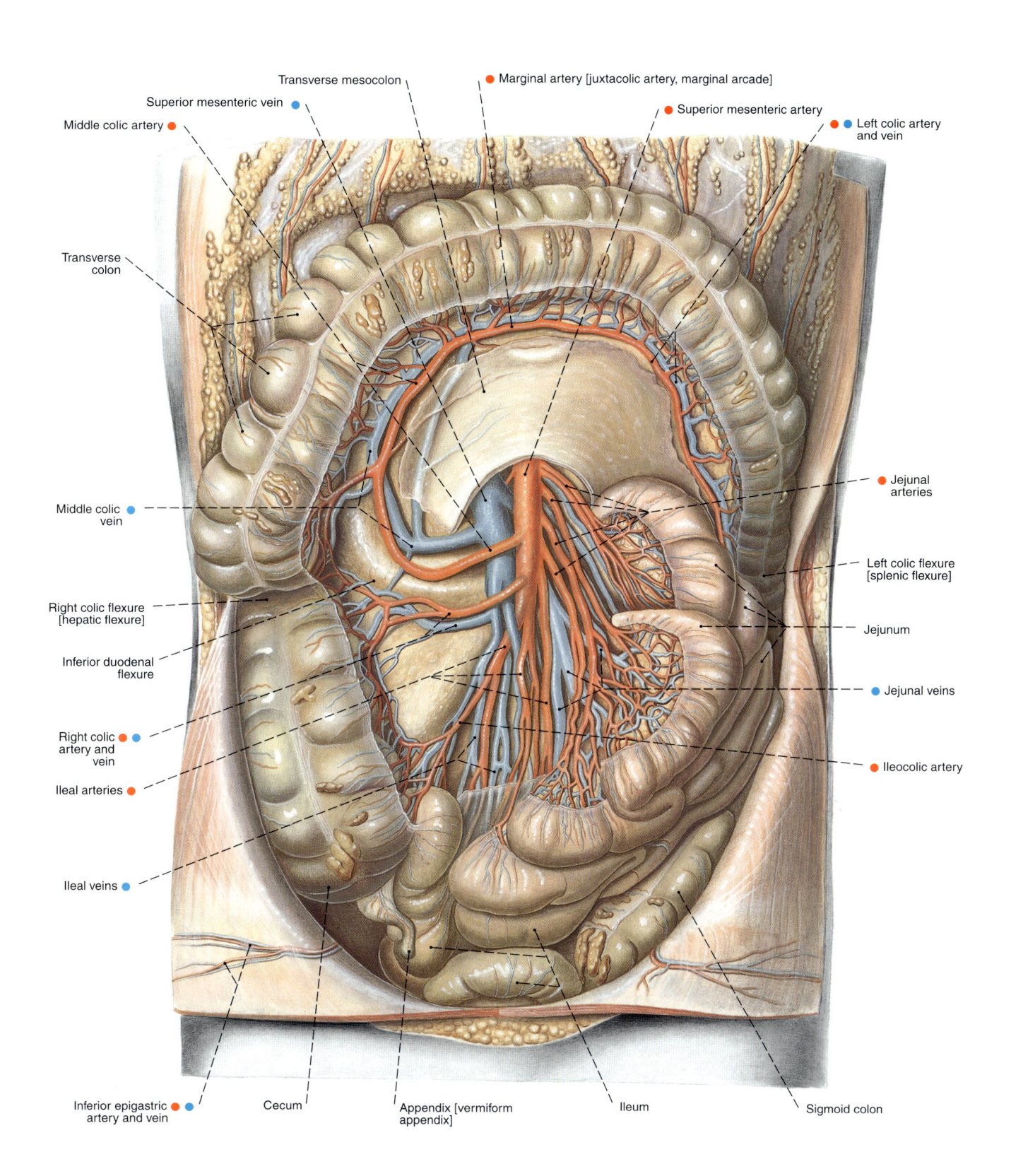

Fig. 1021 Blood vessels of the lower abdomen; greater omentum and transverse colon retracted cranially; small intestine displaced to the left and visceral peritoneum partially removed to expose the blood vessels; ventral aspect. The arteries of the small intestine form arcades.

Abdominal viscera

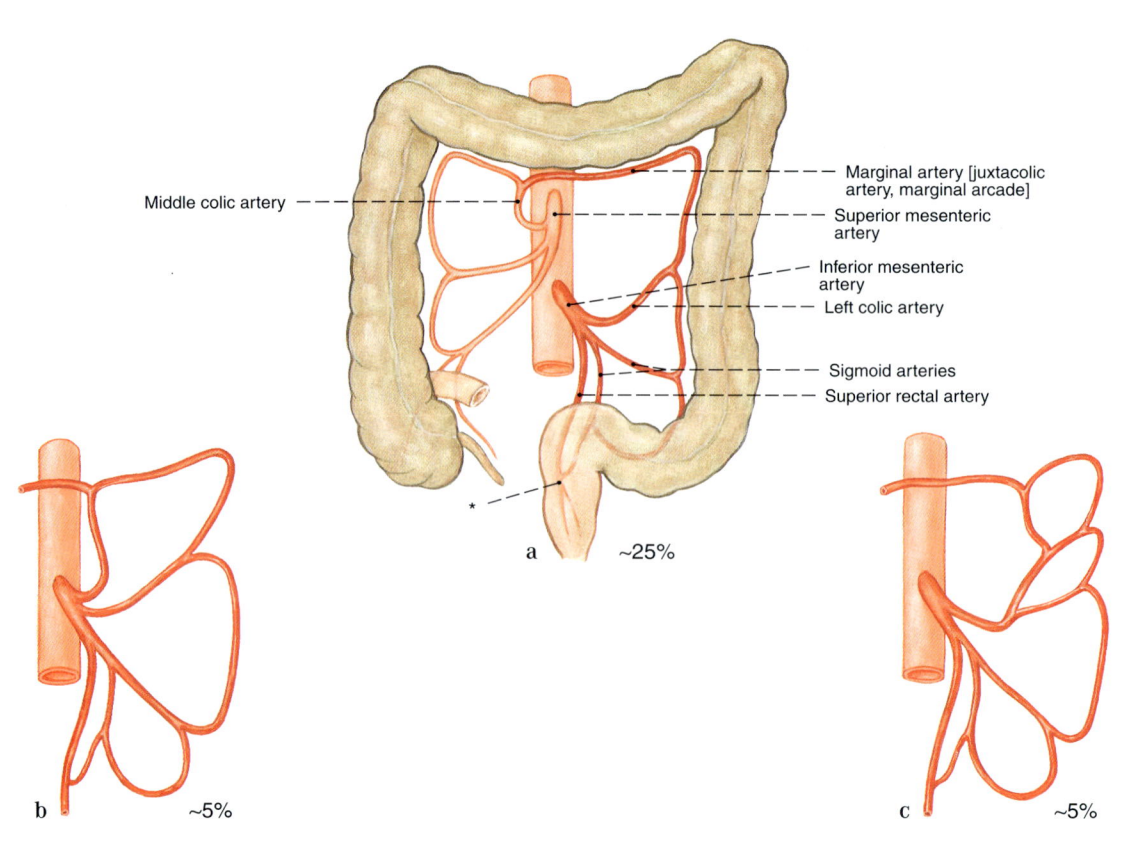

Fig. 1022 a–c Variations in the branches of the inferior mesenteric artery.
    a   Trifurcating trunk supplying the descending colon, the sigmoid colon, and the rectum
    b   Accessory middle colic artery from the inferior mesenteric artery
    c   Accessory middle colic artery from the left colic artery
* Clinically: critical point of SUDECK.

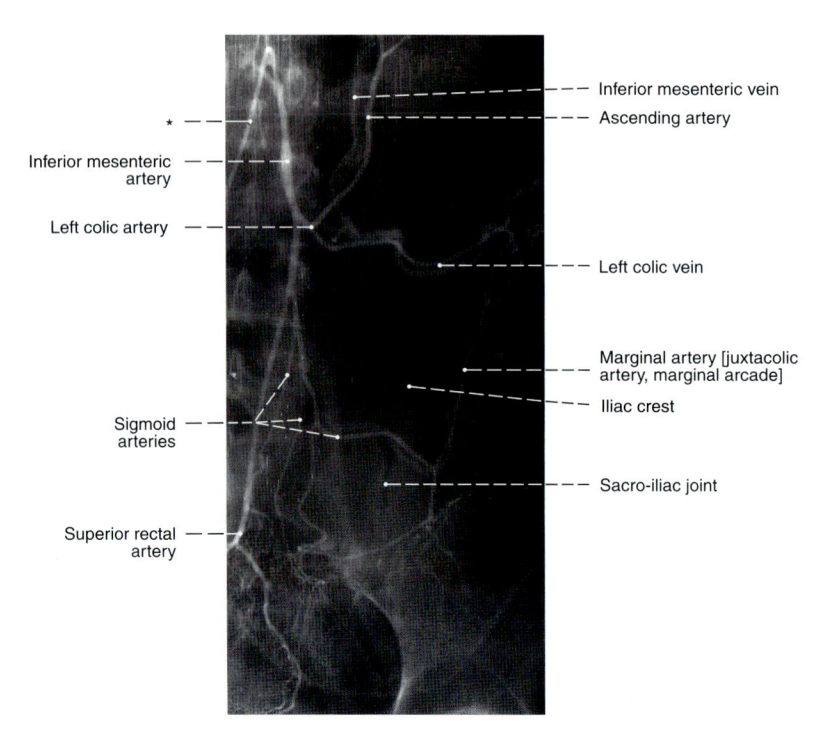

Fig. 1023 Inferior mesenteric artery; AP radiograph after selective injection of contrast medium into the beginning of the inferior mesenteric artery; ventral aspect. The contrast medium partially runs off the colon already; therefore, the veins are also visible.
   * Catheter in aorta.

Inferior mesenteric artery and vein 175

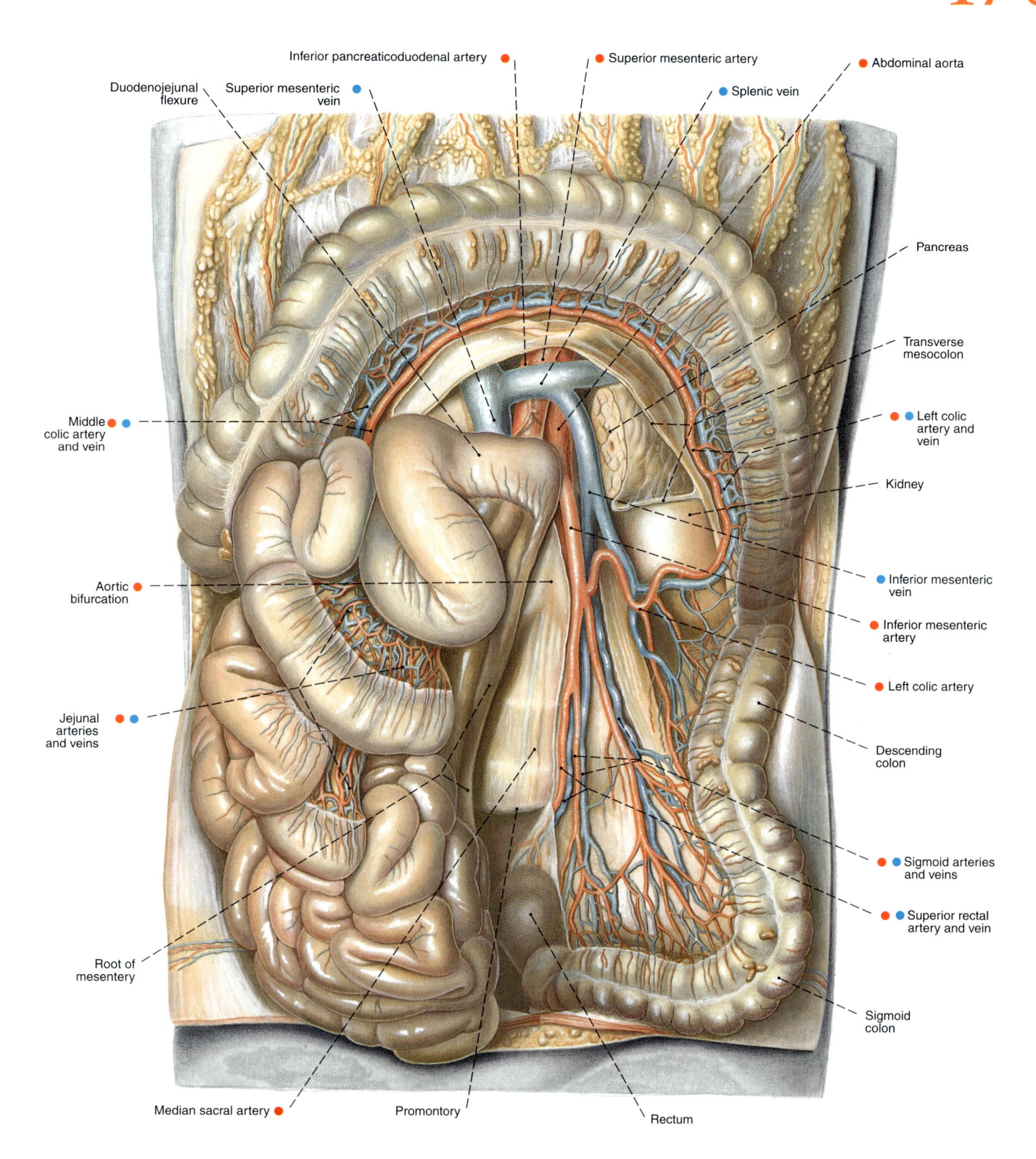

Fig. 1024 Inferior mesenteric artery and vein; small intestine displaced to the right; transverse colon retracted cranially; peritoneum removed to expose the blood vessels of descending and sigmoid colon; ventral aspect.

The connections of the left and middle colic arteries is accomplished by the marginal artery [juxtacolic artery, marginal arcade].

176 Abdominal viscera

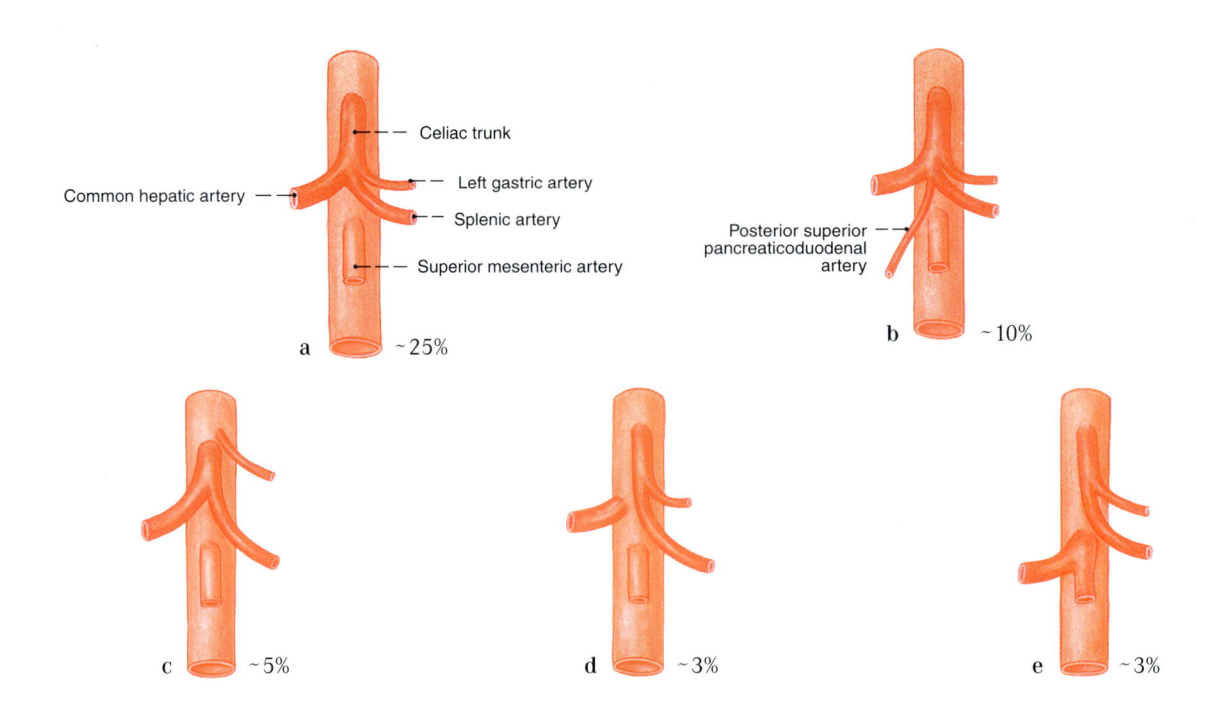

Fig. 1025 a–e Variations of the celiac trunk.
a "Normal textbook case", trifurcating trunk
b Division into four branches
c Formation of a hepatosplenic trunk
d Formation of a gastrosplenic trunk
e Formation of a gastrosplenic trunk and a hepatomesenteric trunk

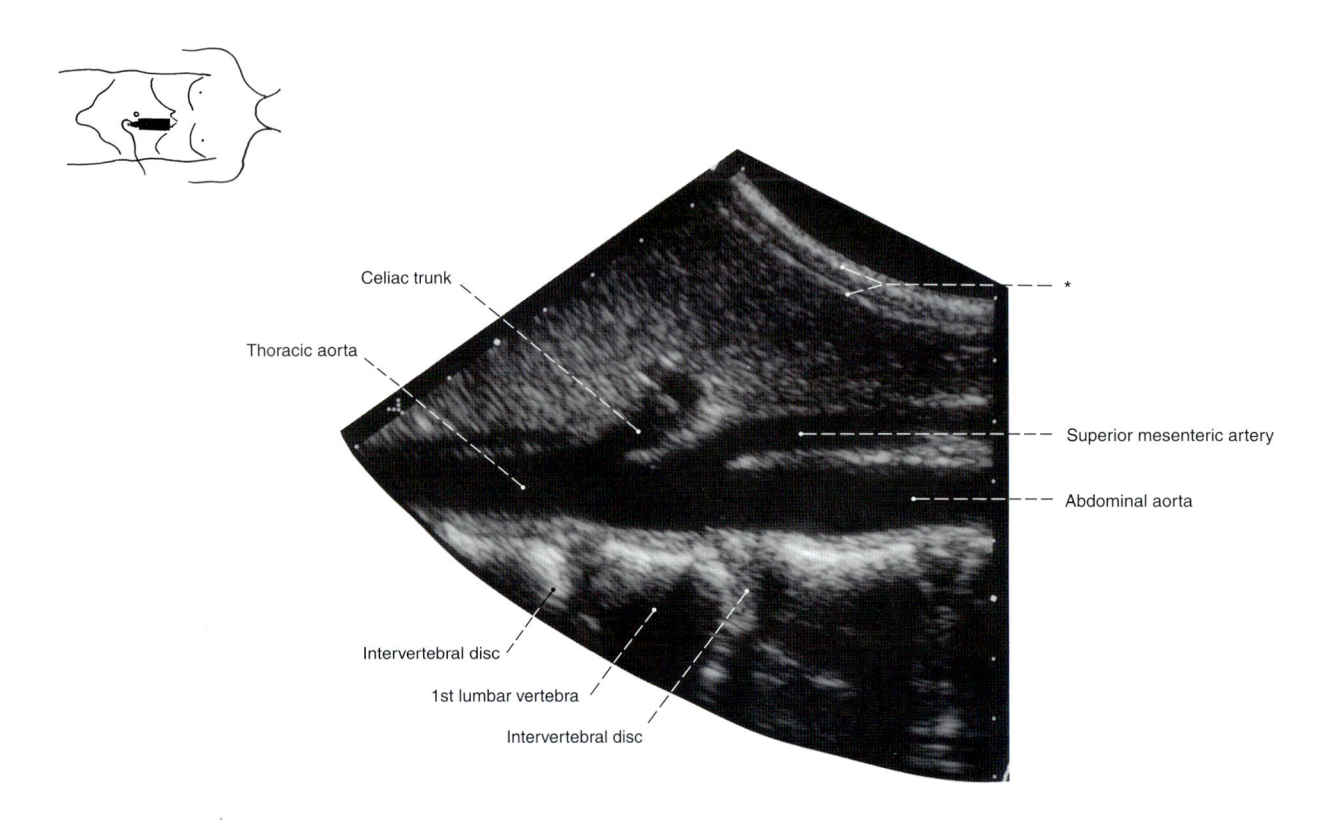

Fig. 1026 Abdominal aorta; ultrasound scan in nearly sagittal plane. Note the short distance between celiac trunk and superior mesenteric artery, which runs partially parallel to the abdominal aorta.

* Abdominal wall.

Position of retroperitoneal organs

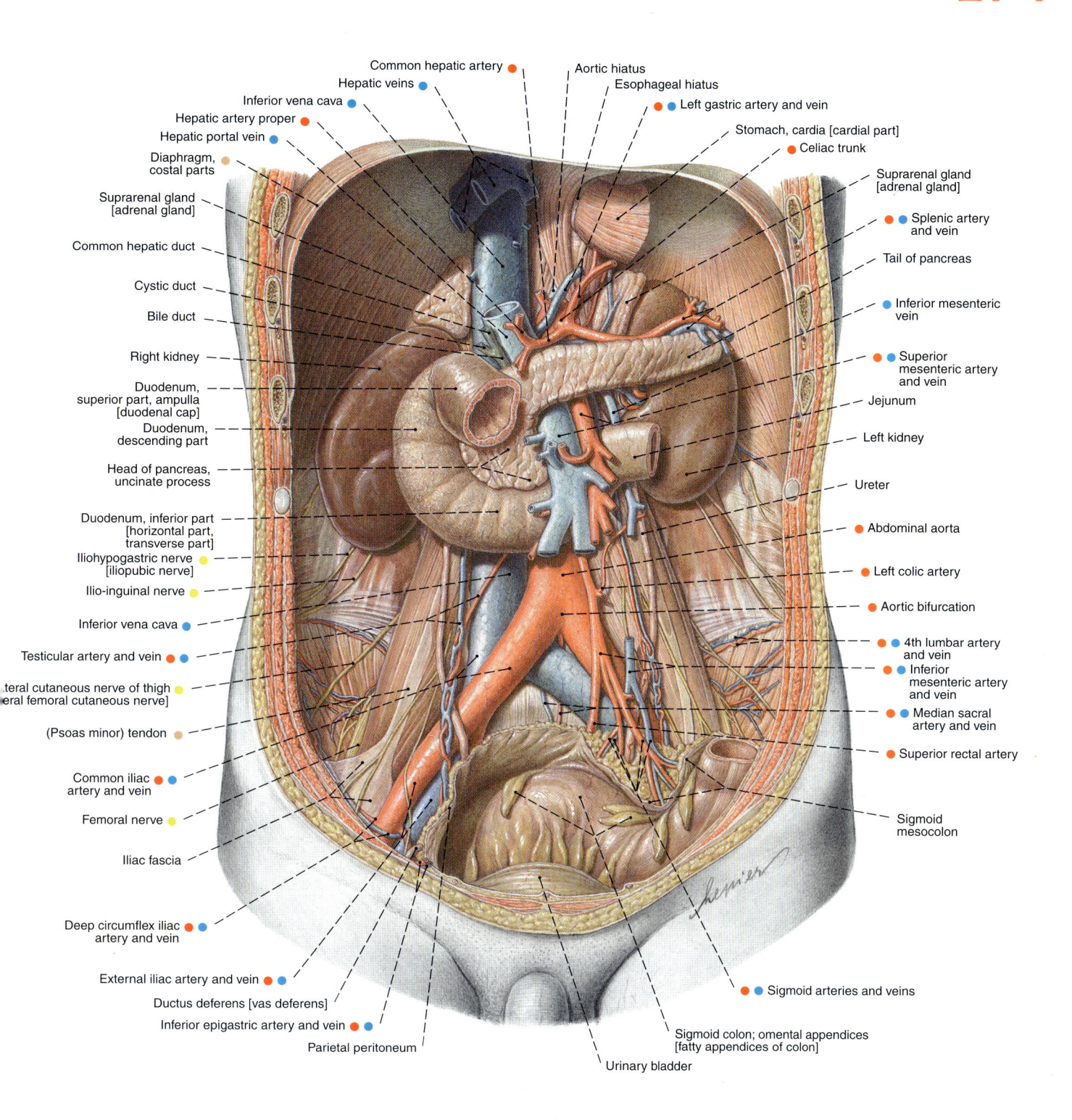

Fig. 1027 Retroperitoneal space in the male; parietal peritoneum extensively removed; ventral aspect.

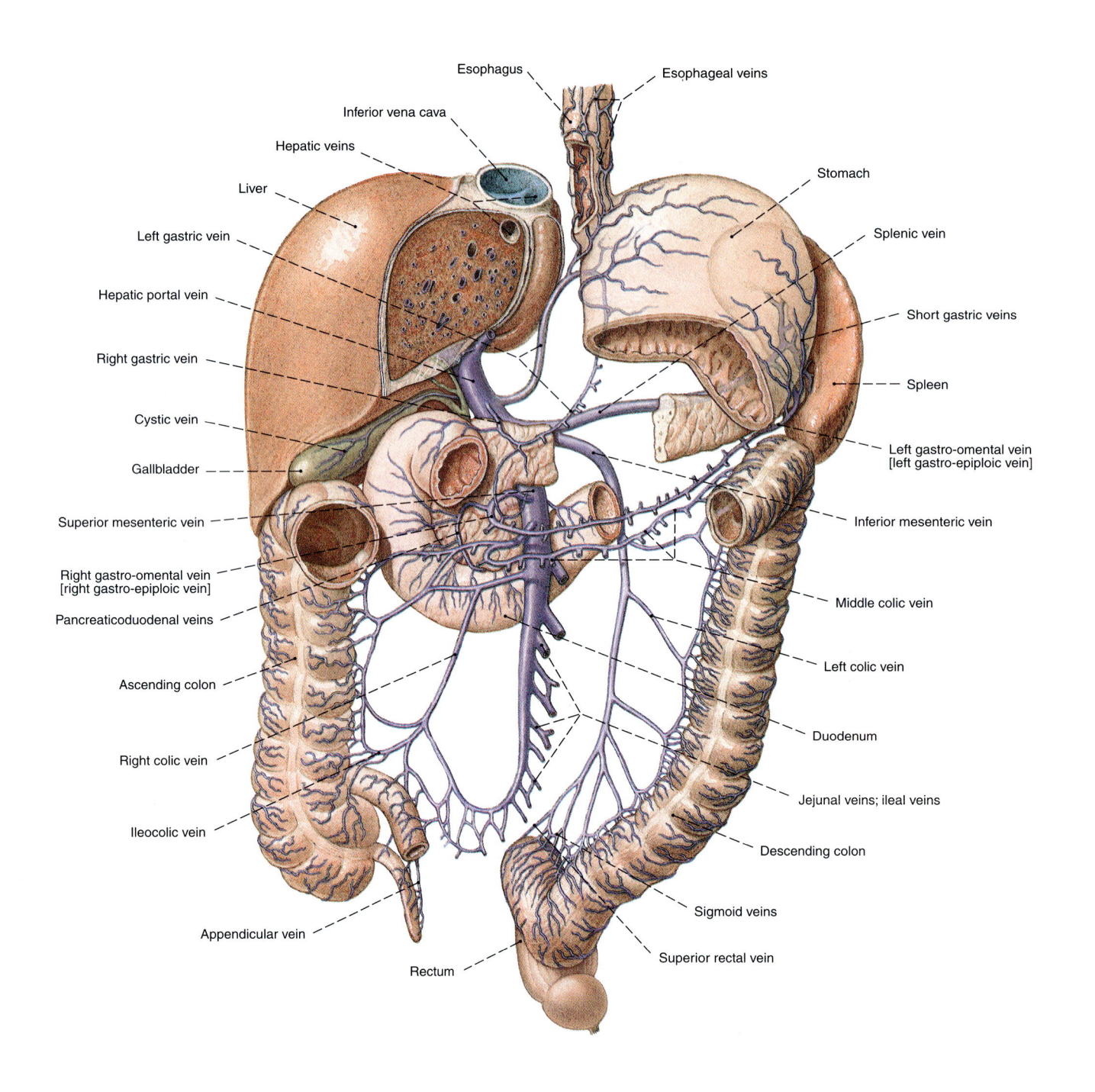

Fig. 1028 Tributaries of hepatic portal vein; parts of stomach and transverse colon and also larger parts of jejunum and ileum removed; ventral aspect.

Hepatic portal vein, inferior vena cava

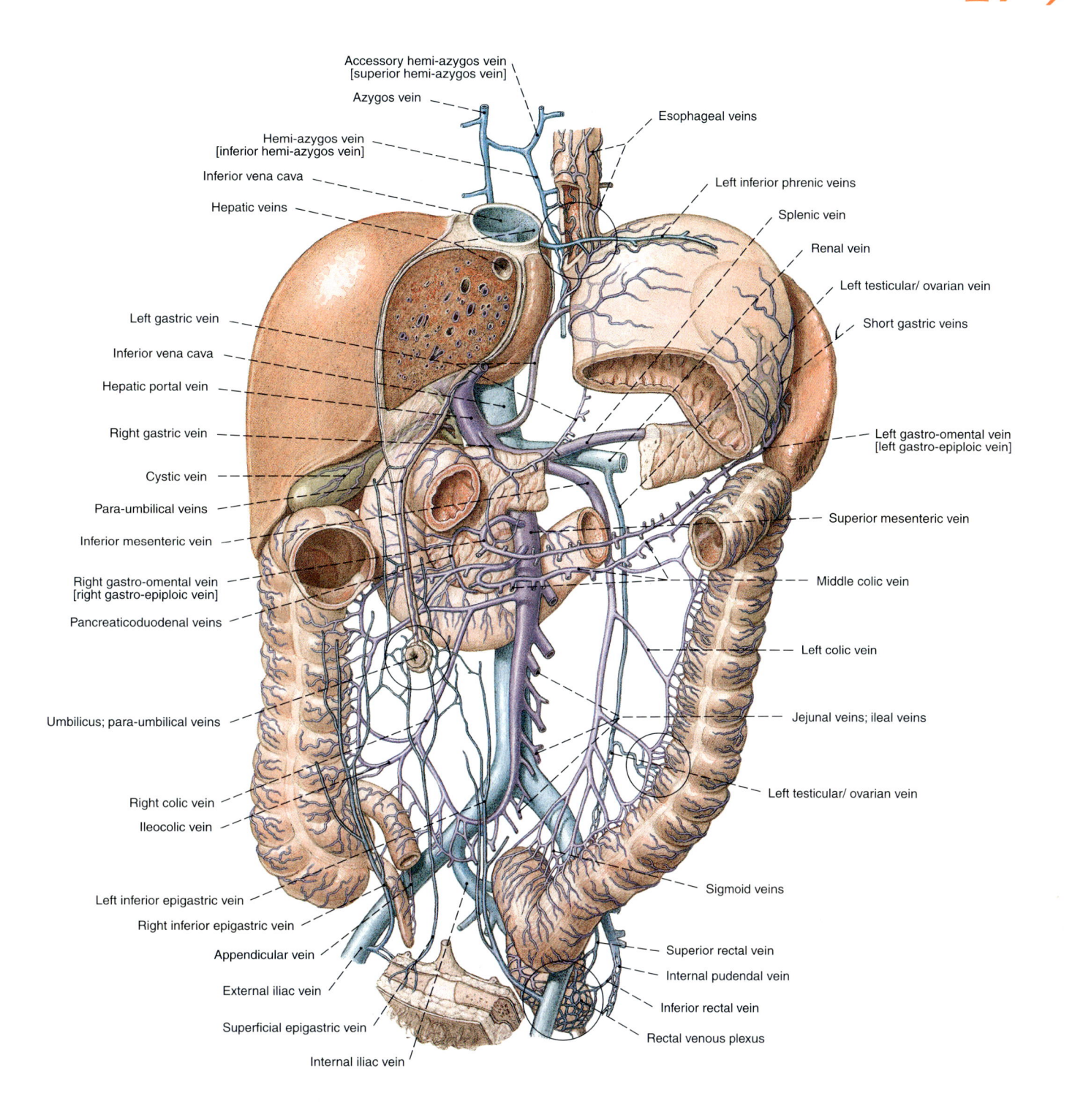

Fig. 1029 Connections between tributaries of hepatic portal vein and inferior vena cava; ventral aspect. These connections—indicated by circles—are called "portocaval anastomoses."

180 *Abdominal viscera*

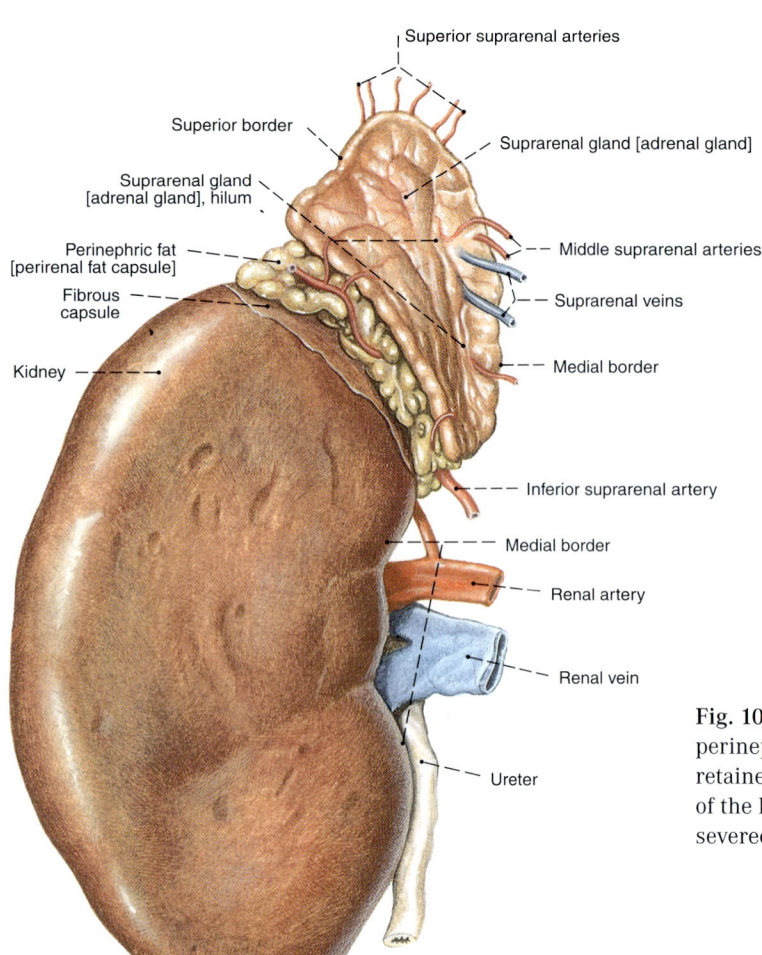

Fig. 1030   Right kidney; suprarenal gland [adrenal gland]; perinephric fat [perirenal fat capsule] and fibrous capsule retained at the superior pole [superior extremity] of the kidney; renal artery and vein, as well as ureter, severed close to the hilum of kidney; ventral aspect.

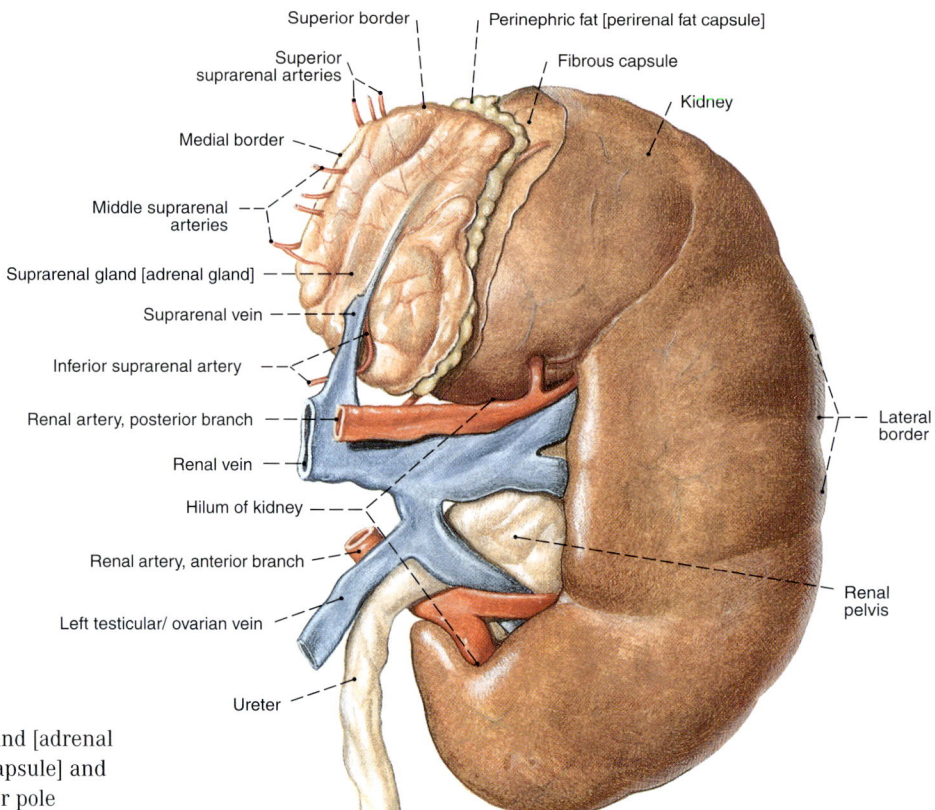

Fig. 1031   Left kidney; suprarenal gland [adrenal gland]; perinephric fat [perirenal fat capsule] and fibrous capsule retained at the superior pole [superior extremity] of the kidney; ventral aspect.

Kidney 181

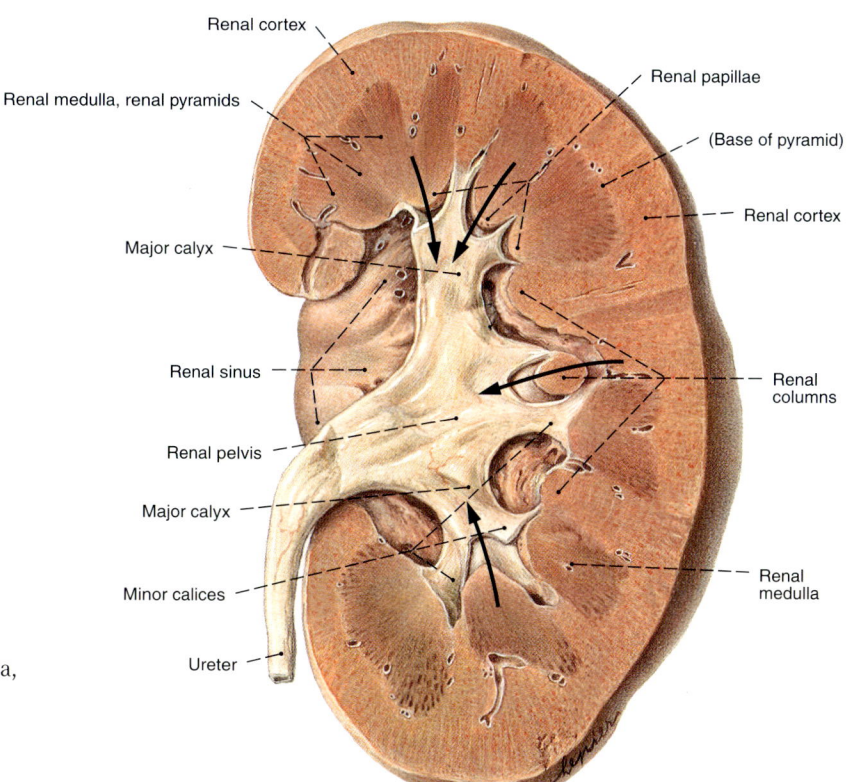

Fig. 1032 Left kidney; oblique vertical hemisection showing renal cortex, renal medulla, and renal pelvis after removal of blood vessels and fat body of the renal sinus; ventral aspect.
Arrows point from the renal pyramids toward the calices.

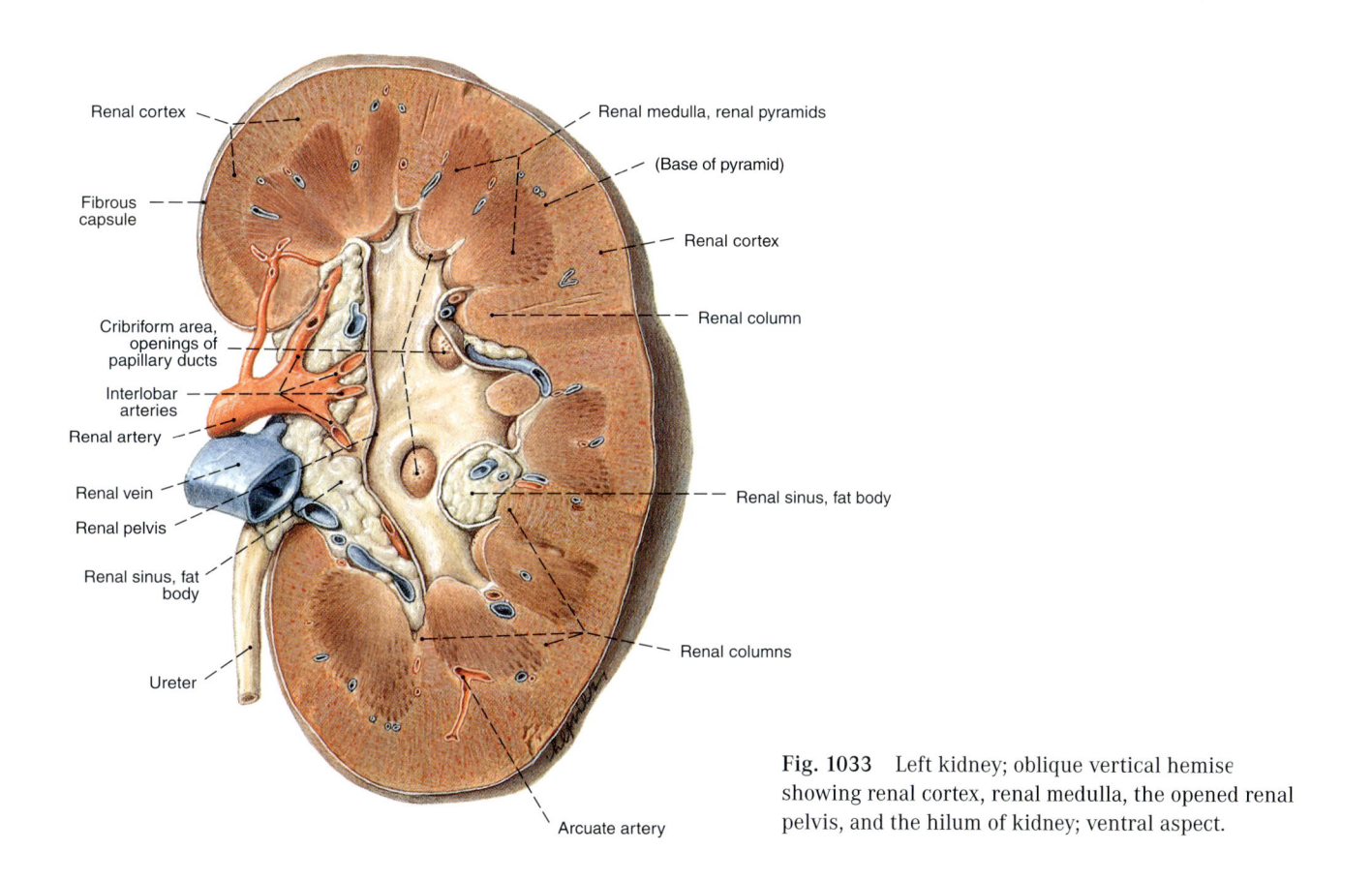

Fig. 1033 Left kidney; oblique vertical hemisection showing renal cortex, renal medulla, the opened renal pelvis, and the hilum of kidney; ventral aspect.

182 Abdominal viscera

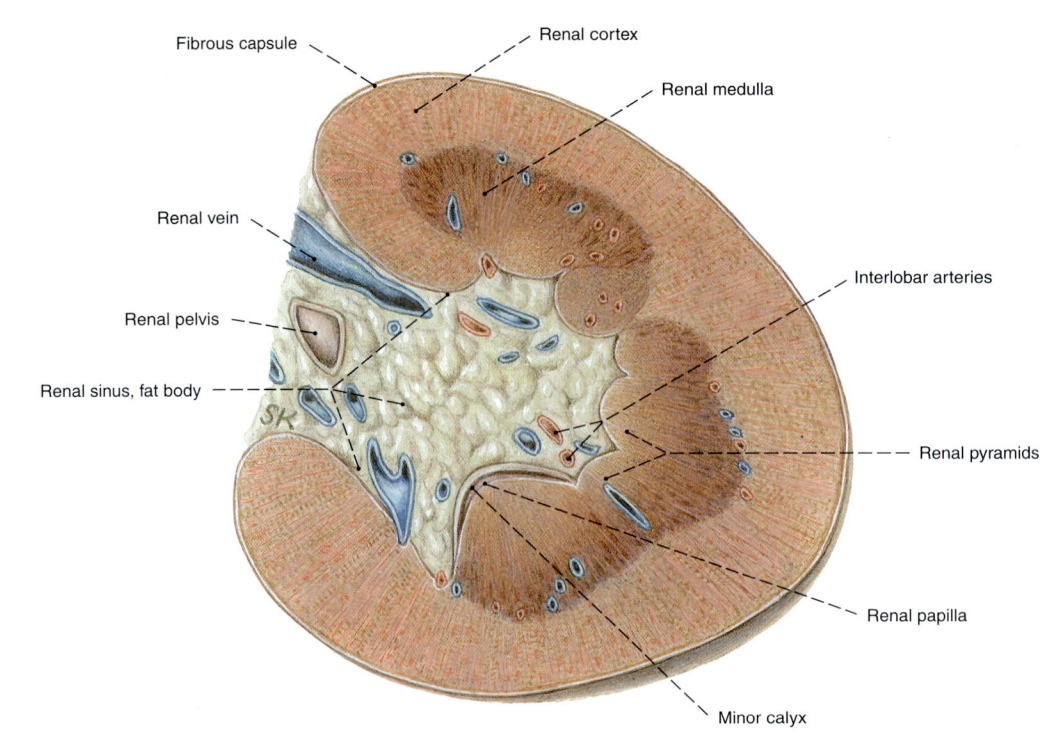

Fig. 1034 Left kidney; transverse section showing the renal sinus; caudal aspect.

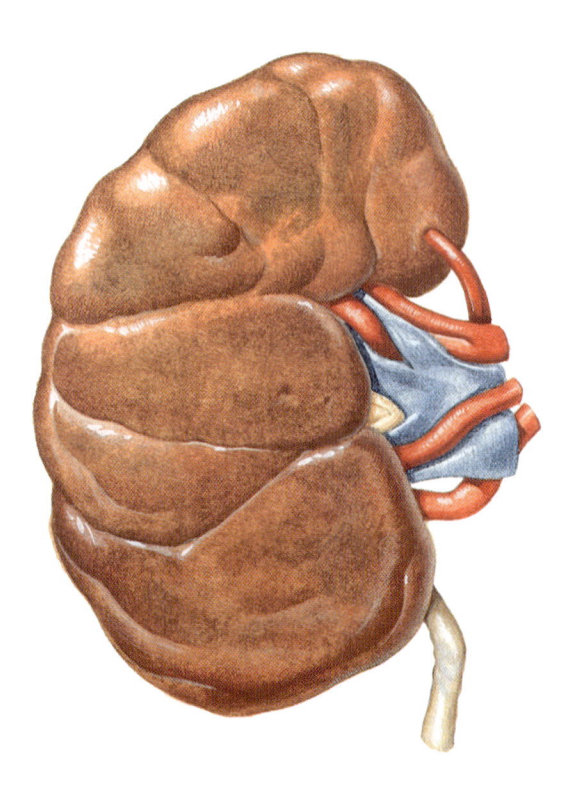

Fig. 1035 Right kidney; ventral aspect.
In this adult specimen the fetal lobulation is retained. Compare Fig. 1037.

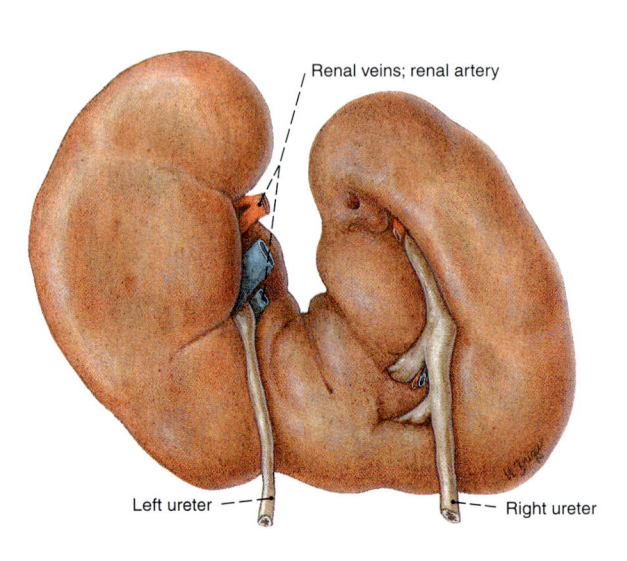

Fig. 1036 Kidney; dorsal aspect.
The inferior poles [inferior extremities] of both kidneys are fused (= horseshoe kidney).

Kidney 183

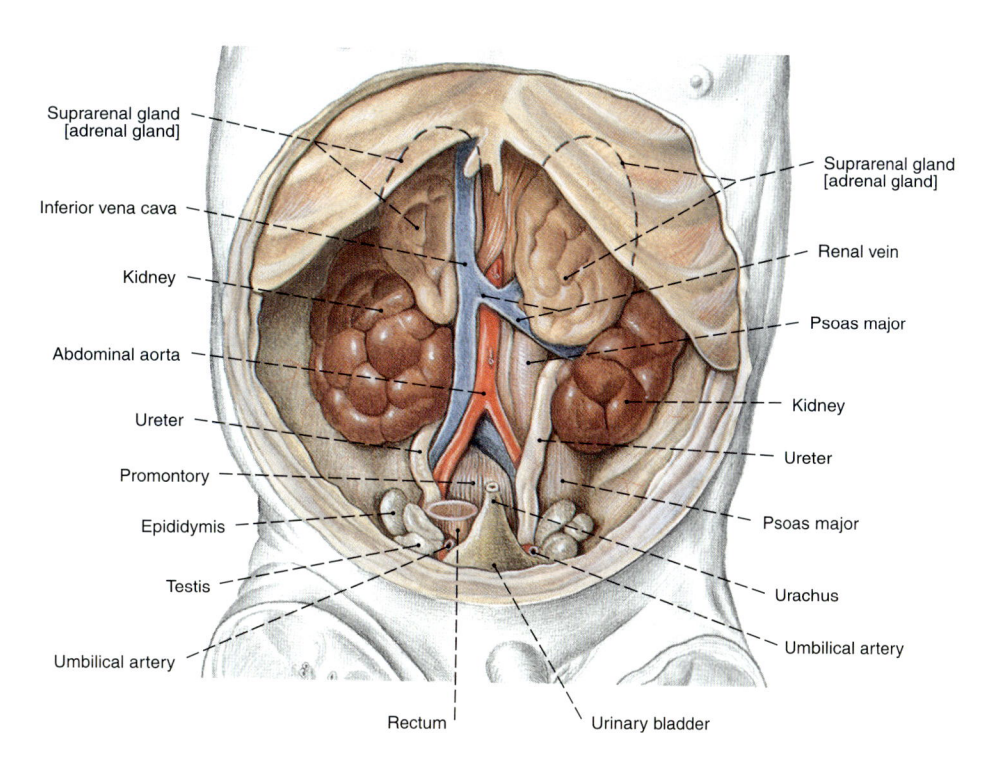

Fig. 1037 Kidney and suprarenal gland [adrenal gland] of an approximately 5-month-old fetus; abdominal wall, stomach, intestine, and liver removed; ventral aspect.
In this developmental stage the lobulation of the kidneys, the size relation of suprarenal glands [adrenal glands] and kidneys, the position of the testes and epididymides in the small pelvis [true pelvis], and the cranially conical passage of the urinary bladder into the urachus are typical.

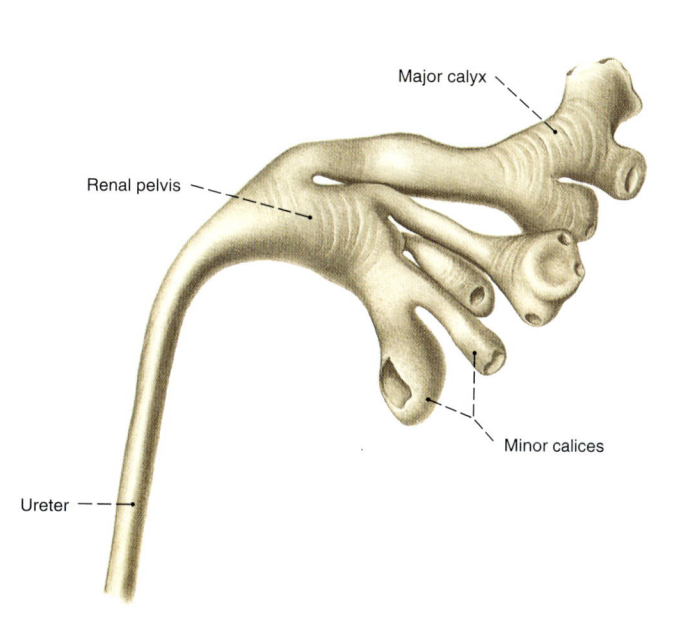

Fig. 1038 Left renal pelvis; injection cast; ventral aspect.
The form of the renal pelvis is very variable. The calices may be long and have a tree-like branching pattern (branching type), as in the figure, or they may be short and terminate in a wide, pouch-like renal pelvis (ampullary type). Many other shapes in between those two main types are possible.

184 *Abdominal viscera*

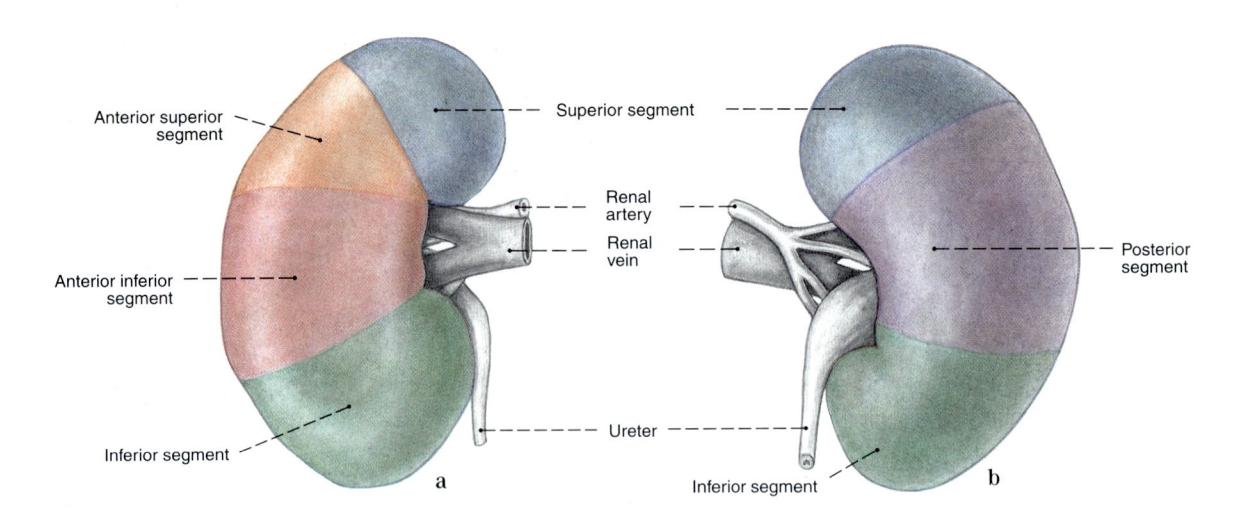

Fig. 1039 a, b Renal segments of right kidney; individual segments are indicated by same colors.

a Ventral aspect
b Dorsal aspect

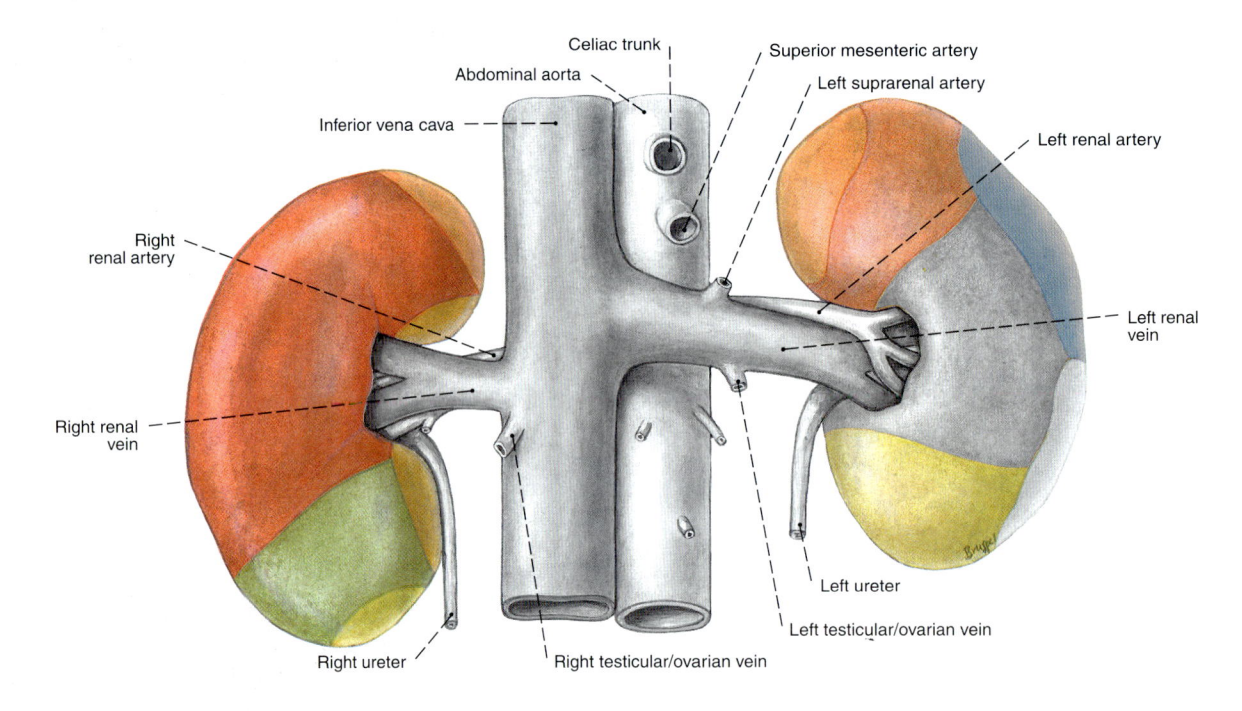

Fig. 1040 Kidney and neighboring organs on the ventral surface; ventral aspect.

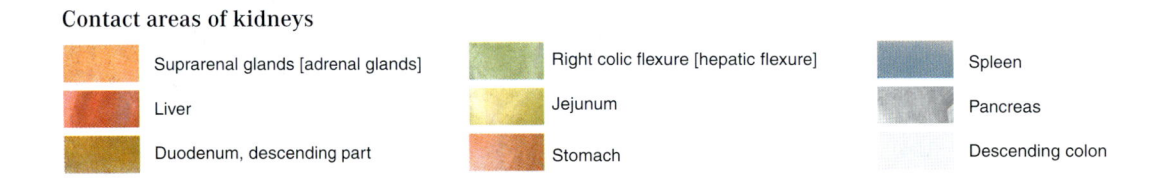

Contact areas of kidneys

- Suprarenal glands [adrenal glands]
- Liver
- Duodenum, descending part
- Right colic flexure [hepatic flexure]
- Jejunum
- Stomach
- Spleen
- Pancreas
- Descending colon

Kidney 185

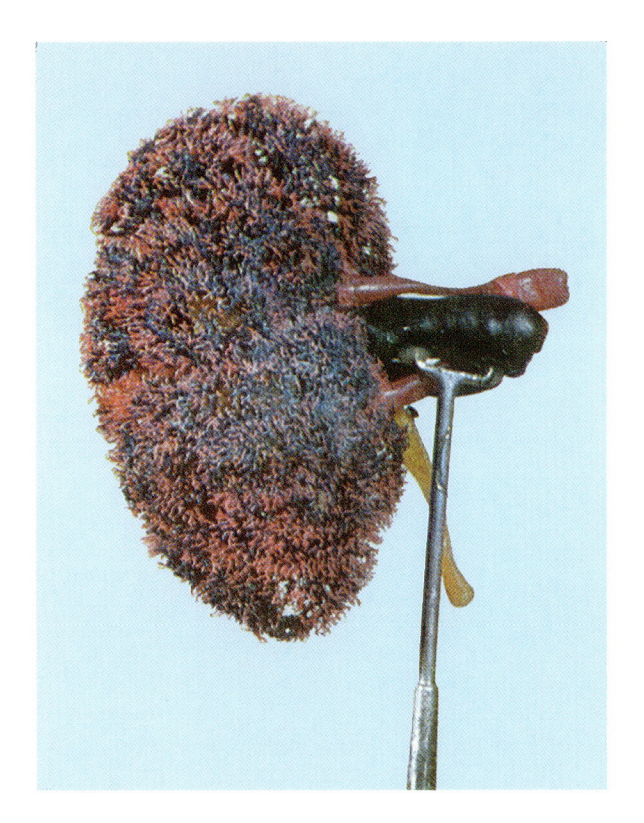

Fig. 1041 Right renal arteries and veins; renal pelvis; corrosion cast after injection of colored polymer into the renal blood vessels and into the renal pelvis (arteries: red, veins: blue, renal pelvis: yellow); ventral aspect.

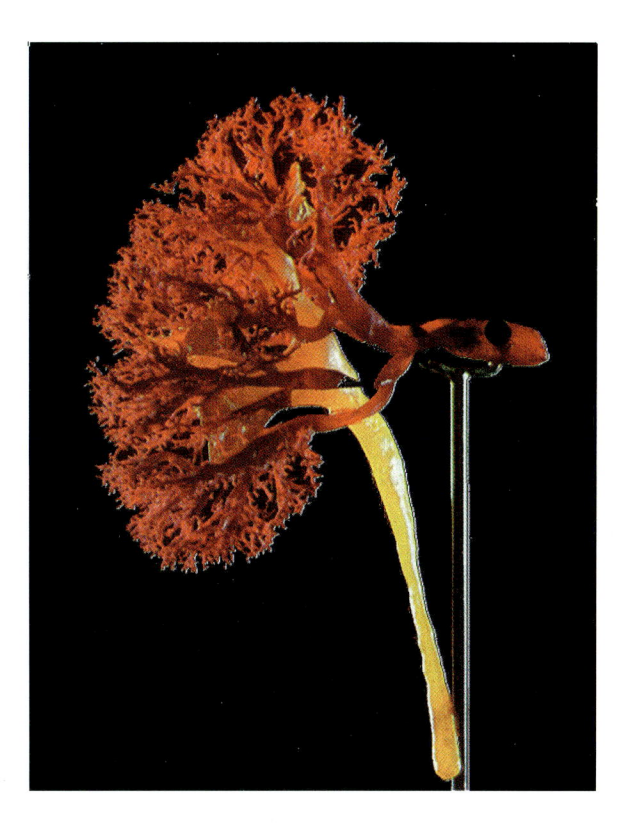

Fig. 1042 Right renal arteries and renal pelvis; corrosion cast after injection of red polymer into the renal arteries and yellow polymer into the ureter; ventral aspect.

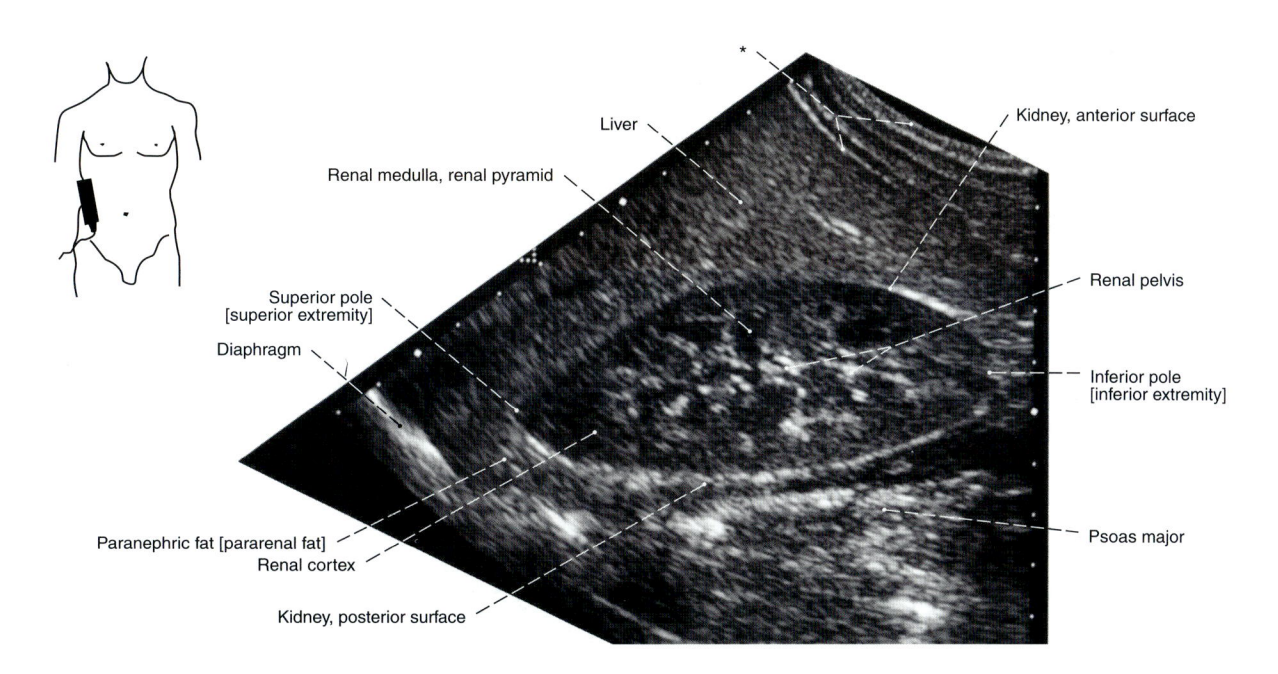

Fig. 1043 Right kidney; ultrasound scan; transducer directed from ventrocaudal to dorsocaudal; lateral aspect.

In addition to the renal pelvis, both the renal cortex and the renal medulla are distinguishable.

* Abdominal wall.

Abdominal and pelvic viscera

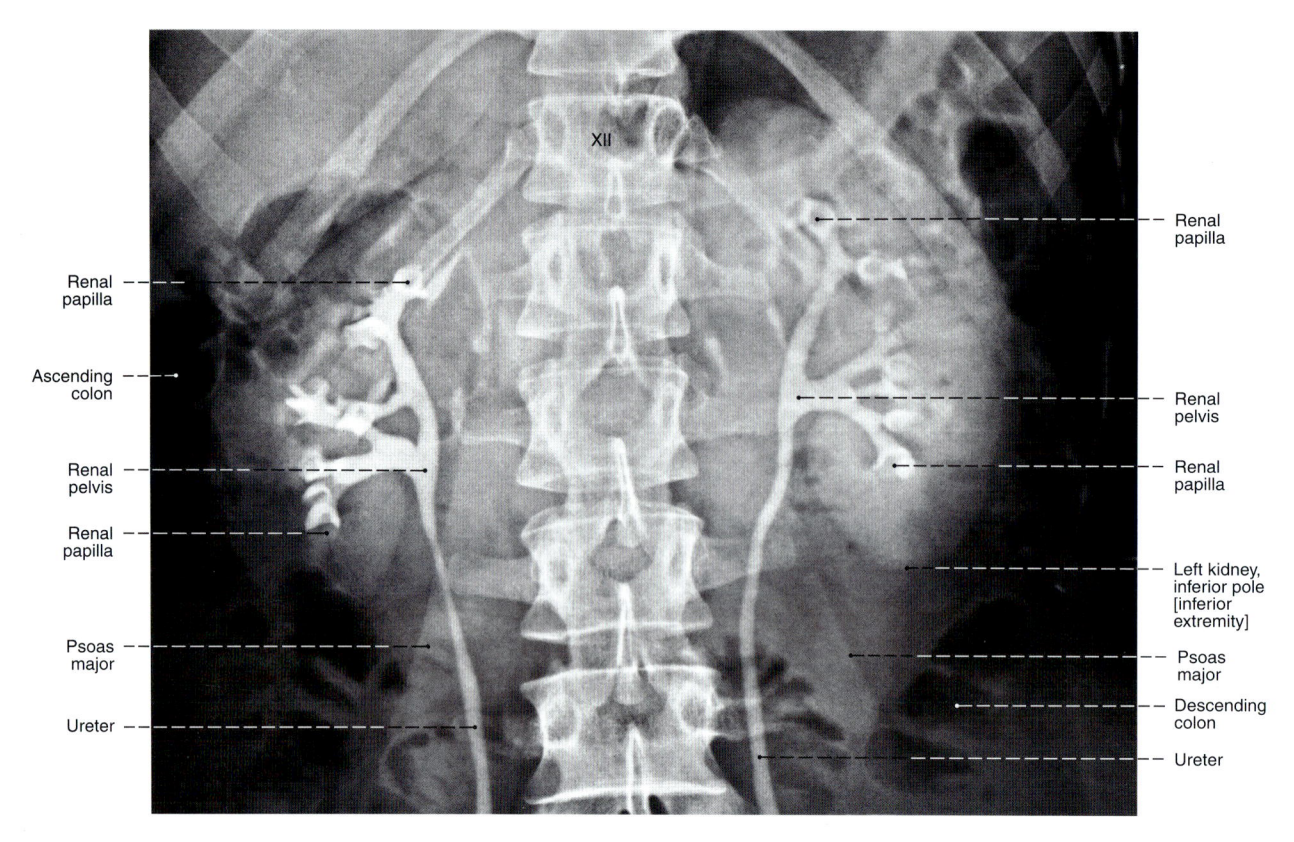

Fig. 1044 Kidney; renal pelvis; ureter; AP radiograph after retrograde injection of contrast medium via both ureters, visualizing also the urine-draining systems within the kidneys; ventral aspect.
XII = 12th thoracic vertebra.

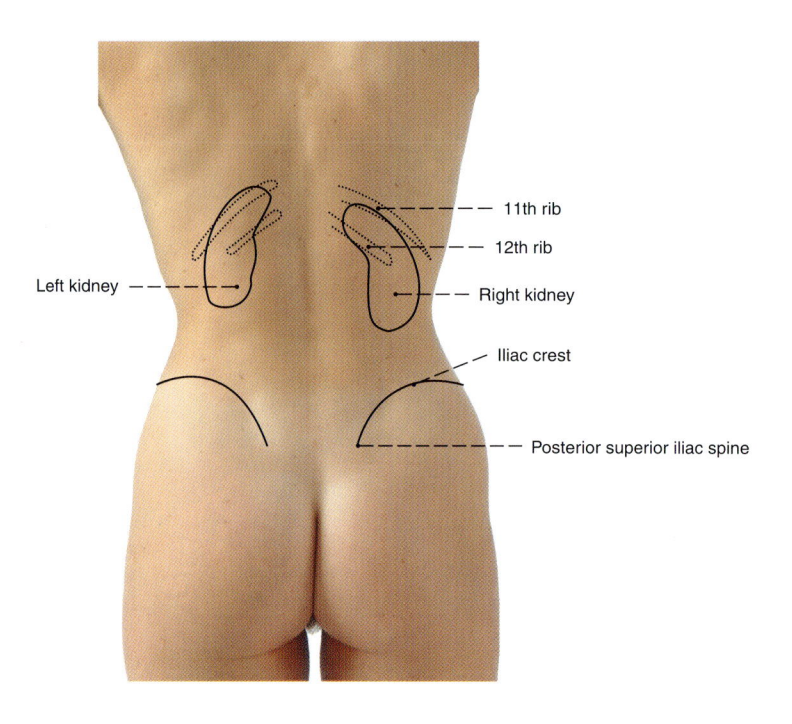

Fig. 1045 Projection of kidneys onto the back. The longitudinal axes of the kidneys diverge caudolaterally. The right kidney is usually more caudal than the left. Compare Fig. 1092.

Suprarenal gland [adrenal gland] and urinary bladder

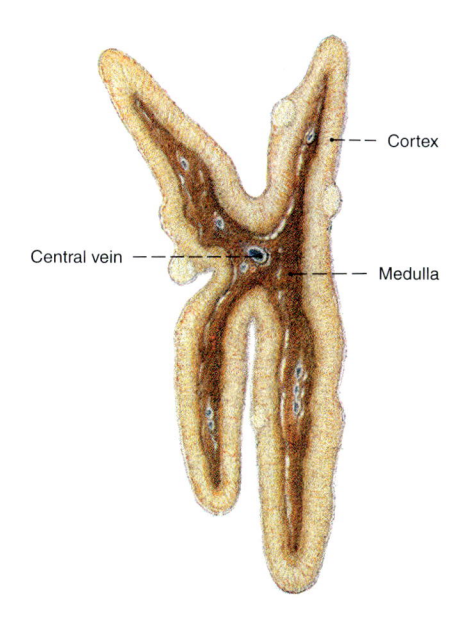

Fig. 1046 Right suprarenal gland [adrenal gland]; sagittal section; lateral aspect.

The figure has been drawn from a fresh specimen. In fixed specimen color differentiation between cortex and medulla are less distinct.

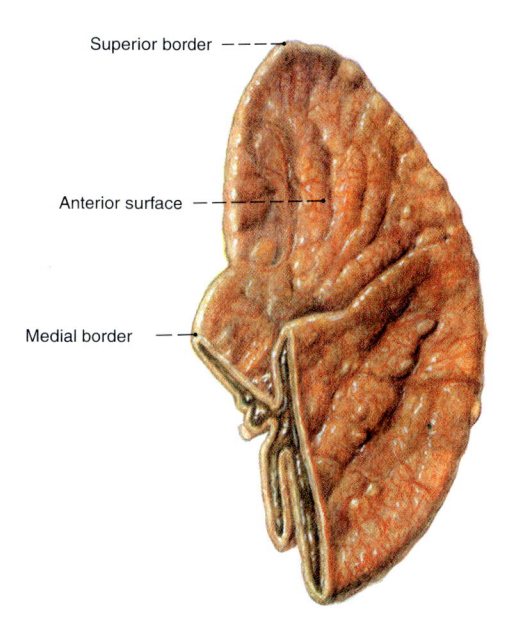

Fig. 1047 Right suprarenal gland [adrenal gland]; the lower part sectioned sagittally; ventral aspect. See also remarks for Fig. 1046.

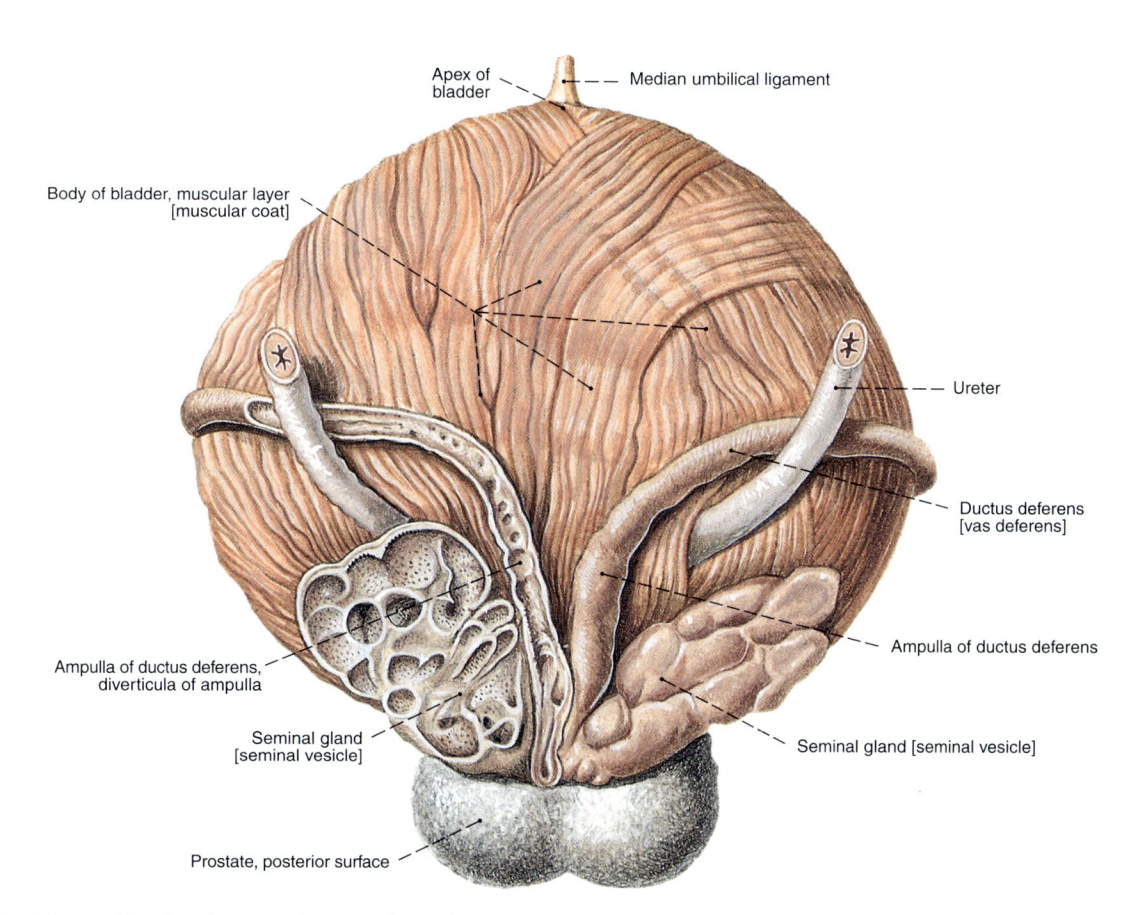

Fig. 1048 Urinary bladder; ductus deferentes [vasa deferentia]; seminal glands [seminal vesicles]; prostate; external muscular layer of urinary bladder dissected; left seminal gland [seminal vesicle] and ductus deferens [vas deferens] cut open.

Pelvic viscera

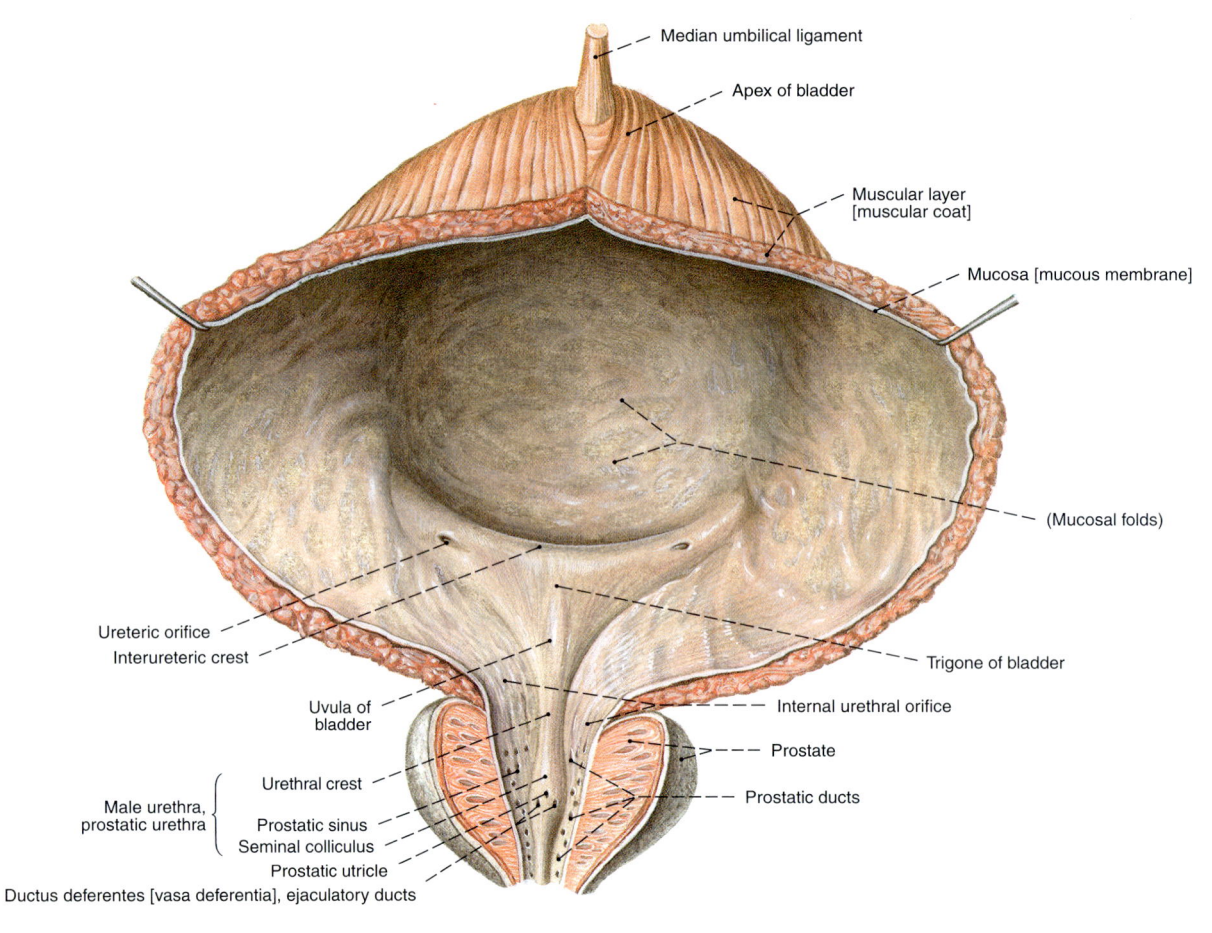

Fig. 1049 Urinary bladder; prostate; urethra; opened by a longitudinal median section; external muscular layer of urinary bladder dissected; ventral aspect.

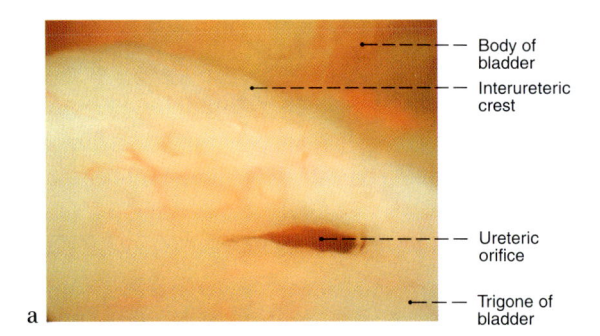

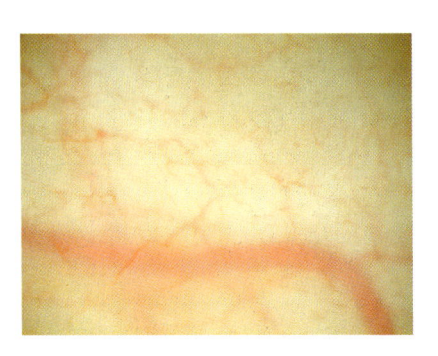

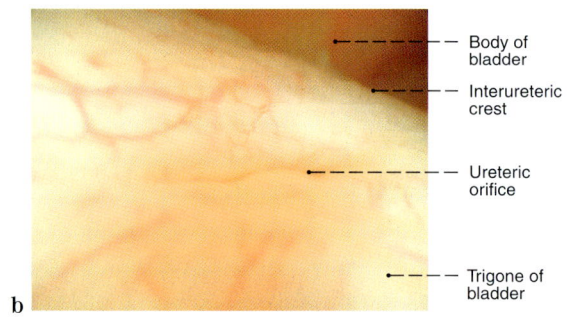

Fig. 1050 a, b Urinary bladder; ureteric orifice visualized by an endoscope introduced through the urethra (cystoscopy).
a ureteric orifice open, a peristaltic wave has transported urine into the urinary bladder
b ureteric orifice closed

Fig. 1051 Urinary bladder; endoscopic view (cystoscopy) of mucosa [mucous membrane] of the body of bladder; inferior aspect.
   In a full, healthy bladder no mucosal folds are visible.

Male urogenital organs 189

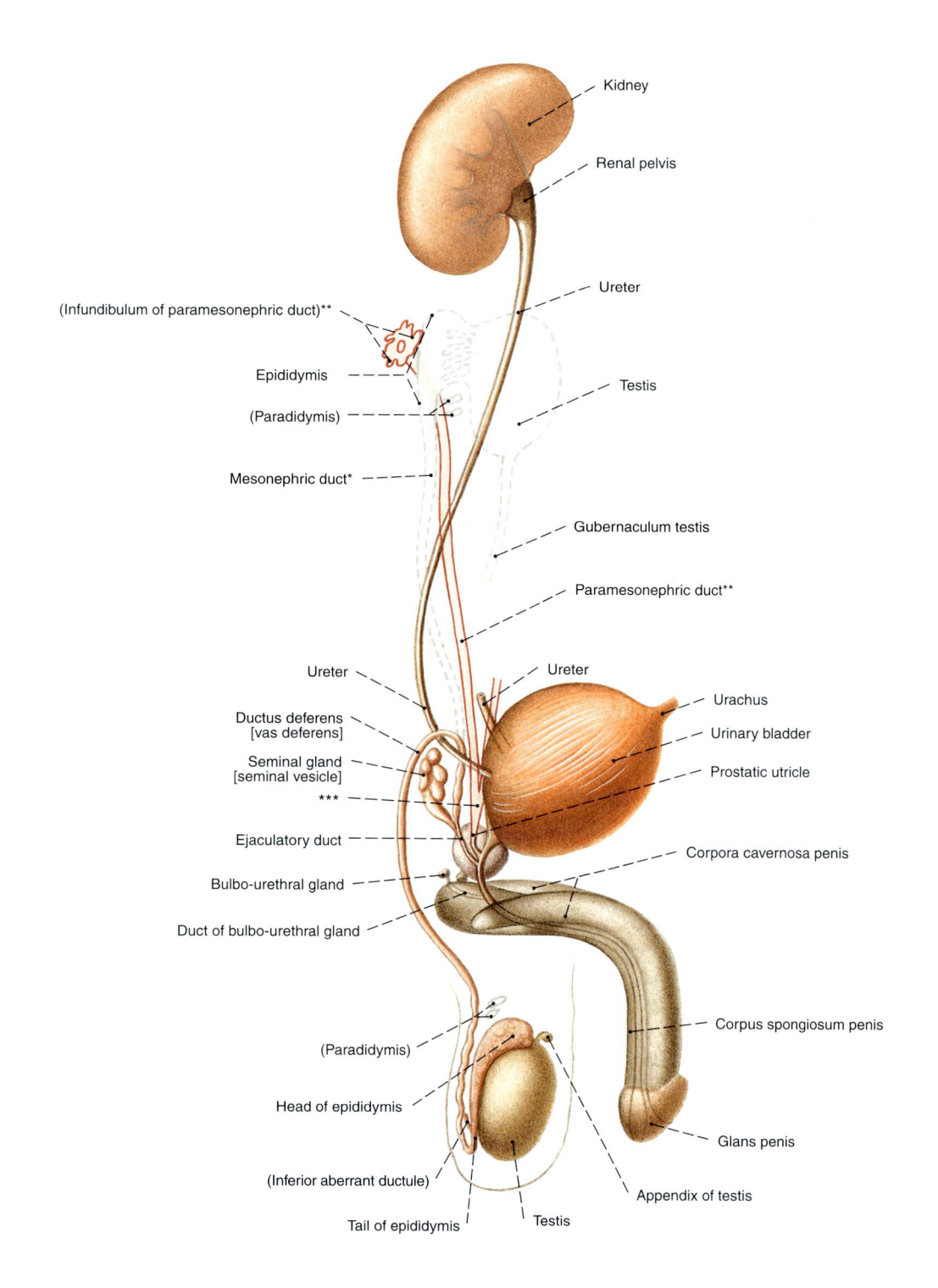

Fig. 1052 Male urogenital organs; diagram of the development: degenerating parts: pale pink, positions before descensus testis in dotted lines; lateral aspect.

  Epididymis = genital part of mesonephros
  Paradidymis = renal part of mesonephros

* WOLFFIAN duct
** MUELLERIAN duct
*** junction of paramesonephric ducts (MUELLERIAN ducts)
Compare fig. 1062, development in the female.

Pelvic viscera

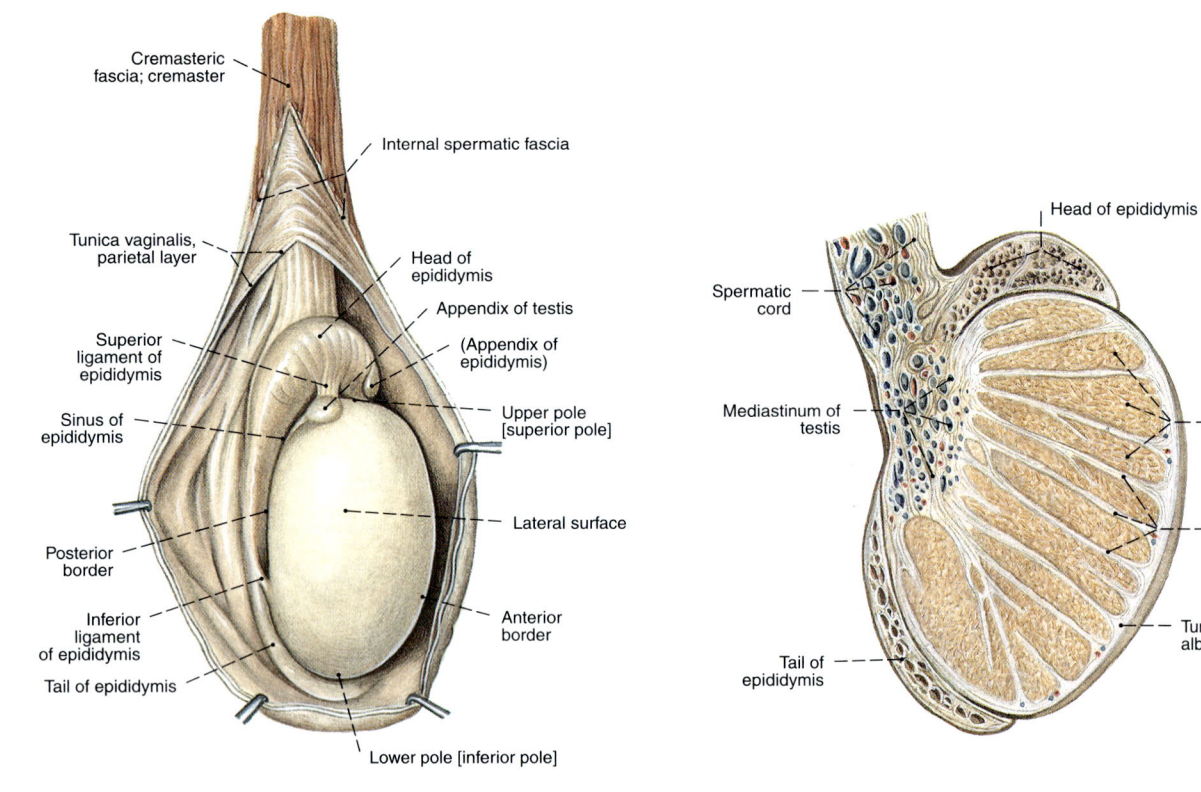

Fig. 1053 Right testis; epididymis; layers of scrotum opened stepwise; lateral aspect.

Fig. 1054 Right testis; epididymis; sagittal section; lateral aspect.

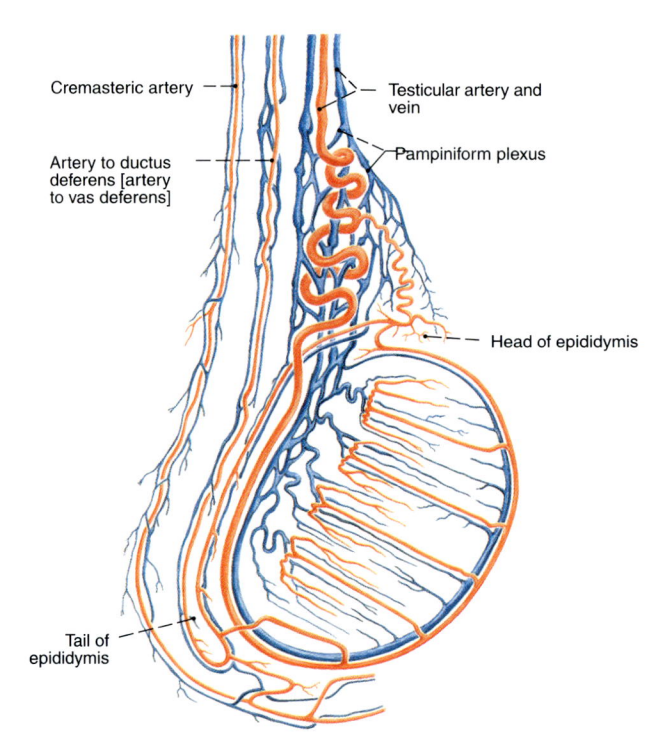

Fig. 1055 Blood vessels of testis; epididymis, and spermatic cord; lateral aspect.
The arteries form anastomoses.

Testis and epididymis

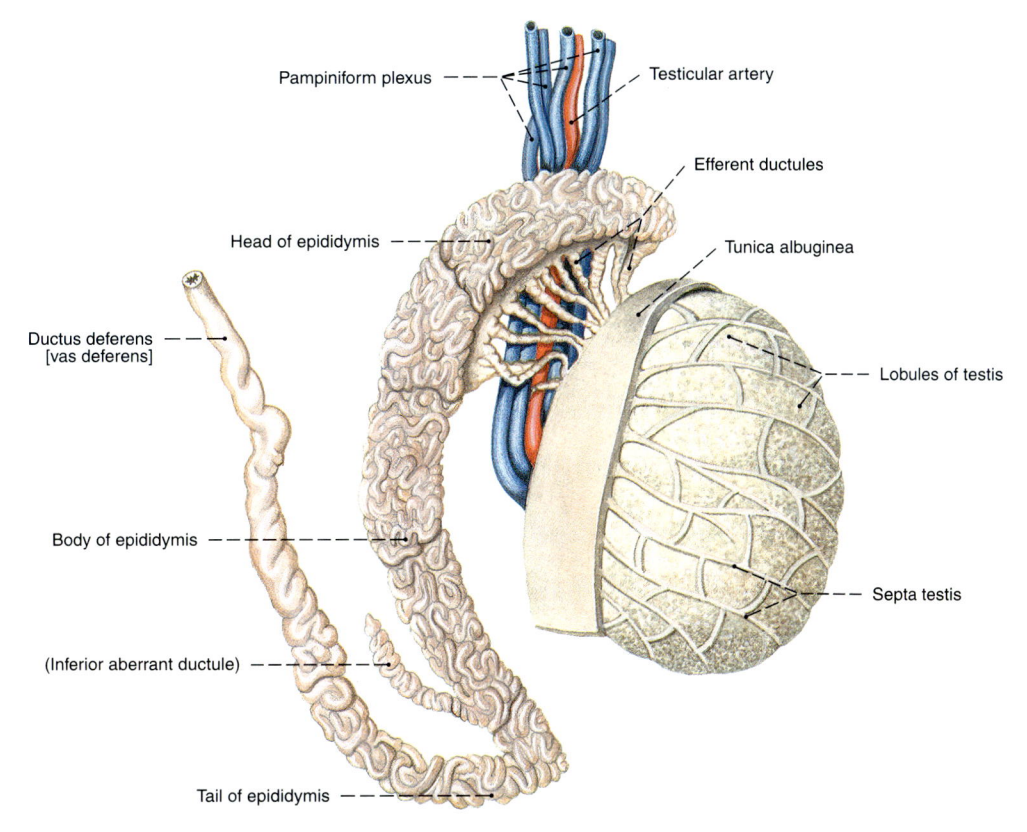

Fig. 1056 Testis; epididymis; ductus deferens [vas deferens]; tunica albuginea extensively removed to expose septa testis; epididymis retracted from testis and duct of epididymis dissected to show its tortuous course (length 5-6 m); lateral aspect.

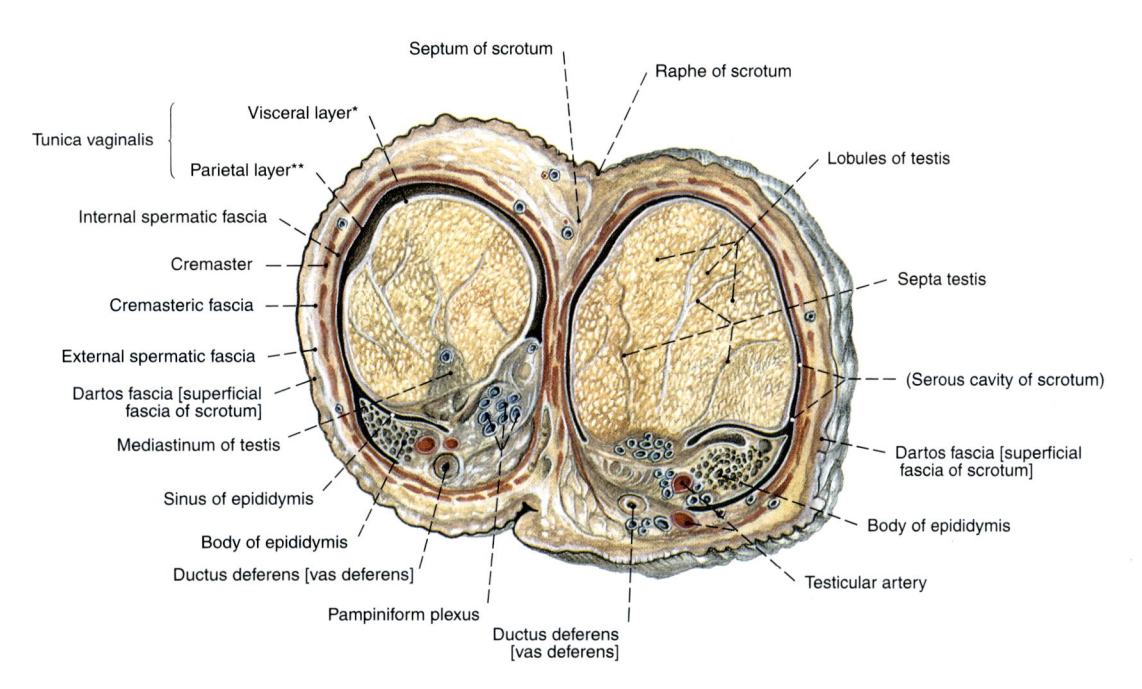

Fig. 1057 Testis; epididymis; scrotum; transverse section to expose the layers of scrotum and sheaths of testis; cranial aspect.

The cross sections are different in size because the testes generally do not lie at the same level in the scrotum.

* also: eporchium
** also: periorchiumAuch: Periorchium

Pelvic viscera

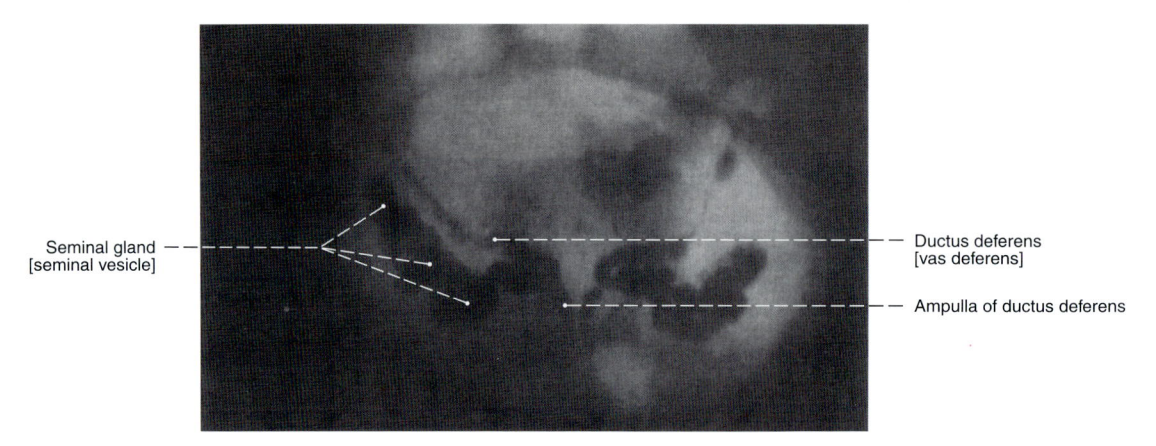

Fig. 1058 Ductus deferentes [vasa deferentia]; seminal glands [seminal vesicles]; AP radiograph after injection of contrast medium via the ejaculatory ducts; ventral aspect.

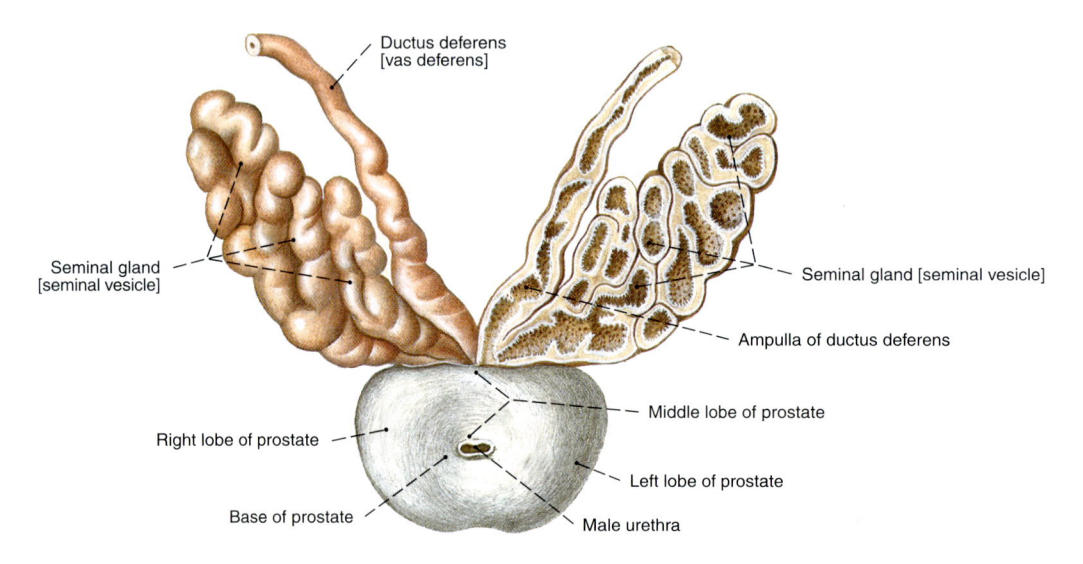

Fig. 1059 Ductus deferentes [vasa deferentia]; seminal glands [seminal vesicles]; prostate; exposure of prostate by sectioning the urethra below the urinary bladder; left ductus deferens [vas deferens] and seminal gland [seminal vesicle] opened with a longitudinal section; cranial aspect.

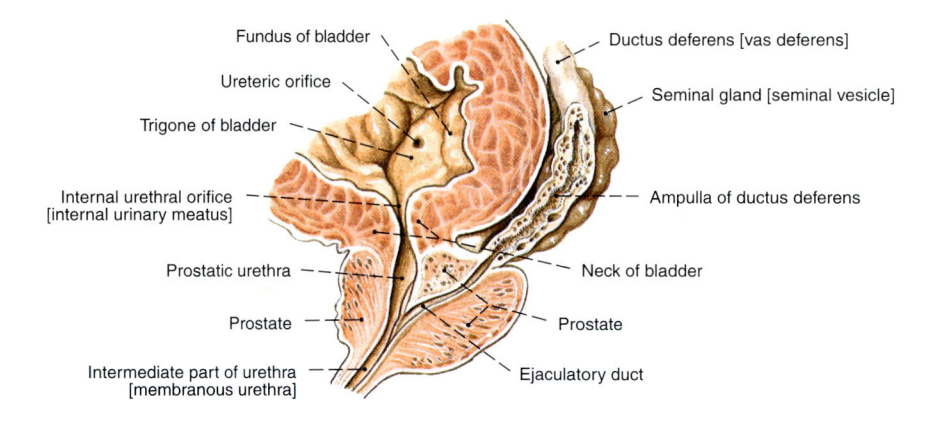

Fig. 1060 Urinary bladder; prostate; ductus deferentes [vasa deferentia]; seminal glands [seminal vesicles]; oblique section to expose opening of left ejaculatory duct into the urethra; left lateral aspect.

The thickness of the muscular layer [muscular coat] of the bladder indicates a contracted empty bladder.

Male urogenital organs

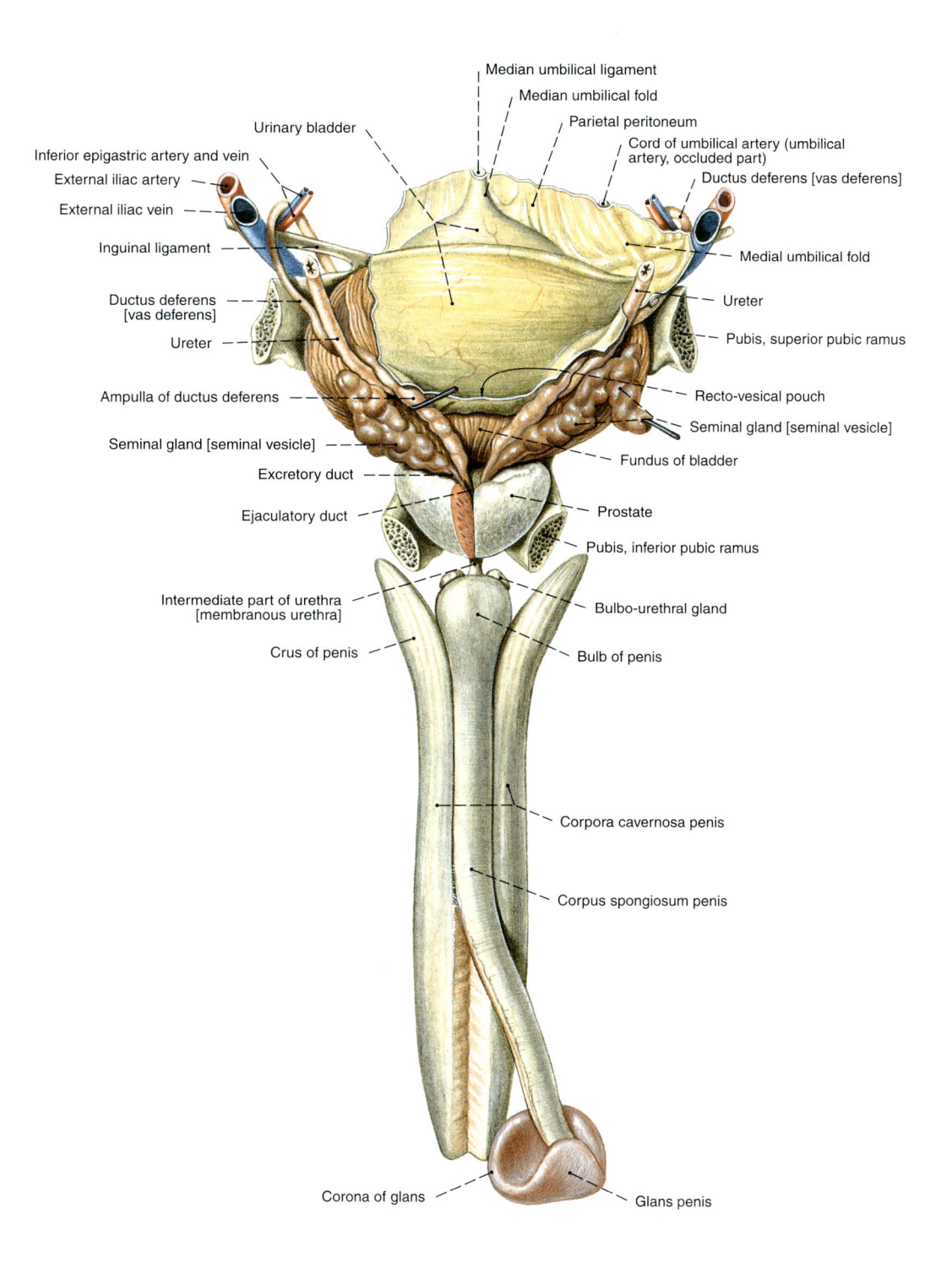

Fig. 1061 Urinary bladder; ductus deferentes [vasa deferentia]; seminal glands [seminal vesicles]; prostate; male urethra; parts of pubis retained; a wedge-shaped part of the prostate removed to expose the left ejaculatory duct; distal part of corpus spongiosum penis retracted dorsally; dorsal aspect.

Pelvic viscera

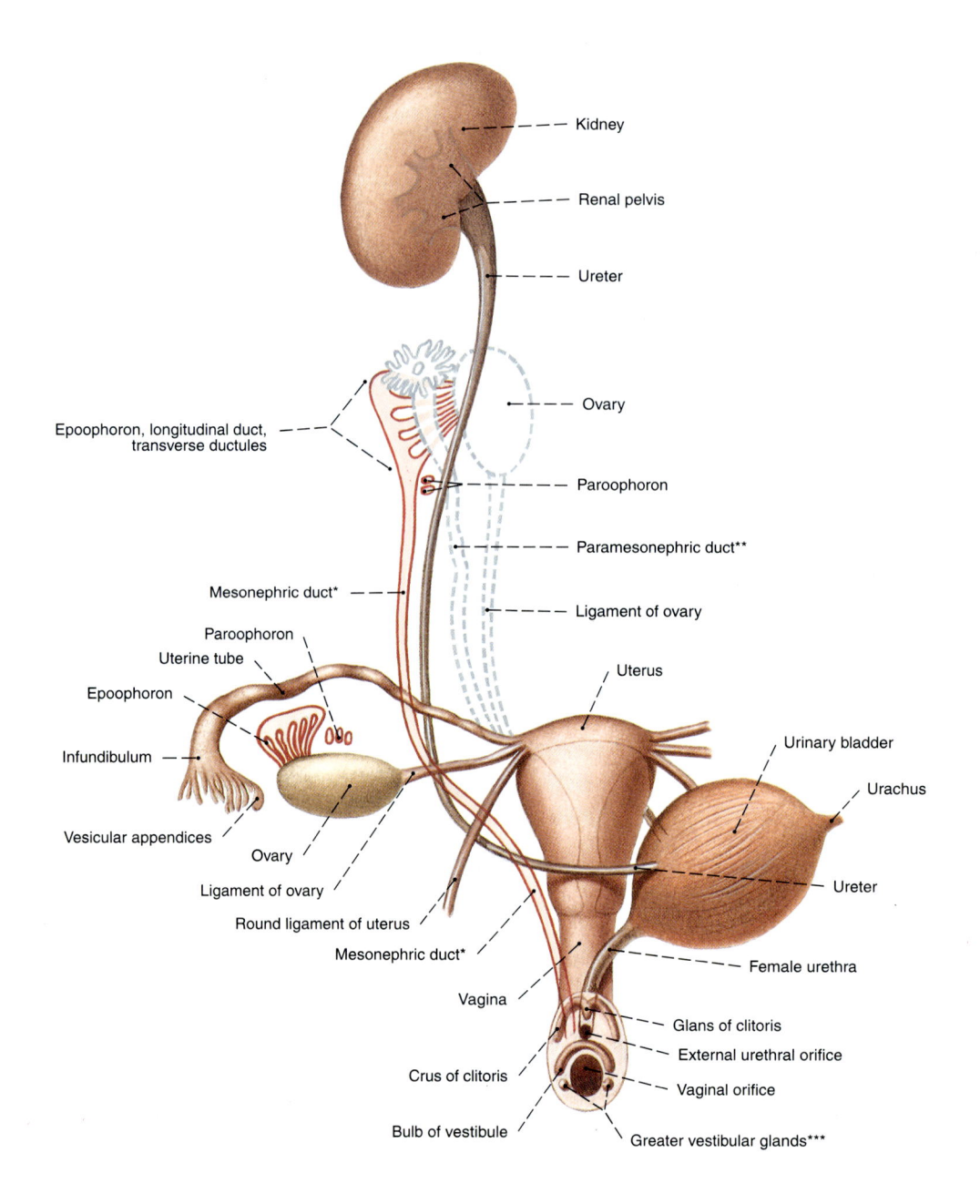

Fig. 1062 Female urogenital organs; diagram of the development: degenerating parts: pale pink, positions before descensus ovarii in dotted lines; urinary bladder retracted laterally; ventral aspect.

* WOLFFIAN duct.
** MUELLERIAN duct.
*** BARTHOLIN's glands.

Compare Fig. 1052, development in the male.

Epoophoron = genital part of mesonephros.
Paroophoron = renal part of mesonephros.

Female internal genitalia 195

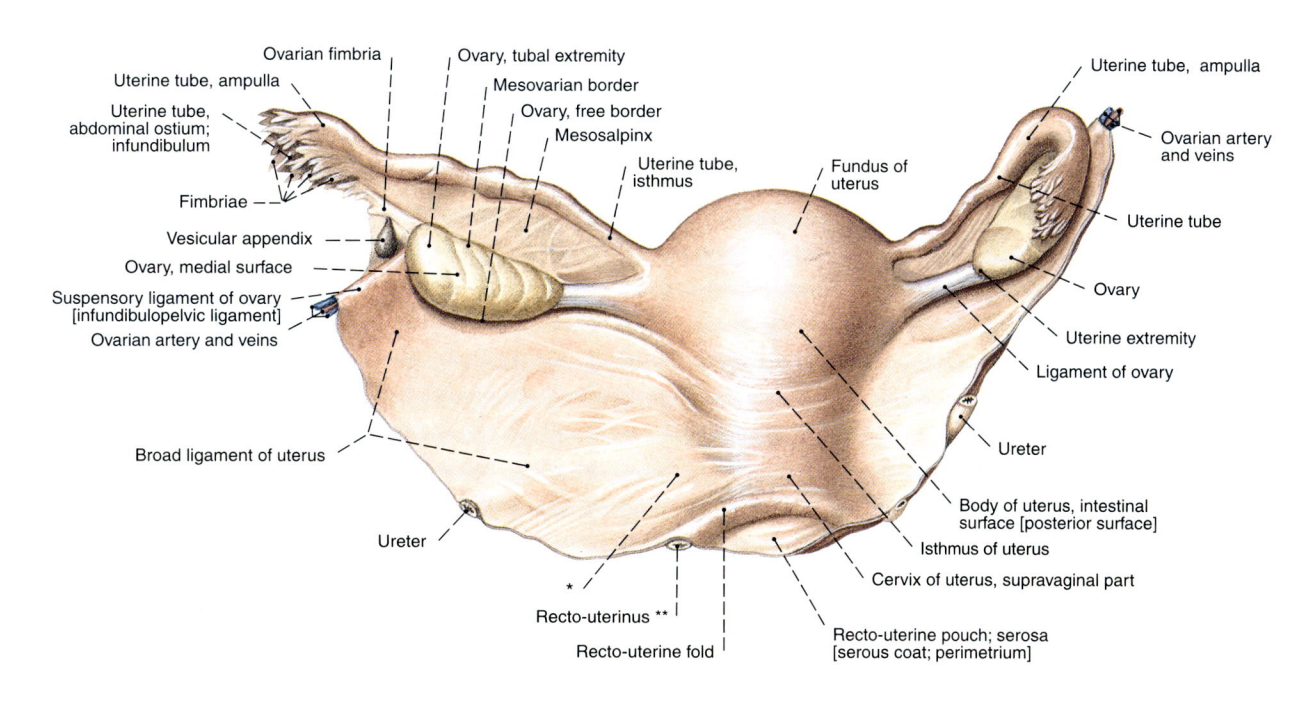

Fig. 1063　Female internal genitalia; dorsal aspect.

* Clinically: cardinal ligament; see Fig. 1070.
** Clinically: uterosacral ligament.

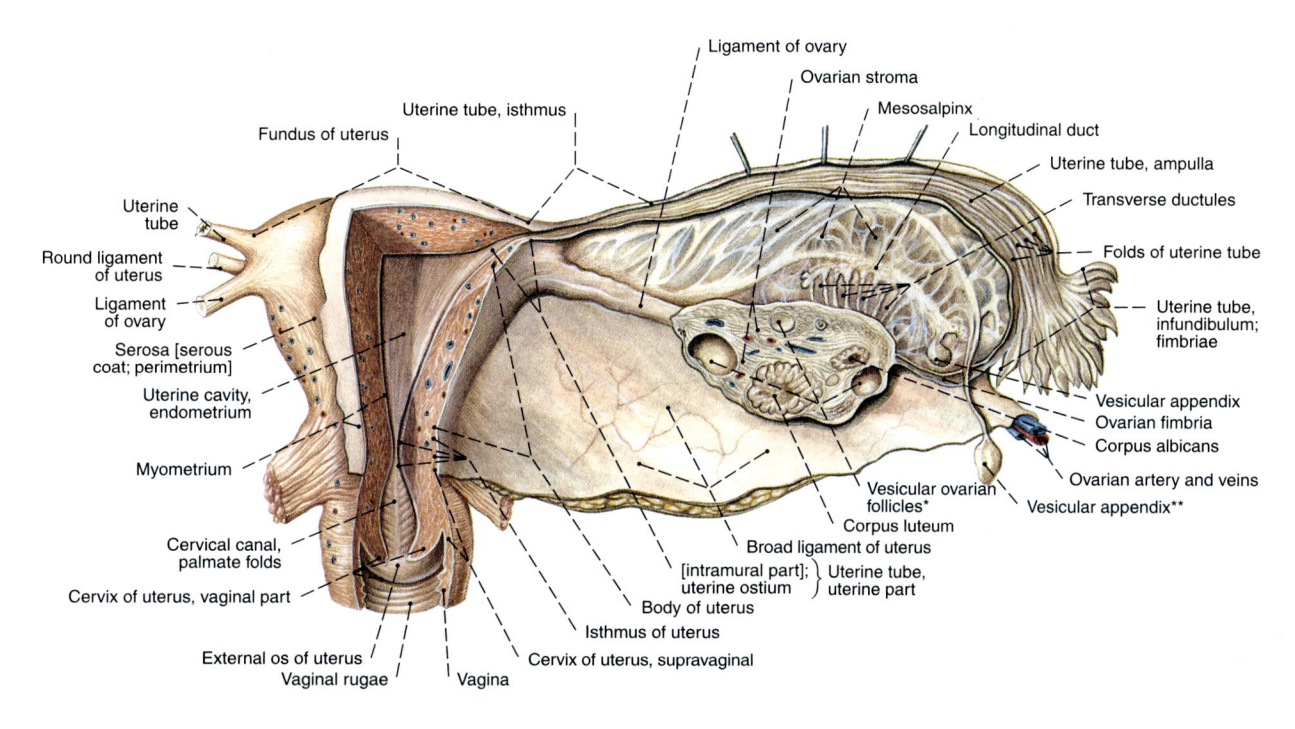

Fig. 1064　Female internal genitalia; female in reproductive age; image of lumen of vagina, uterus, and right uterine tube; ovary sectioned frontally and peritoneum removed from mesosalpinx; dorsal aspect.

* Clinically: GRAAFian follicle.
** Stalked hydatid.

Pelvic viscera

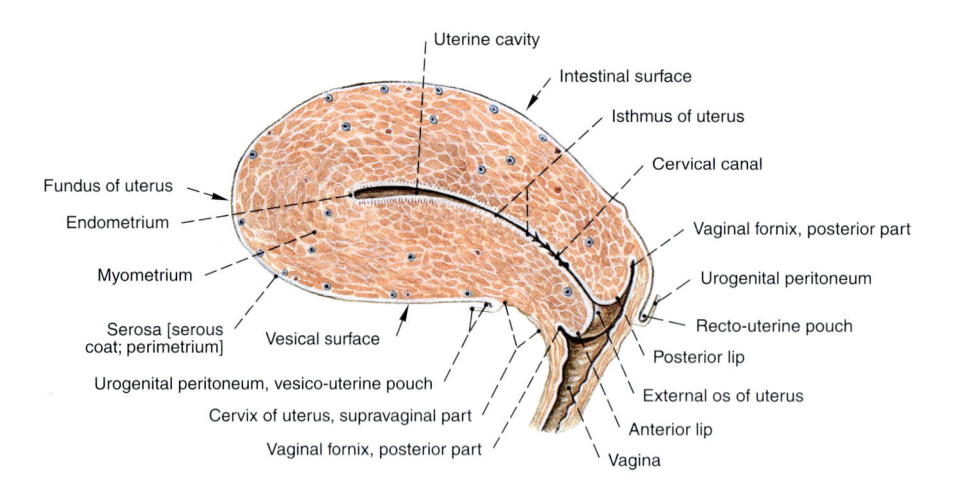

Fig. 1065 Uterus; vagina; female in reproductive age; median section exposing the lumen; lateral aspect.

Fig. 1066 Uterus; vagina; normal angles between vagina, cervix of uterus, and body of uterus; schematic median section; lateral aspect.

* Longitudinal axis of vagina.
** Longitudinal axis of cervix of uterus.
*** Longitudinal axis of body of uterus.

Angle between vagina and cervix of uterus = version
Angle between cervix and body of uterus = flexion
Normal relationships of uterus: anteversion, anteflexion
Position in relation to median plane = position
(compare Fig. 1067, uterus in dextroposition).

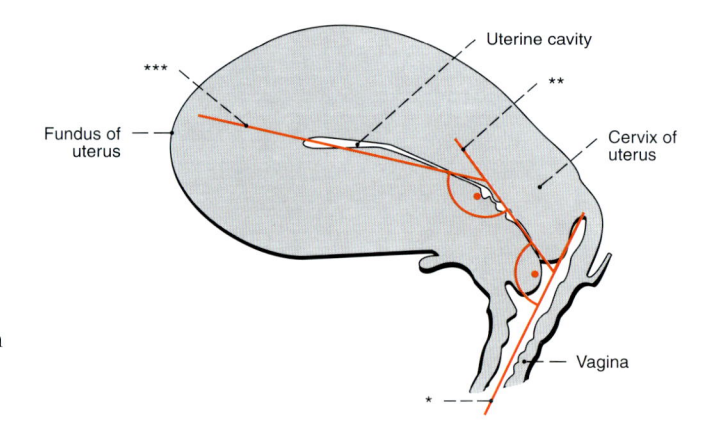

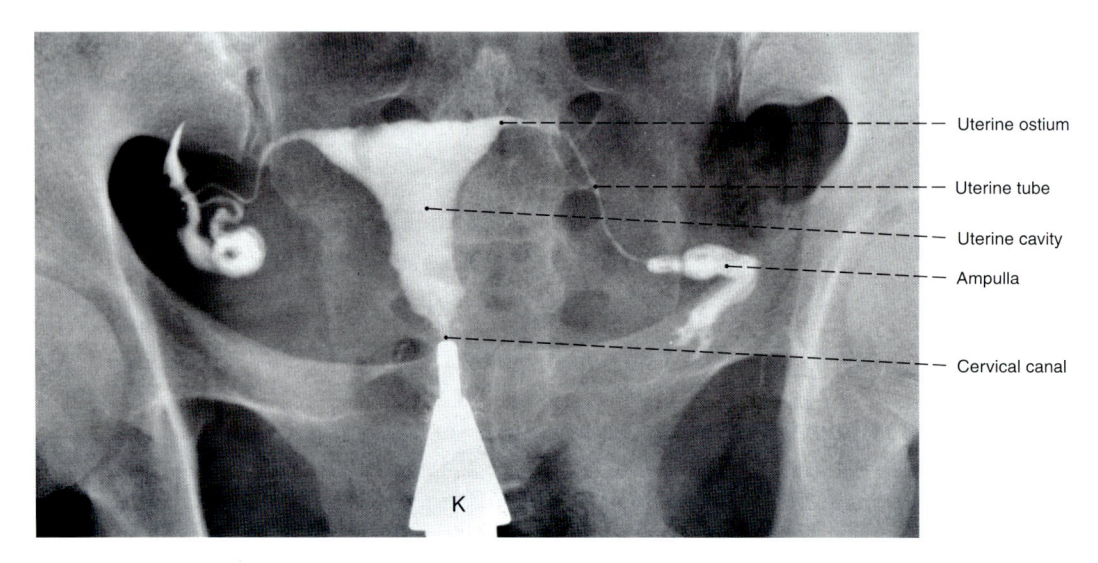

Fig. 1067 Uterus; uterine tube; AP radiograph after injection of contrast medium via the cervix of uterus (hysterosalpingography); ventral aspect.

This previously used clinical method enabled diagnosis of passage of uterine tube.
K = adapter for injection tube for contrast medium.

Female internal genitalia

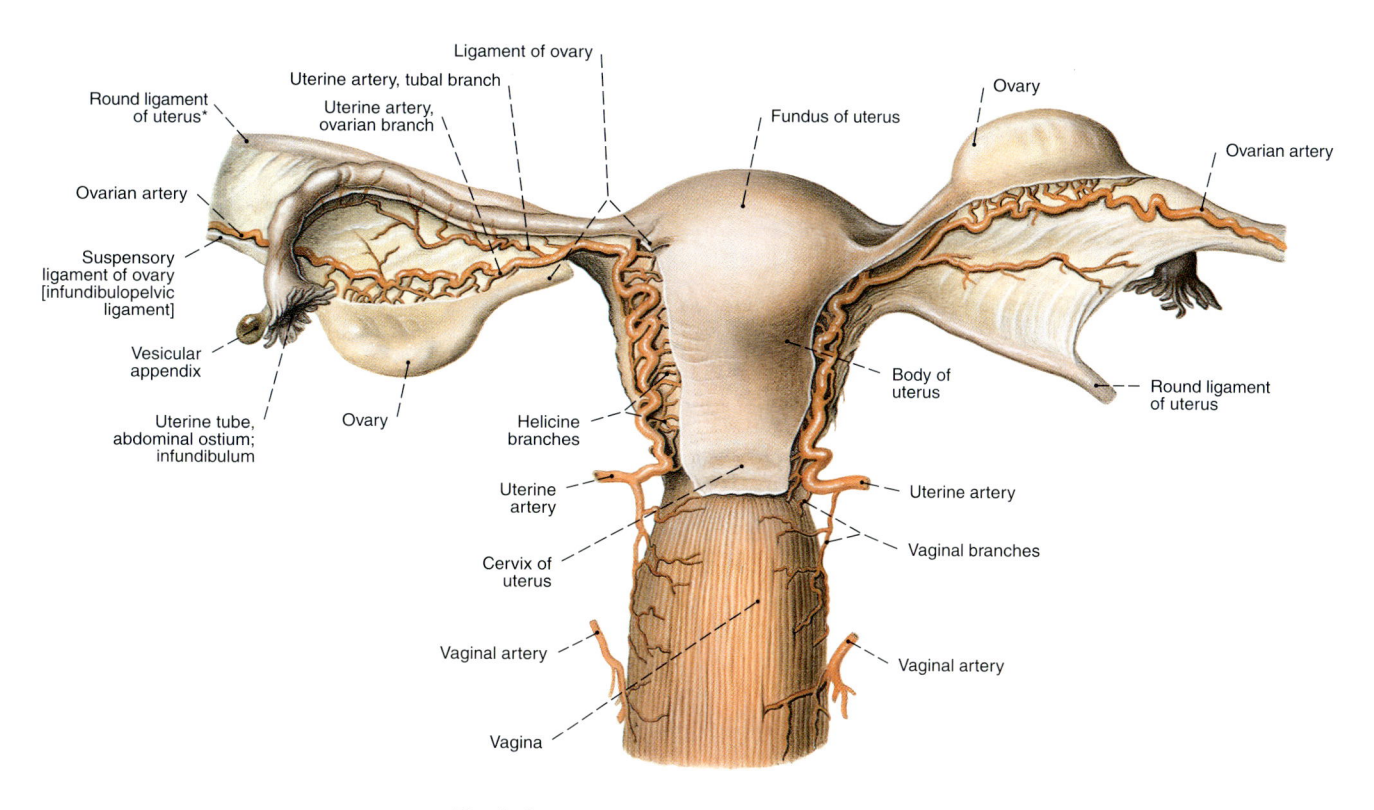

Fig. 1068 Arteries of female internal genitalia; broad ligament of uterus extensively and peritoneum partially removed; part of left ligament of ovary removed; dorsal aspect.

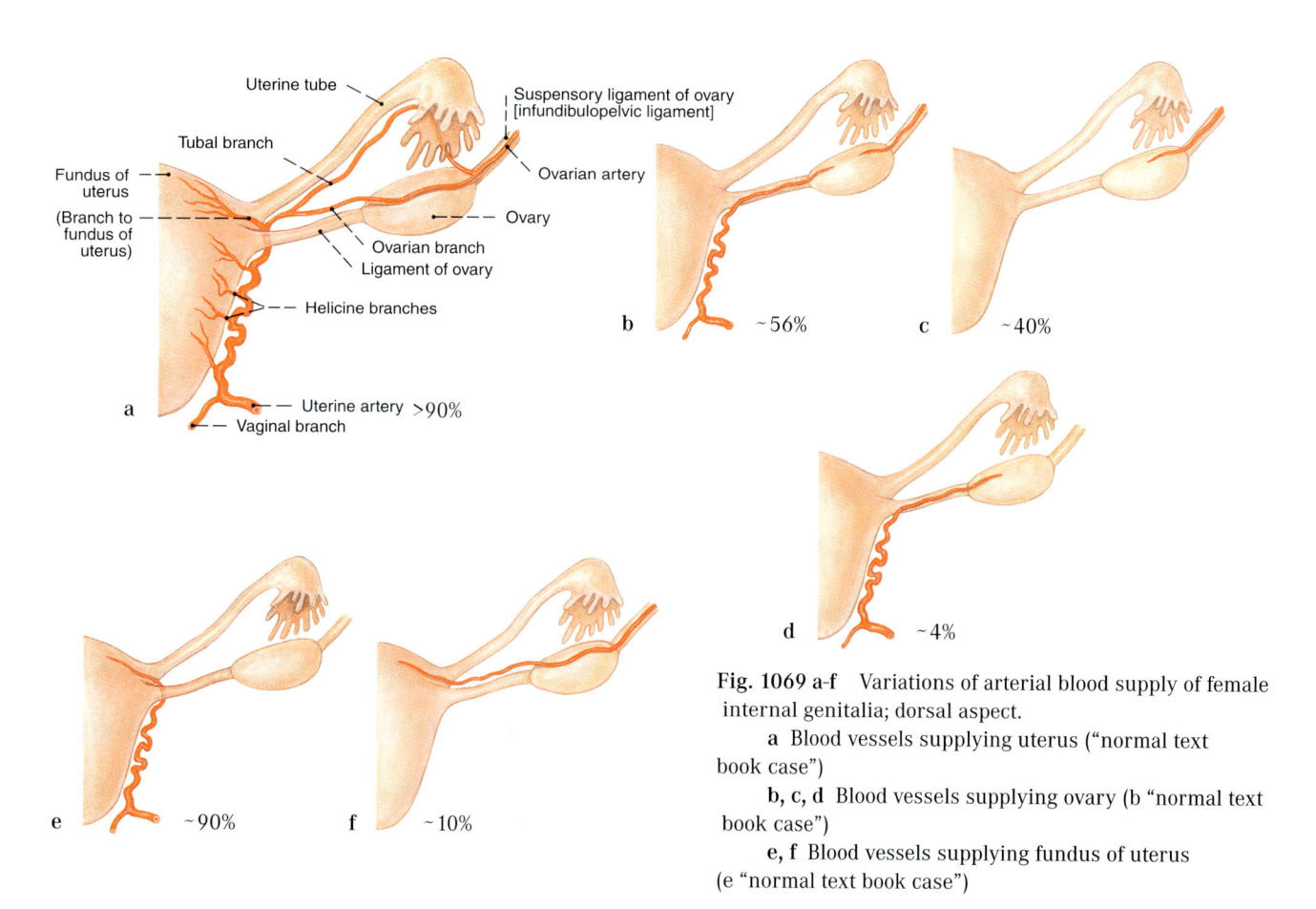

Fig. 1069 a–f Variations of arterial blood supply of female internal genitalia; dorsal aspect.
    a Blood vessels supplying uterus ("normal text book case")
    b, c, d Blood vessels supplying ovary (b "normal text book case")
    e, f Blood vessels supplying fundus of uterus (e "normal text book case")

Pelvic viscera

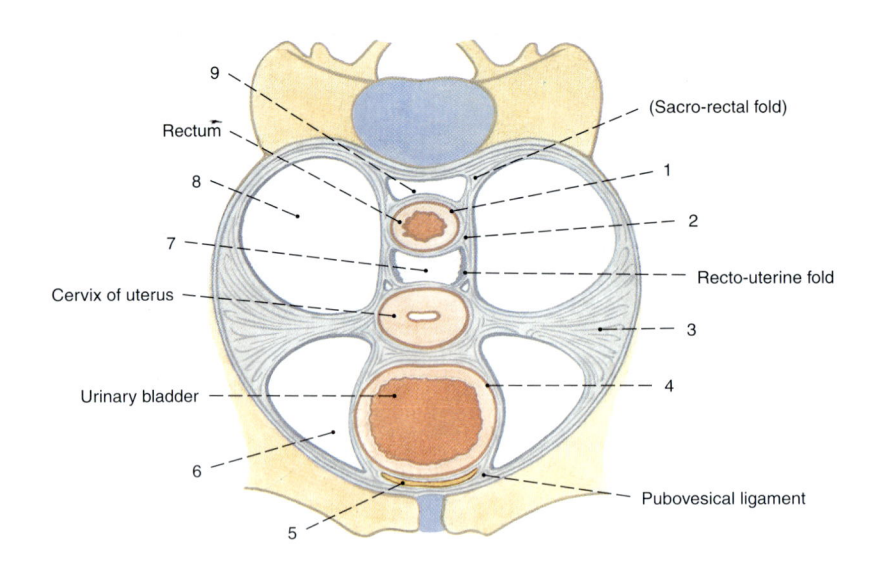

Fig. 1070 Uterus; diagram of ligaments and fascial spaces in the lesser pelvis [true pelvis]; transverse section at level of cervix of uterus; superior aspect.

Recent anatomical studies raise the question about the existence of ligaments from the uterus to the lateral wall of the pelvis, which have been called cardinal ligament of uterus.

1 = rectal fascia
2 = uterosacral ligament
3 = cardinal ligament, parametrium
4 = vesical fascia
5 = retropubic space (prevesical cave of RETZIUS)
6 = paravesical space, paracystium
7 = recto-uterine pouch (pouch of DOUGLAS)
8 = pararectal space, paraproctium
9 = retrorectal space

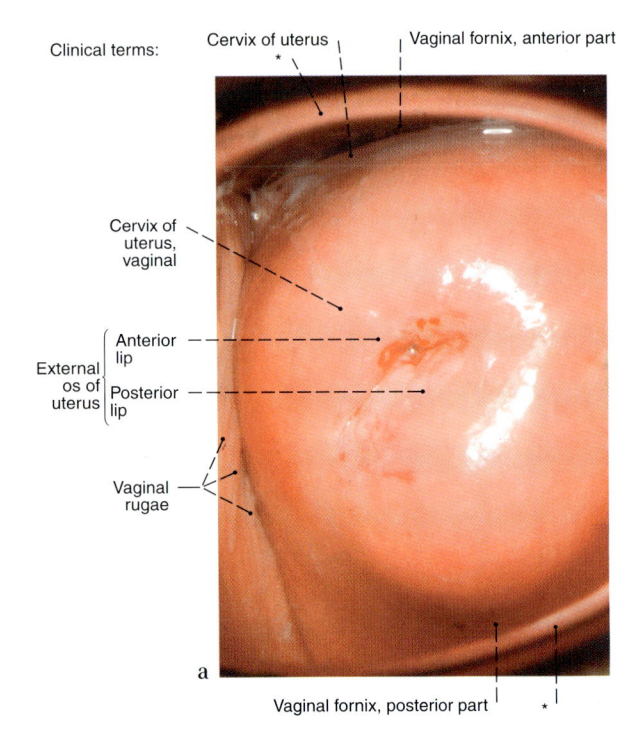

Fig. 1071 a, b Cervix of uterus, vaginal part.
    a Photo of a young female, who has not born a child before (nulliparous)
    b Photo of a young female who has born two children

Inspection of the vaginal part of cervix is enabled by spreading the normally slit-like vagina with two specula (*); caudal aspect. The vaginal part of cervix projects clearly into the vagina.

Uterus, pregnancy   199

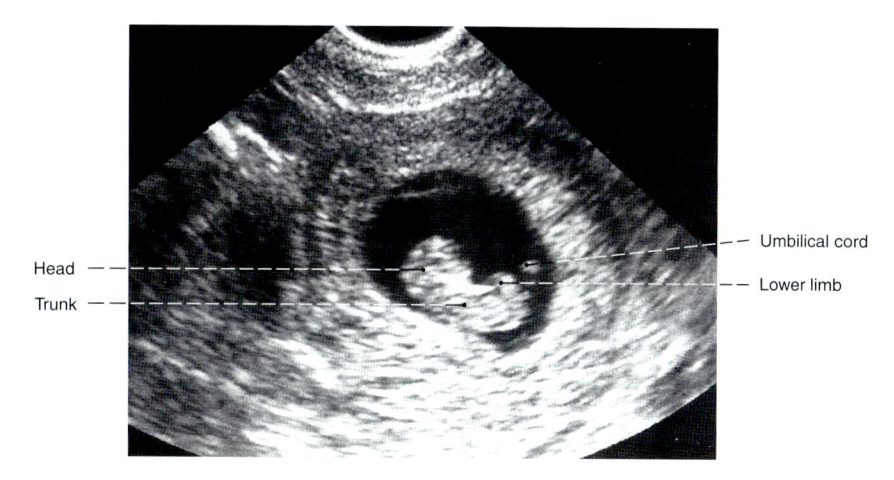

Fig. 1072 Uterus with embryo; ultrasound scan in the 10th week of pregnancy, scanned through the abdominal wall; right lateral aspect.

The embryo swims in the amniotic fluid of the chorionic cavity.

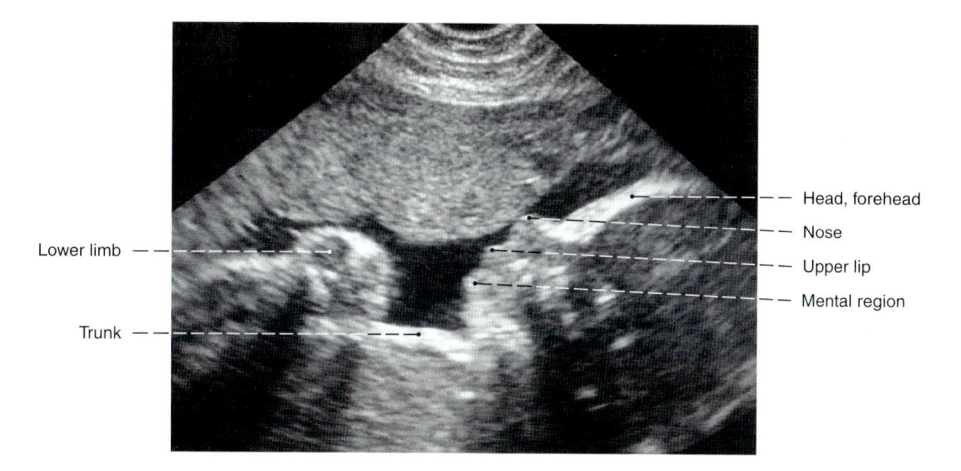

Fig. 1073 Uterus with fetus; ultrasound scan in the 28th week of pregnancy, scanned through the abdominal wall; left lateral aspect.

During ultrasonography movements of the limbs and opening of the mouth can be examined.

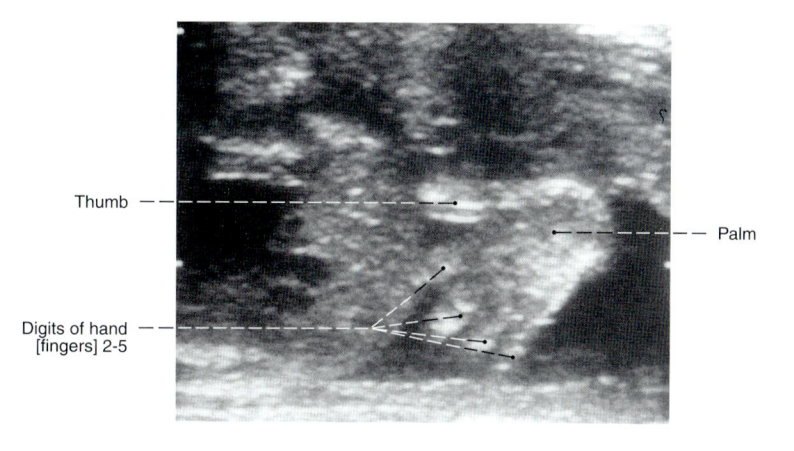

Fig. 1074 Hand of a fetus; ultrasound scan in the 24th week of pregnancy; details such as the fingers can be studied; lateral aspect.

Pelvic viscera

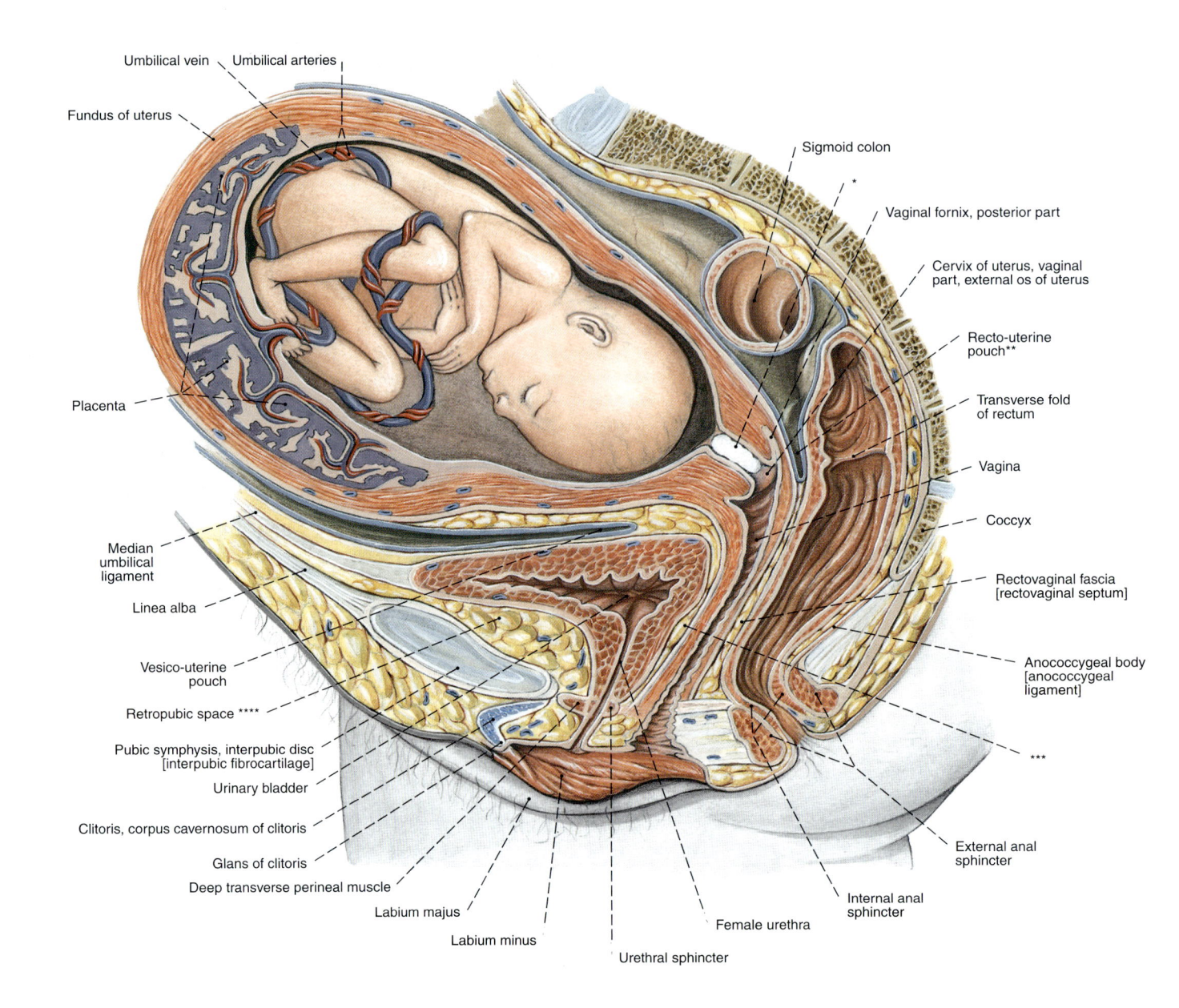

Fig. 1075 Uterus with fetus; pelvis sectioned in the median plane; left lateral aspect.
The wall of uterus becomes even thinner at the end of pregnancy.

* Mucous plug (of KRISTELLER) in the cervical canal of uterus.
** Pouch of DOUGLAS.
*** Vesicovaginal septum.
**** Cave of RETZIUS.

Uterus, pregnancy 201

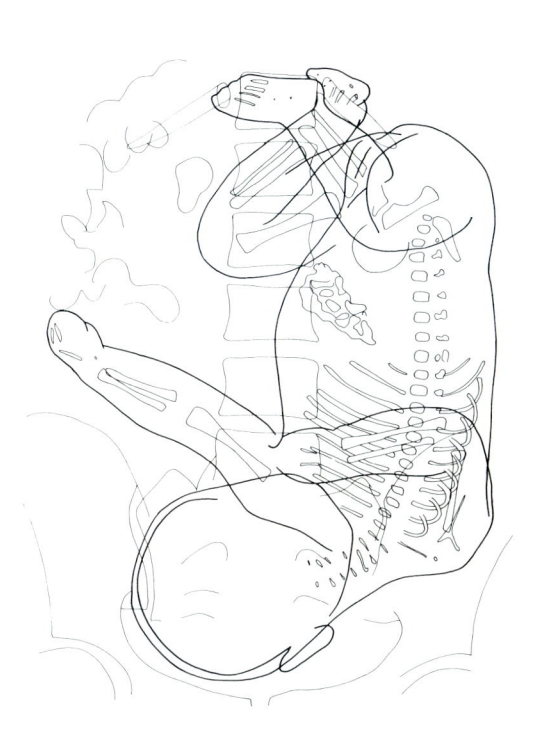

Fig. 1076 Fetus; AP radiograph shortly before birth; ventral aspect.

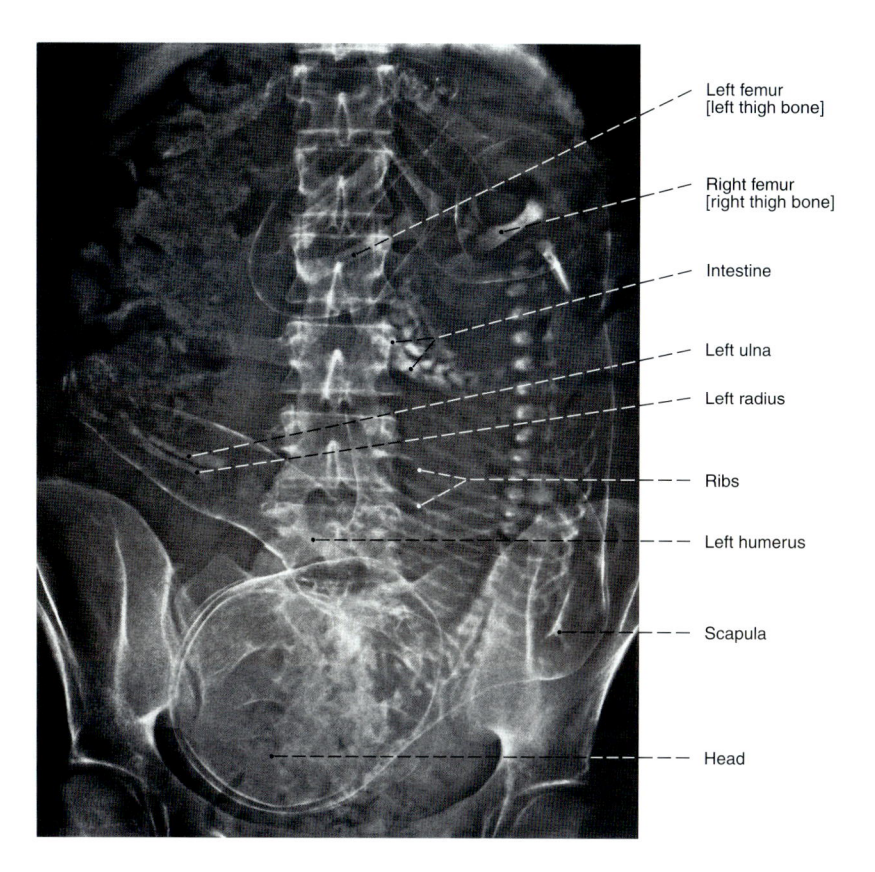

Previously this method was occasionally used to measure the size of the head of the fetus in relation to the pelvis of the female.

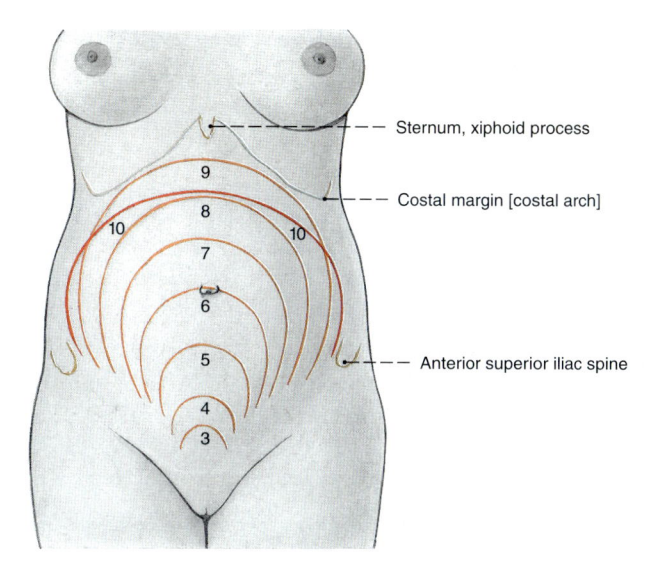

Fig. 1077 Uterus; sizes during pregnancy; numerals indicate the end of the respective month of pregnancy (28 days); in the last month the fundus of uterus goes down again.

Pelvic viscera

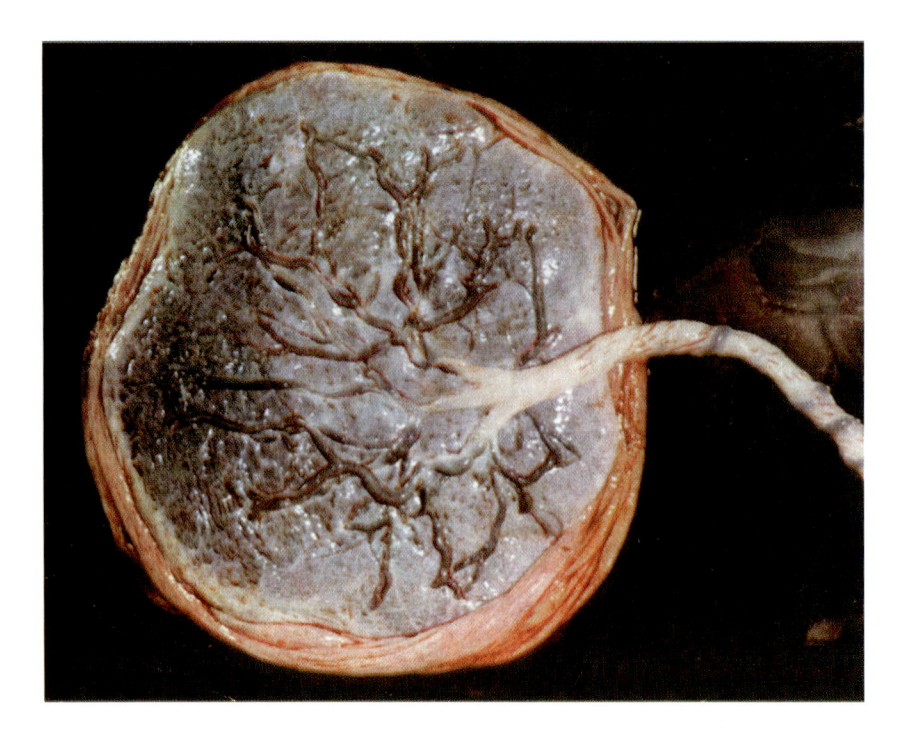

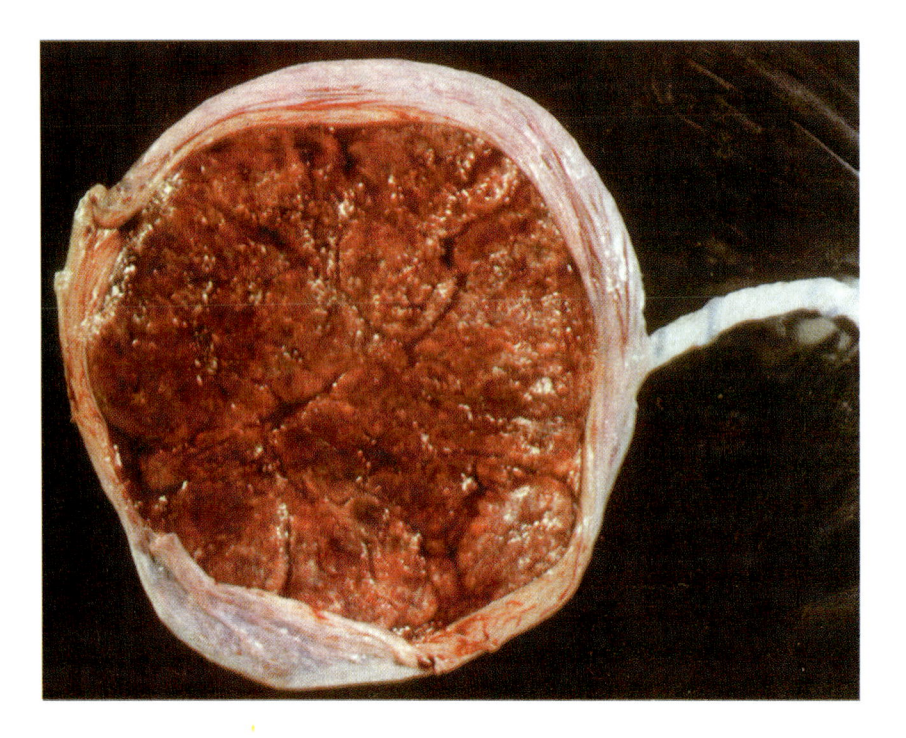

Fig. 1078 a, b   Placenta; umbilical cord.
a   View of fetal surface
b   View of maternal surface of a parturient placenta

The fetal surface is shiny and smooth because of the amnion; the maternal surface is divided into lobes (= cotyledons) by deep grooves and colored blood red.

Female internal genitalia

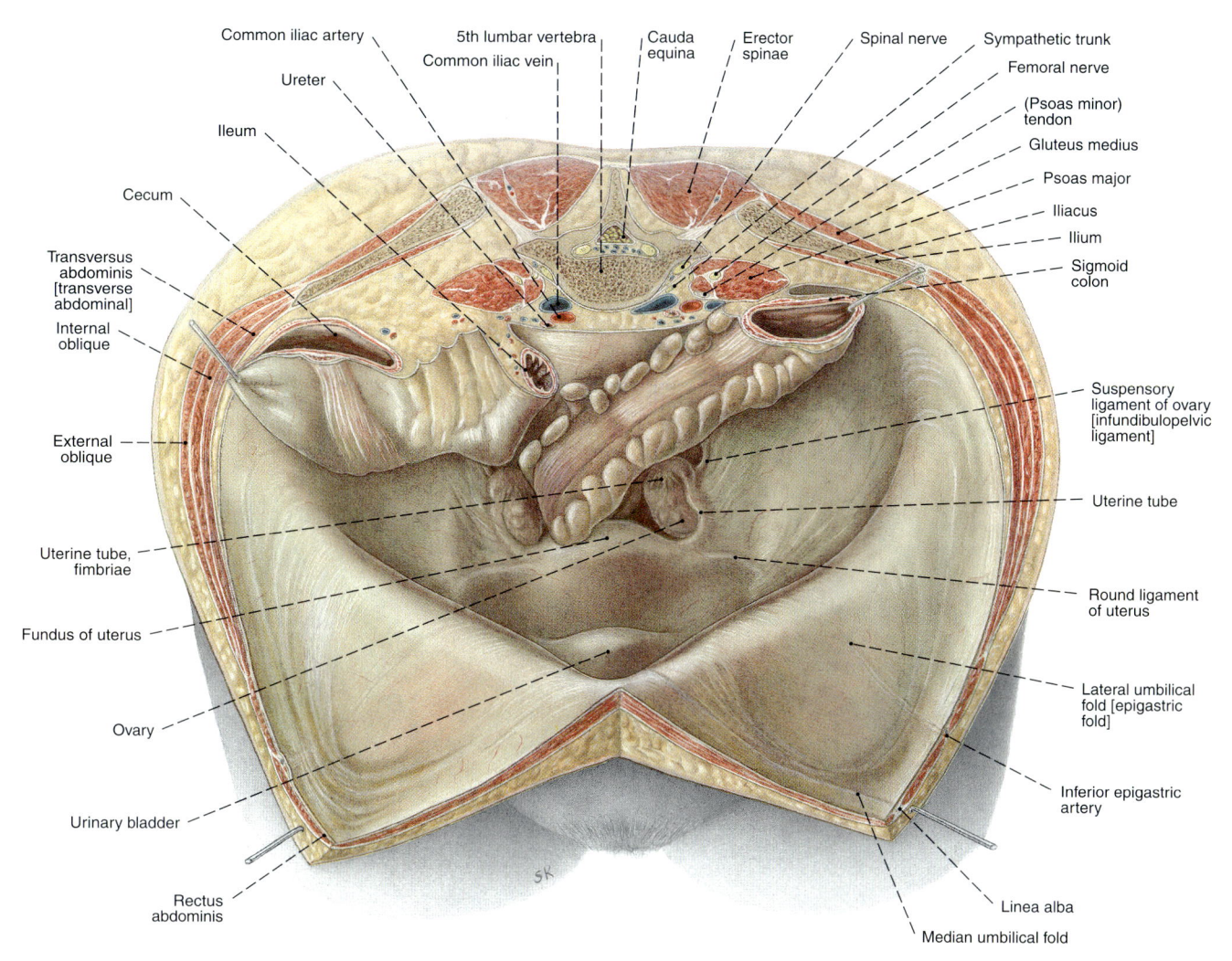

Fig. 1079 Female internal genitalia; horizontal section at level of 5th lumbar vertebra; anterior abdominal wall sectioned longitudinally in the right rectus abdominis and retracted laterally by hooks; cecum and sigmoid colon retracted cranially by a hook; ventral superior aspect.

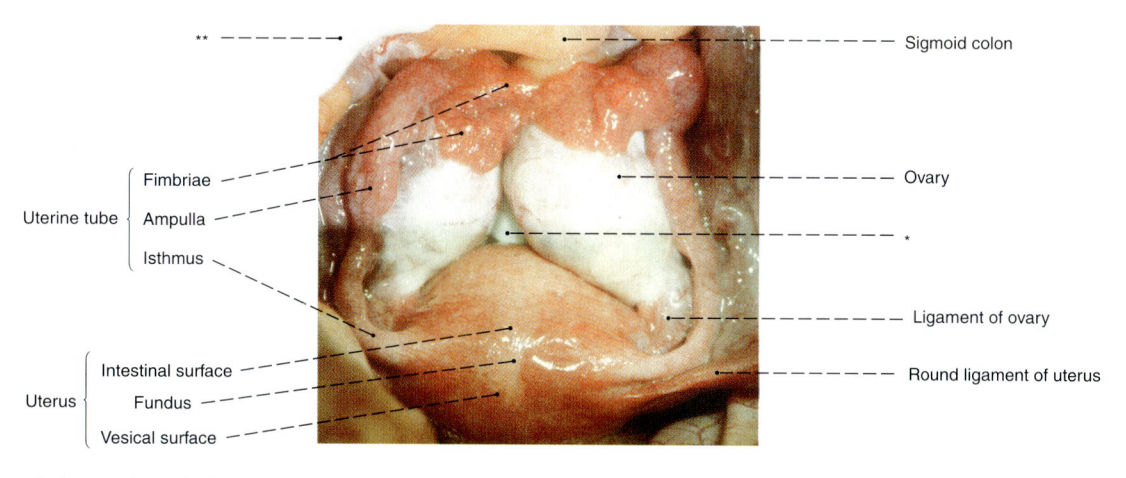

Fig. 1080 Female internal genitalia; surgical exposure of a young female; ovaries are displaced superomedially by compresses (*) in the pouch of DOUGLAS; ventral superior aspect.
** Swab.

Pelvic viscera

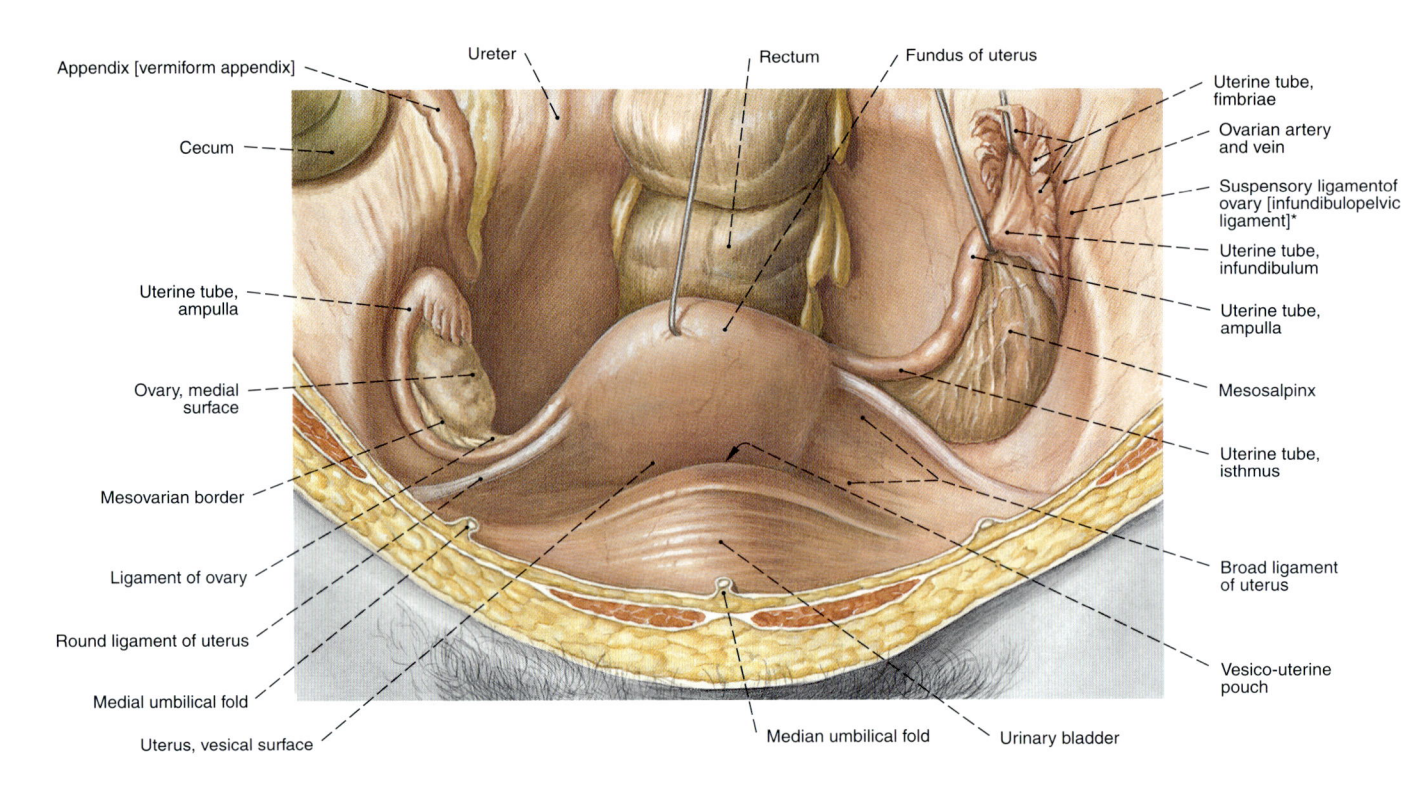

Fig. 1081 Female internal genitalia; uterus retracted by a hook to expose vesico-uterine pouch and broad ligament of uterus; left uterine tube retracted cranially to expose mesosalpinx; ventral aspect.
The close relationship of the appendages (ovary and uterine tube) with the appendix [vermiform appendix] may cause differential diagnostic problems in the case of inflammations.

* Clinically: infundibulopelvic ligament.

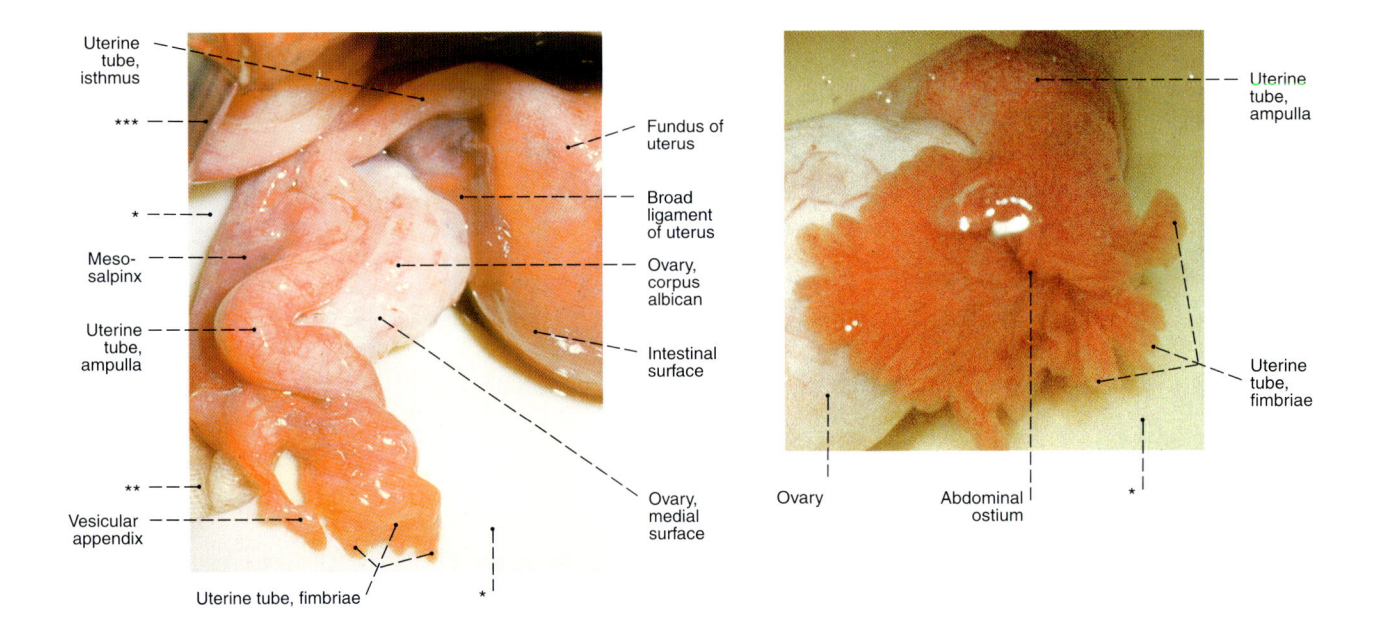

Fig. 1082 Uterine tube, ovary; surgical exposure in a young female; dorsal superior aspect.
* Plastic tray to elevate ovary and uterine tube.
** Swab.
*** Surgical hook.

Fig. 1083 Abdominal ostium of uterine tube, ovary; surgical exposure in a young female; the pelvic cavity filled with saline to expose the fimbriae; dorsal superior aspect.
* Plastic tray to elevate uterine tube.

Rectum 205

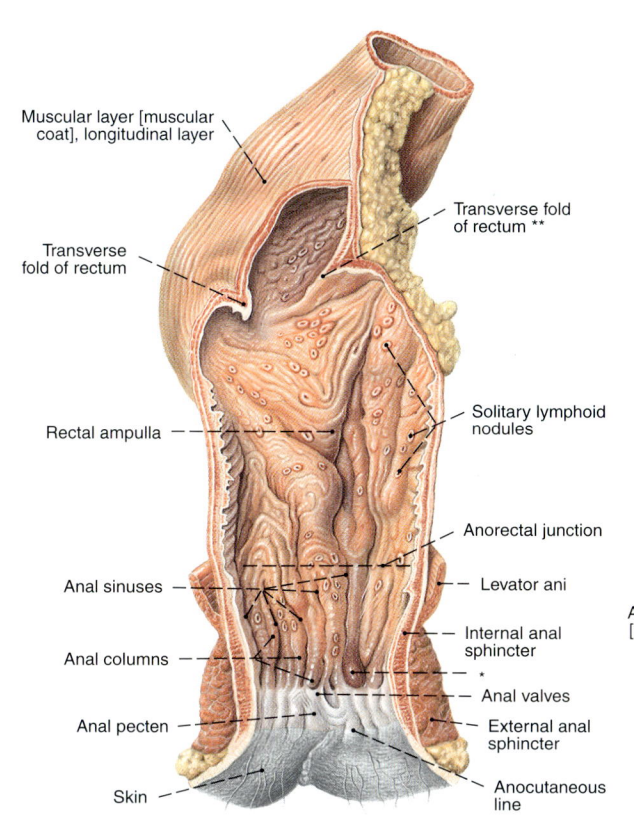

Fig. 1084 Rectum; anus; frontal section exposing mucosa [mucous membrane] and sphincters; ventral aspect.

* Hemorrhoidal node.
** KOHLRAUSCH's fold.

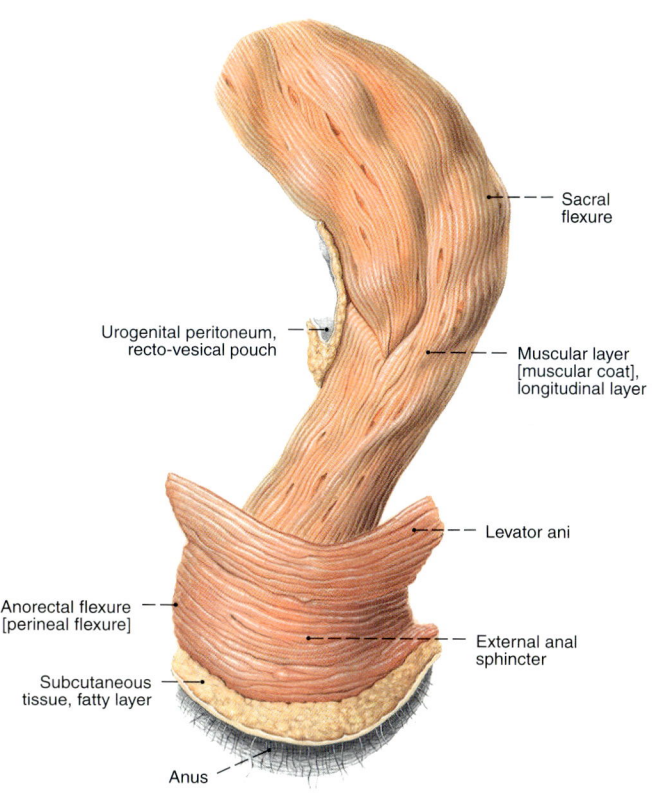

Fig. 1085 Rectum; anus; surrounding tissue extensively removed to expose muscular layer [muscular coat]; right lateral aspect.

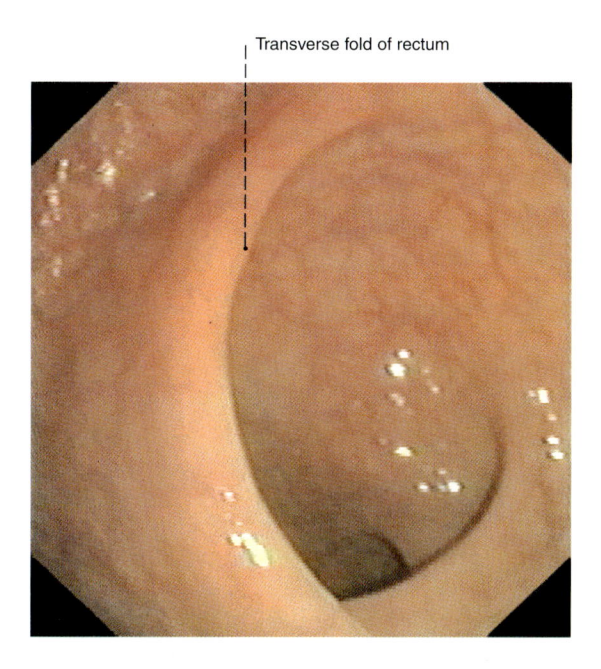

Fig. 1086 Rectum; anus; rectoscopic view of rectal ampulla by an endoscope inserted through the anal canal to examine the mucosa [mucous membrane]; inferior aspect.

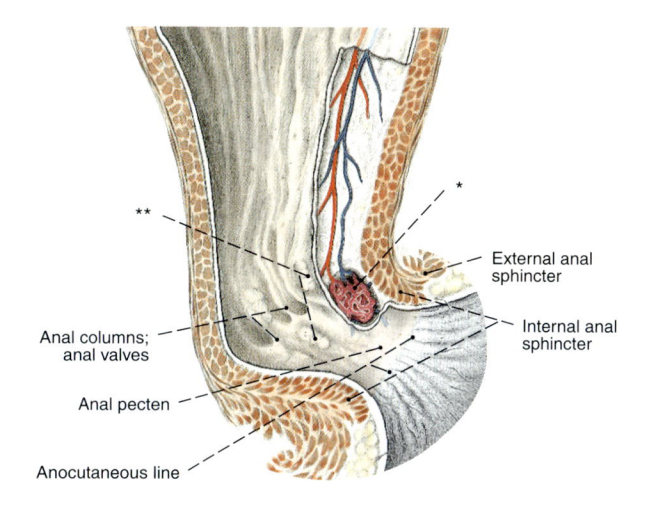

Fig. 1087 Rectum; anus; median section exposing arteriovenous anastomoses in the anal columns; mucosa [mucous membrane] partially removed; left lateral aspect. Closure of the anus is achieved by muscles (internal and external anal sphincters, levator ani), mucosal folds, and erectile-type arteriovenous anastomoses.

* Rectal glomerulus, numerous arteriovenous anastomoses in the anal columns.
** Clinically: hemorrhoidal zone.

206 *Pelvic viscera*

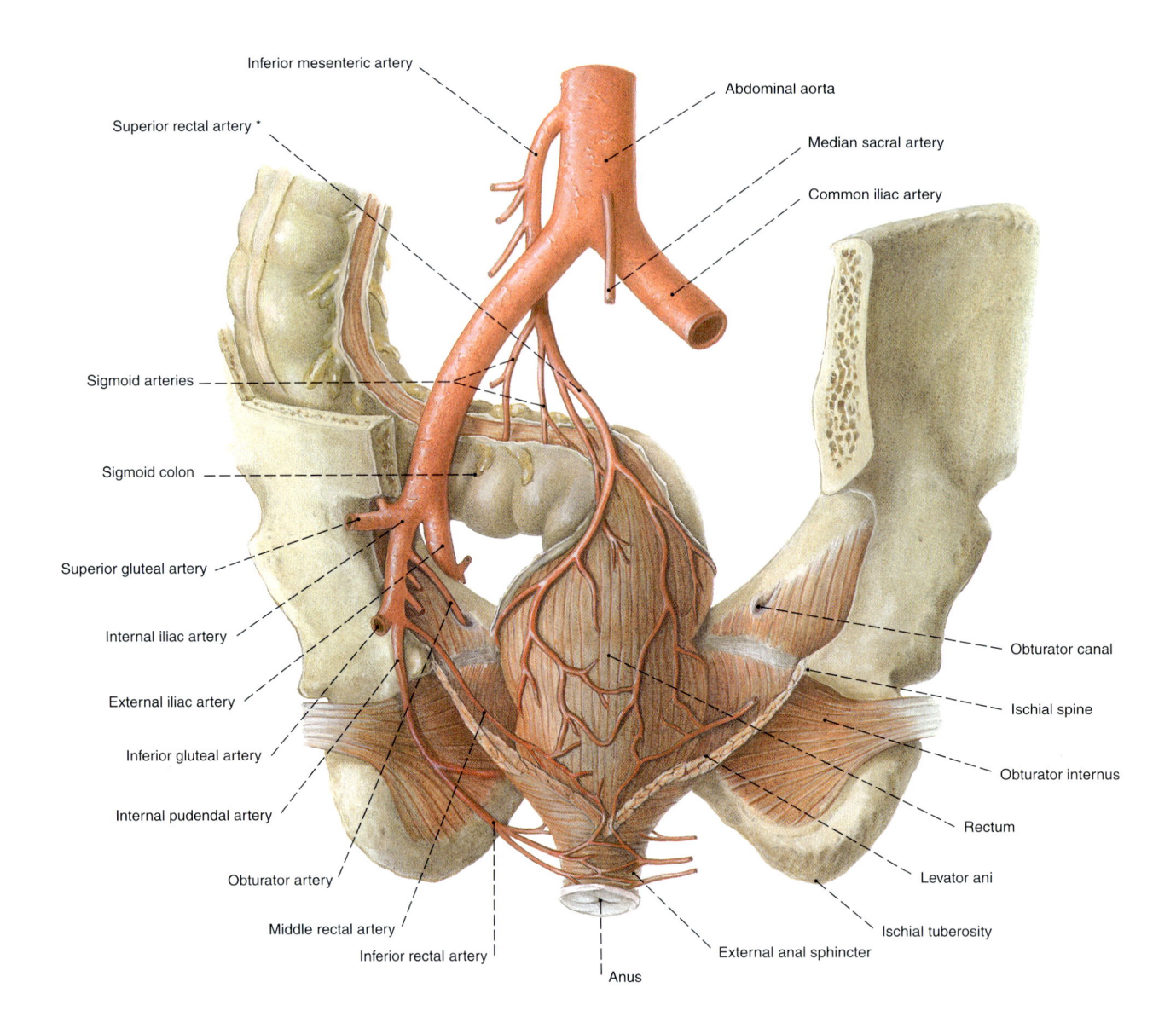

Fig. 1088 Arteries of rectum; figure showing the most important branches of the iliac artery only on the left dorsal aspect.

* Clinically: critical point of SUDECK (from there no further anastomoses to the sigmoid arteries).

Rectum

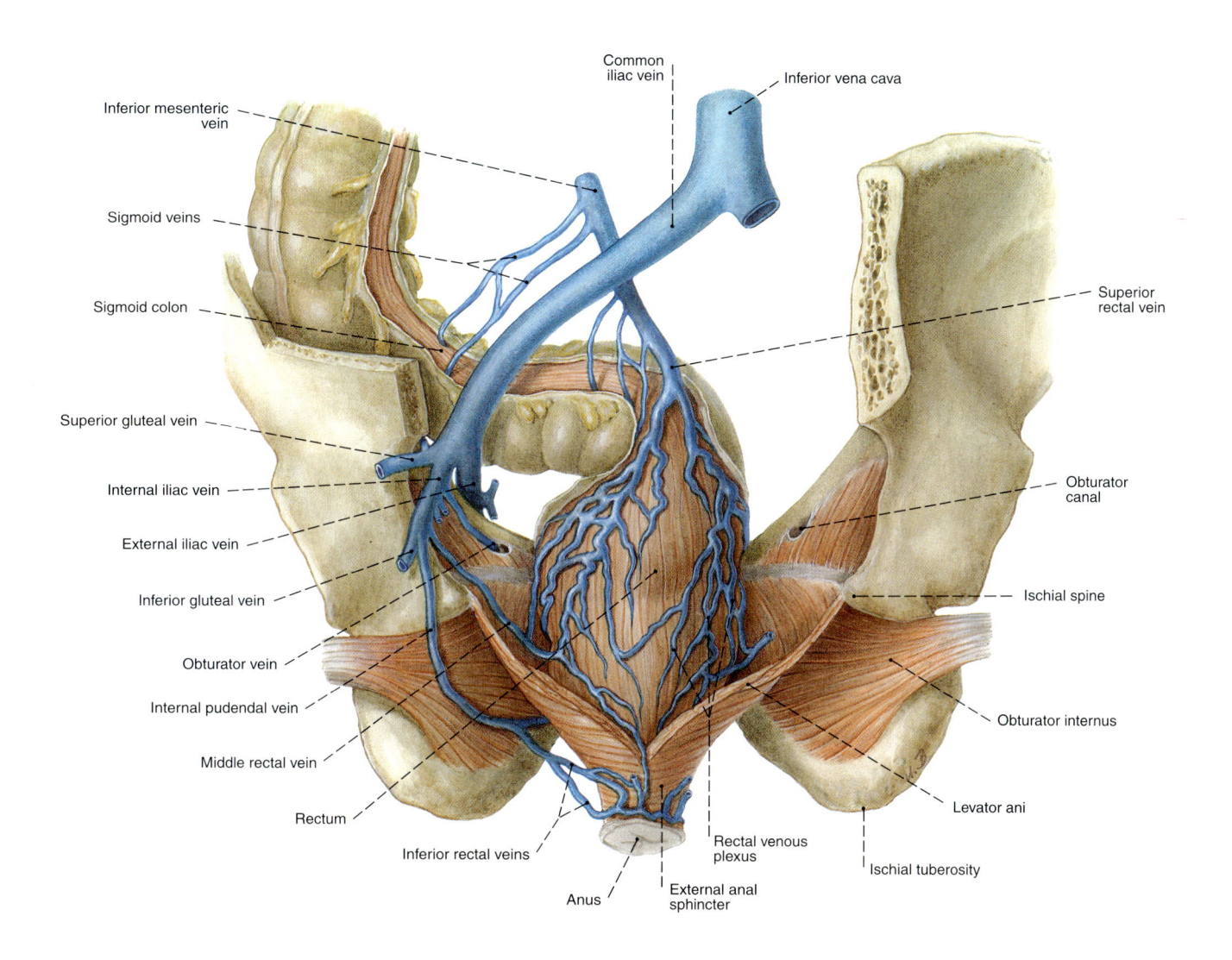

Fig. 1089 Veins of rectum; diagram with parts of pelvis and pelvic diaphragm [pelvis floor]; dorsal aspect. Many of the small veins are in fact doubled; however they are drawn only as single veins for clearness of the figure. The venous network beneath the rectal mucosa is not shown. There are numerous connections between veins draining into the hepatic portal vein (superior rectal vein) and the veins draining into the inferior vena cava (middle and inferior rectal veins). These belong to the so-called portocaval anastomoses and are of significant clinical relevance.

208 Pelvic viscera

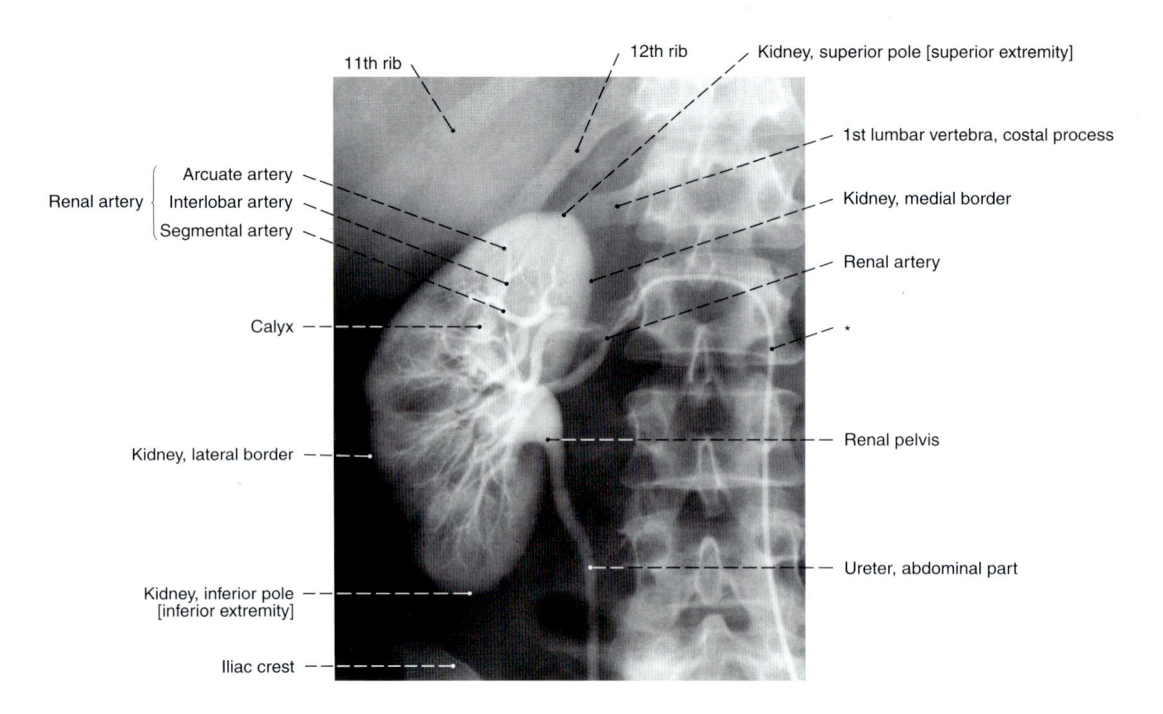

Fig. 1090 Kidney; AP radiograph after intravenous injection of contrast medium, which is excreted via the kidney (i.v. pyelography) to visualize renal pelvis and ureter; simultaneous visualization of arteries by injection of contrast medium into the renal artery through a catheter* introduced via the aorta (arteriography).

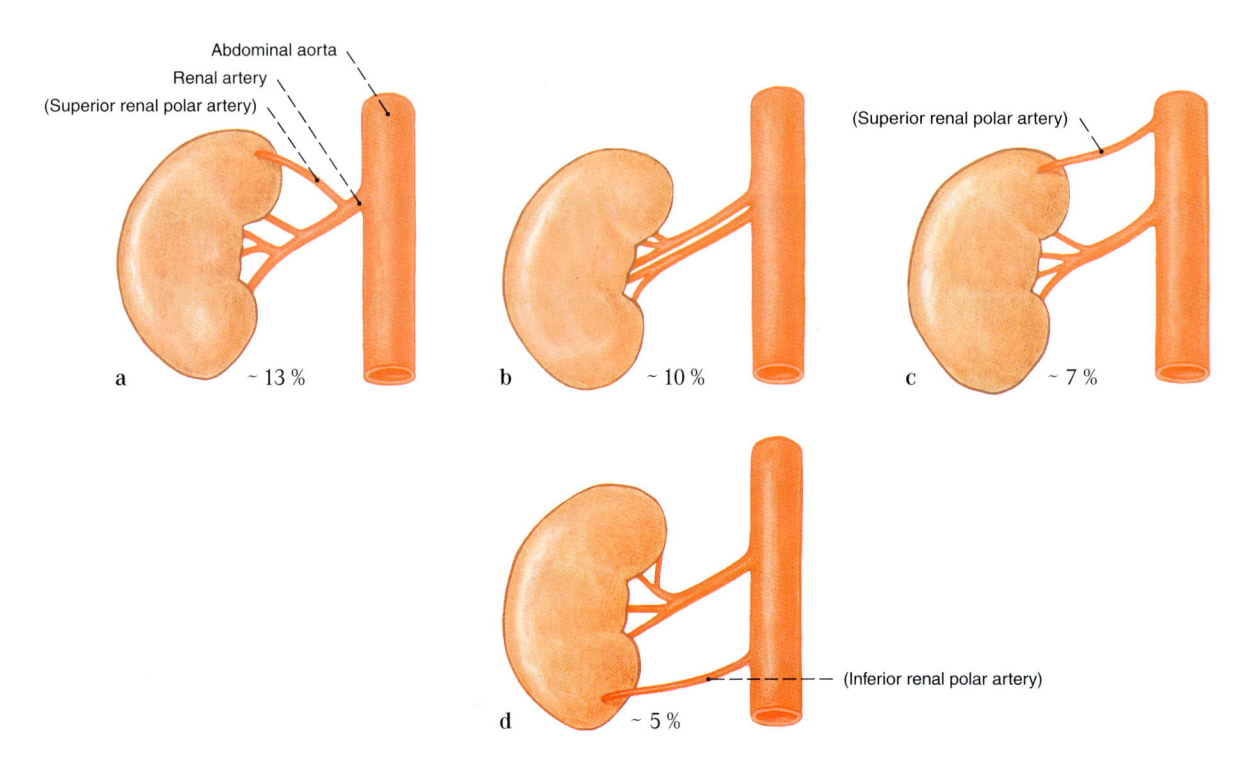

Fig. 1091 a–d Variations in the arterial blood supply of the kidney.

a Renal artery with a branch to the superior pole [superior extremity]
b Two renal arteries to hilum of kidney
c Accessory artery to the superior pole [superior extremity]
d Accessory artery to the inferior pole [inferior extremity]

Position of retroperitoneal viscera 209

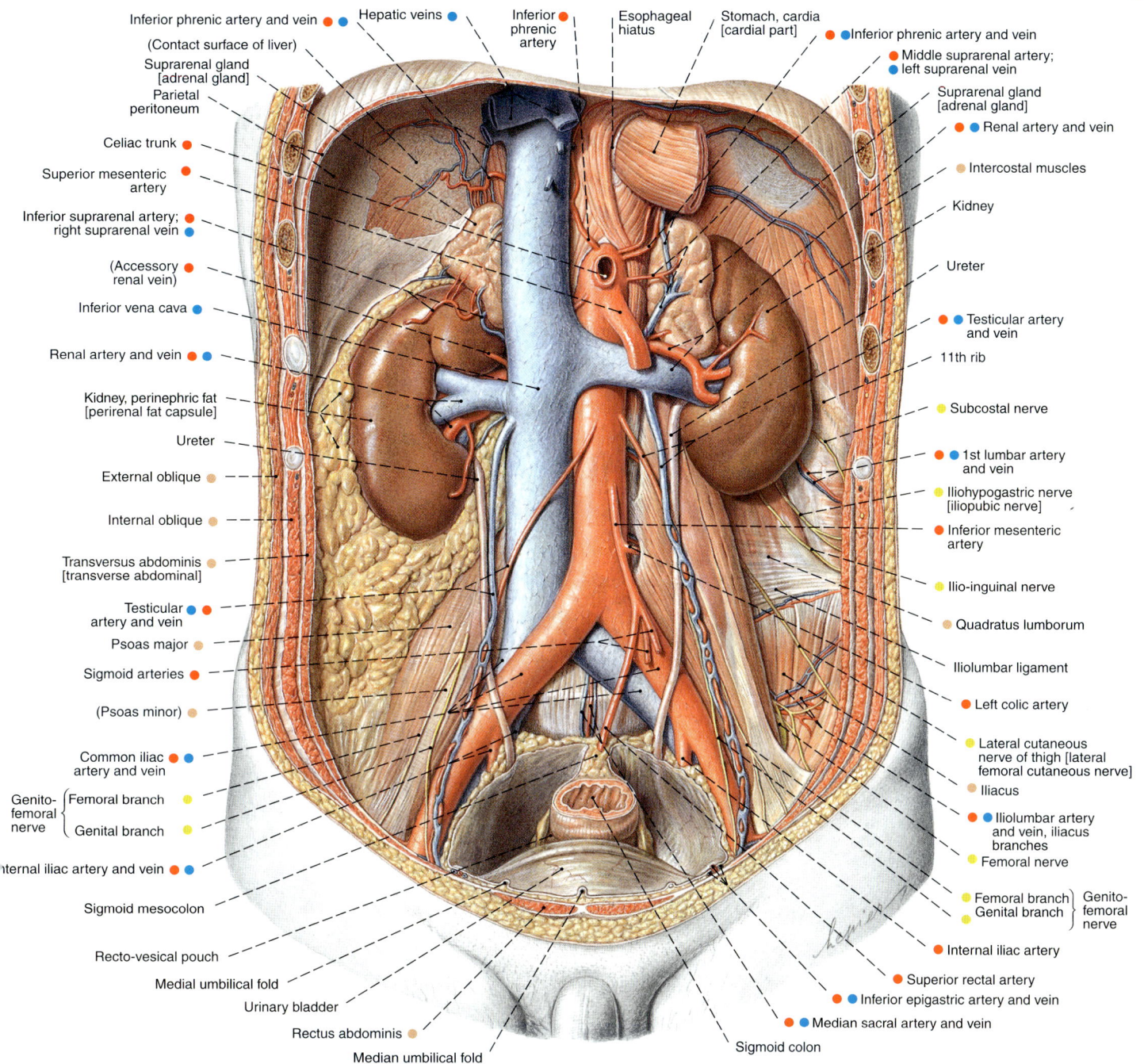

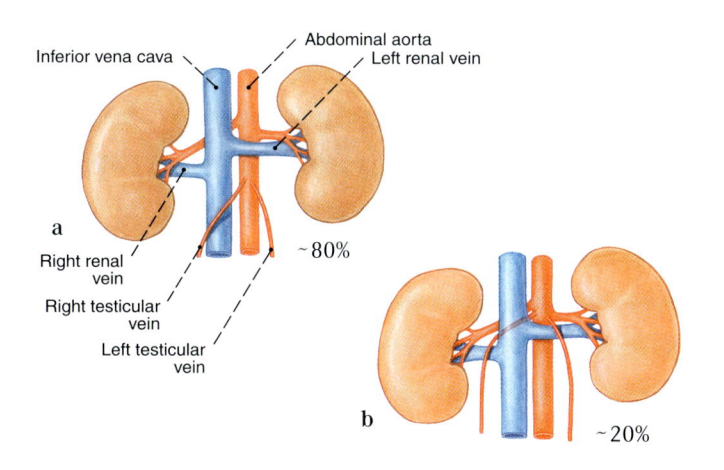

Fig. 1092 Position of retroperitoneal organs in the male; intestine, liver, pancreas, and spleen removed; ventral aspect. While the left testicular vein drains into the left renal vein, the right testicular artery drains directly into the inferior vena cava. Similar relationships apply for the ovarian veins.

Fig. 1093 a, b Variations of the course of the testicular arteries.

a "Normal textbook case"
b Both testicular arteries originating superior to the renal veins; right testicular artery dorsal to inferior vena cava, left testicular artery ventral to renal vein

210 Abdominal viscera

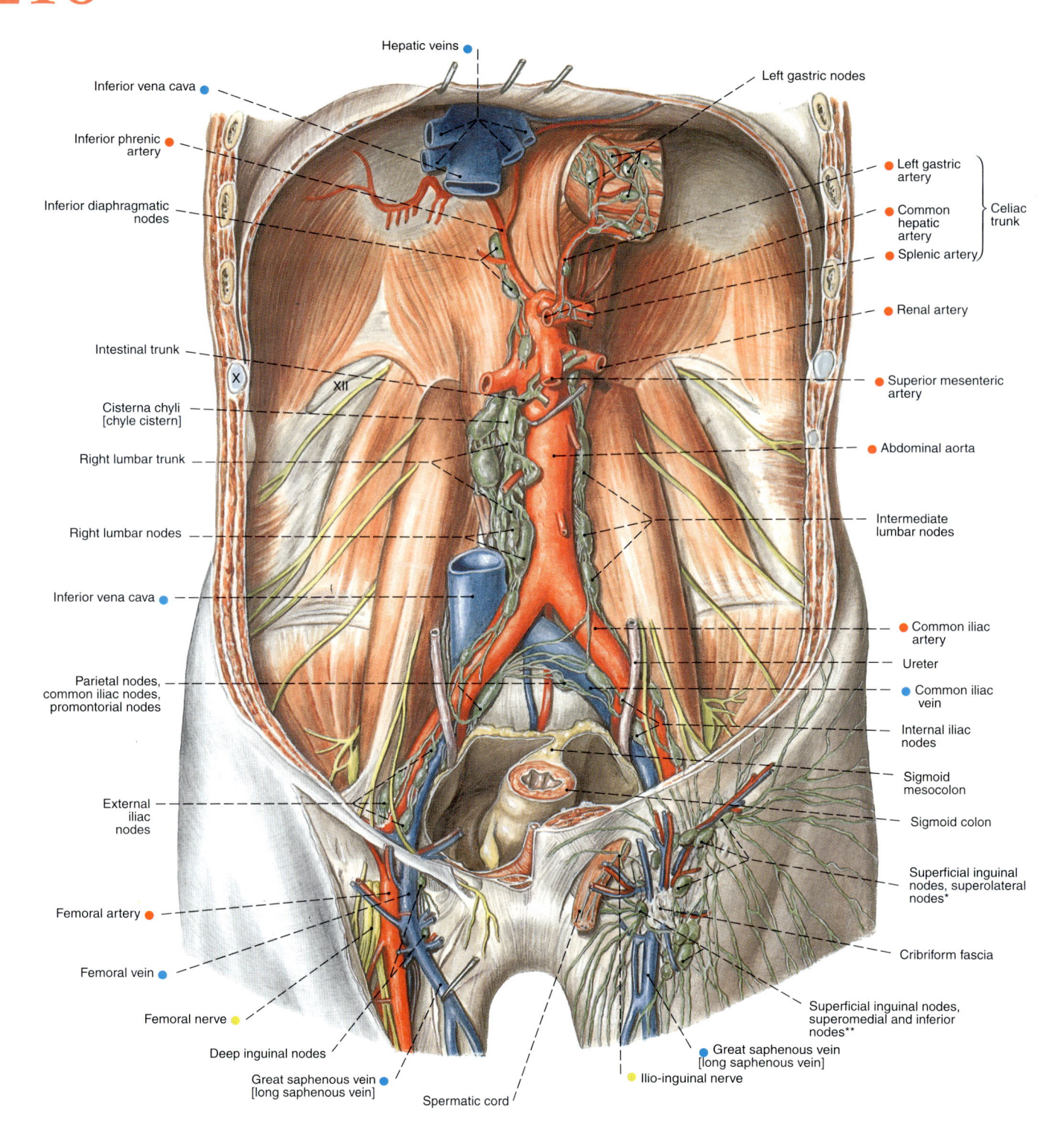

Fig. 1094
Lymph nodes and lymphatic vessels of the posterior abdominal wall and the groin [inguinal region]; all organs of the abdominal cavity, retroperitoneal fat, and parts of skin of thigh removed; ventral aspect.

Roman numerals I–XII indicate the ribs.
* Clinically: "horizontal chain"; tributary: lower abdominal wall, gluteal region, perineum, and external genitalia.
** Clinically: "vertical chain"; tributary: lower limb.

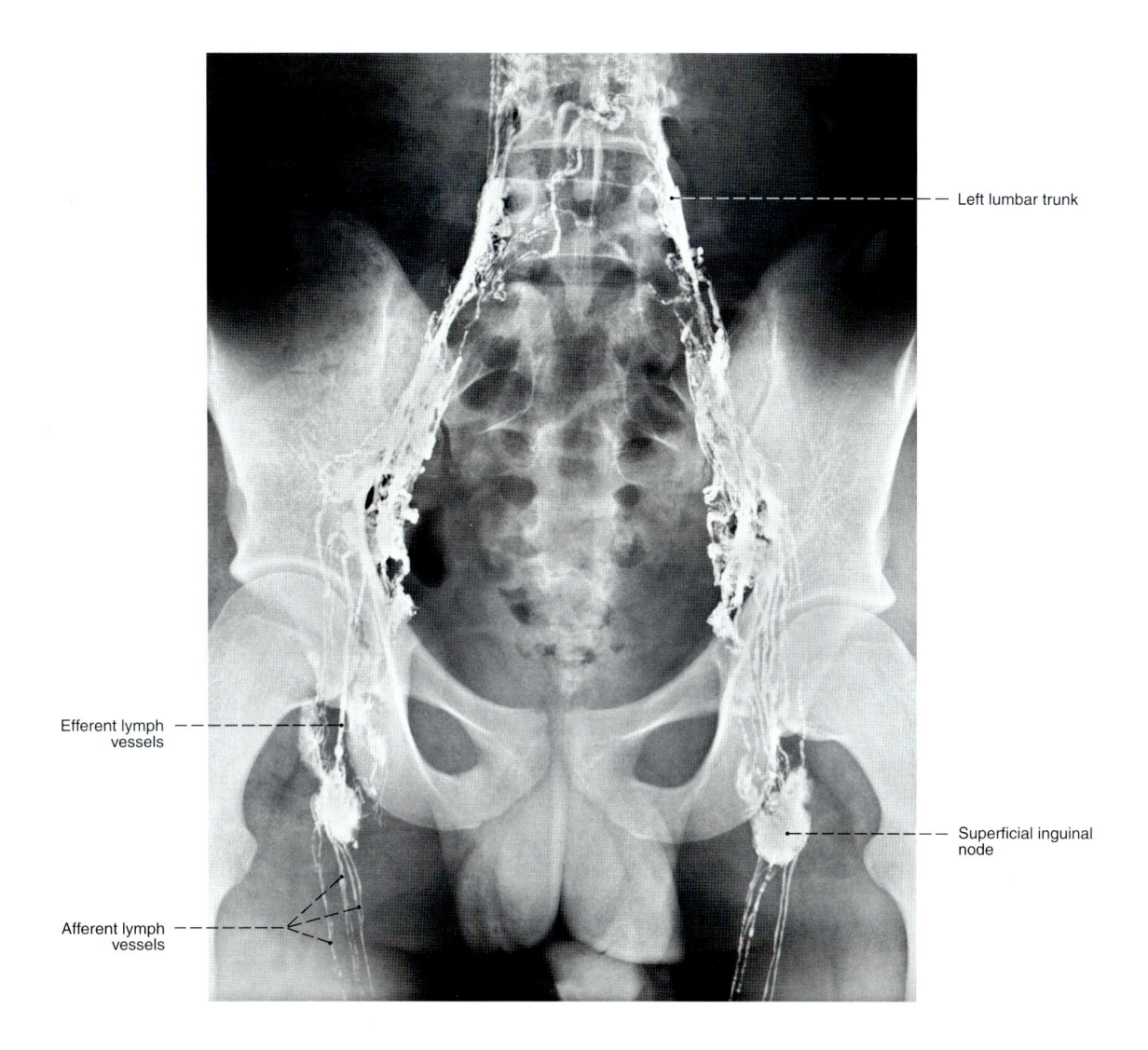

Fig. 1095 Lymphatic vessels and lymph nodes of the groin [inguinal region], the pelvis, and the lumbar region; AP radiograph after injection of contrast medium into the lymphatic vessels of both feet (lymphography). The pearl chain-like distensions of the lymphatic vessels are valvular segments. Storage of contrast medium starts in the inguinal nodes.

Abdominal viscera

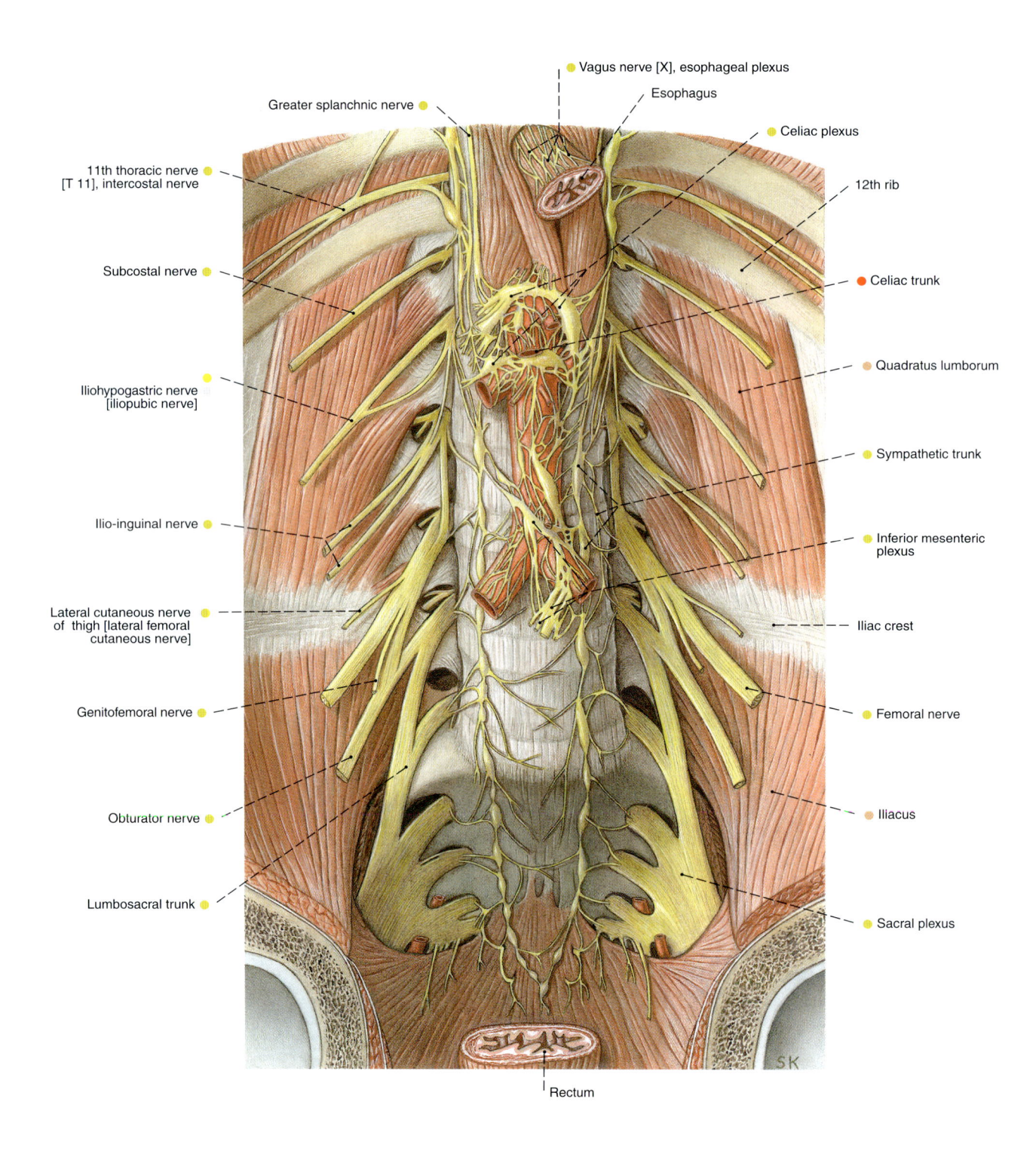

Fig. 1096 Nerves of the posterior abdominal wall, lumbosacral plexus, and abdominal part of autonomic division [autonomic part of peripheral nervous system]; viscera, blood vessels, and psoas major removed; ventral aspect.

Position of retroperitoneal viscera 213

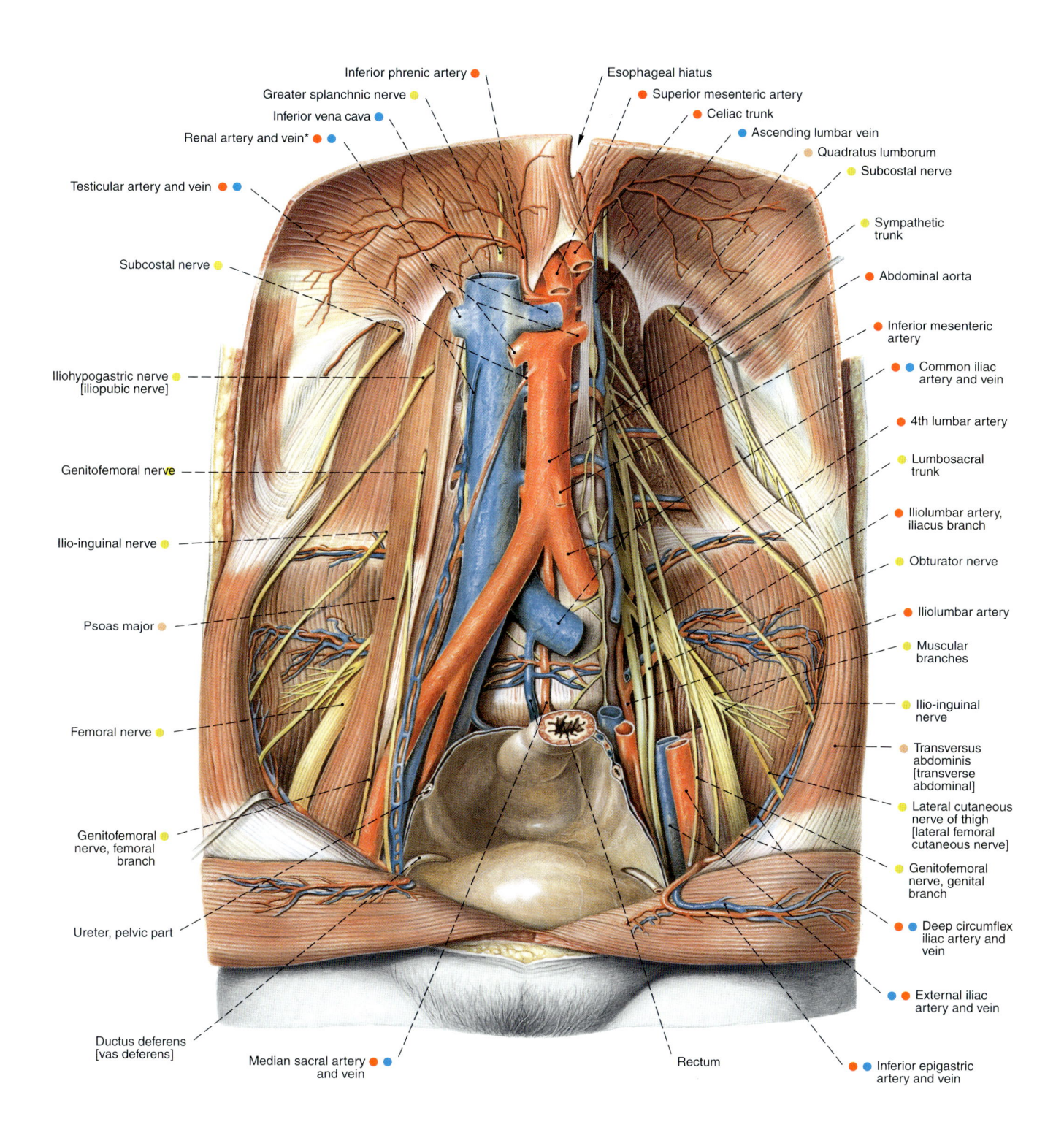

Fig. 1097 Blood vessels and nerves of the posterior abdominal wall in the male; left psoas major and iliac artery and vein extensively removed to expose lumbar plexus; ventral aspect.

* In approximately 10% the left renal vein passes dorsal to the aorta.

Pelvic viscera

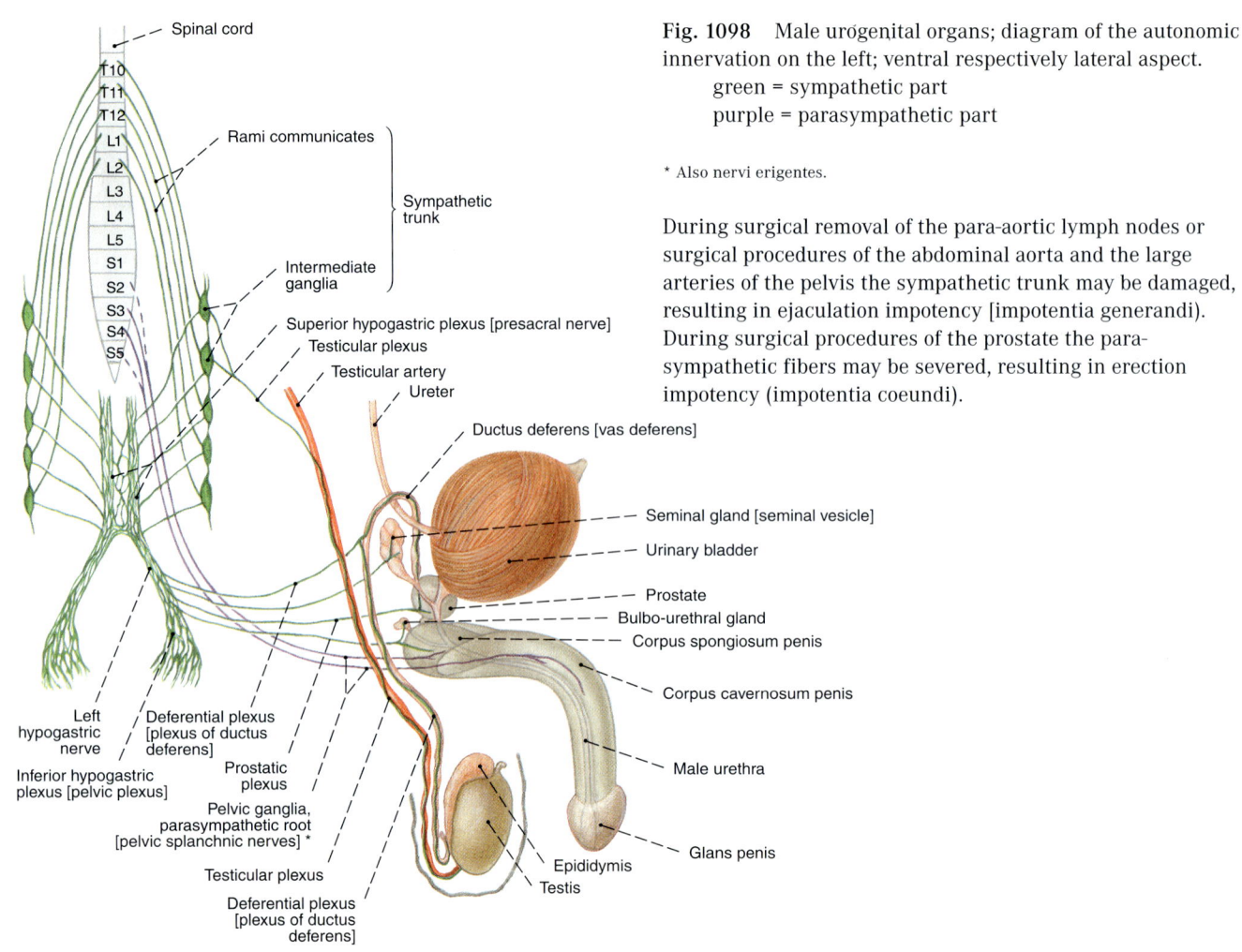

Fig. 1098 Male urogenital organs; diagram of the autonomic innervation on the left; ventral respectively lateral aspect.
green = sympathetic part
purple = parasympathetic part

* Also nervi erigentes.

During surgical removal of the para-aortic lymph nodes or surgical procedures of the abdominal aorta and the large arteries of the pelvis the sympathetic trunk may be damaged, resulting in ejaculation impotency [impotentia generandi]. During surgical procedures of the prostate the parasympathetic fibers may be severed, resulting in erection impotency (impotentia coeundi).

Innervation of male genitals

	Origin	Course	Organ	Function
Parasympathetic part	Spinal cord, sacral part (S 2- S 4)	Pelvic ganglia, parasympathetic root [pelvic splanchnic nerves]	Penis Corpora cavernosa and spongiosum	Vasodilatation Erection
Sympathetic part	Spinal cord, thoracic part (T 10 - T 12) Spinal cord, lumbar part (L 1 - L 2)	Superior and inferior mesenteric plexus ↓ Sympathetic trunk ↓ Testicular plexus ↓ Superior hypogastric plexus ↓ Hypogastric nerve ↓ Inferior hypogastric plexus	Testis Bulbo-urethral gland Ductus deferens [vas deferens] Seminal gland [seminal vesicle] Prostate	Regulation of blood flow Secretion Contraction, transportation of sperm into urethra Ejaculation into urethra
Somatic efferent Somatic afferent	Spinal cord, sacral part (S 2- S 4)	Pudendal nerve Posterior scrotal nerves Dorsal nerve of penis	(Sphincter of bladder) Ischiocavernosus Bulbospongiosus Skin of scrotum Skin of penis	Closure of bladder prevents retrograde ejaculation into the bladder Expulsion of ejaculate from urethra

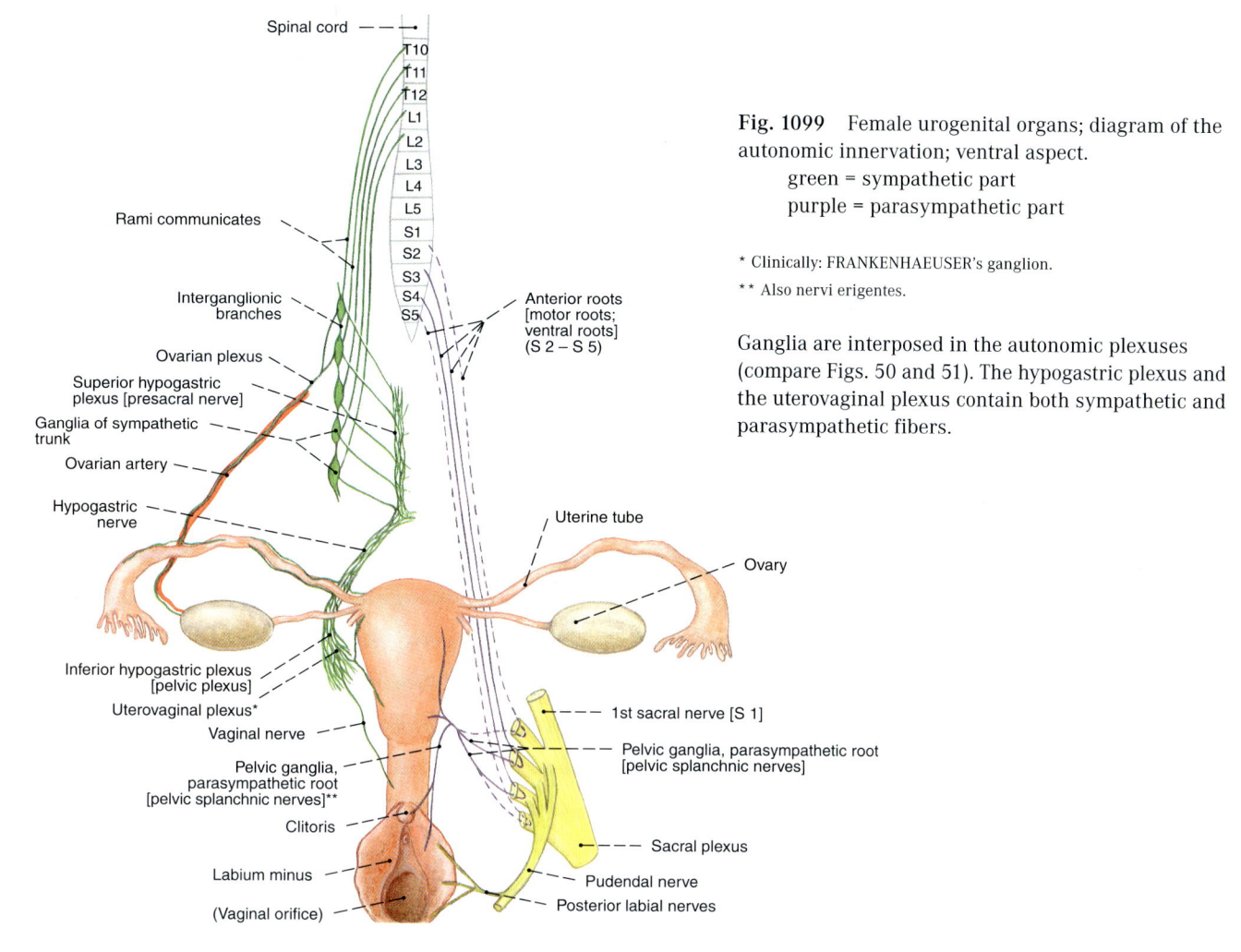

Female genitalia, innervation

Fig. 1099 Female urogenital organs; diagram of the autonomic innervation; ventral aspect.
- green = sympathetic part
- purple = parasympathetic part

* Clinically: FRANKENHAEUSER's ganglion.
** Also nervi erigentes.

Ganglia are interposed in the autonomic plexuses (compare Figs. 50 and 51). The hypogastric plexus and the uterovaginal plexus contain both sympathetic and parasympathetic fibers.

Innervation of female genitalia

	Origin	Course	Organ	Function
Parasympathetic part	Spinal cord, sacral part (S 2- S 4) Spinal cord, thoracic part (T 10 - T 12)	Pelvic ganglia, parasympathetic root [pelvic splanchnic nerves] ↓ Cavernous nerves of clitoris	Uterine tube Uterus Vagina Clitoris	Vasodilatation Vasodilatation Transudation Erection
Sympathetic part	Spinal cord, lumbar part (L 1 - L 2) Spinal cord, sacral part (S 2- S 4)	Superior mesenteric plexus ↓ Ovarian plexus ↓ Renal plexus Sympathetic trunk ↓ Superior hypogastric plexus ↓ Hypogastric nerve ↓ Inferior hypogastric plexus ↓ Uterovaginal plexus (FRANKENHAEUSER's ganglion)	Ovary Uterine tube Uterus Vagina	Vasoconstriction Contraction
Somatic efferent Somatic afferent		Pudendal nerve Dorsal nerve of clitoris Posterior labial nerves	Clitoris Labia majora Ischiocavernosus Bulbospongiosus	Contraction

216 *Pelvic viscera*

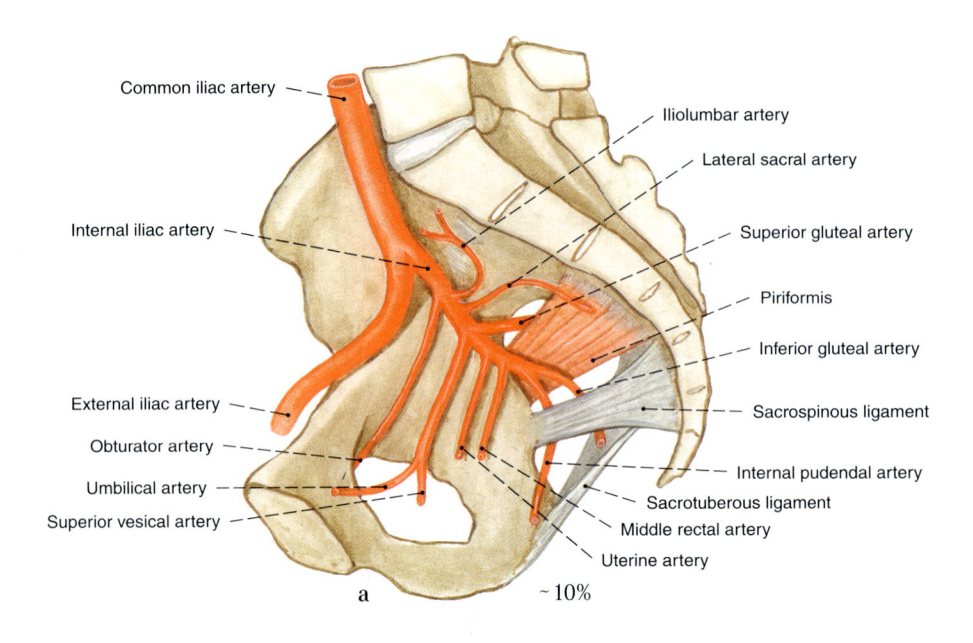

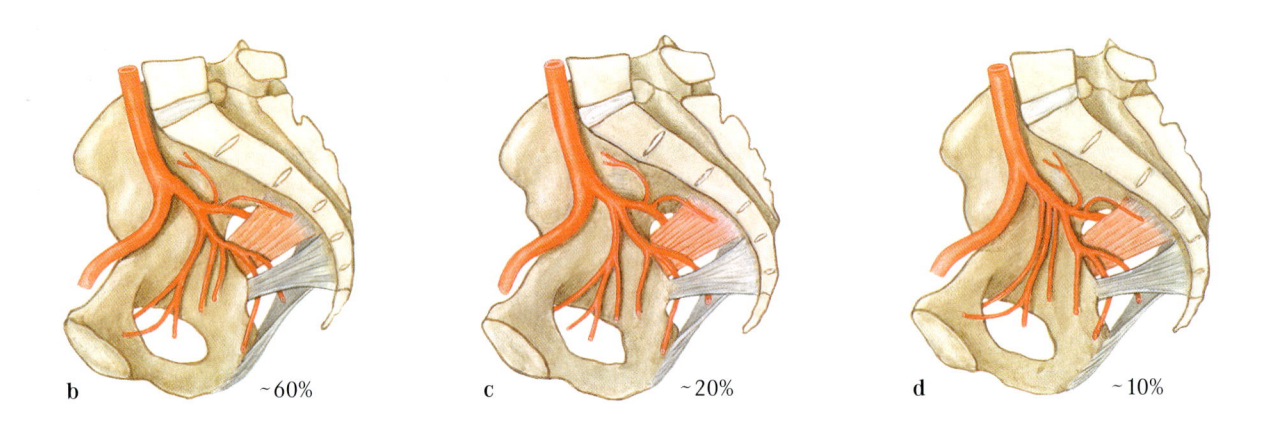

Fig. 1100 a–d   Variations of branching pattern of internal iliac artery; right lateral aspect.

- **a** Origin of all branches from the trunk of the internal iliac artery
- **b** Division of the internal iliac artery into two main branches ("normal textbook case")
- **c** Division of the internal iliac artery into three main branches
- **d** Division of the internal iliac artery into more than three main branches

Internal iliac artery

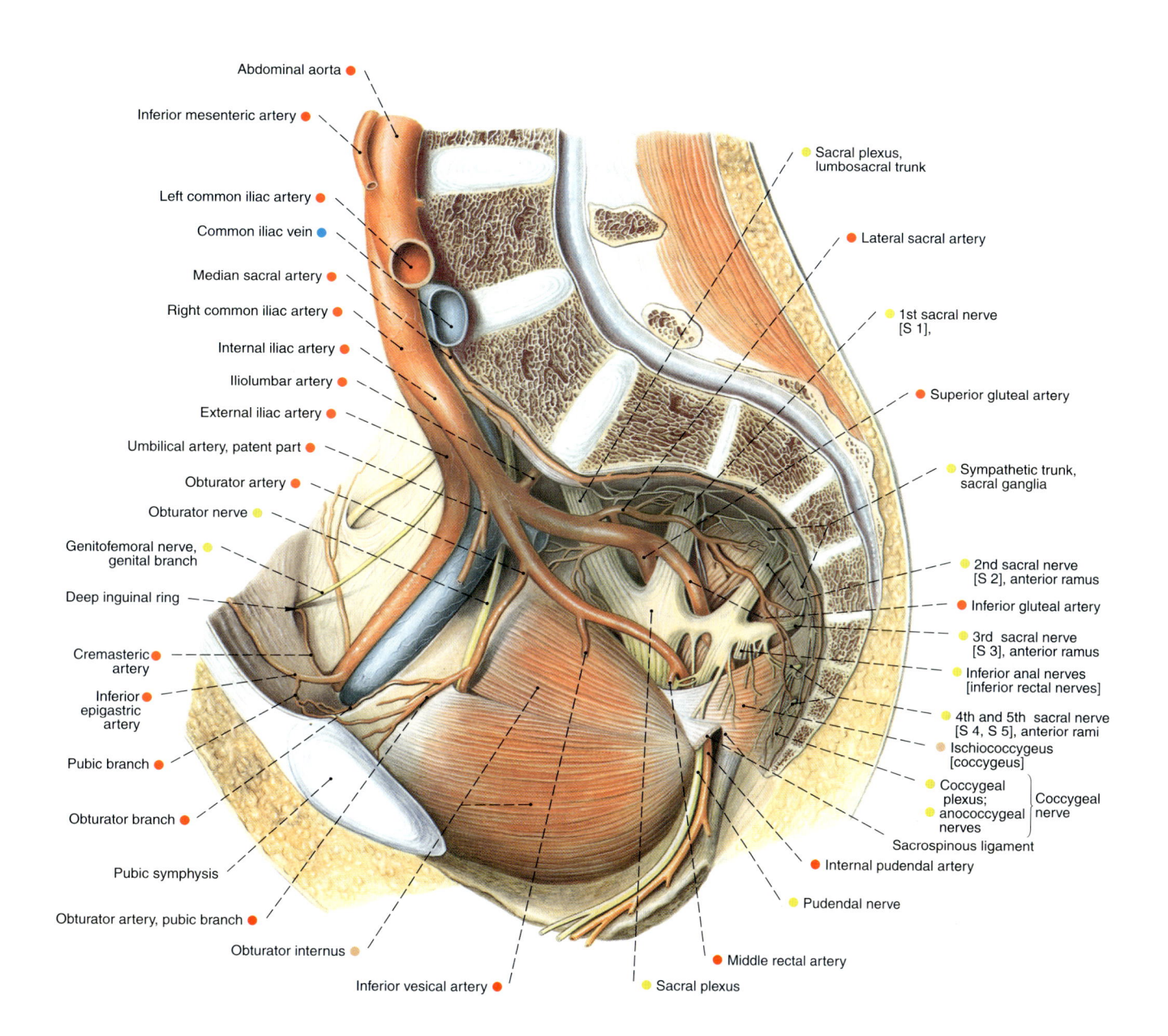

Fig. 1101 Internal iliac artery; sacral plexus; demonstration of the branches after removal of all pelvic viscera and fascias in a median sectioned pelvis: sacrospinous ligament incised to demonstrate the course of the internal pudendal artery; right lateral aspect. Compare Fig. 1100.

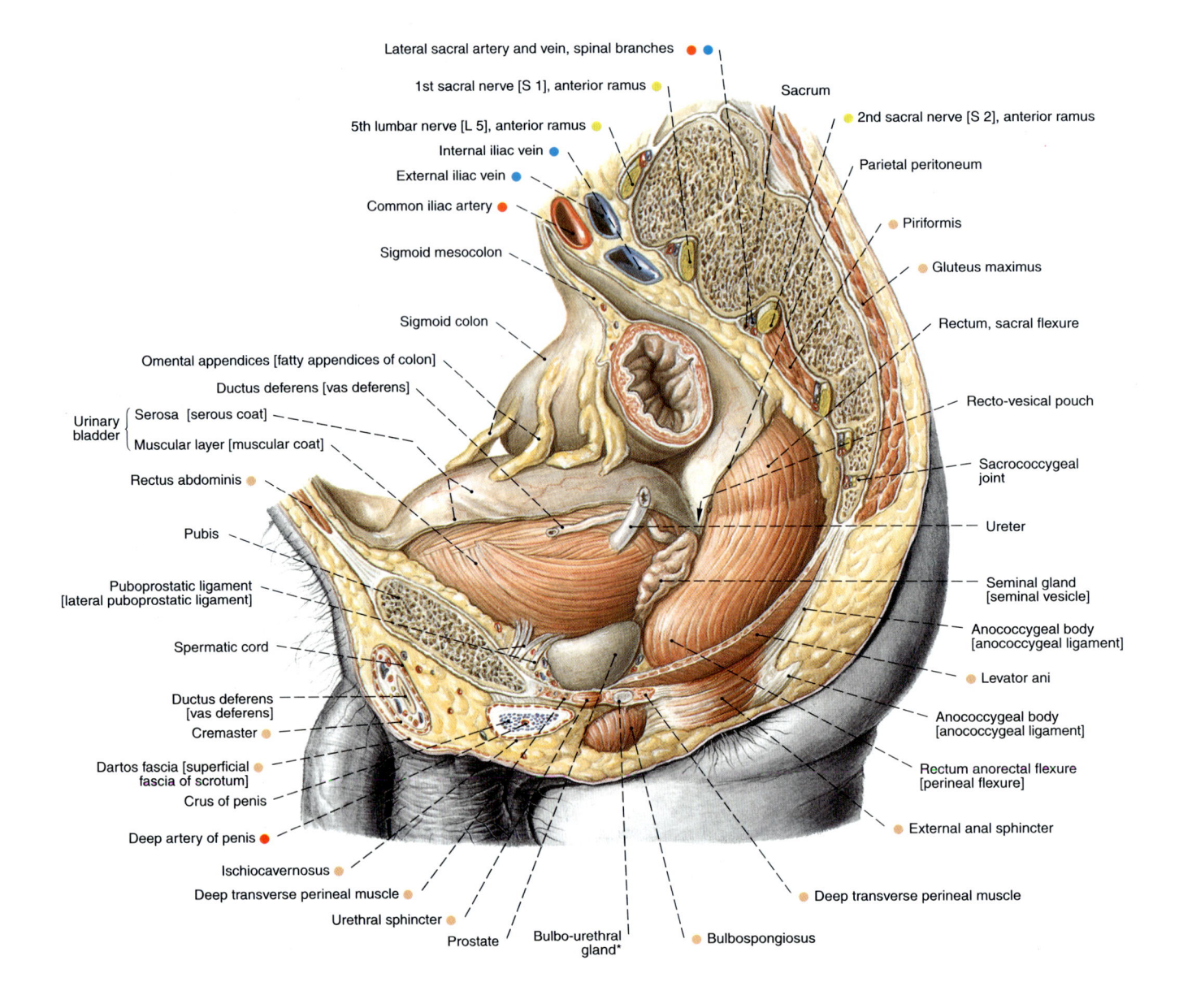

Fig. 1102 Male pelvic viscera; left paramedian section of the pelvis; peritoneum of lateral surface of urinary bladder partially removed to expose the course of ureter and ductus deferens [vas deferens]; right lateral aspect.
* Clinically also COWPER's gland.

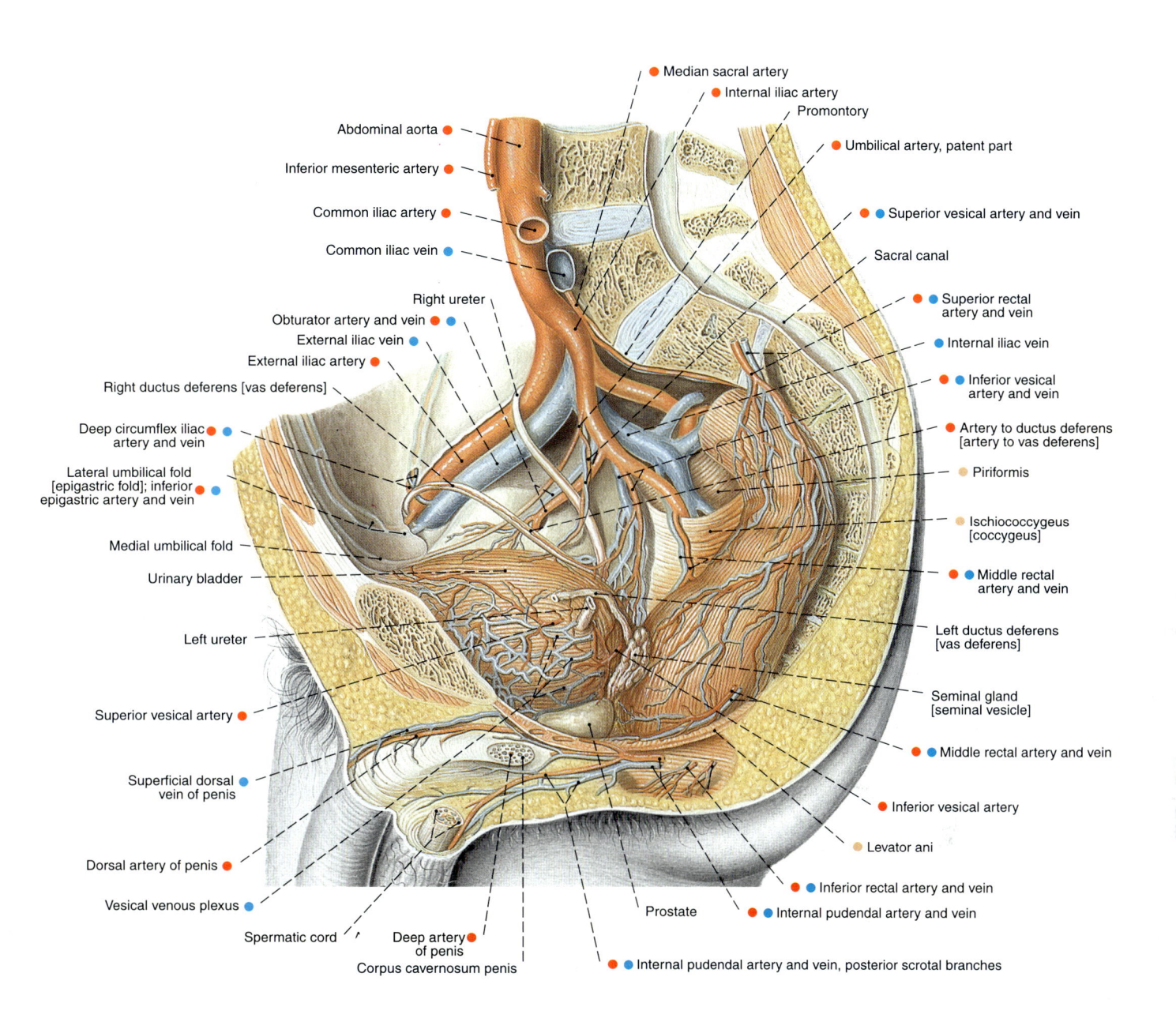

Fig. 1103 Blood supply of the male pelvic viscera; left paramedian section of the pelvis; peritoneum extensively removed; right lateral aspect.

220 *Pelvic viscera*

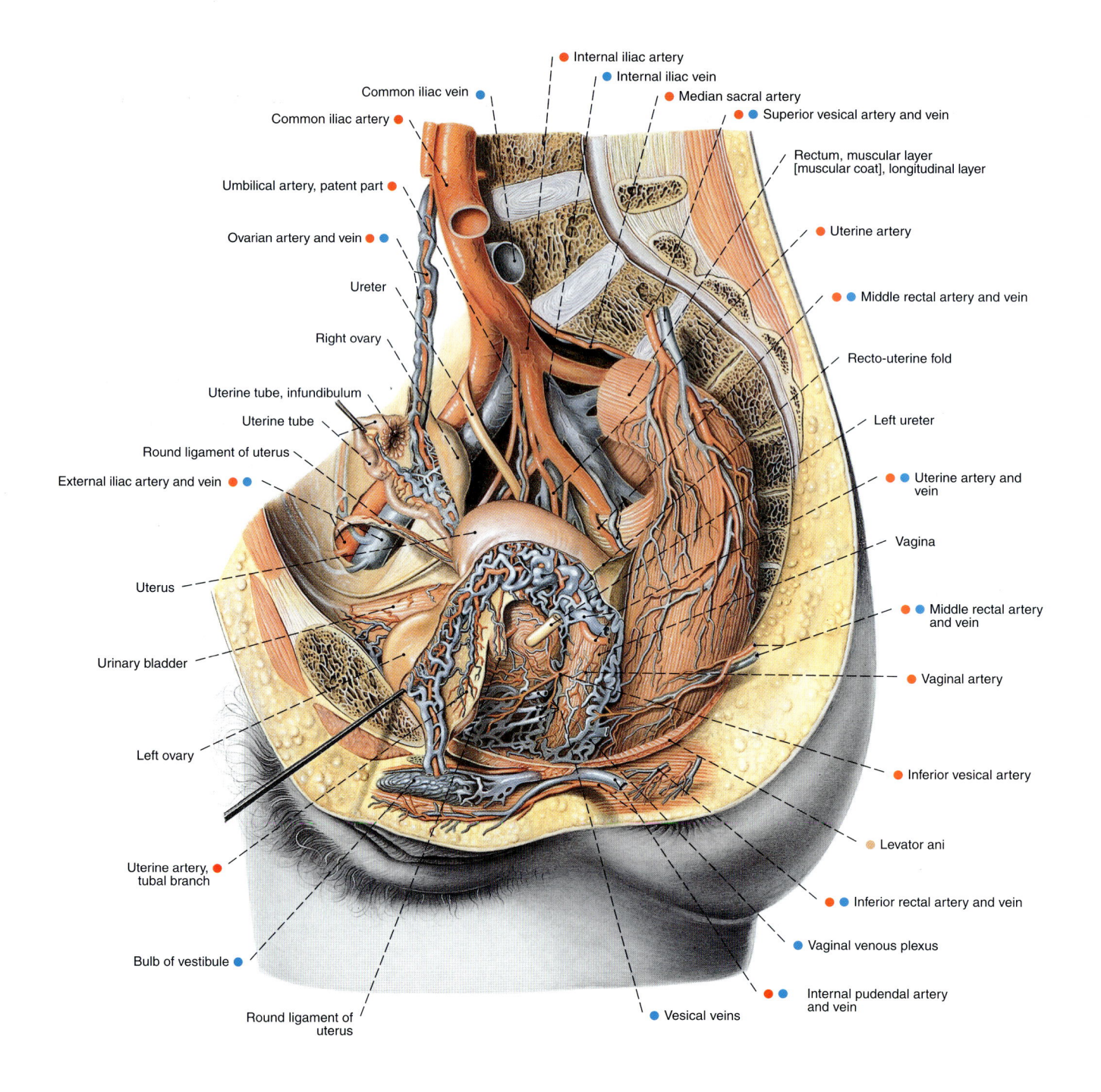

Fig. 1104 Blood supply of the female pelvic viscera; left paramedian section of the pelvis; intestine extensively and peritoneum partially removed; right ovary retracted cranially and left ovary retracted ventrocaudally to expose the blood vessels; right lateral aspect.

Well-developed venous plexuses surround the pelvic viscera. In elderly females the ovarian artery is frequently atrophic and, thus, difficult to dissect.

Lymphatic vessels and obturator artery 221

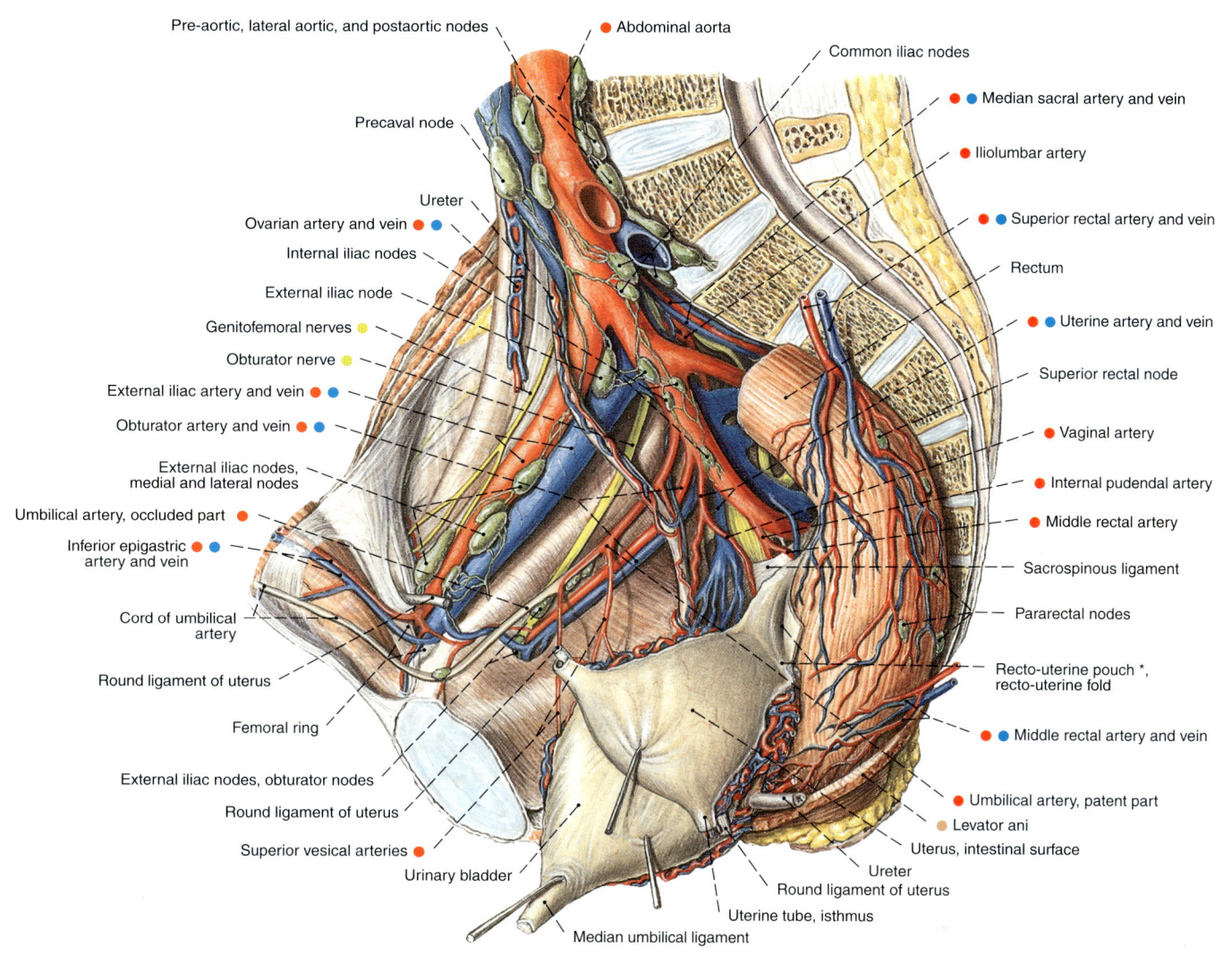

Fig. 1105 Lymphatic vessels and lymph nodes of the right pelvic wall in the female; median section of the pelvis; uterus retracted anteriorly to the left and peritoneum extensively removed; lateral aspect.

The lymph nodes are generally much smaller than shown, but always present. Via lymphatic vessels of the round ligament of uterus tumor cells may invade from the uterus to the inguinal lymph nodes.

* Clinically: pouch of DOUGLAS.

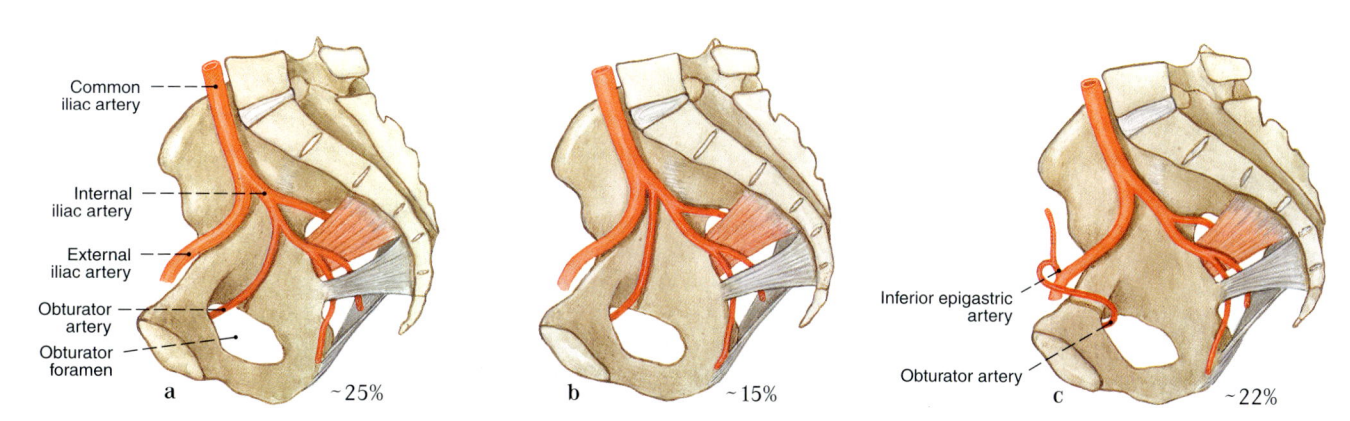

Fig. 1106 a–c Variations in the origin of obturator artery; right lateral aspect.
a Origin from ventral branch of internal iliac artery ("normal textbook case")
b Separate origin from internal iliac artery
c Origin from external iliac artery
Only in 75% the obturator artery is a branch of the trunk of the internal iliac artery.

Pelvic diaphragm [pelvic floor] and urogenital diaphragm [superficial and deep perineal spaces] (Figs. 1107, 1108, 1115-1118, 1126, 1128)

The pelvic floor comprises two muscles that overlie each other partially. The pelvic diaphragm includes the levator ani and the ischiococcygeus [coccygeus].
Between both inferior pubic rami stretches a triangular plate, the urogenital diaphragm. Its fibers are directed transversally and they close the urogenital hiatus. Amongst others it comprises the deep transverse perineal muscle, the urethral sphincter (both together also called urethral compressor), and the superficial transverse perineal muscle. In the male only the urethra, in the female both urethra and vagina penetrate the urogenital diaphragm.

Muscle / innervation	Origin	Insertion	Function
1. **Levator ani** *Branches of sacral nerve (S 3 and S 4)* Comprises: Pubococcygeus, puboprostaticus [levator prostatae], pubovaginalis puborectalis, iliococcygeus	**Pubococcygeus:** pubis (inner surface nest to pubic symphysis), tendinous arch of levator ani, ischial spine **Iliococcygeus:** tendinous arch of levator ani (posterior third)	Perineal body (prerectal fibers), in the male into the prostatic fascia (levator prostatae), in the female into the vaginal wall (pubovaginalis), merges with the external anal sphincter, surrounds the anus (puborectalis), anococcygeal body, coccyx	Surrounds the rectum dorsally; the medial free border forms the urogenital hiatus, in the male for passing of the urethra, in the female for passing of urethra and vagina; suspension band for the pelvic floor
2. **Ischiococcygeus [coccygeus]** *Branches of sacral nerve (S 4 and S 5)*	Ischial spine (inner surface; blends with the sacrospinous ligament)	Sacrum (lateral border of lower segments), coccyx	Supports pelvic floor
3. **External anal sphincter** *Pudendal nerve (sacral plexus)*	**Subcutaneous part:** dermis [corium] and subcutaneous tissue surrounding anus **Superficial part:** Perineal body **Deep part:** Ring-like fibers up to levator ani	Dermis [corium] and subcutaneous tissue surrounding anus, anococcygeal ligament	External sphincter of anus
4. **Deep transverse perineal muscle** *Pudendal nerve (sacral plexus)*	Ramus of ischium, adventitia of internal pudendal vessels (obliquely over pubic arch, resp. subpubic angel, completed by inferior pubic ligament and transverse perineal ligament)	Trapezoid muscle plate with openings for urethra in the male, respectively urethra and vagina in the female	Secures urogenital hiatus
5. **Superficial transverse perineal muscle** *Pudendal nerve (sacral plexus) (inconstant muscle)*	Superficial part of deep perineal transverse muscle	Blends with perineal body	Supports deep perineal transverse muscle
6. **Urethral sphincter** *Pudendal nerve (sacral plexus) embraces the intermediate part of urethra [membranous urethra]*	Ring muscle	Ring muscle	Secures urogenital hiatus; assists urinary continence; closes urinary bladder during ejaculation
7. **Ischiocavernosus** *Pudendal nerve (sacral plexus)*	Ramus of ischium	Tunica albuginea of corpus spongiosum	Fixes crura of penis in the male, respectively crura of clitoris in the female to the ischiopubic ramus and to the urogenital diaphragm; assist ejaculation respectively orgasm
8. **Bulbospongiosus** *Pudendal nerve (sacral plexus)* Embraces the bulb of penis in the male and the bulb of vestibule in the female	Perineal body, in the male also from the inferior surface of the corpus spongiosum penis (raphe of penis)	In the male it courses laterally to the corpus spongiosum of penis to the inferior urogenital fascia and to the dorsum of penis; in the female the fibers are attached to the corpus cavernosum of clitoris and to the inferior urogenital fascia	Fixes bulb of penis in the male, respectively bulb of vestibule in the female to the urogenital diaphragm; assists ejaculation in the male, respectively orgasm in the female

Pelvic diaphragm [pelvic floor] 223

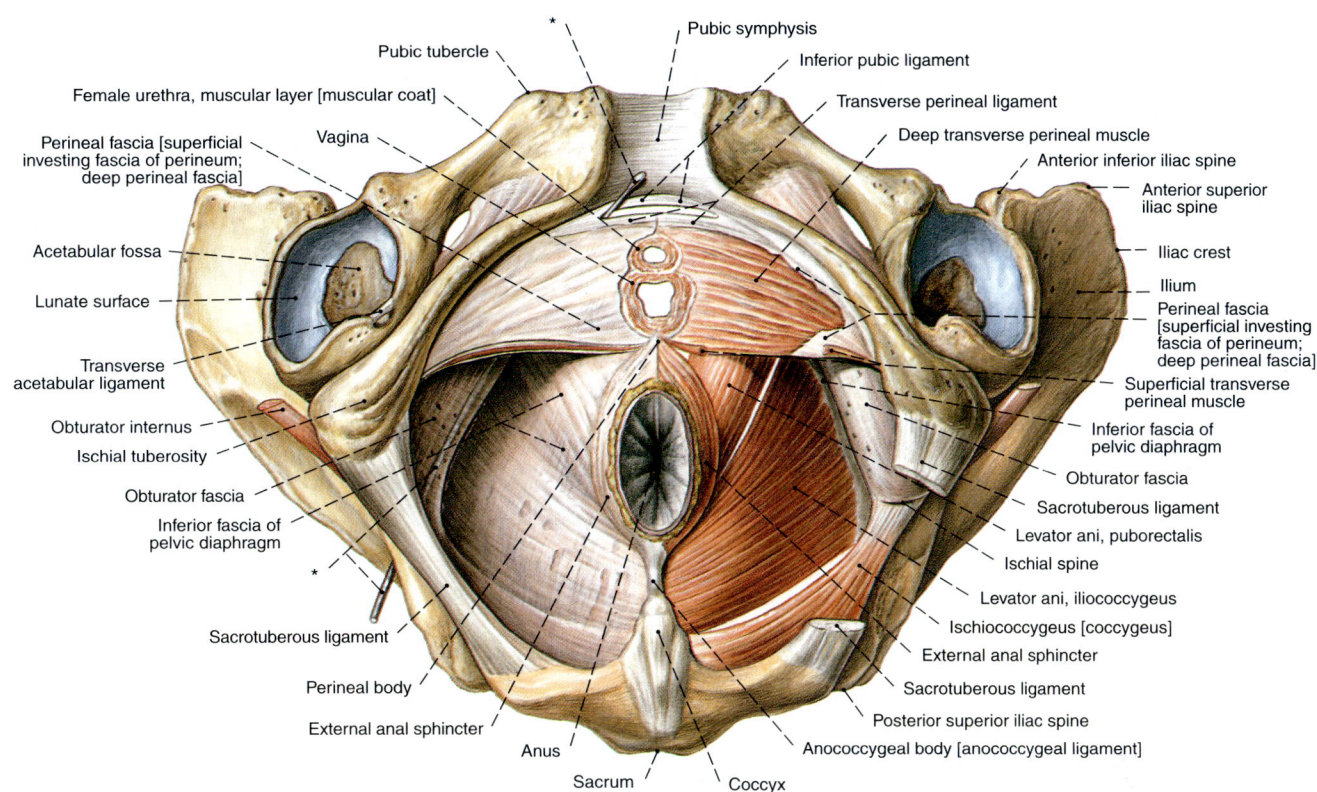

Fig. 1107 Perineal muscles and pelvic diaphragm [pelvic floor] in the female; left sacrotuberous ligament partially removed to expose ischiococcygeus [coccygeus]; caudal aspect.

In the elderly female the superficial transverse perineal muscle frequently contains only a few muscle fibers.

* Probe in pudendal canal (ALCOCK's canal).

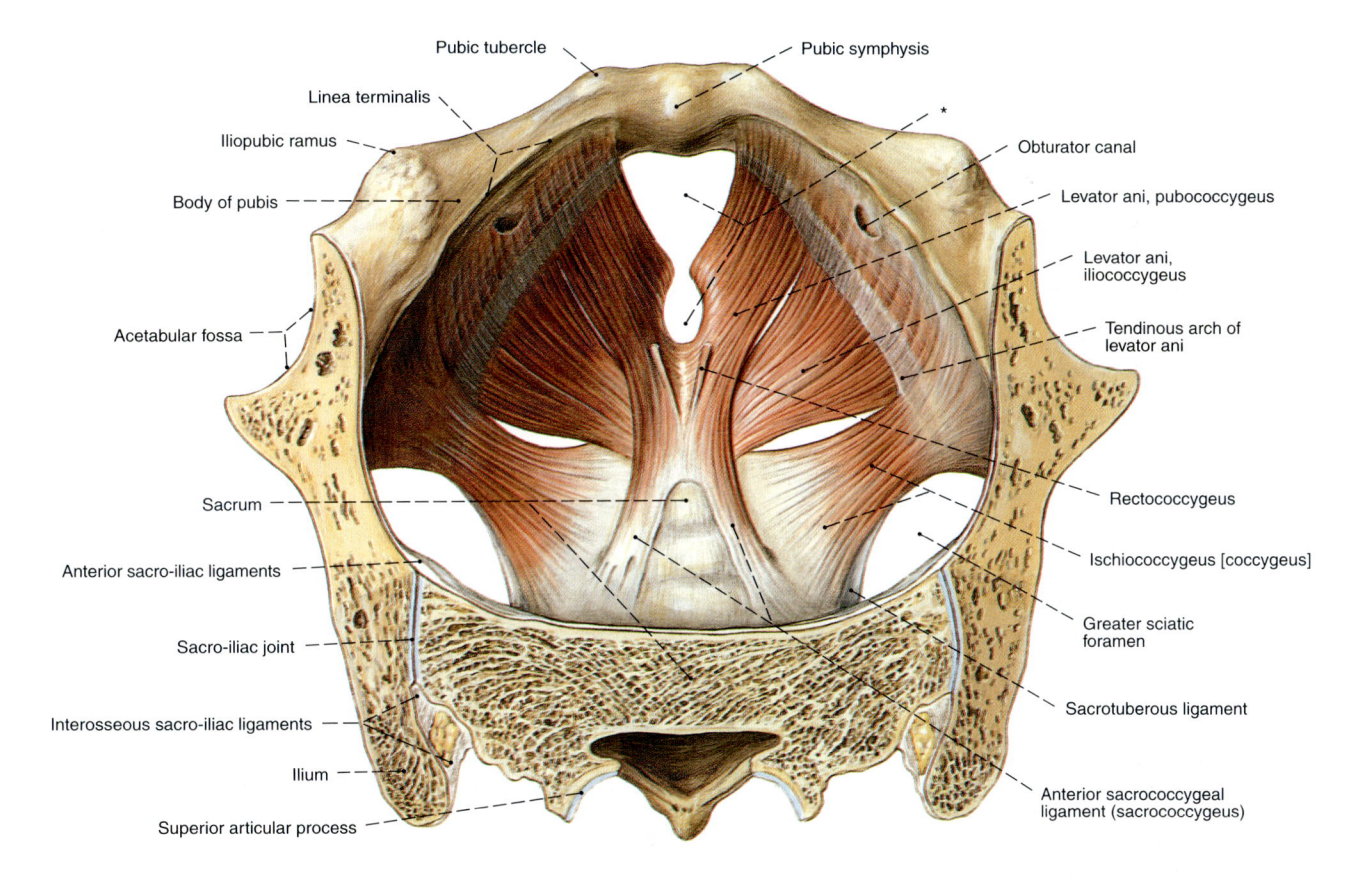

Fig. 1108 Pelvic diaphragm [pelvic floor] in the female; upper part of pelvic girdle sectioned in the transverse plane; cranial aspect.

Ischiococcygeus [coccygeus] and sacrococcygeus frequently contain only a few muscle fibers which cover the corresponding ligaments.

* Clinically: urogenital hiatus.

224 Pelvic viscera

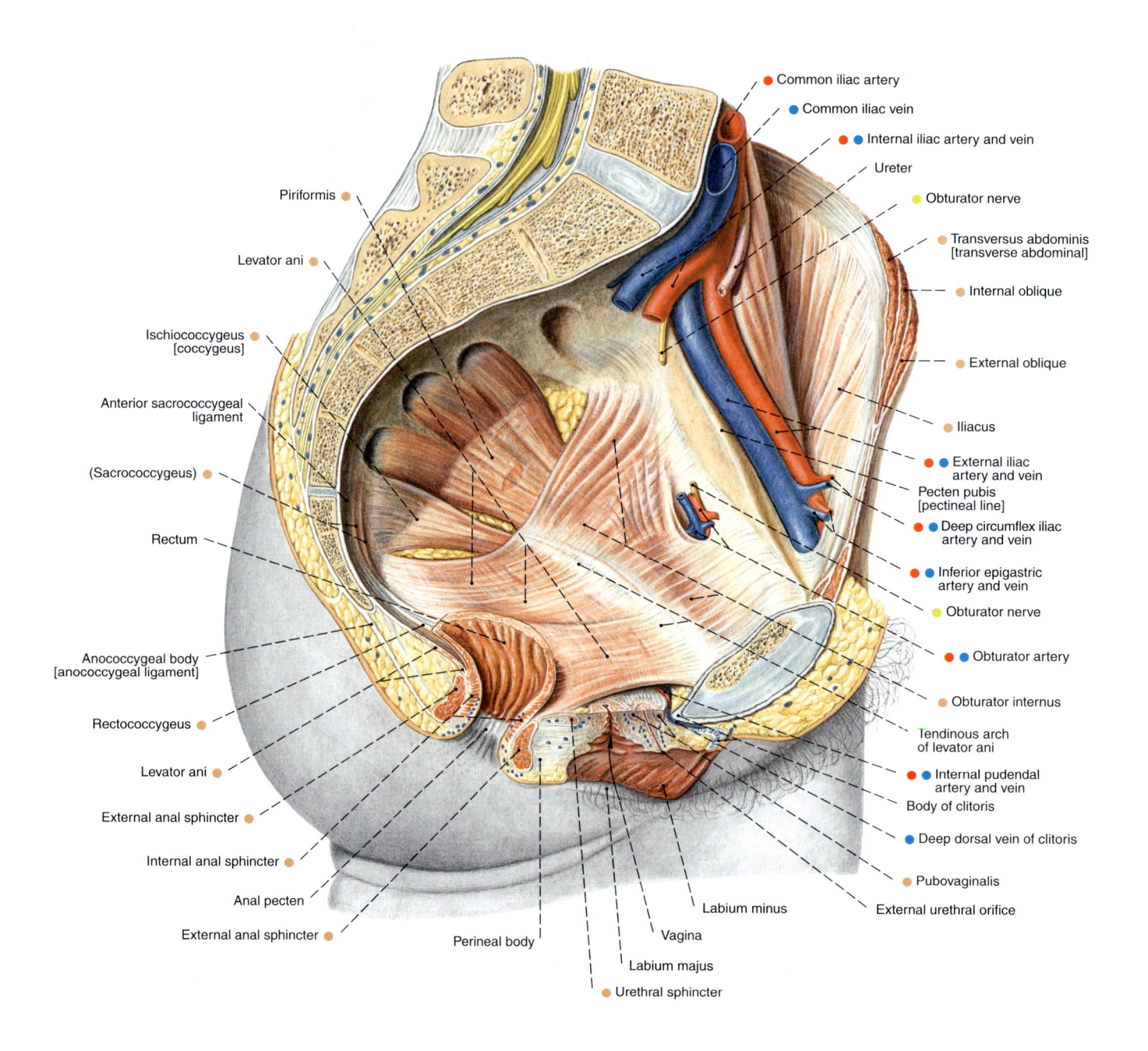

Fig. 1109 Muscles of pelvic diaphragm [pelvic floor] in the female; median section of the pelvis; organs entirely and most of the nerves and blood vessels removed to expose musculature; left lateral aspect.

Rectum 225

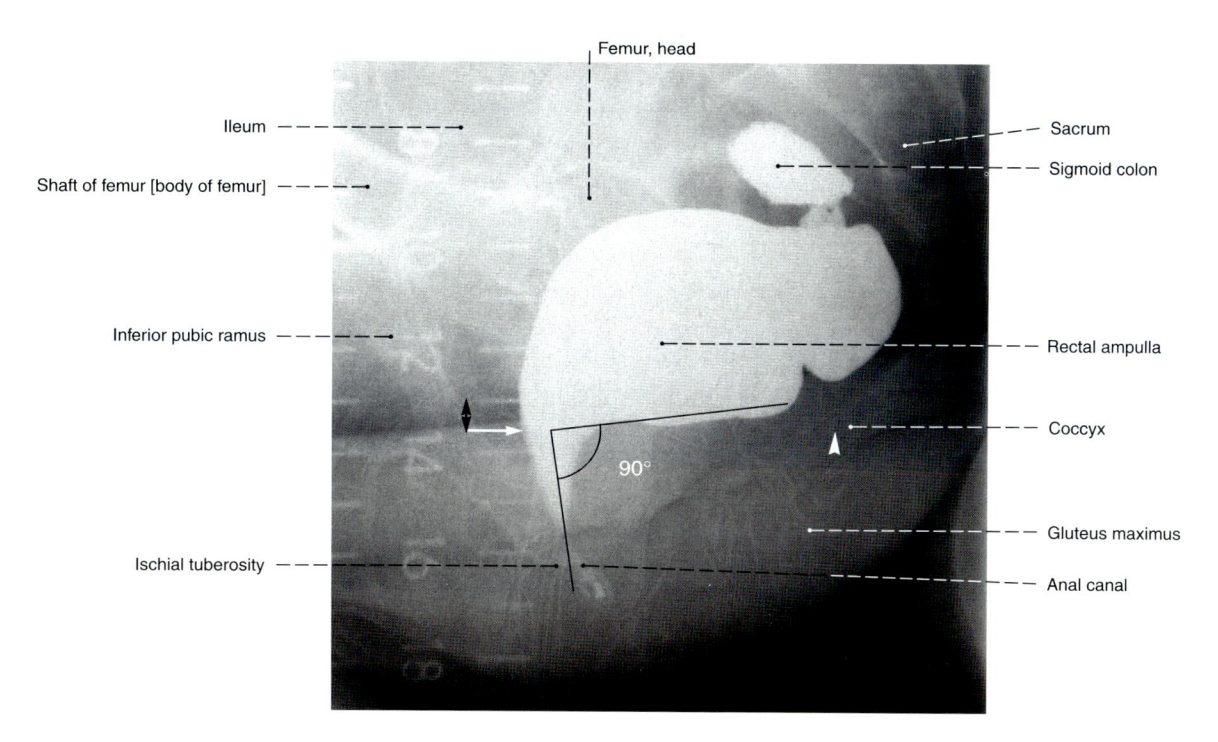

Fig. 1110 Rectum; lateral radiograph after filling with contrast medium and voluntary closure of anus (defecography). The junction between anus and rectum (arrow) is located at the tip of the coccyx (white arrowhead). The angle between anal and rectal axes is 90°. This angle is caused by the loop of levator ani (puborectalis). Scale in cm.

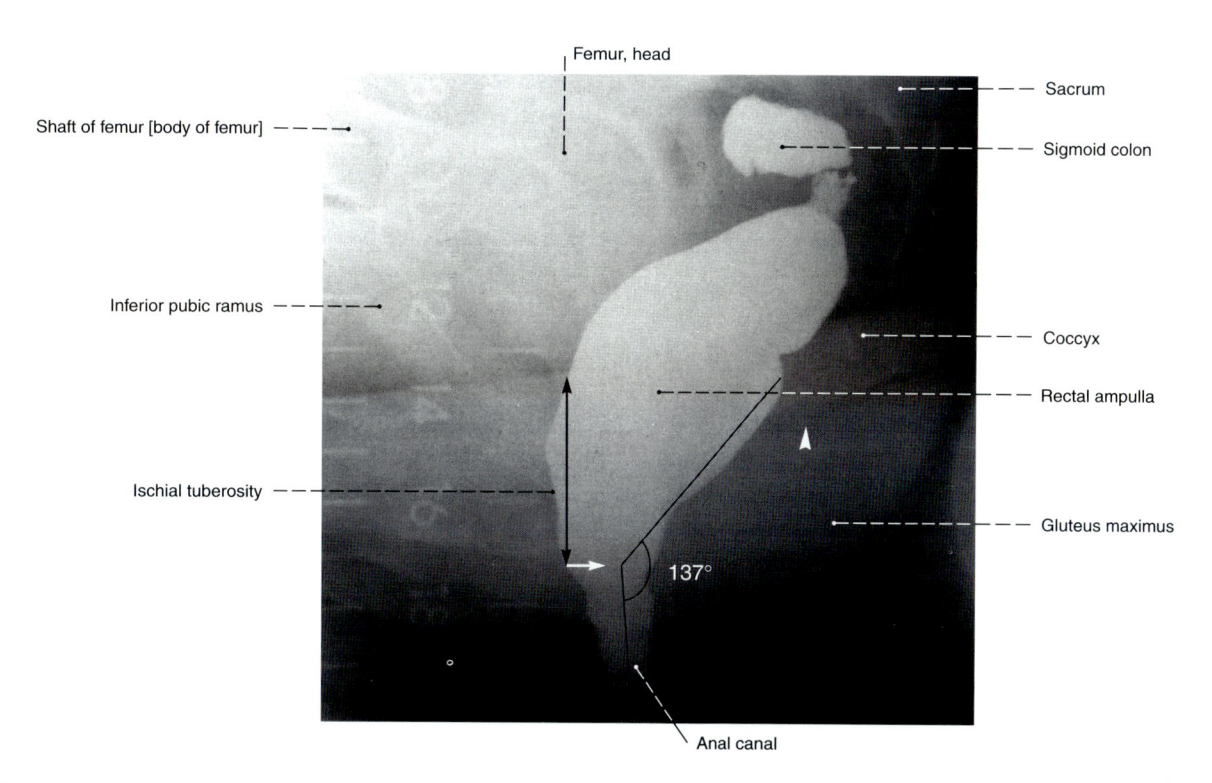

Fig. 1111 Rectum; lateral radiograph after filling with contrast medium during defecation (defecography). Compared to Fig. 1110 the anorectal junction has descended, and the angle has increased to 137° due to relaxation of the loop of levator ani. The bend that acts like a valve is now straightened, and the column of feces presses directly upon the anal canal for defecation.

226 *Pelvic viscera*

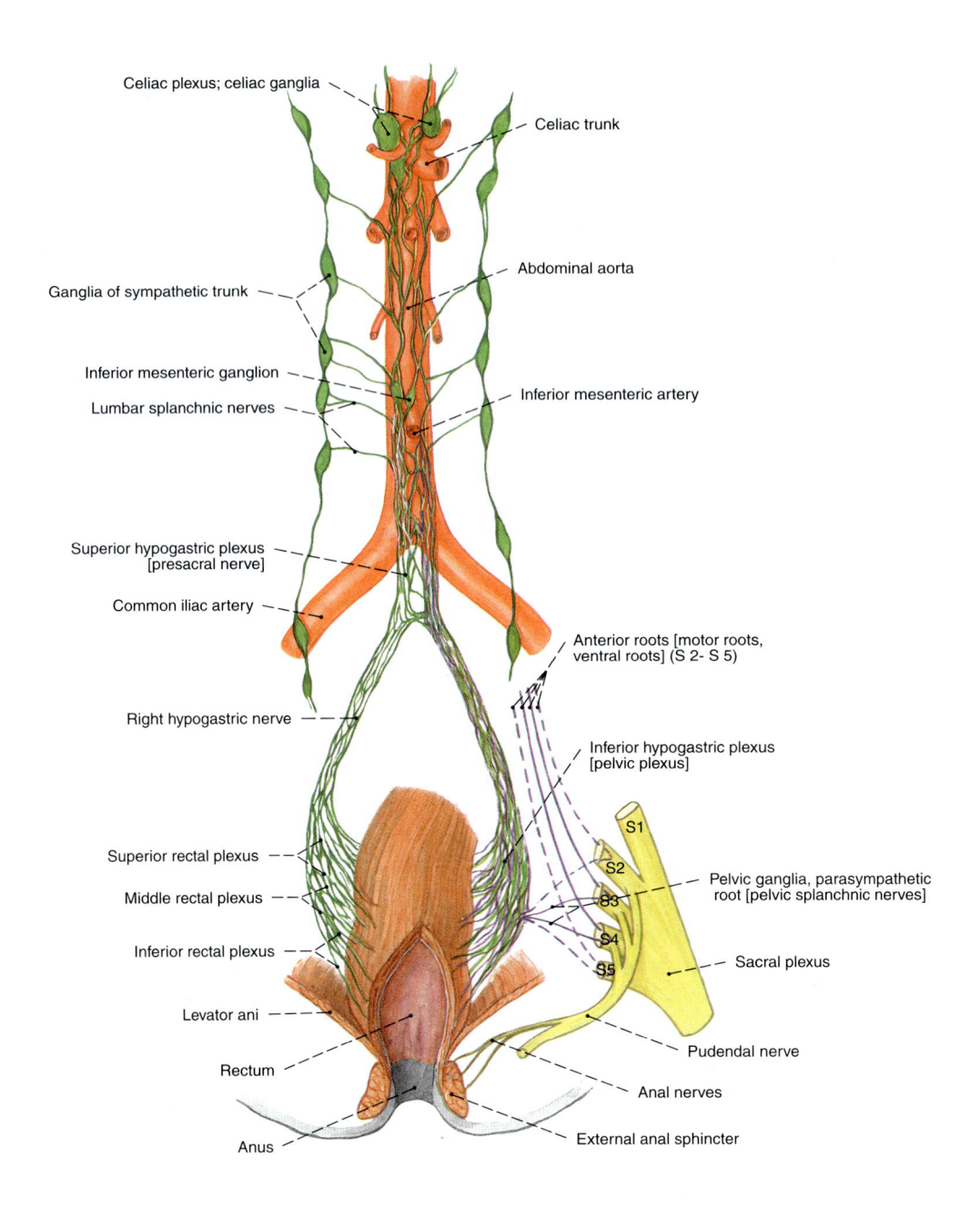

Fig. 1112 Rectum; diagram of innervation; ventral aspect.
green = sympathetic part
purple = parasympathetic part

Parasympathetic fibers course through the hypogastric plexus [presacral nerve] to the pelvic viscera and also cranially via the hypogastric nerve. The inferior hypogastric plexus [pelvic plexus] contains both sympathetic and parasympathetic fibers and ganglia (pelvic ganglia).

Glureal region 227

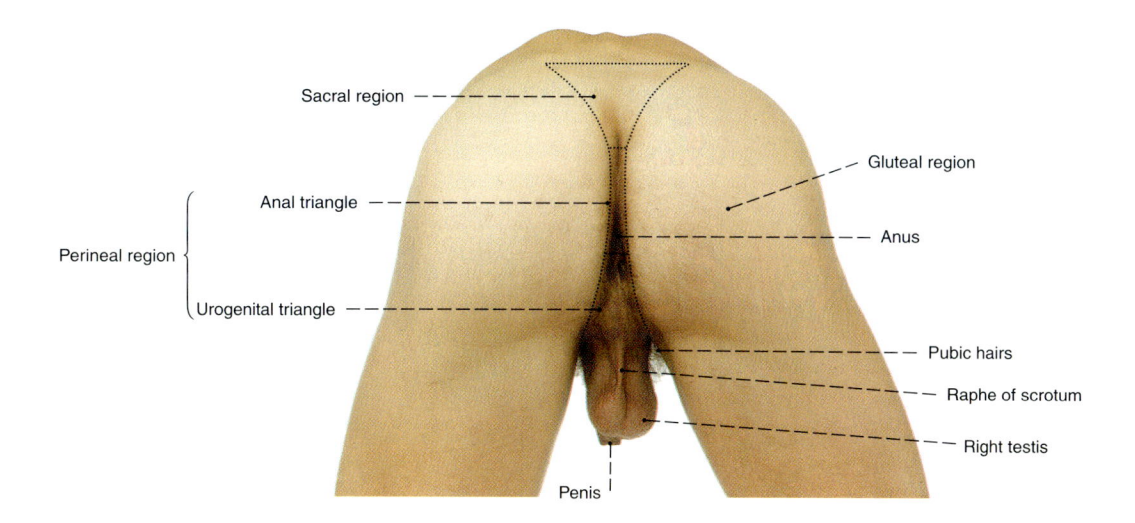

Fig. 1113 Gluteal and perineal region in the male; dorsal aspect.
In the cold the cremaster pulls the scrotum toward the perineum.

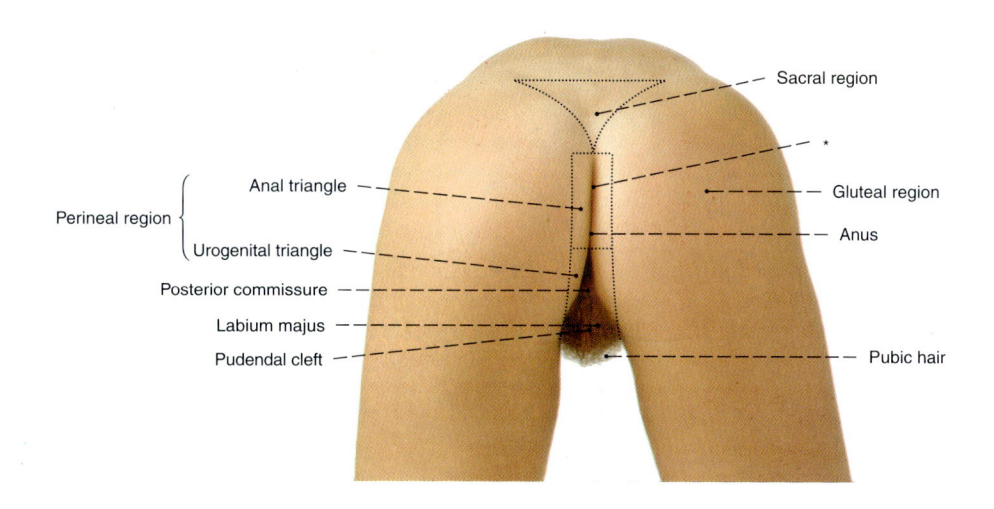

Fig. 1114 Gluteal and perineal region in the female; dorsal aspect.
*Clinically: anal cleft.

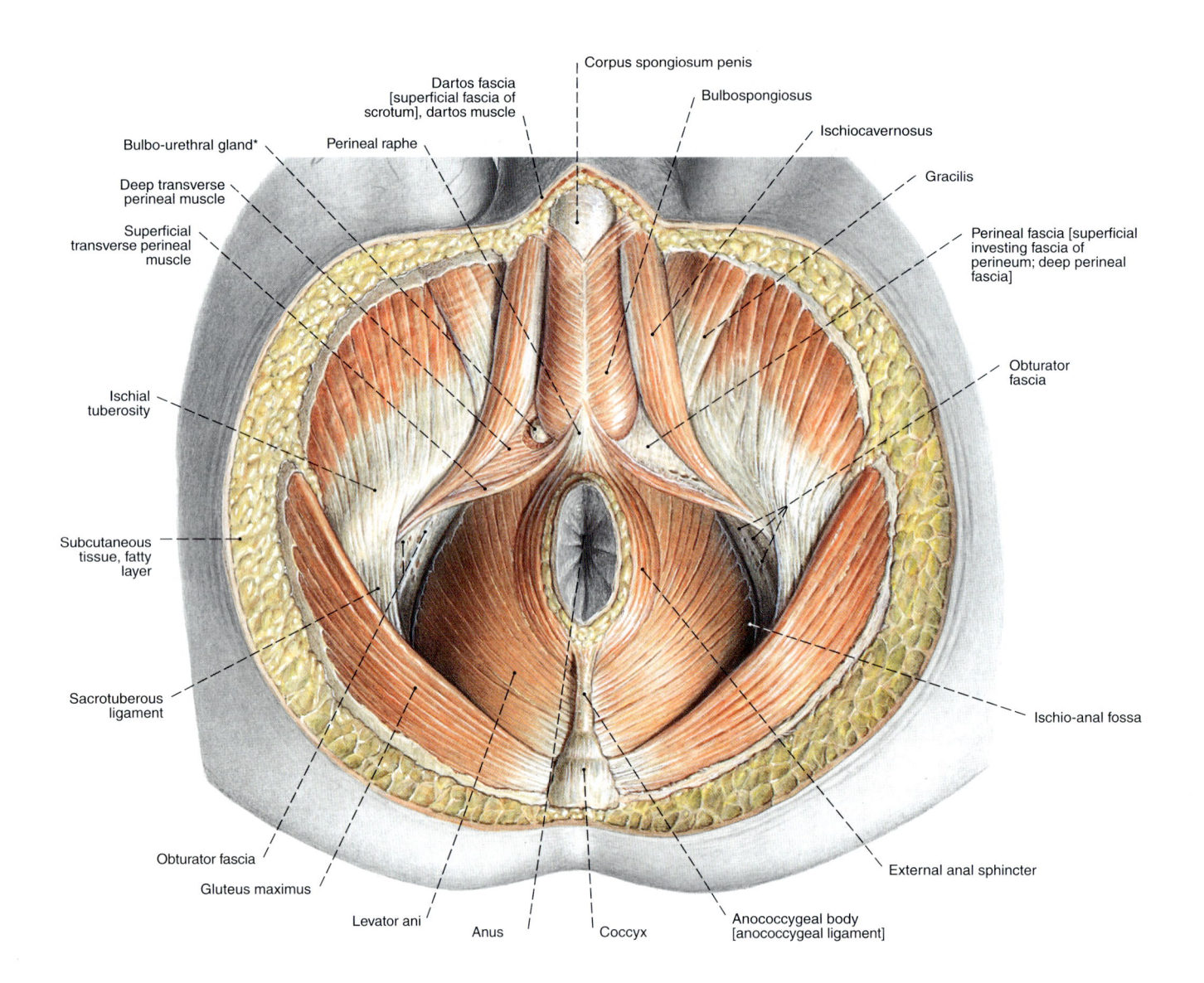

Fig. 1115 Perineum and pelvic diaphragm [pelvic floor] in the male; fat body of ischio-anal fossa removed; inferior fascia of urogenital diaphragm removed on the right and bulbo-urethral gland exposed; caudal aspect.
* Also COWPER's gland.

Pelvic diaphragm [pelvic floor] 229

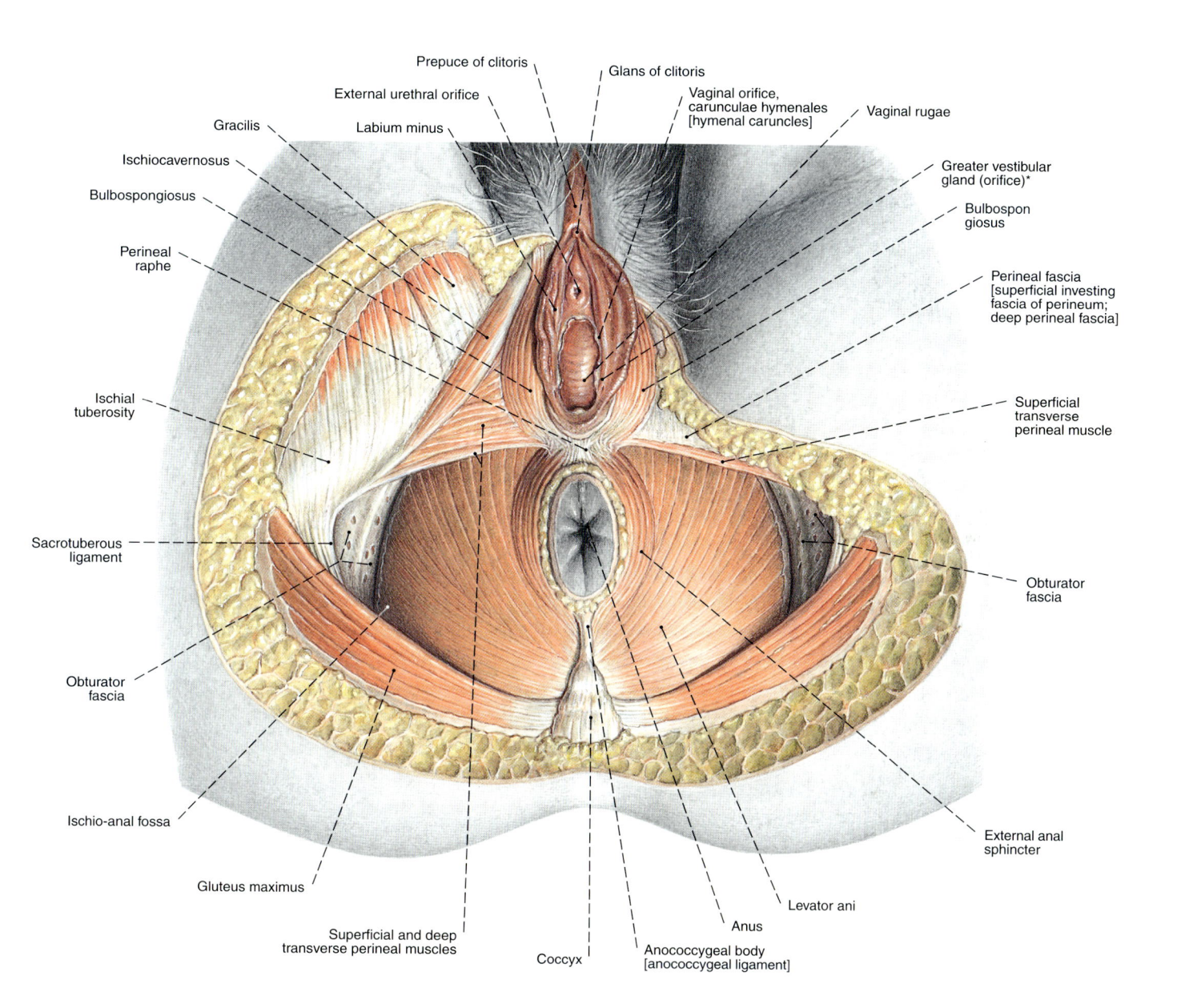

Fig. 1116 Perineum; pelvic diaphragm [pelvic floor]; female external genitalia; fat body of ischio-anal fossa removed; caudal aspect.

* Also BARTHOLIN's gland.

Vaginal orifice and anus are situated close to each other. During parturition both skin and muscles of the perineum may be lacerated up to the anal sphincter muscles (1st–3rd grade perineal lacerations). These can be avoided by a prior lateral or median incision (lateral or median episiotomy).

Pelvic viscera

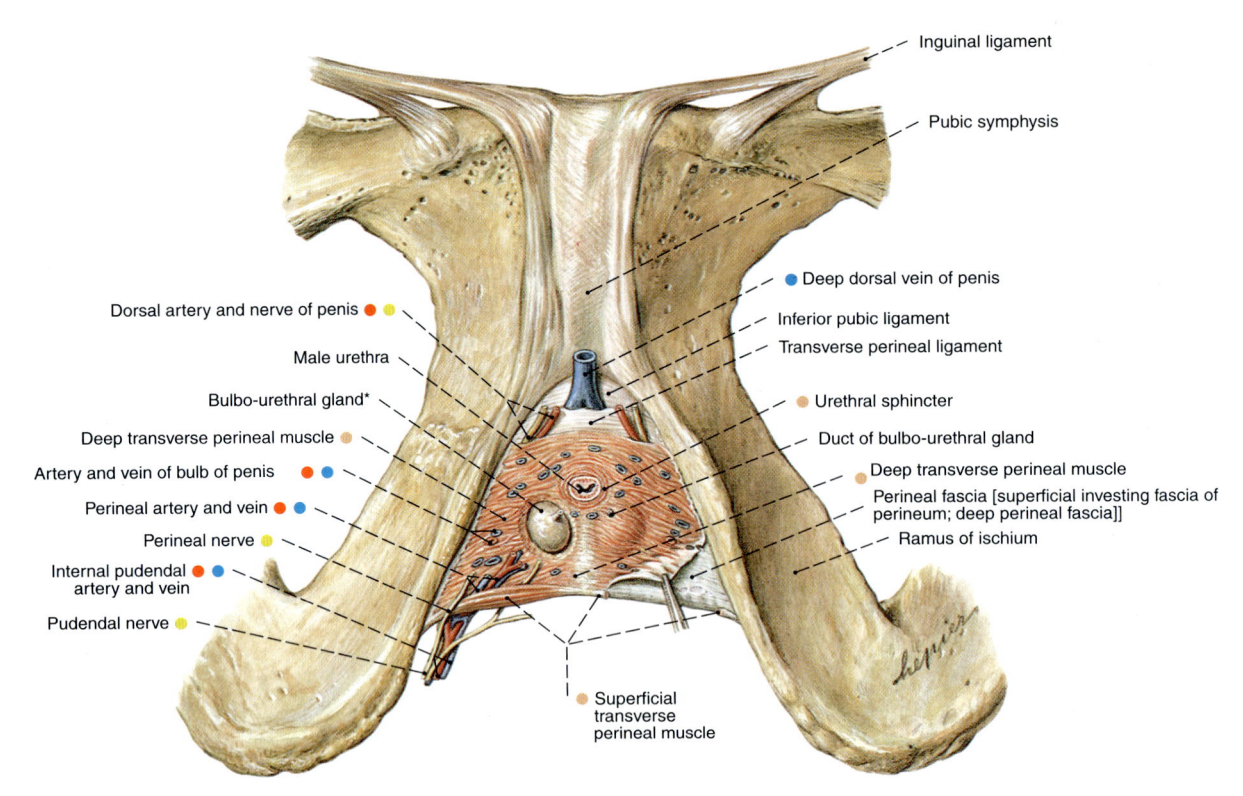

Fig. 1117 Urogenital diaphragm in the male; inferior fascia extensively removed; right bulbo-urethral gland dissected; caudal aspect. Compare Fig. 1118.

* Clinically: COWPER's gland.

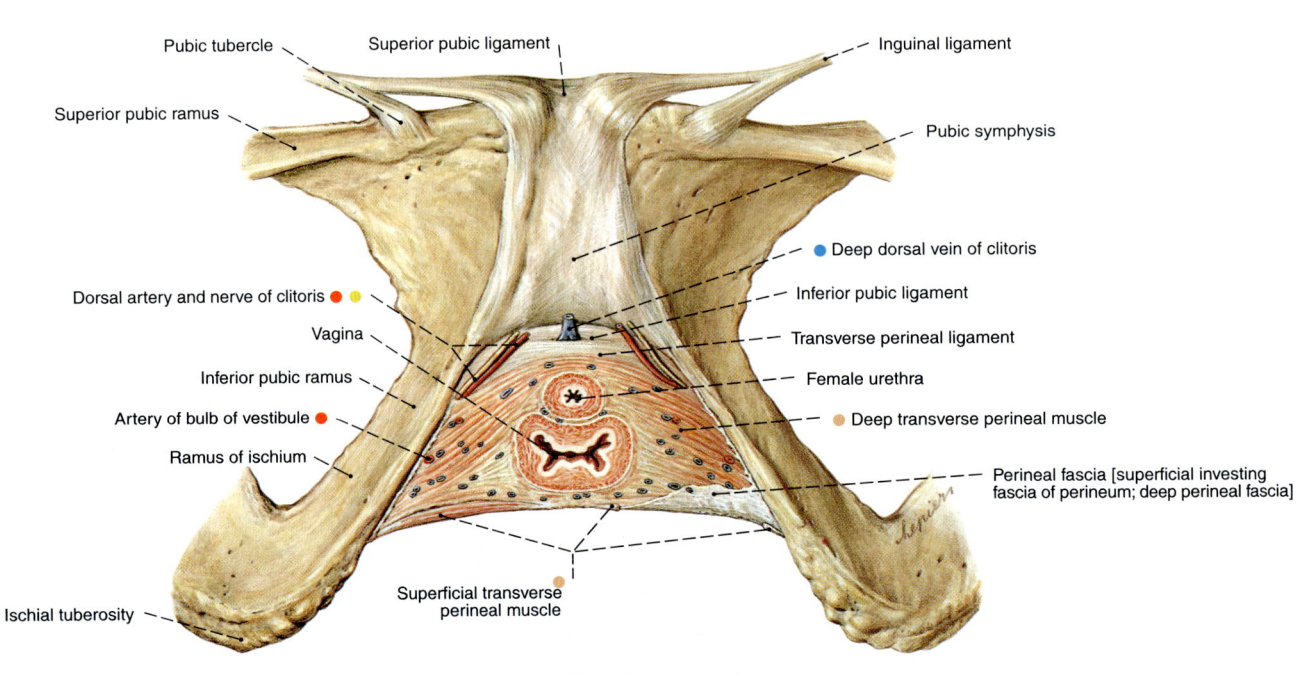

Fig. 1118 Urogenital diaphragm in the female; inferior fascia extensively removed; caudal aspect. Compare Fig. 1117.

Male genitalia 231

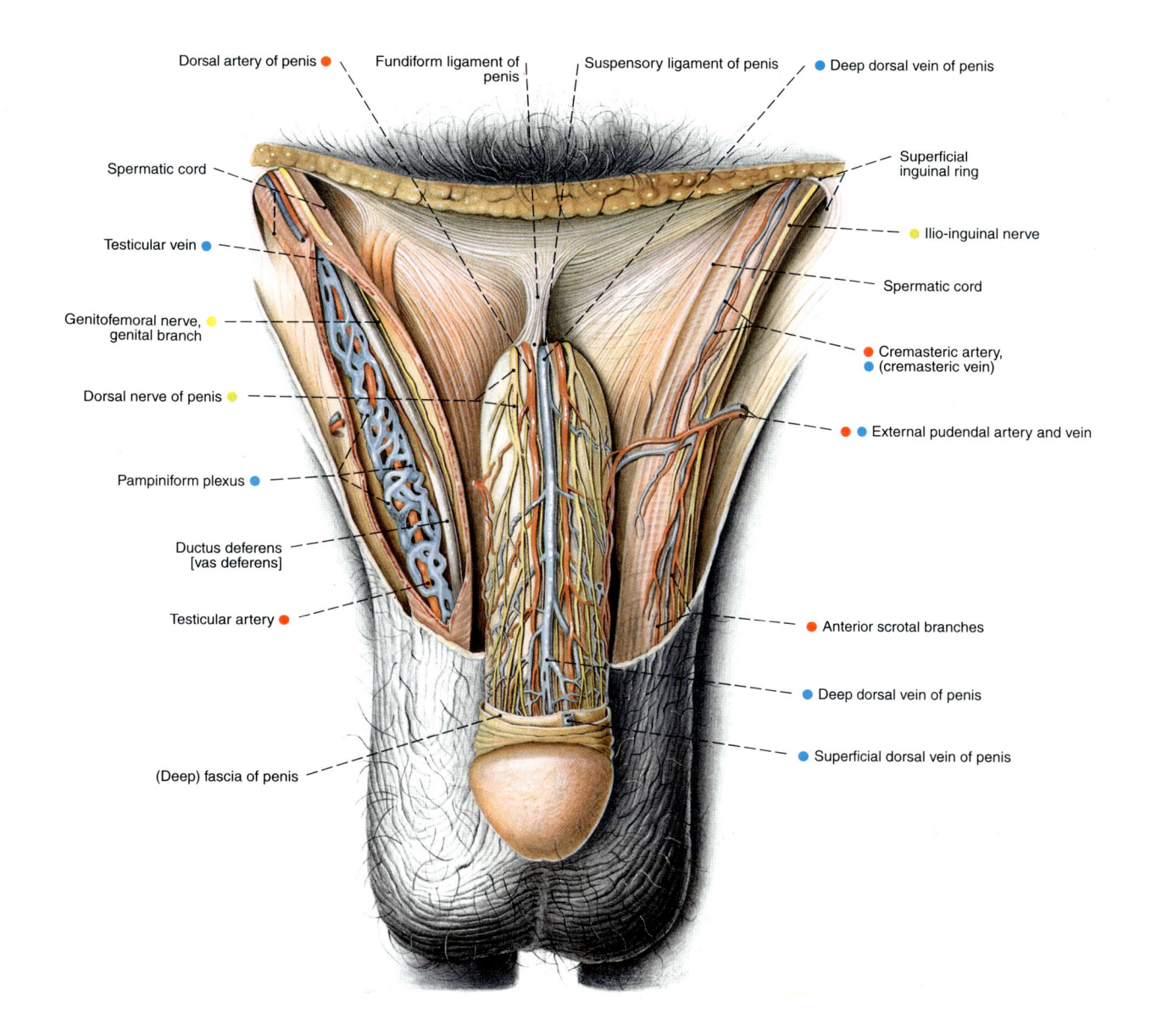

Fig. 1119 External male genitalia; demonstration of nerves and blood vessels by extensive removal of skin and superficial fascia of penis; layers of spermatic cord incised on the right; ventral aspect.

The venous plexus (pampiniform plexus) surrounding the testicular artery is constantly well-developed.

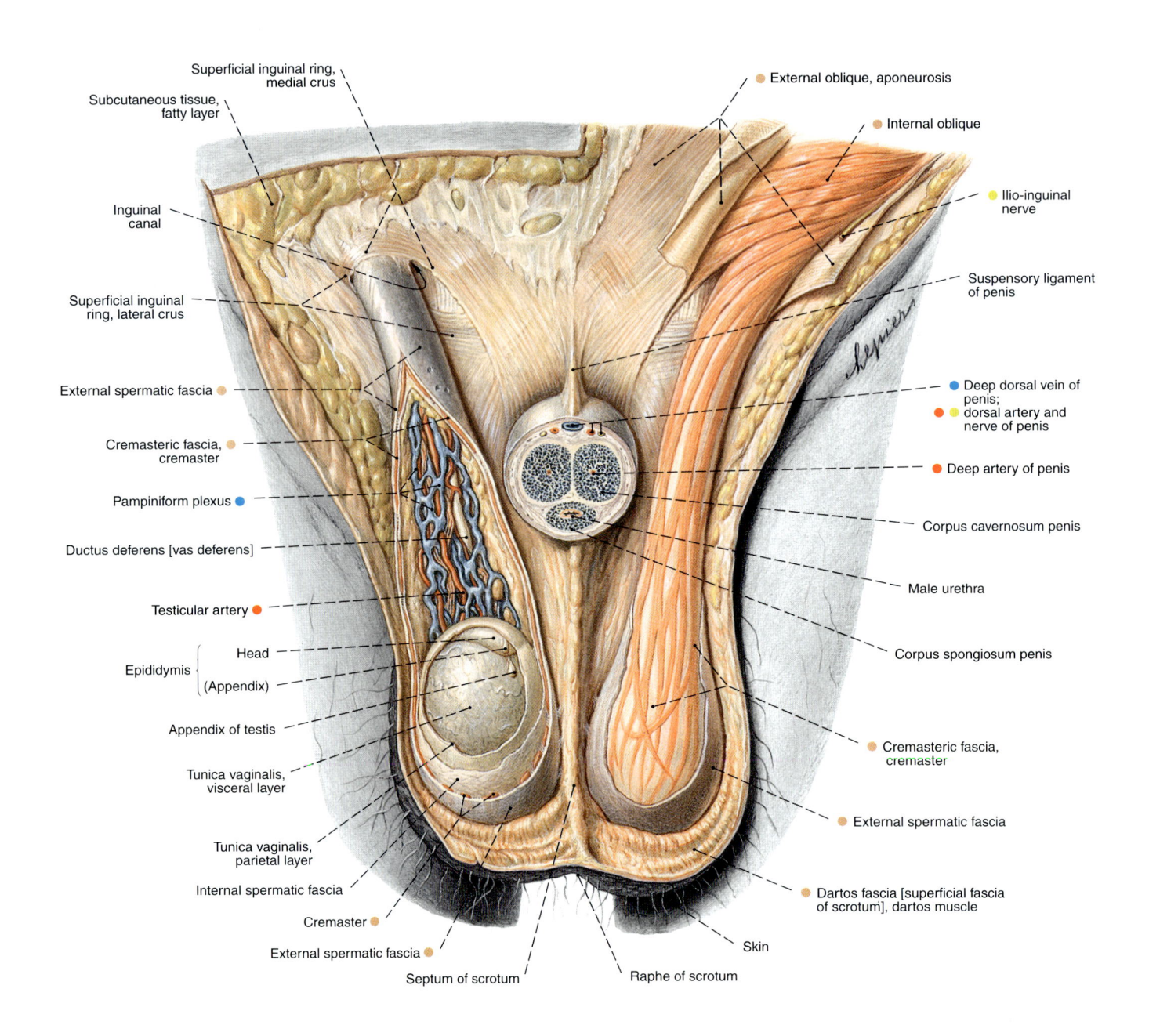

Fig. 1120 Male genitalia; skin of abdomen and parts of skin of scrotum removed; body of penis severed; layers of spermatic cord dissected on the right; ventral aspect.
Compare Figs. 824 and 827, origin of cremaster and fascias from the muscles of the abdominal wall.

Male genitalia 233

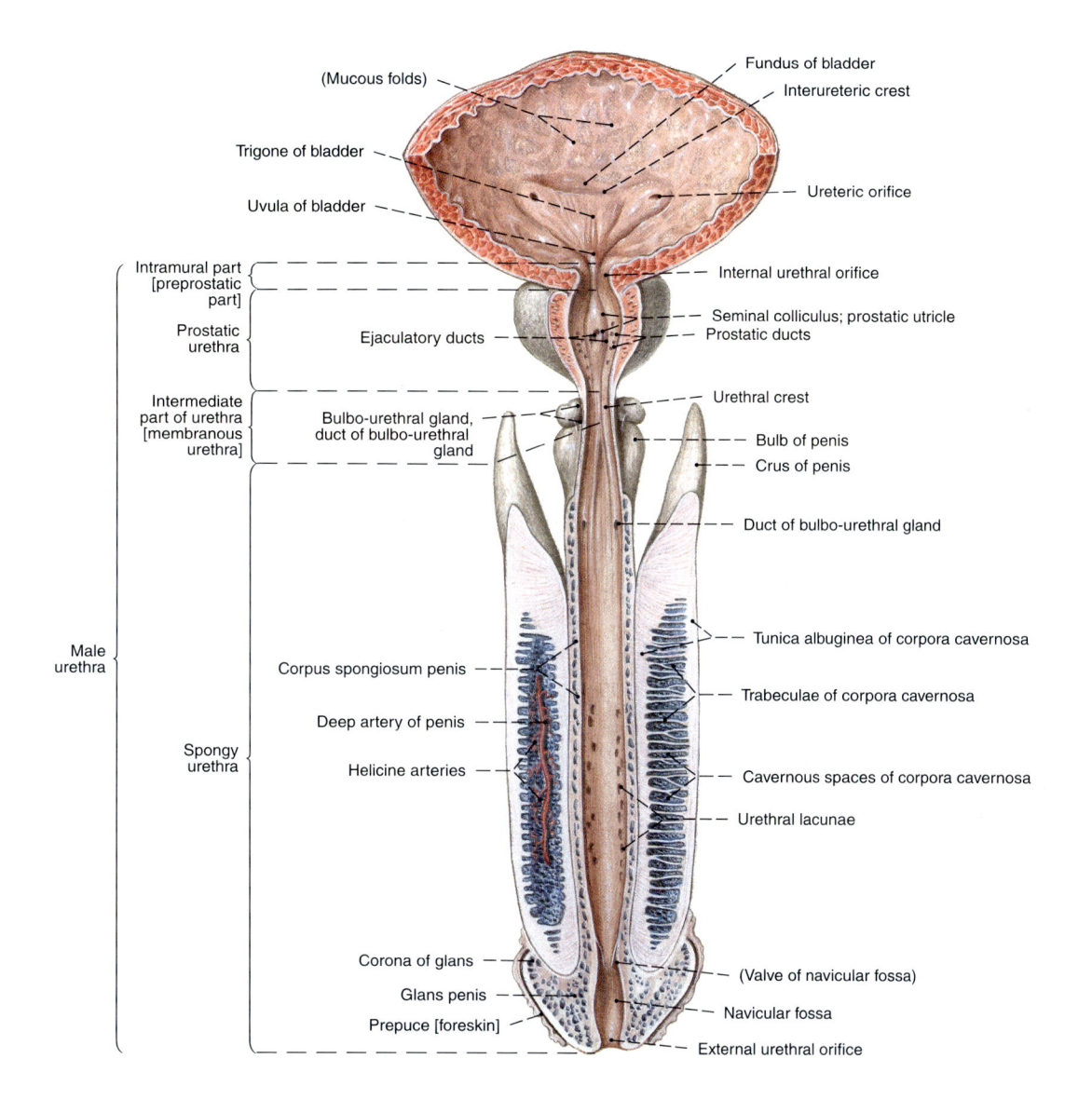

Fig. 1121　Urinary bladder; prostate; male urethra; urinary bladder and urethra opened to expose the lumen; skin of penis extensively removed; ventral aspect.
In its normal position the urethra has an arched course (compare Fig. 1145).

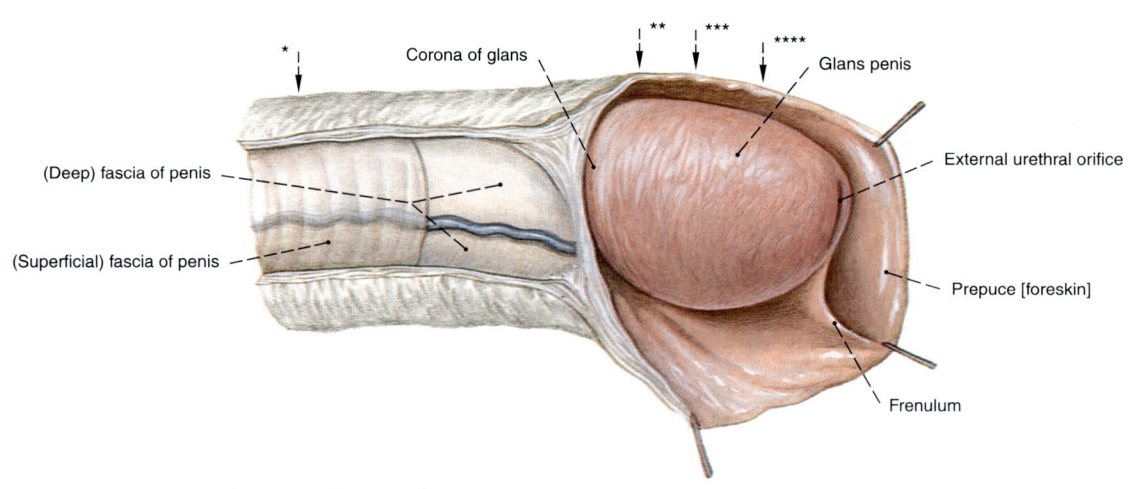

Fig. 1122 Penis with glans and prepuce [foreskin]. Skin and superficial fascia of penis removed layer by layer; lateral aspect.

* Level of cross-section in Fig. 1123a.
** Level of cross-section in Fig. 1123b.
*** Level of cross-section in Fig. 1123c.
**** Level of cross-section in Fig. 1123d.

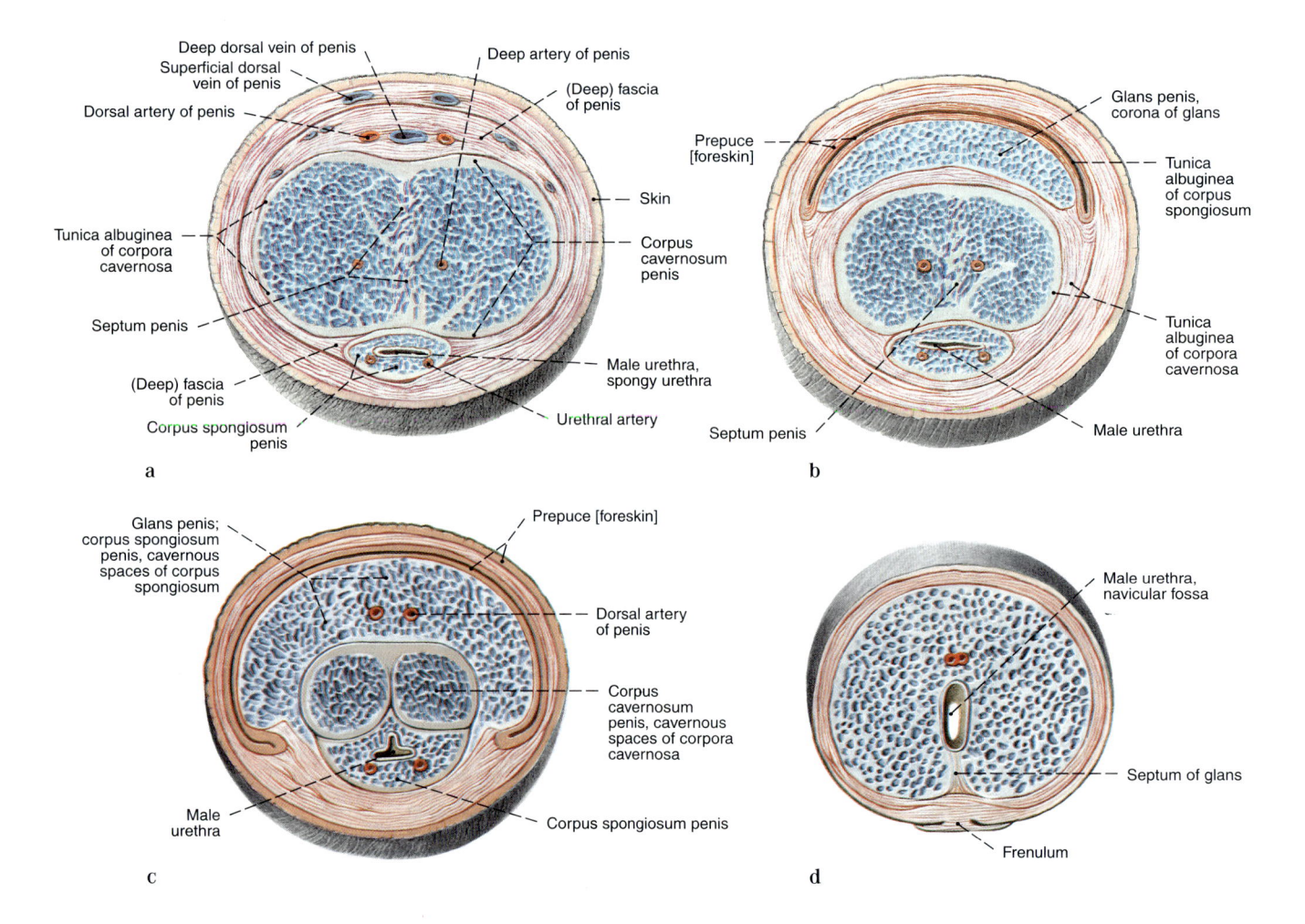

Fig. 1123 a–d Penis; cross-sections; levels of section indicated in Fig. 1122; ventral aspect.
a Cross-section through the middle of body. Both corpora cavernosa are incompletely separated by the septum penis.
b Cross-section at level of proximal circumference of glans penis.
c Cross-section through the middle of glans penis.
d Cross-section at level of distal end of glans penis.

Male genitalia 235

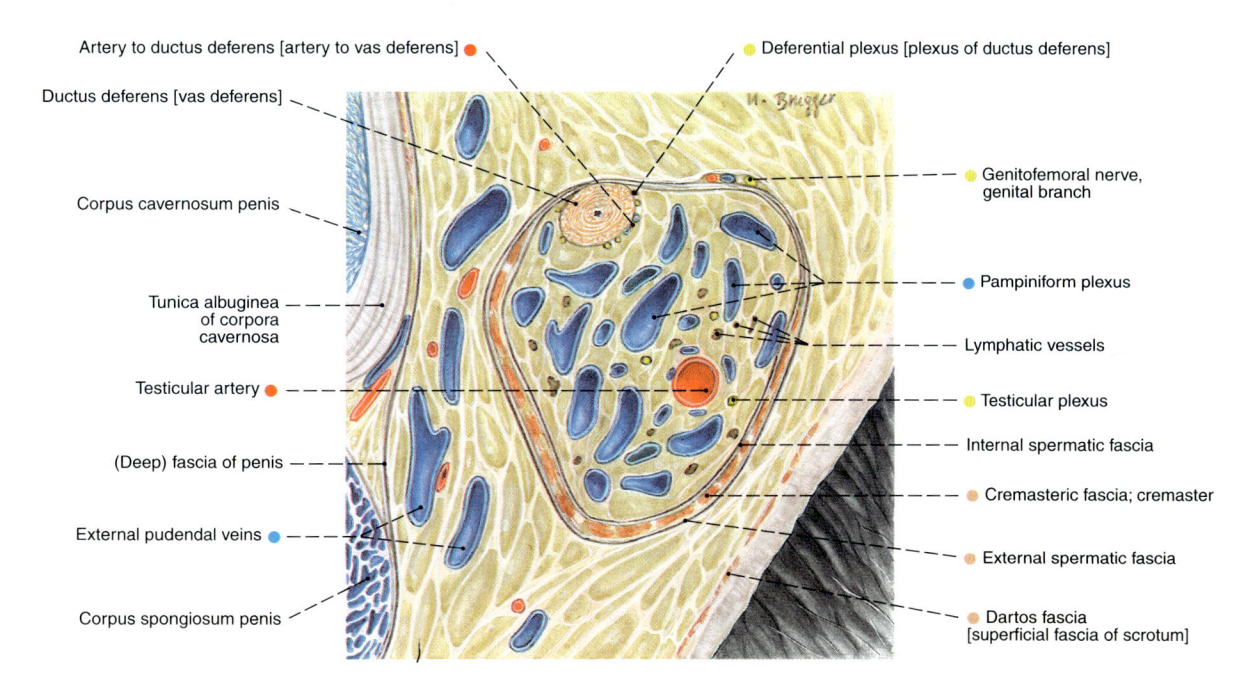

Fig. 1124 Left spermatic cord; frontal section; ventral aspect (250%).
Development of cremaster, pampiniform plexus, and the position of ductus deferens [vas deferens] are highly variable.

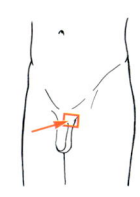

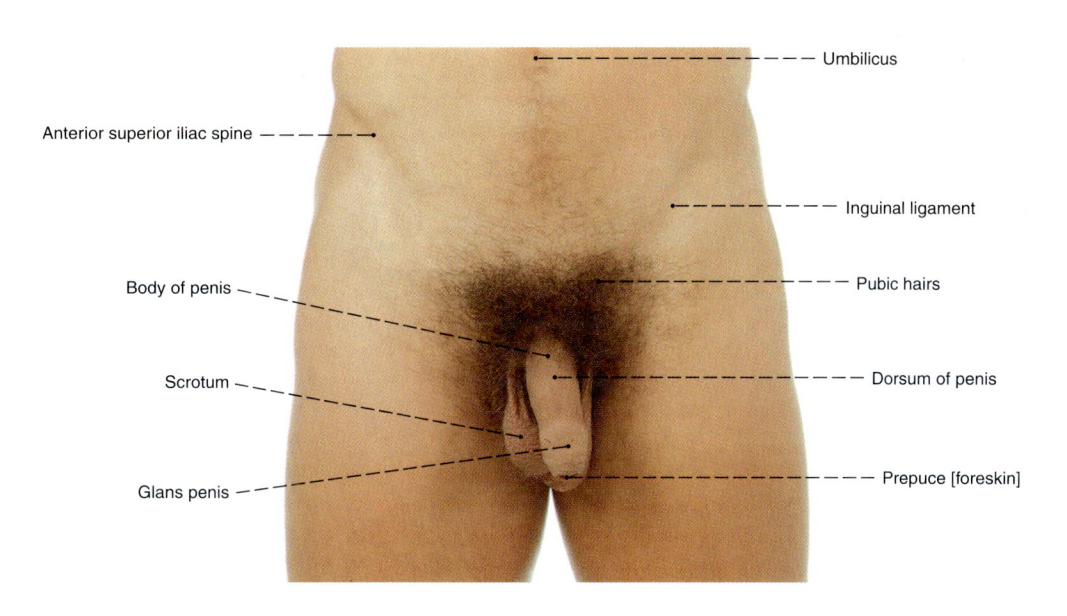

Fig. 1125 External male genitalia; ventral aspect.

236 Pelvic viscera

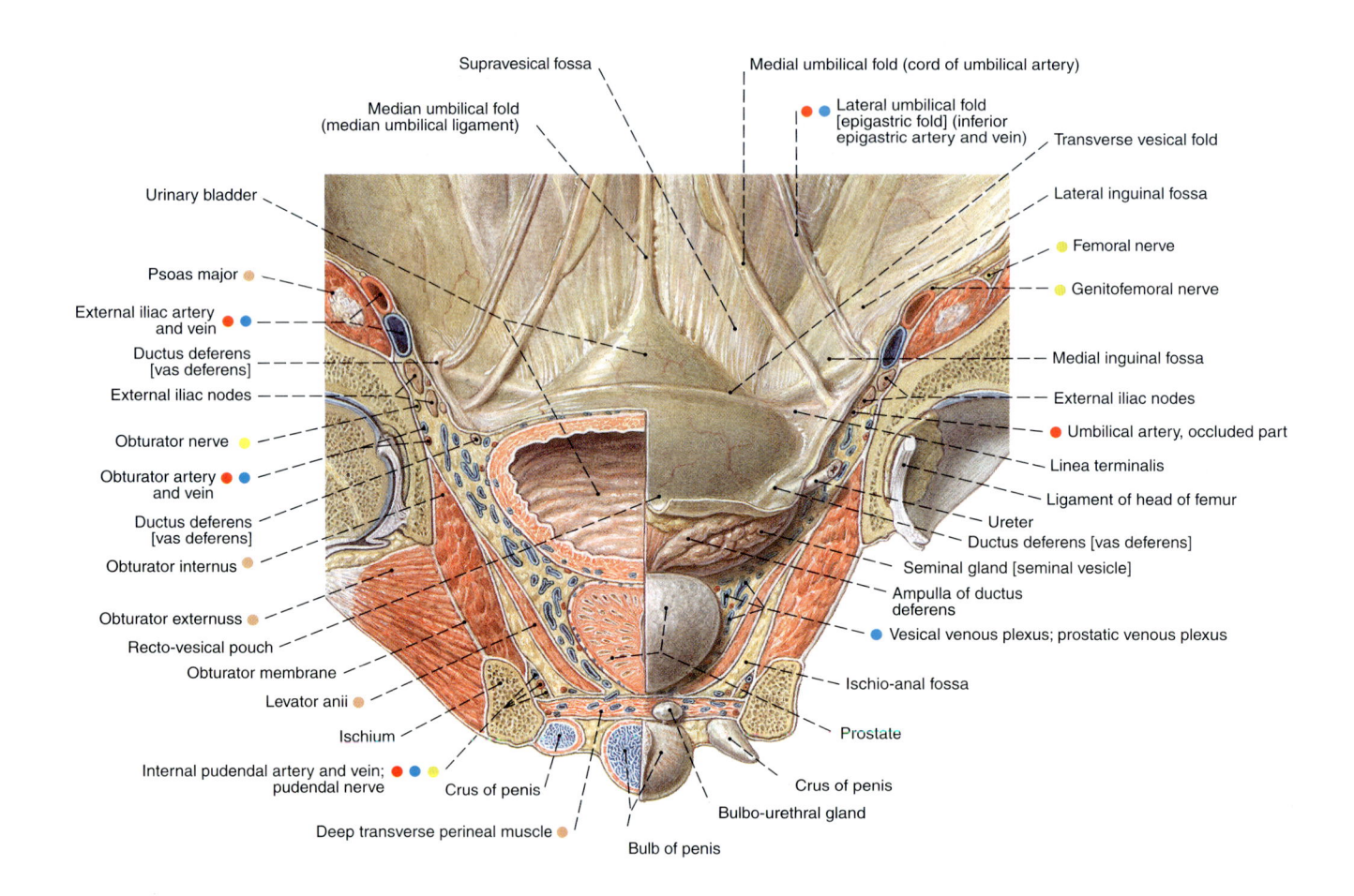

Fig. 1126 Pelvic diaphragm [pelvic floor]; pelvic viscera and anterior abdominal wall in the male; frontal section through the head of femur on the left; urinary bladder and prostate not sectioned on the right; dorsal aspect.

Blood vessels and nerves of perineal region

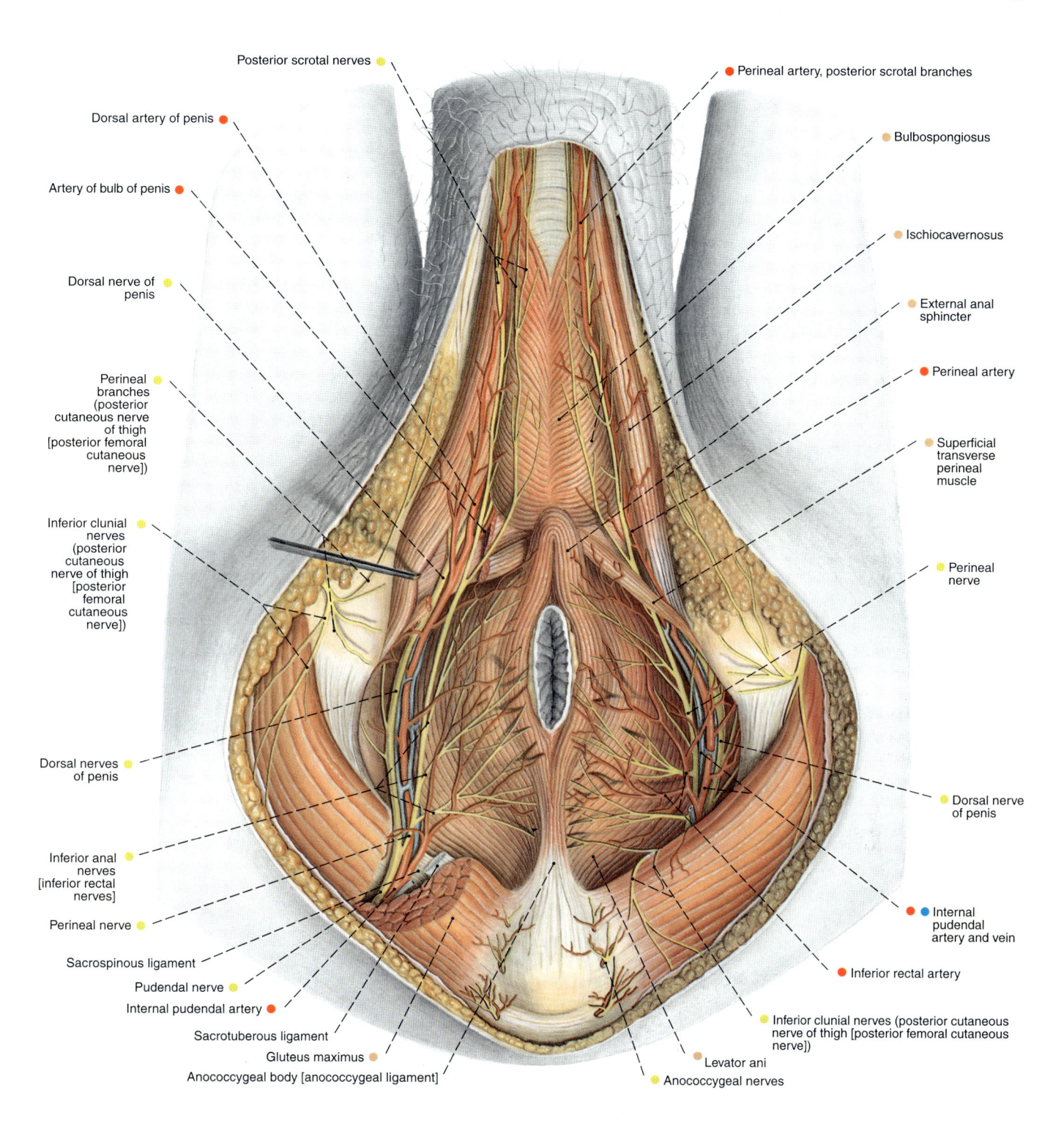

Fig. 1127 Blood vessels and nerves of perineal region and external male genitalia; fat body of ischio-anal fossa removed and gluteus maximus incised to expose the course of pudendal nerve and internal pudendal artery; caudal aspect.

238 Pelvic viscera

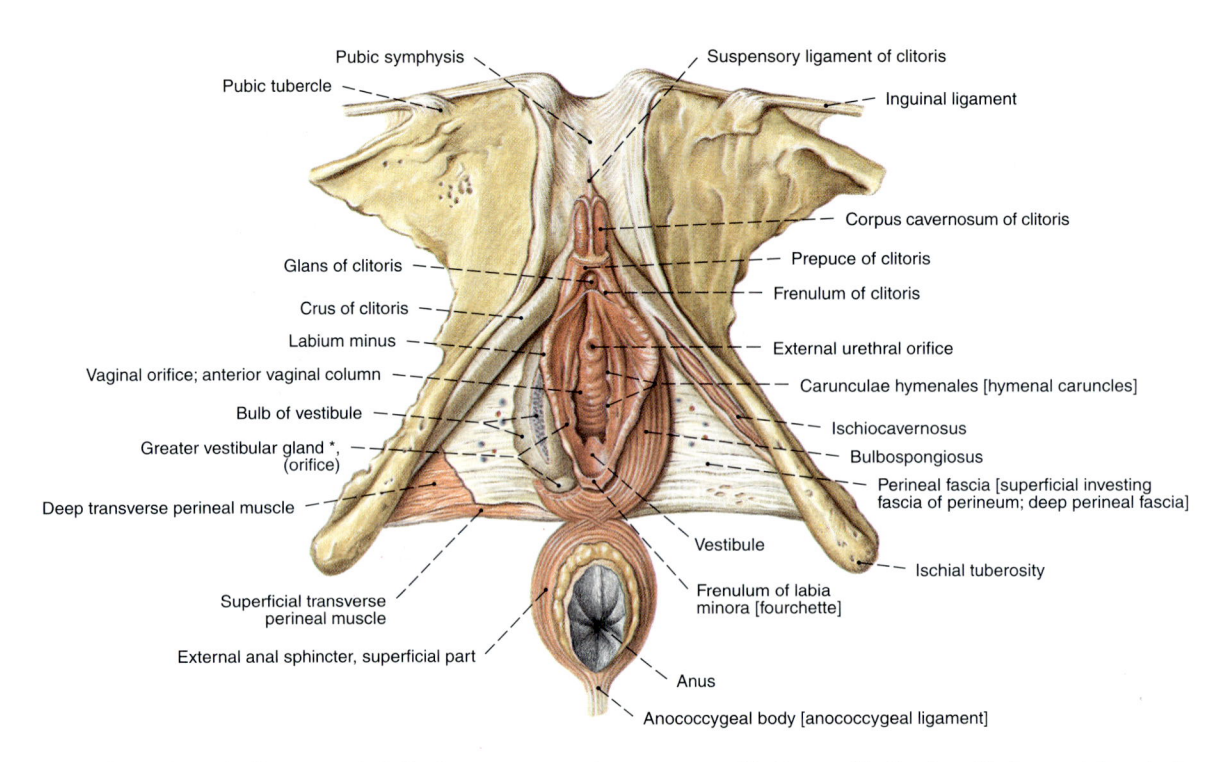

Fig. 1128 External female genitalia; urogenital diaphragm; inferior fascia of urogenital diaphragm extensively removed, ischiocavernosus dissected on the left, bulbospongiosus removed to expose erectile tissue of bulb of vestibule; caudal ventral aspect.

* Clinically: BARTHOLIN's gland.

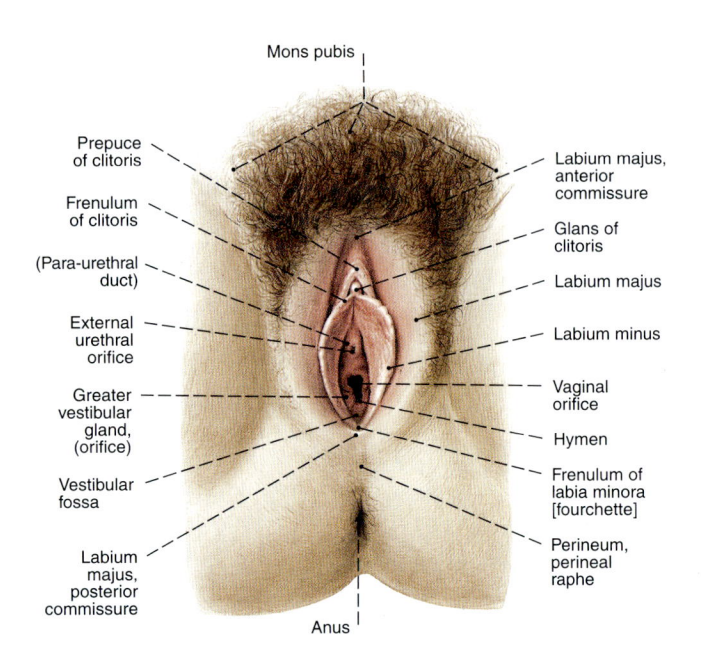

Fig. 1129 External female genitalia; caudal aspect.
View of the vestibule is only possible when labia majora et minora are spread open with specula or the examiner's fingers (not shown).

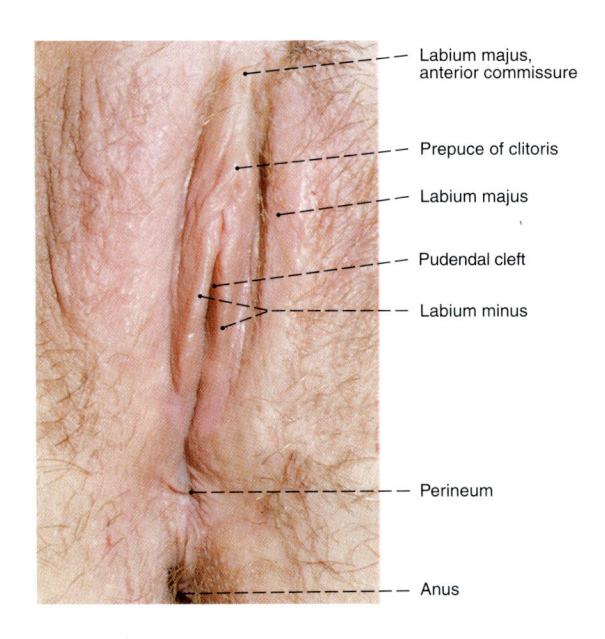

Fig. 1130 External female genitalia; caudal aspect.
Even when the legs are spread apart, the labia minora close the vaginal orifice as shown in this 26-year-old female.

Blood vessels and nerves of perineal region

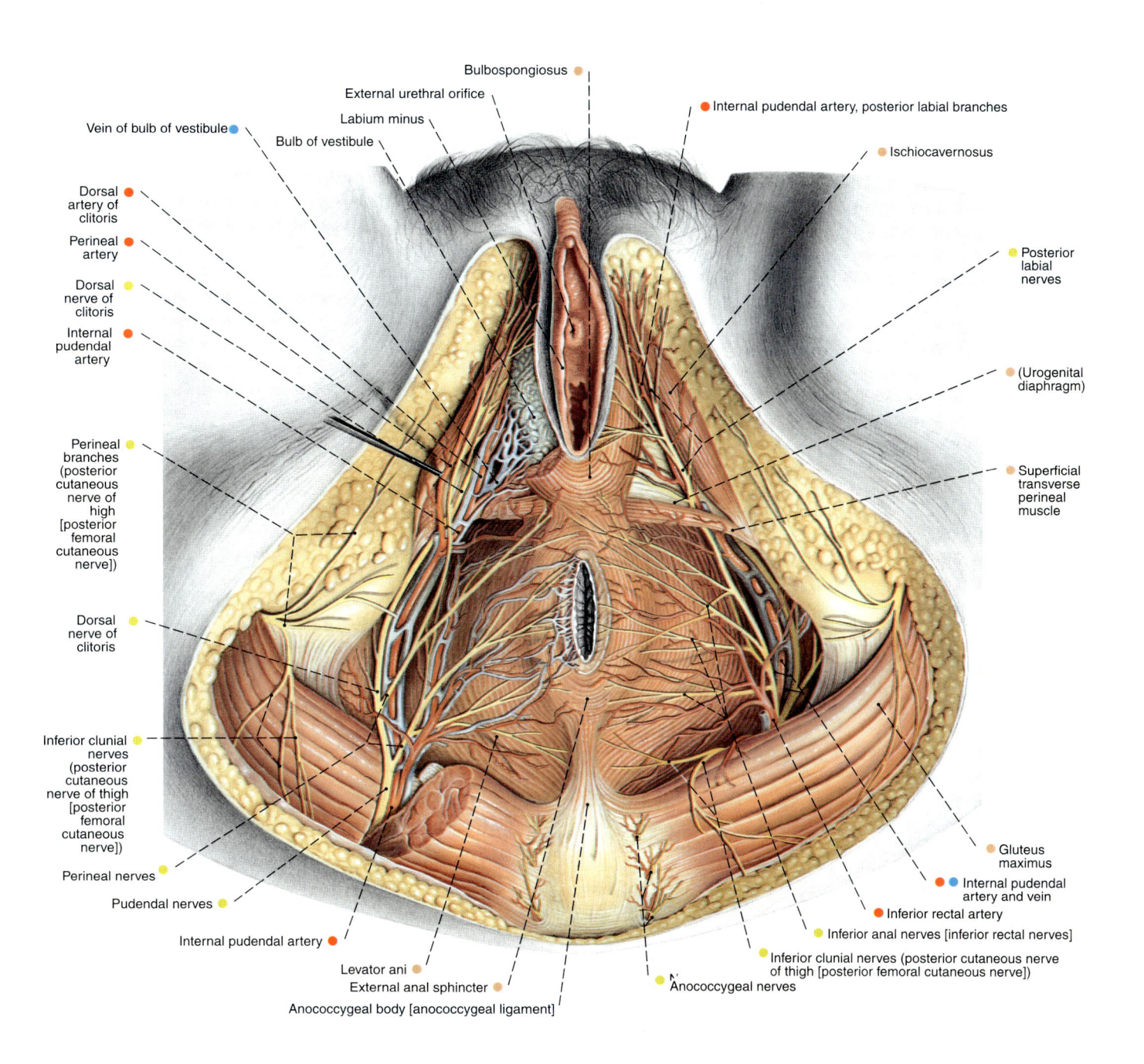

Fig. 1131 Blood vessels and nerves of perineal region and external female genitalia; subcutaneous tissue and fat body of ischio-anal fossa removed and gluteus maximus and deep transverse perineal muscle incised on the right to expose the course nerves and blood vessels; bulbospongiosus removed on the right to expose erectile tissue of bulb of vestibule; caudal aspect.

Pelvic viscera

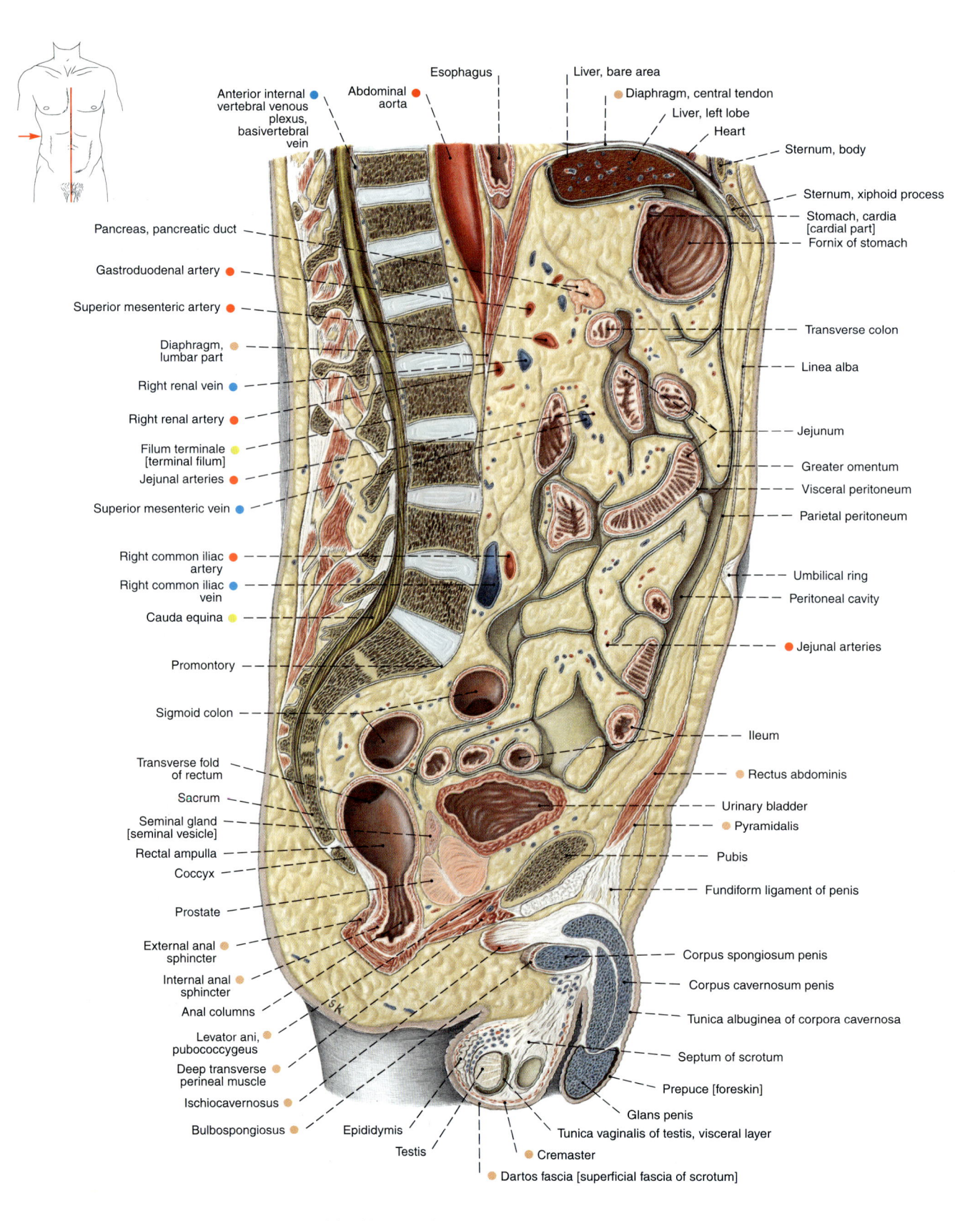

Fig. 1132 Abdomen and pelvis in the male; median section; lateral aspect.
The external male genitalia and the ventral parts of the pelvis are sectioned left to the median plane.

Abdomen and pelvis 241

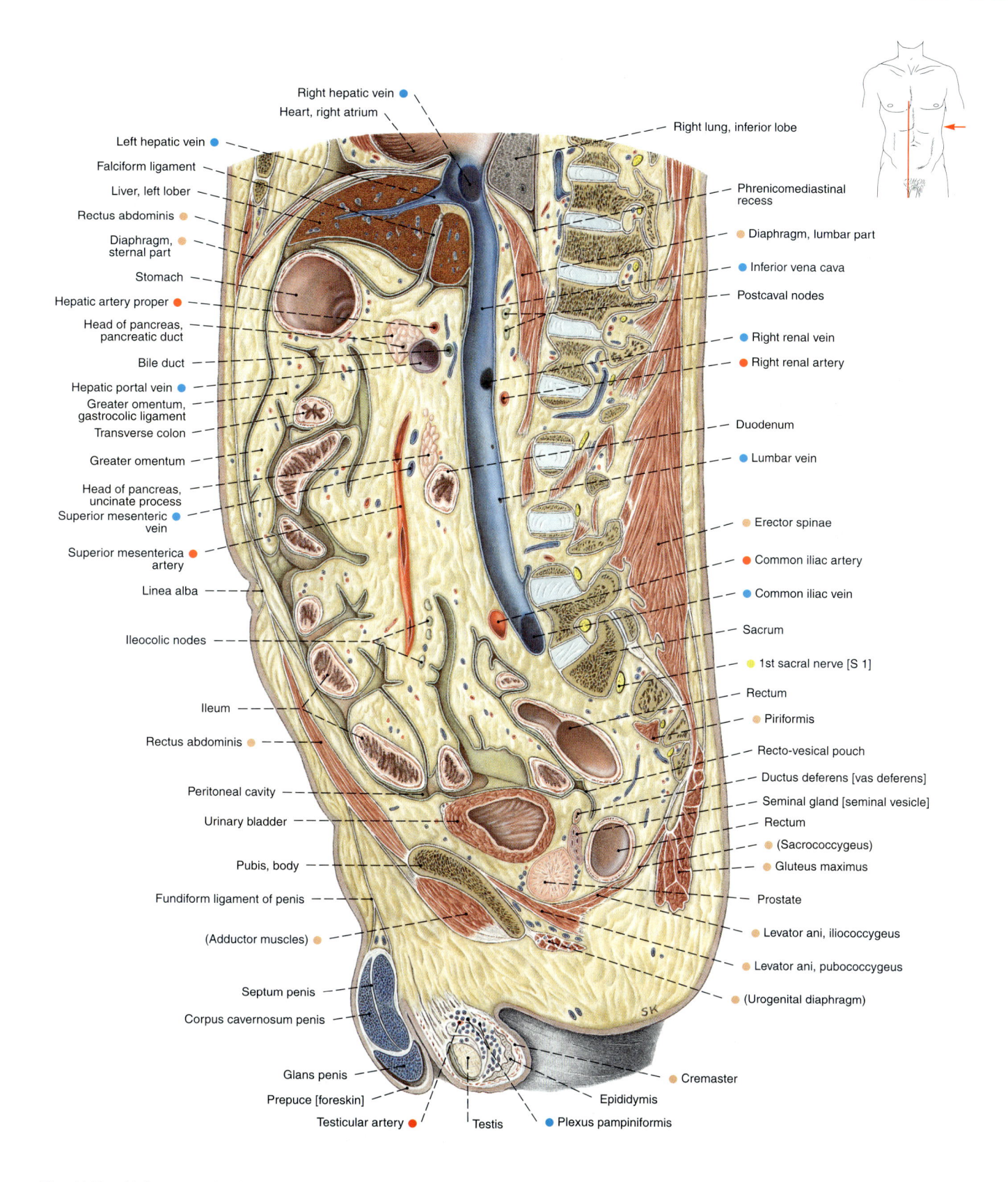

Fig. 1133 Abdomen and pelvis in the male; right paramedian section; right medial aspect.
Due to a lateral curvature (scoliosis) of the lumbar vertebral column, it is sectioned further lateral than the thoracic vertebral column. Compared to the subcutaneous fat more fat is found in the greater omentum.

242 Abdominal and pelvic viscera

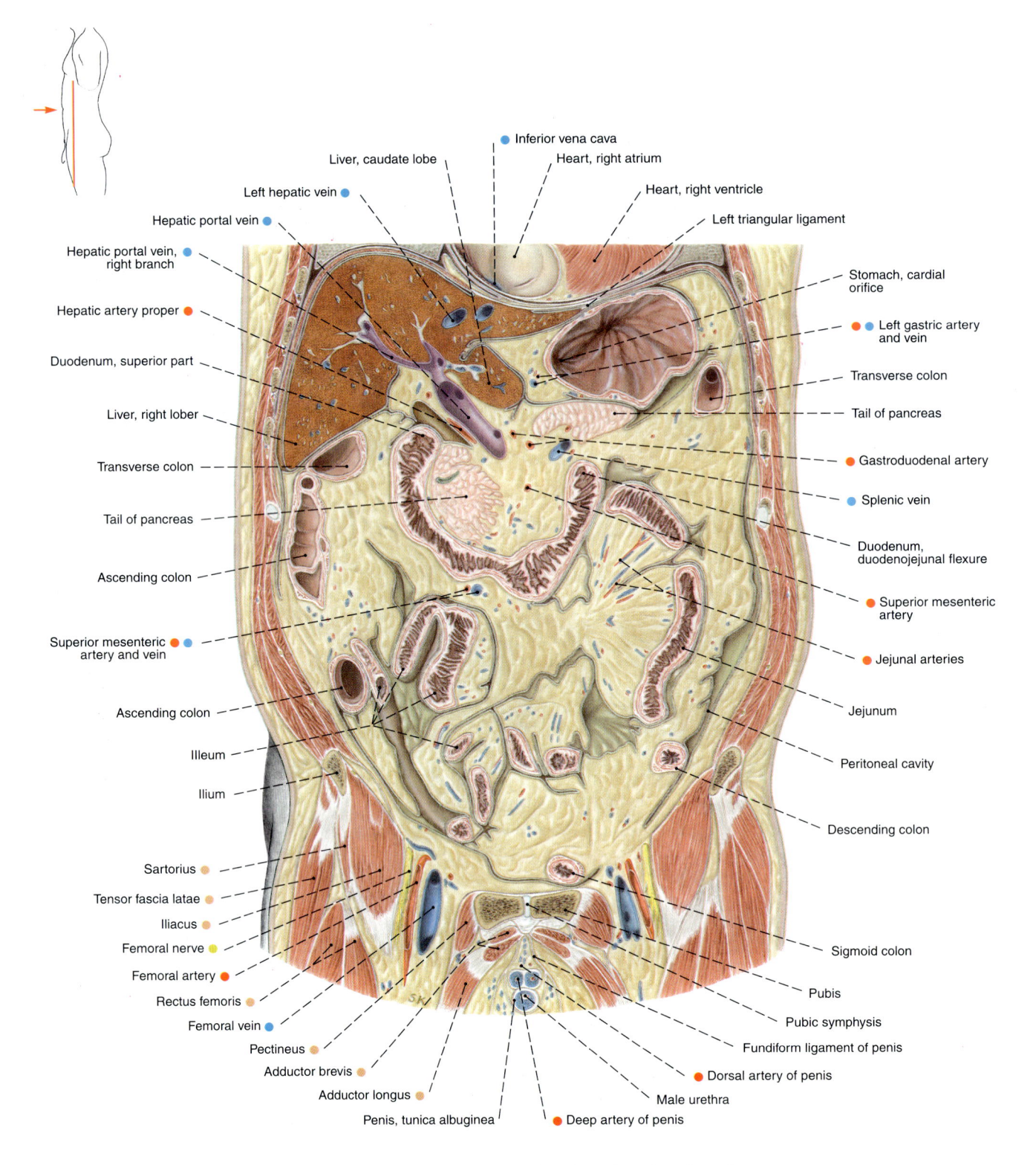

Fig. 1134 Abdomen and pelvis; frontal section through most anterior part of peritoneal cavity; ventral aspect. Muscles, blood vessels, and nerves are labeled in Fig. 837.

Abdomen

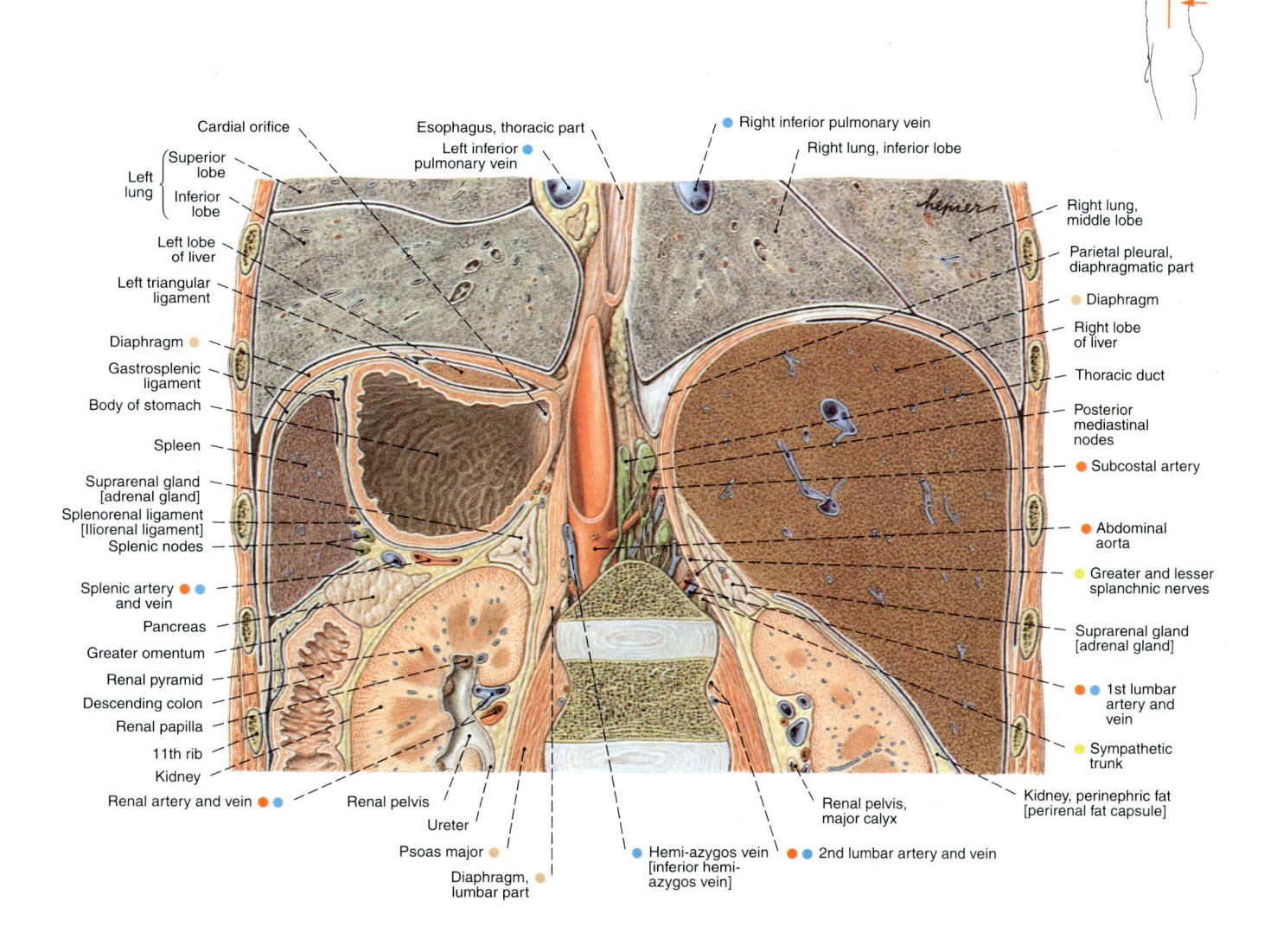

Fig. 1135 Abdomen; frontal section exposing diaphragm, upper abdominal organs and kidneys; dorsal aspect.
Due to the lumbar lordosis the 1st and 2nd lumbar vertebrae are sectioned.

244 Abdominal and pelvic viscera

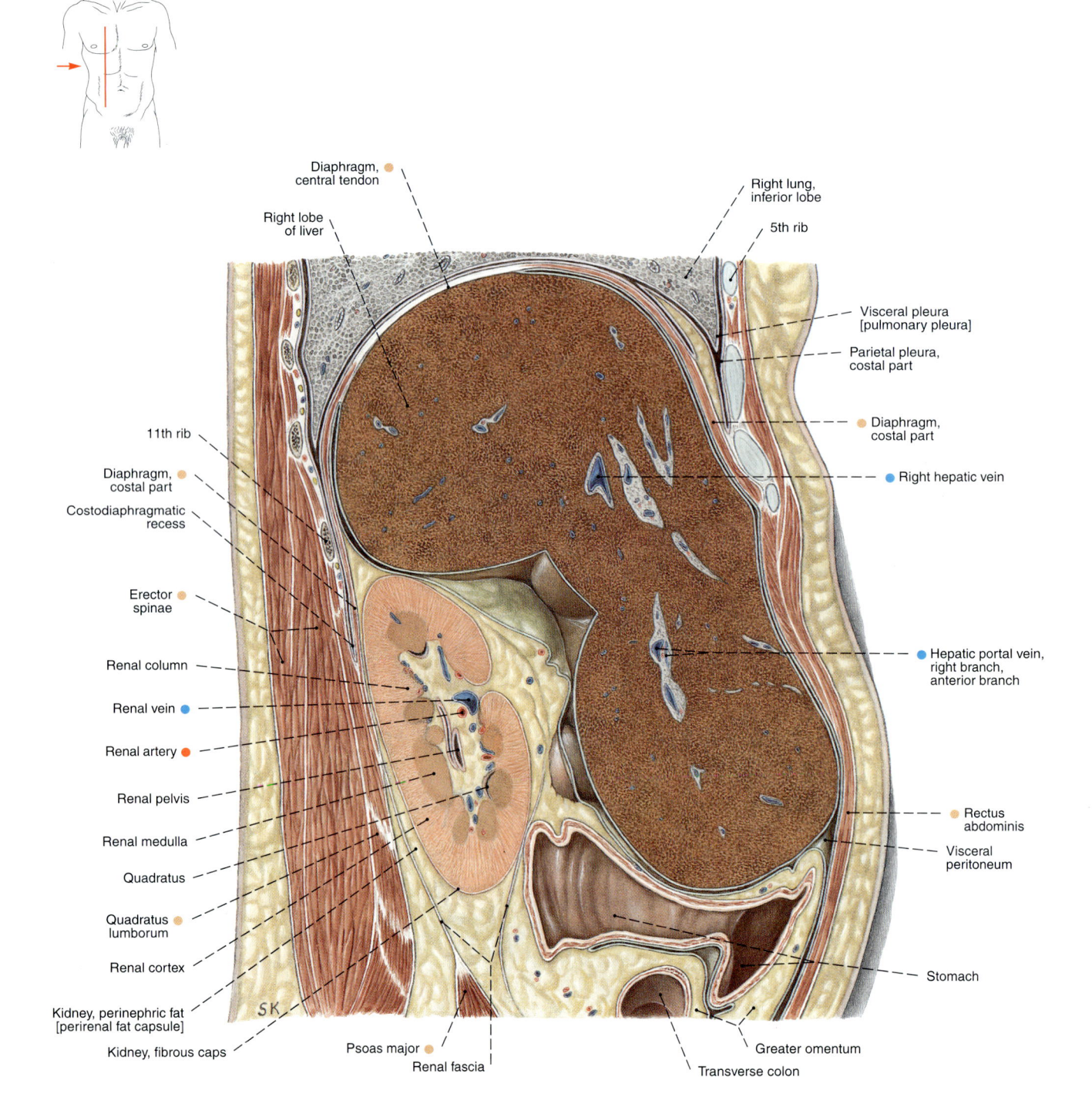

Fig. 1136 Abdomen; sagittal section through the upper abdomen at the level of the right kidney; viewed from the right.

Abdomen 245

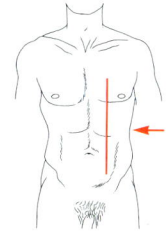

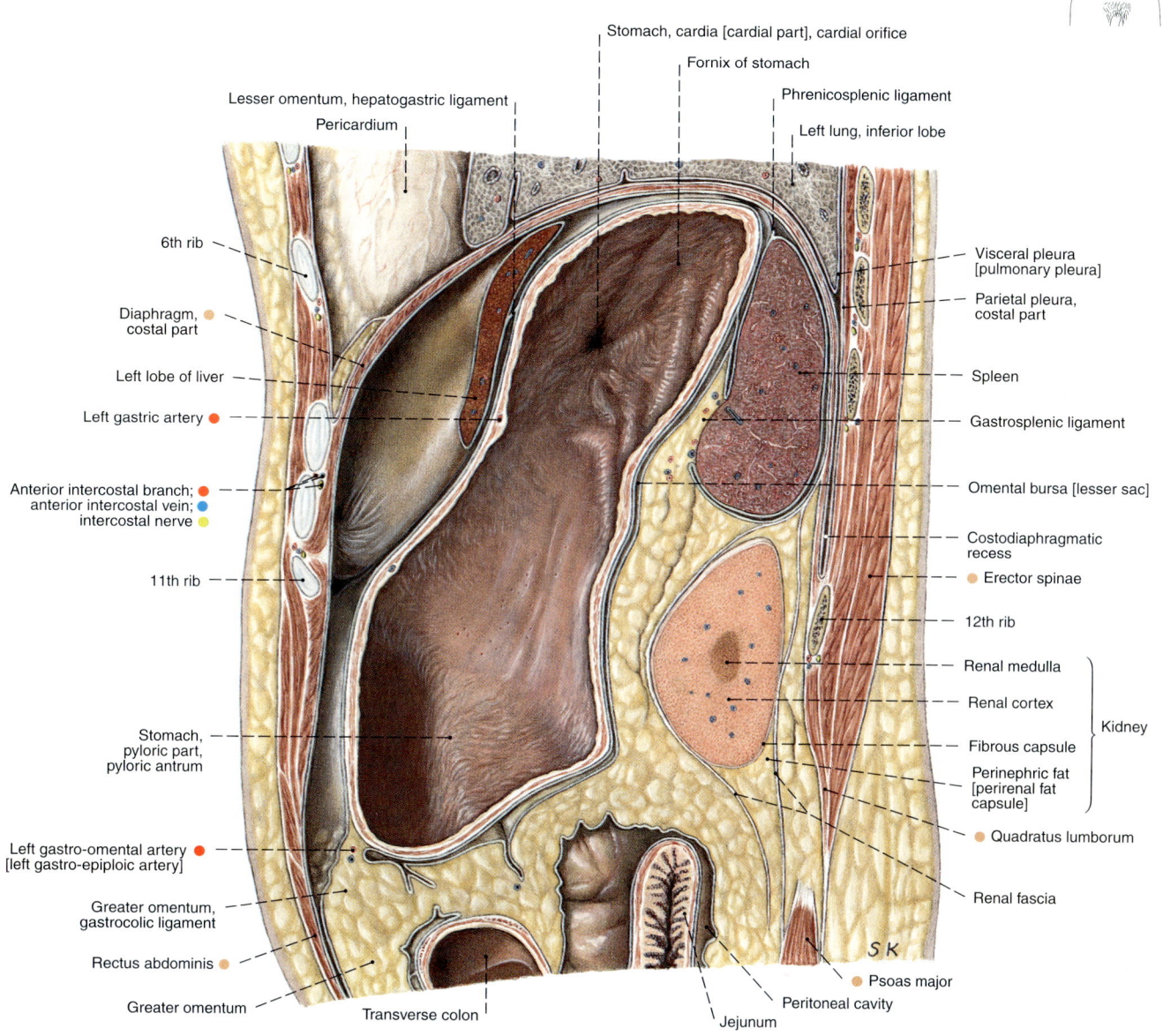

Fig. 1137 Abdomen; sagittal section through the upper abdomen at the level of the spleen; viewed from the left. The capsule of the liver is pathologically thickened.

246   *Abdominal organs*

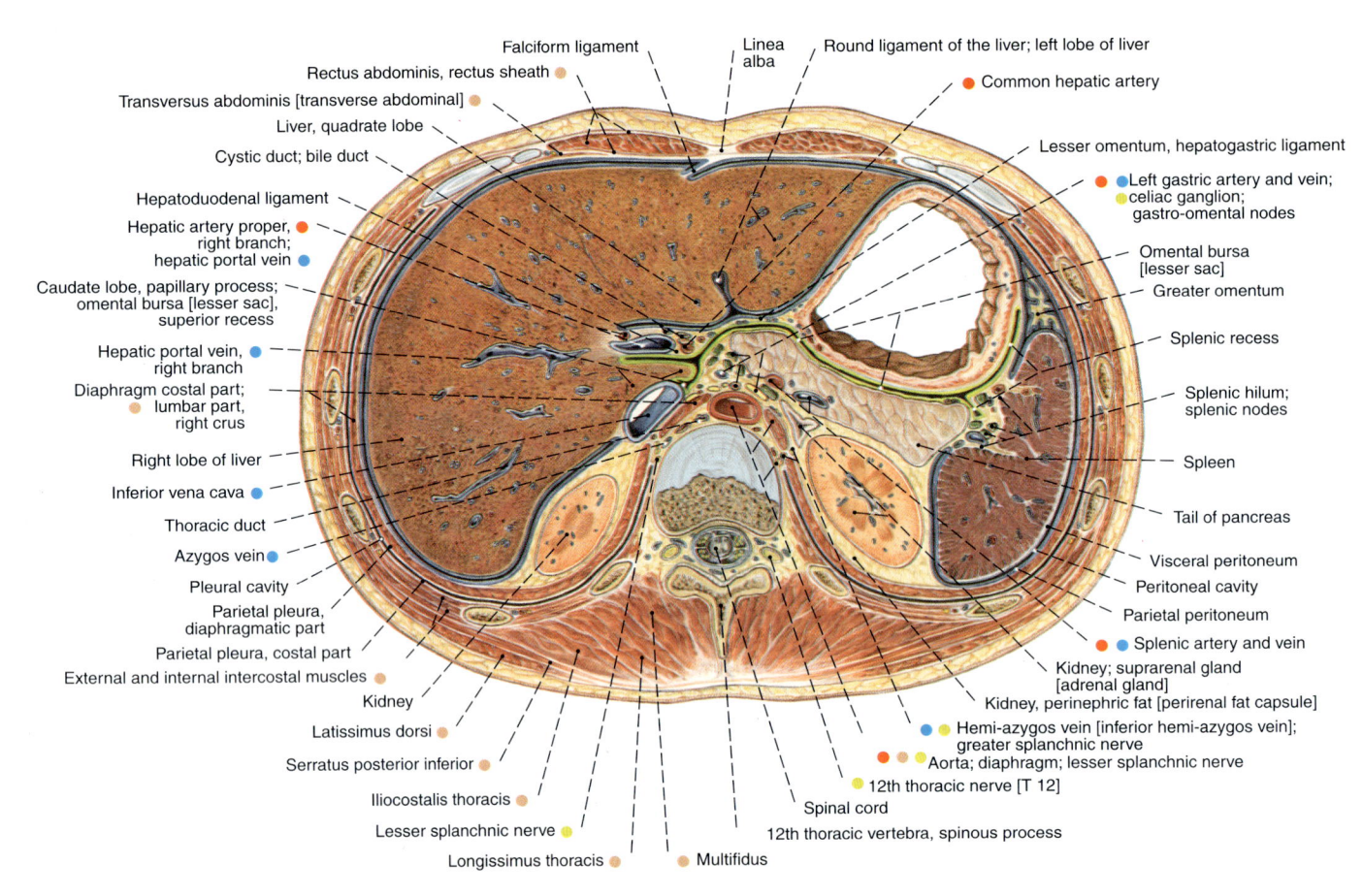

Fig. 1138 Abdomen; transverse section at level of intervertebral disc between 12th thoracic and 1st lumbar vertebra; peritoneum in blue, in the area of the omental bursa [lesser sac] in yellow green; caudal aspect. In this specimen the subcutaneous tissue was poorly developed.

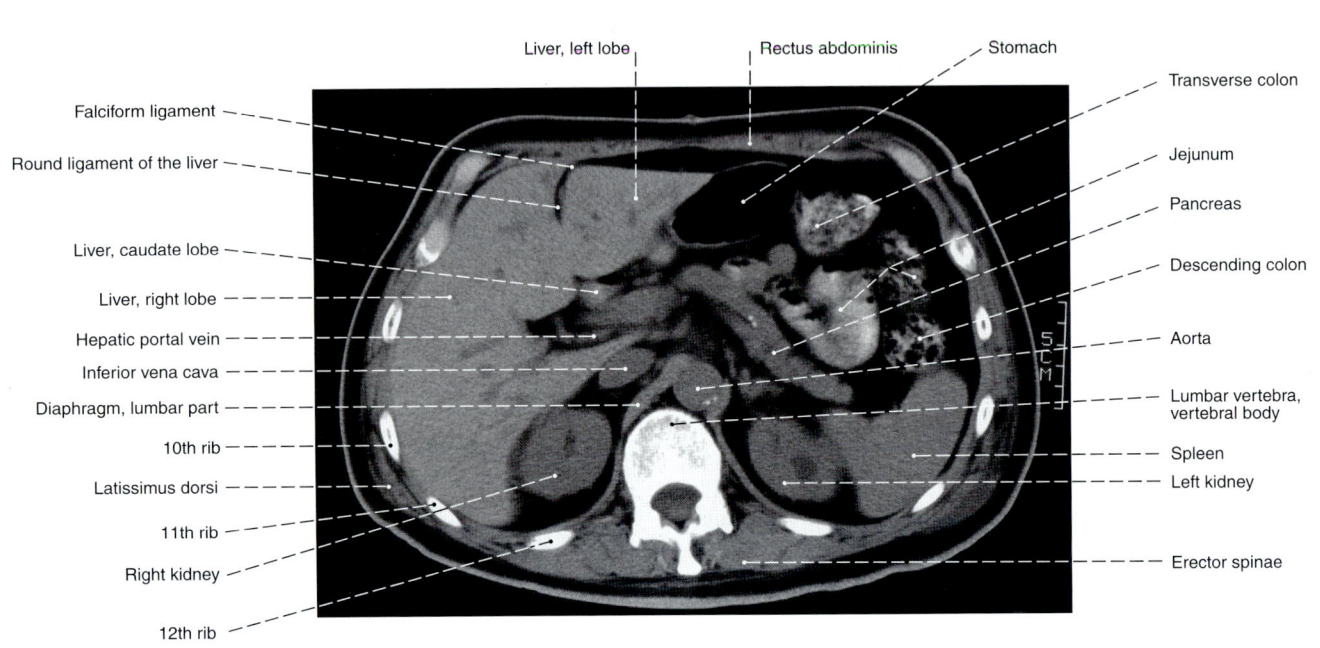

Fig. 1139 Abdomen; computer tomographic transverse section at level of 1st lumbar vertebrae; caudal aspect. Intestine is partially filled with contrast medium.

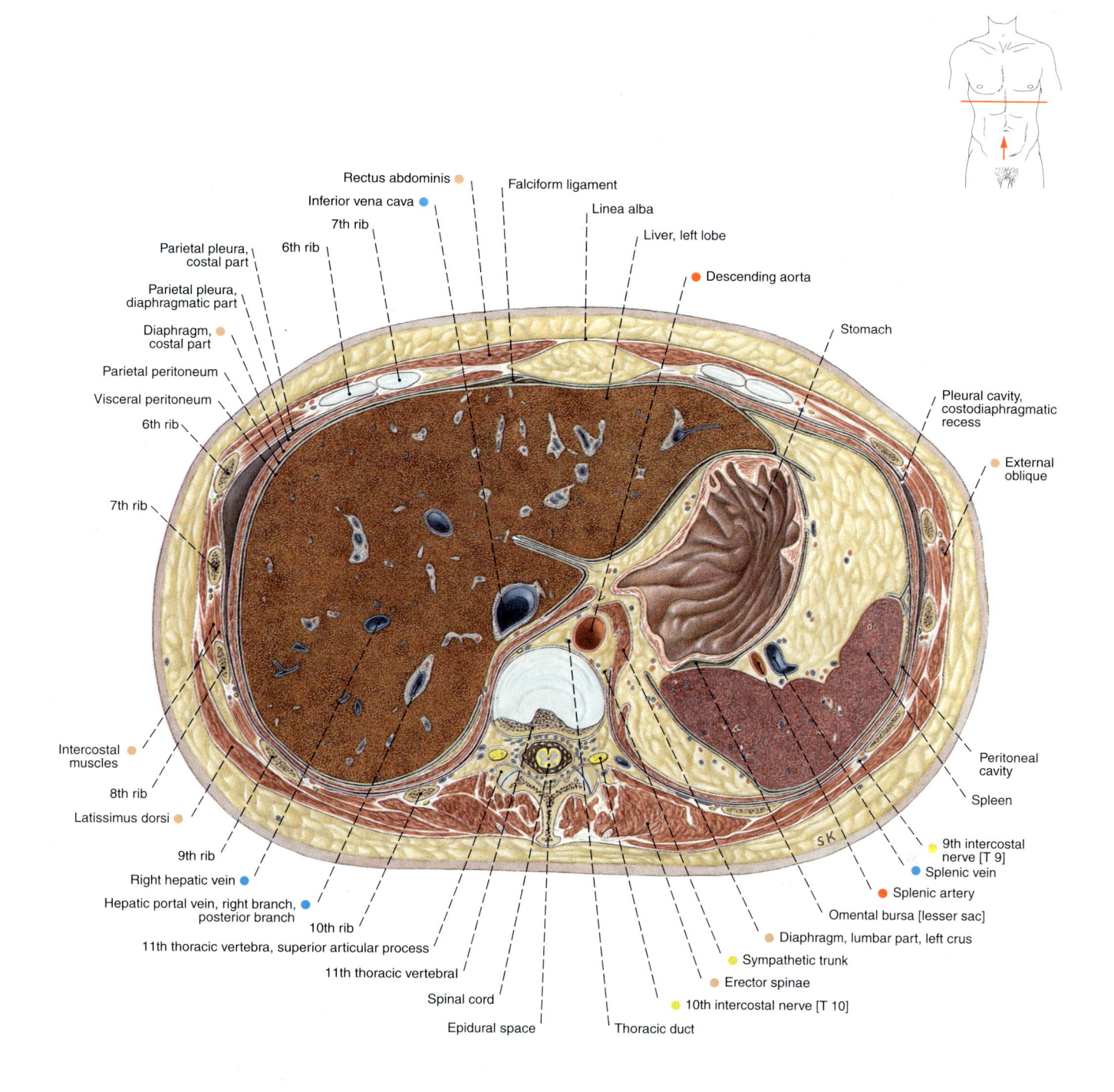

Fig. 1140 Abdomen; transverse section through upper abdomen at level of 11t thoracic vertebra; caudal aspect.

248 Abdominal viscera

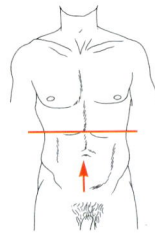

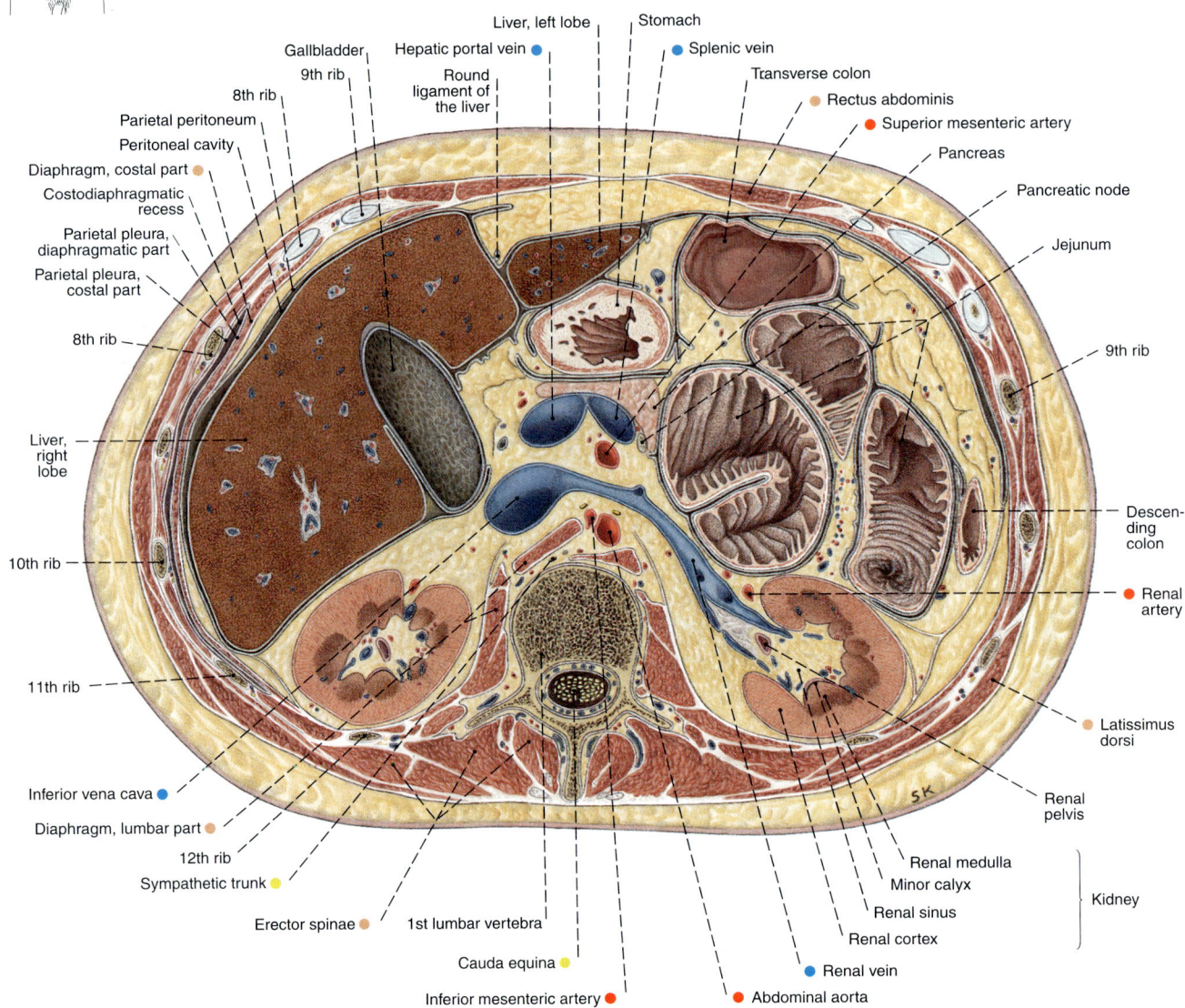

Fig. 1141 Abdomen; transverse section through upper abdomen at level of 1st lumbar vertebra; caudal aspect.
The spinal cord has already become the cauda equina in this case. The stomach is contracted and thus the mucosa [mucous membrane] looks thickened.

Abdomen 249

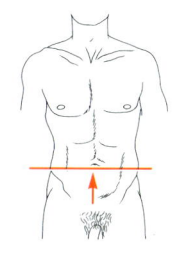

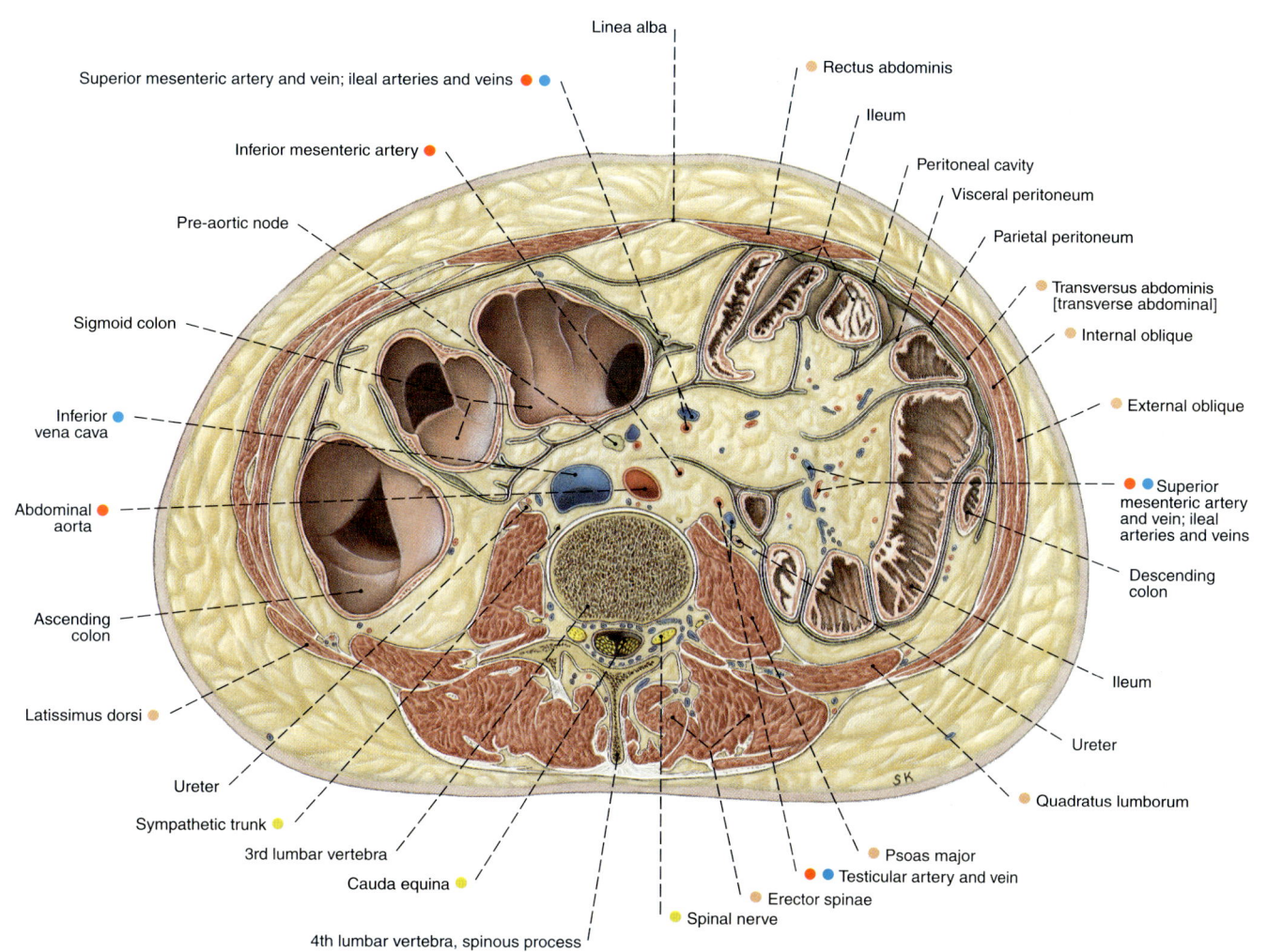

Fig. 1142 Abdomen; transverse section through lower abdomen at level of 3rd lumbar vertebra; caudal aspect. In this case a far cranial extending loop of the sigmoid colon was present, of which both the ascending and descending parts have been sectioned.

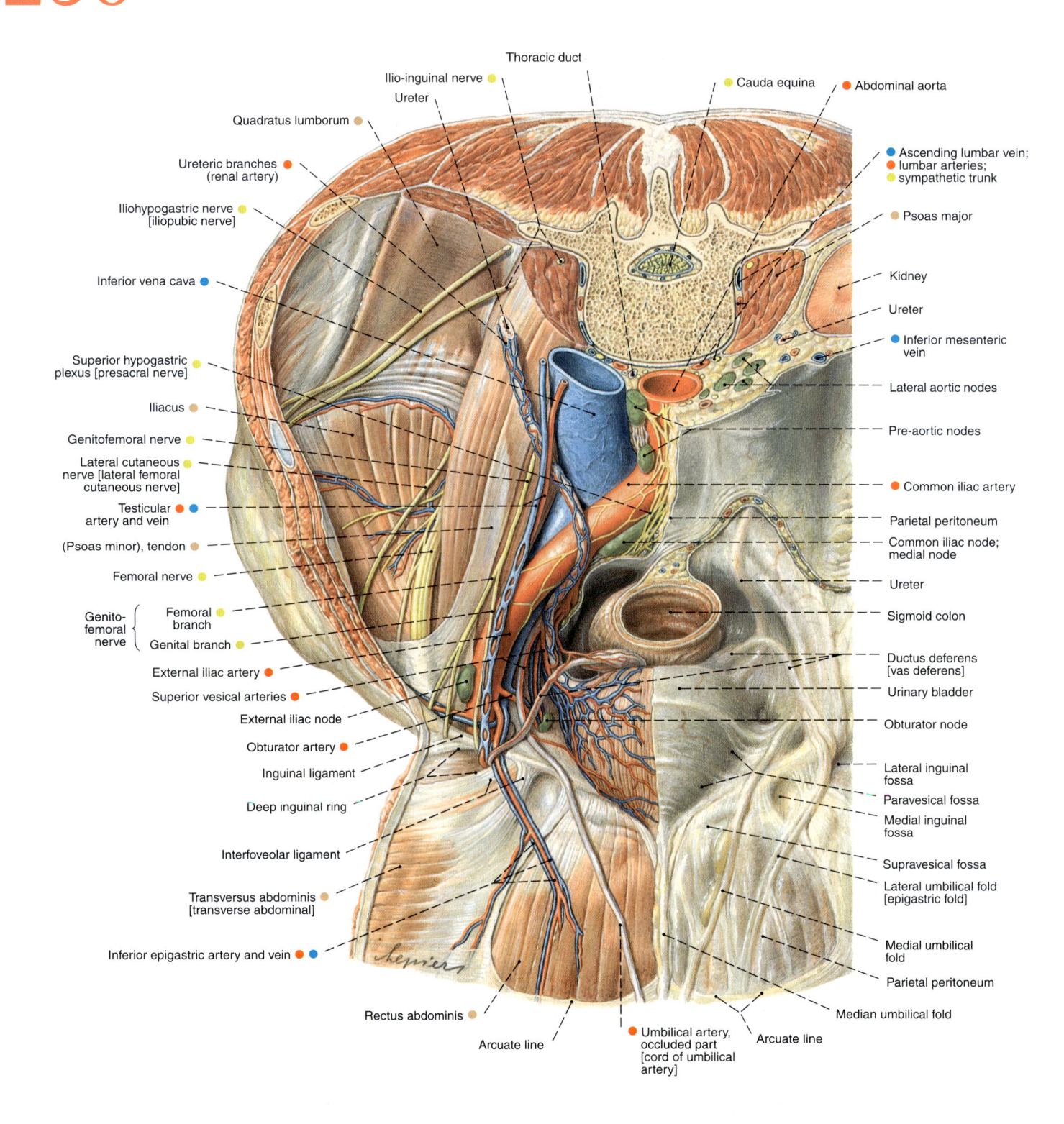

Fig. 1143 Abdominal wall and pelvic viscera in a male; posterior abdominal wall sectioned in the transverse plane; anterior abdominal wall reflected anteriorly; on the right peritoneum removed to expose blood vessels and nerves; cranial aspect.

Pelvis 251

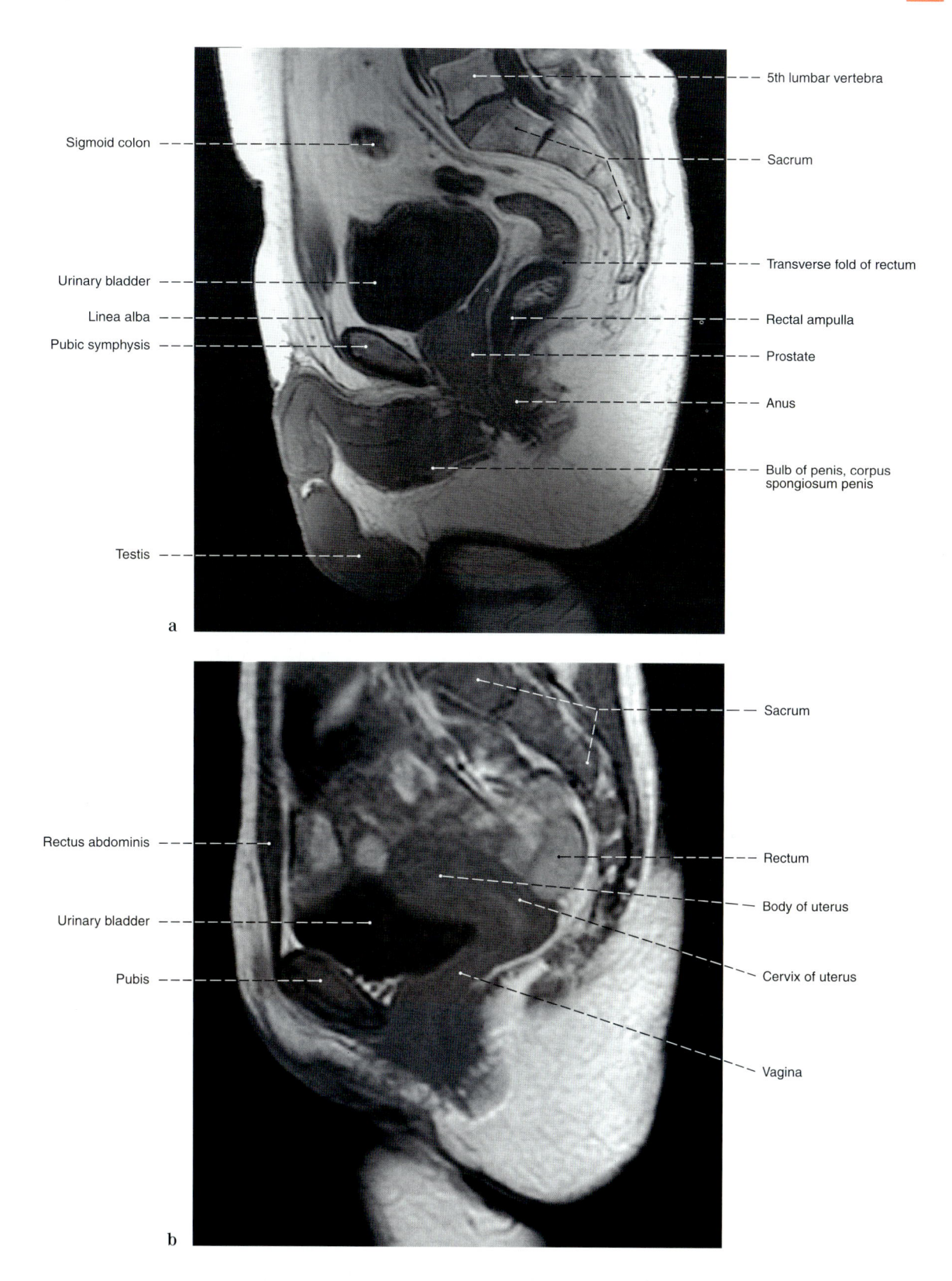

Fig. 1144 a, b Pelvis; magnetic resonance image; paramedian section; viewed from the left.
a In the male
b In the female
Compare to Figs. 1145 and 1146.

252 *Pelvic viscera*

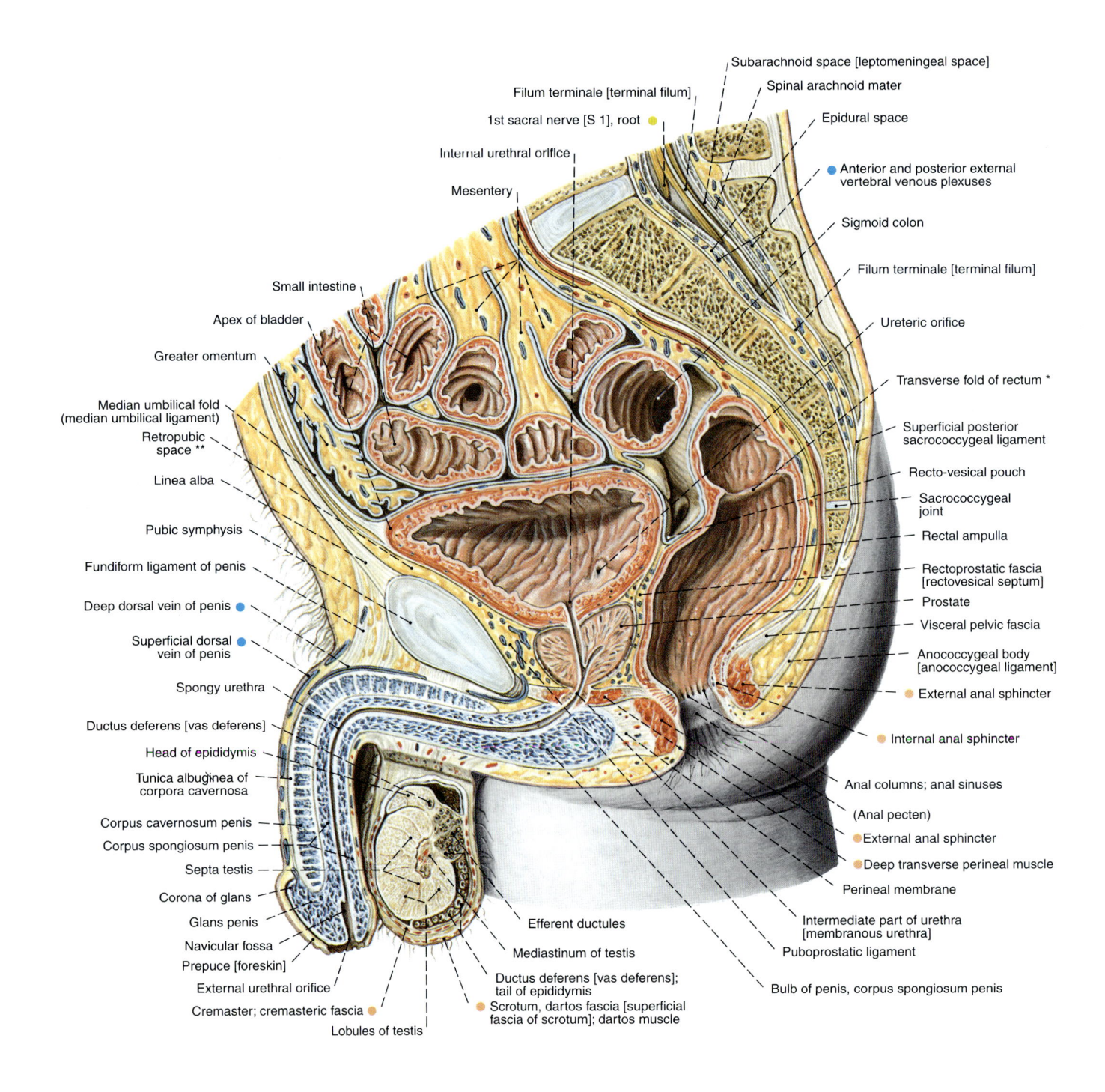

Fig. 1145 Pelvis in the male; median section; right lateral aspect.
* Clinically: KOHLRAUSCH's fold.
** Clinically: cave of RETZIUS.

Pelvis 253

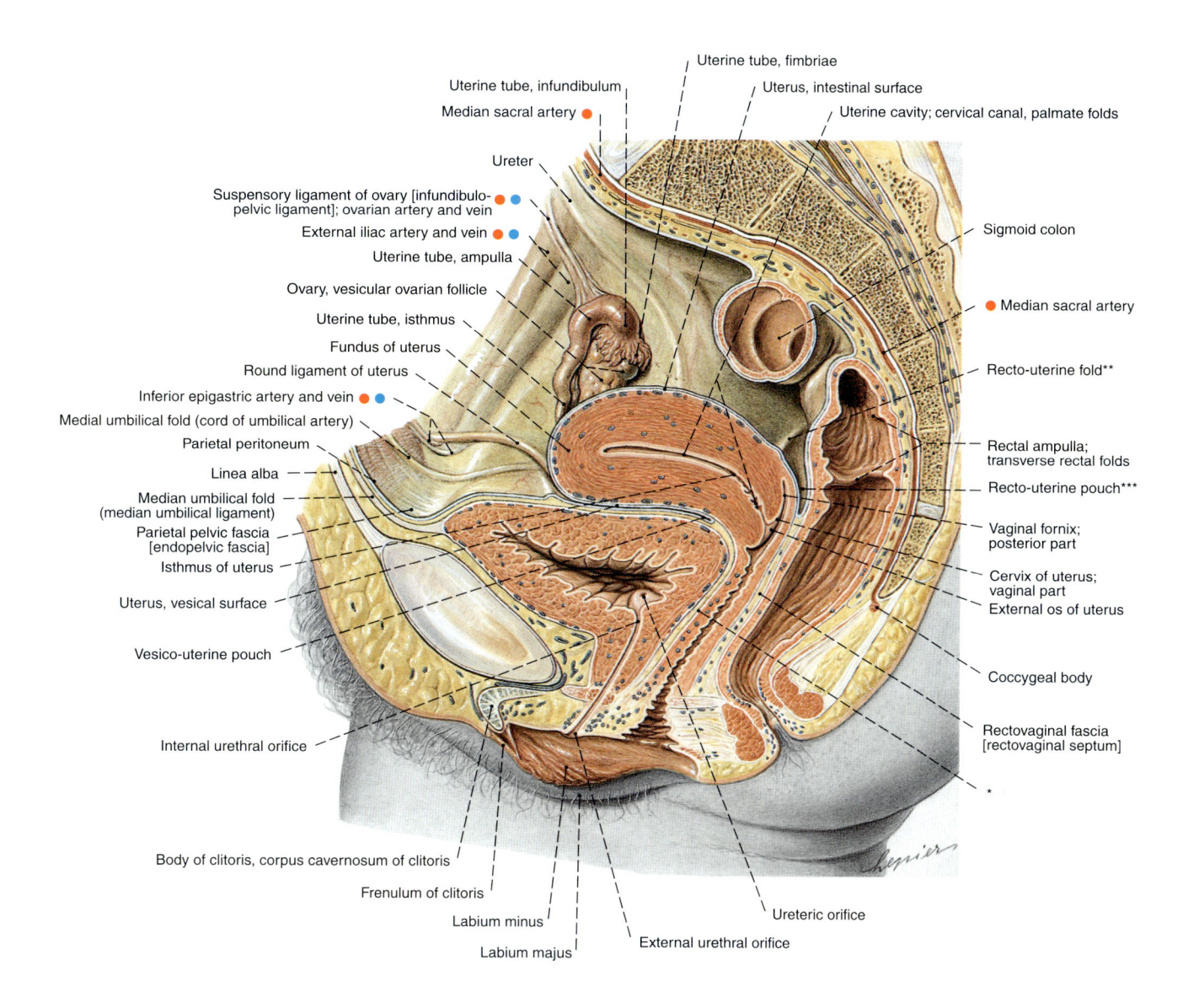

Fig. 1146   Pelvis in the female; median section; small and large intestines removed except for terminal parts of sigmoid colon and rectum; right lateral aspect.

*   Clinically: vesicovaginal septum.
**   Clinically: fold of DOUGLAS, sacro-uterine ligament.
*** Clinically: pouch of DOUGLAS.

254 Pelvic viscera

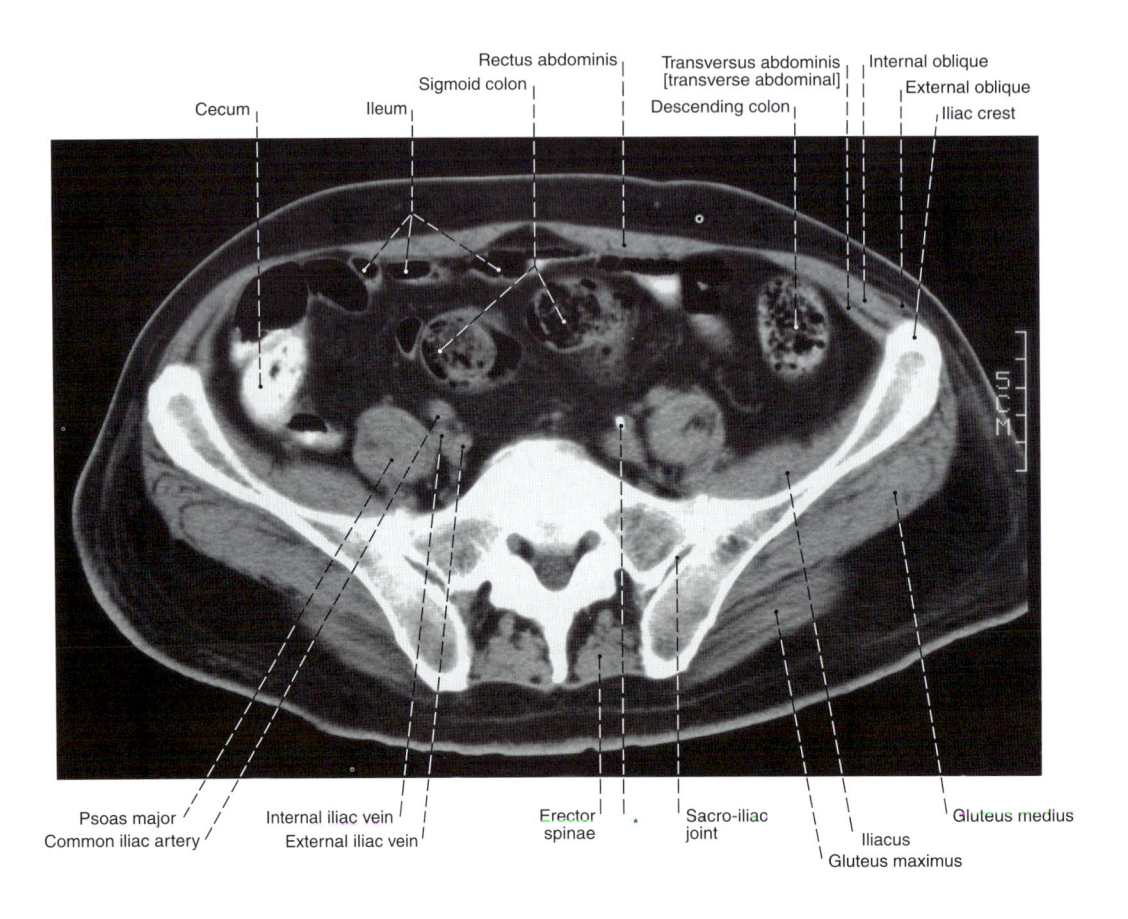

Fig. 1147　Pelvis; computer tomographic cross-section at level of 1st sacral segment after administration of contrast medium into the colon in supine position; caudal aspect.

* Calcification in the wall of the common iliac artery.

The contrast medium has become mixed with intestinal contents in the sigmoid and descending colon, while the cecum is almost entirely filled with contrast medium. The thickness of the subcutaneous fat in the gluteal region is well developed in this patient; this must be considered for intramuscular injections because many medications must only be injected into the musculature and not into the subcutaneous tissue.

Pelvis **255**

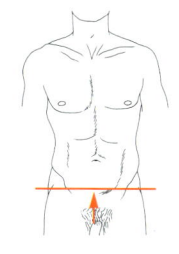

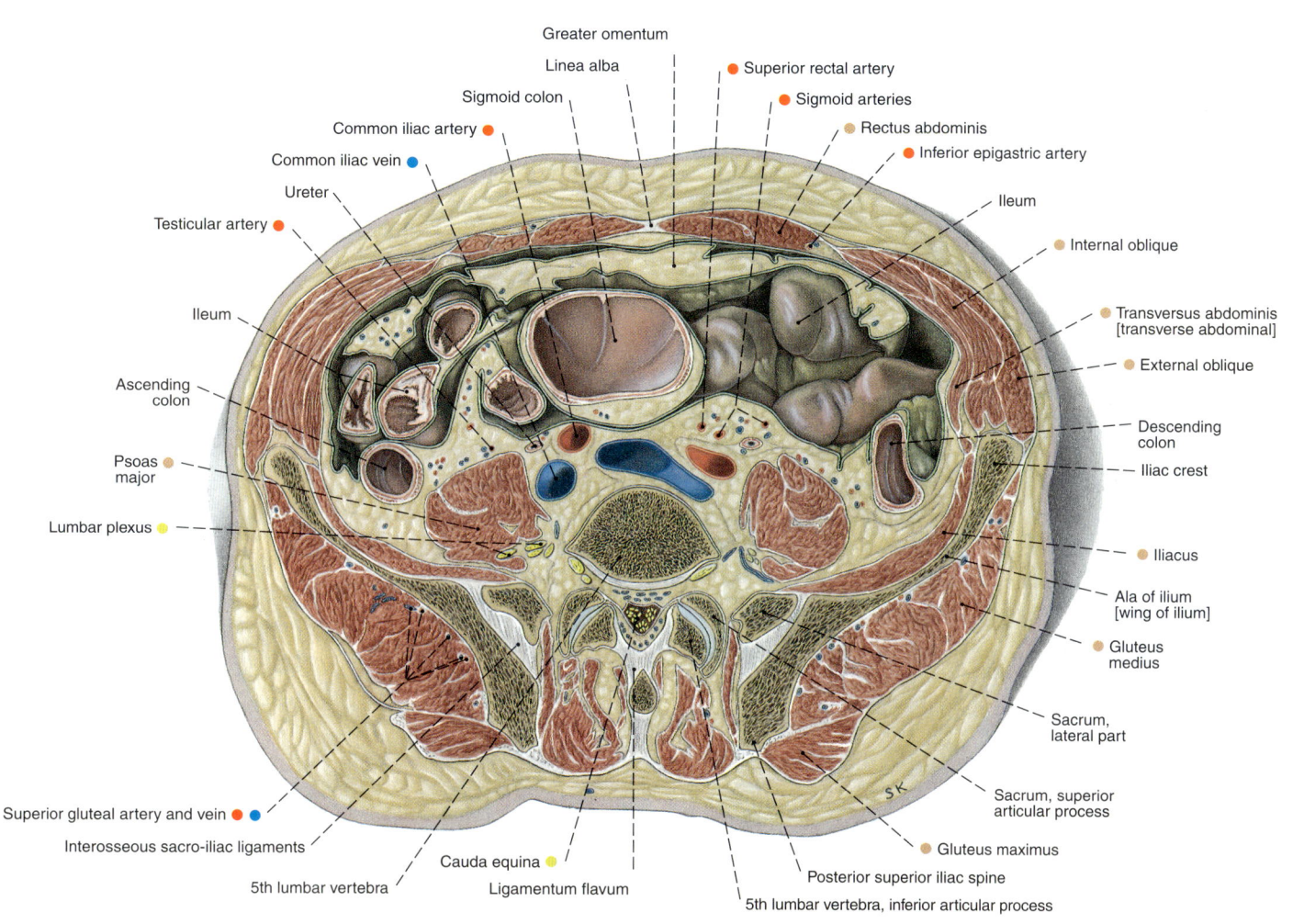

Fig. 1148 Pelvis; transverse section at level of 5th lumbar vertebra; caudal aspect. This section is from another male than were the sections in Figs. 1140-1142. The sigmoid colon extends far cranially; thus, the top of the flexure is sectioned. The thickness of the subcutaneous fat in the gluteal region must be considered for intramuscular injections.

Pelvic viscera

Fig. 1149 Male pelvis; transverse section through lesser pelvis [true pelvis]; caudal aspect.
Due to slight asymmetry of the pelvis the right and left hip joints are sectioned at slightly different levels.

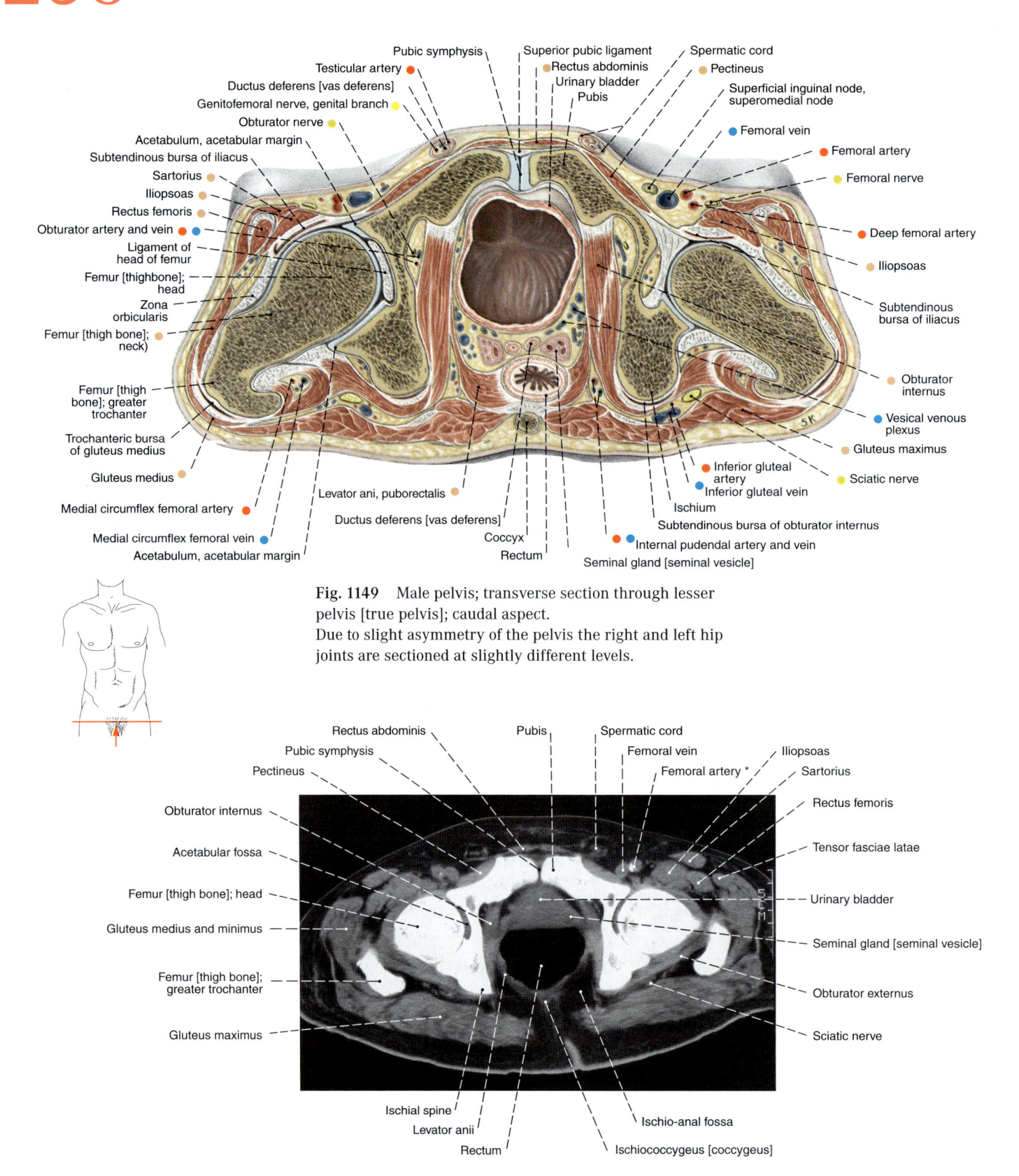

Fig. 1150 Male pelvis; computer tomographic cross-section through lesser pelvis [true pelvis] in supine position at approximately same level as in Fig. 1149; caudal aspect.

* Calcification in medial part of femoral artery.

Pelvis 257

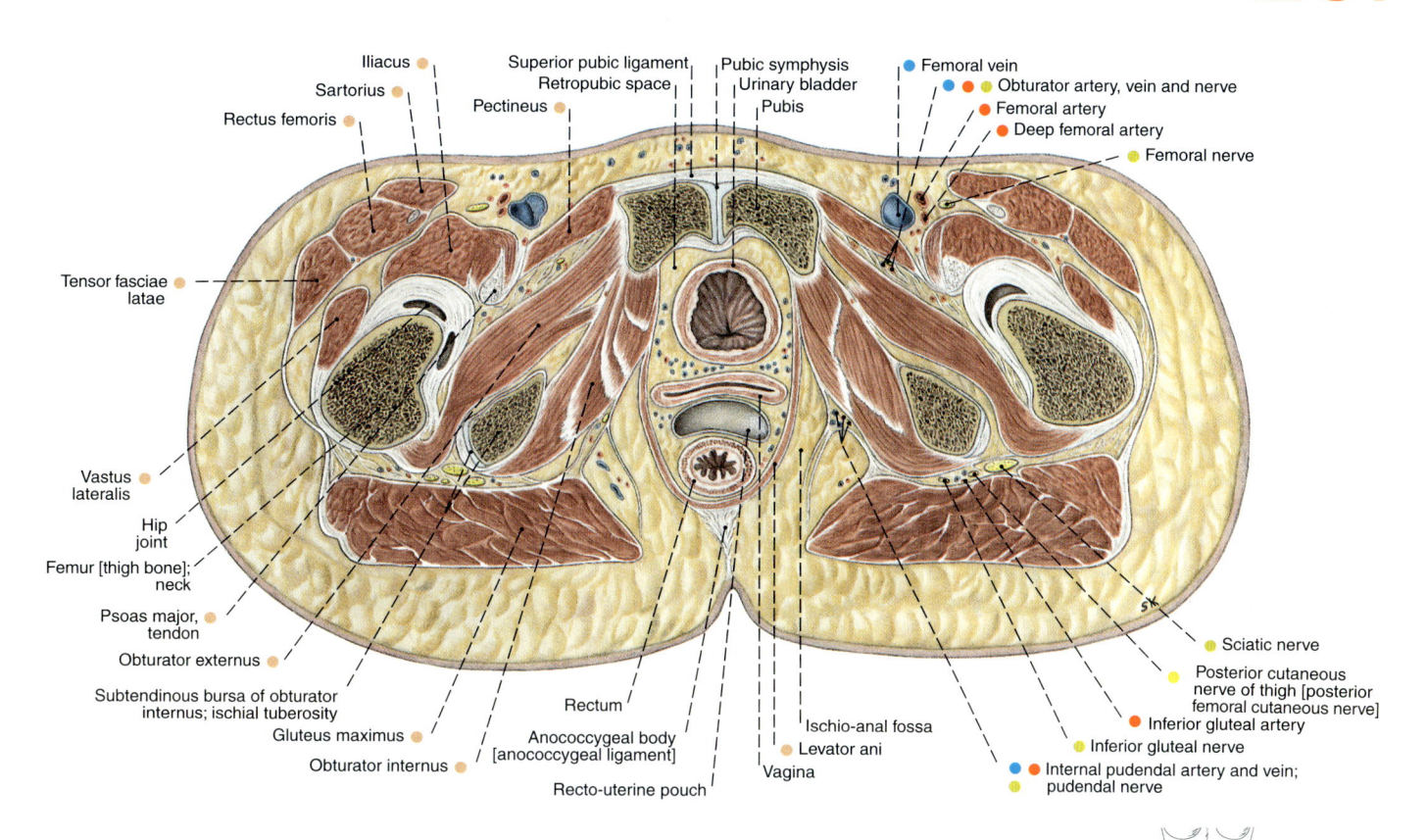

Fig. 1151 Female pelvis; transverse section through lesser pelvis [true pelvis] at level of pubic symphysis; caudal aspect.

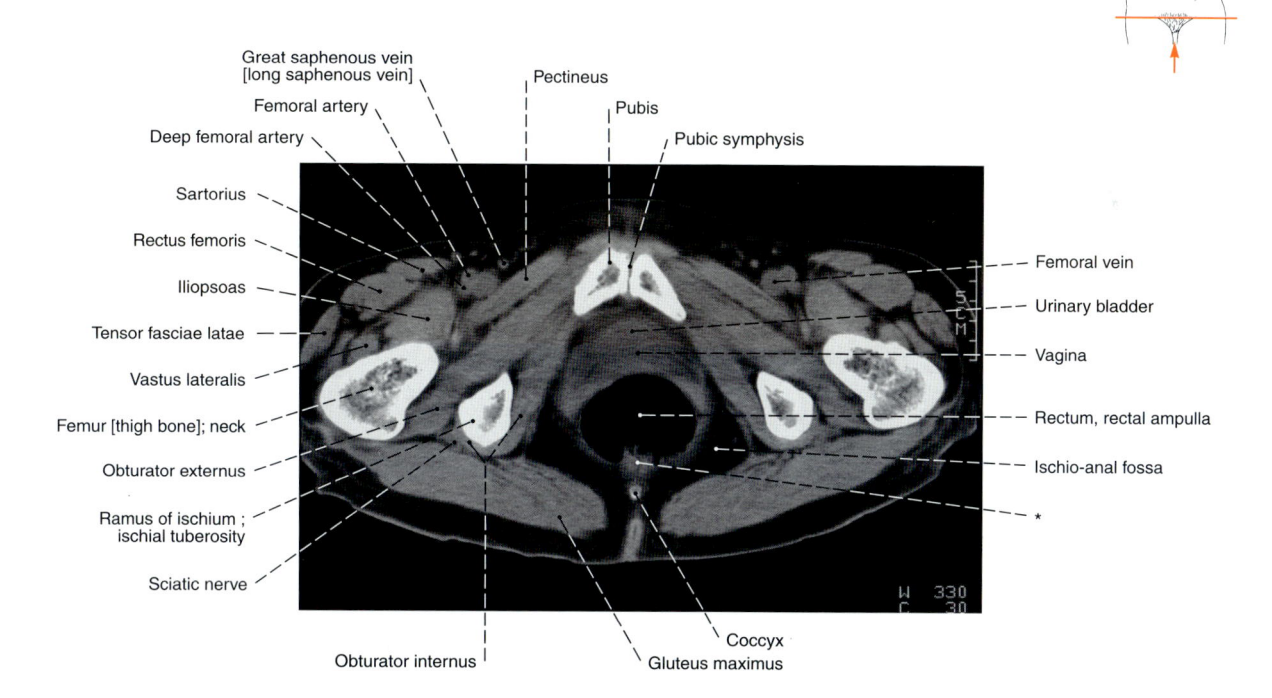

Fig. 1152 Female pelvis; computer tomographic cross-section through lesser pelvis [true pelvis] in supine position at approximately same level as in Fig. 1151; caudal aspect.

* Residua of contrast medium in intestinal contents.

Pelvic viscera

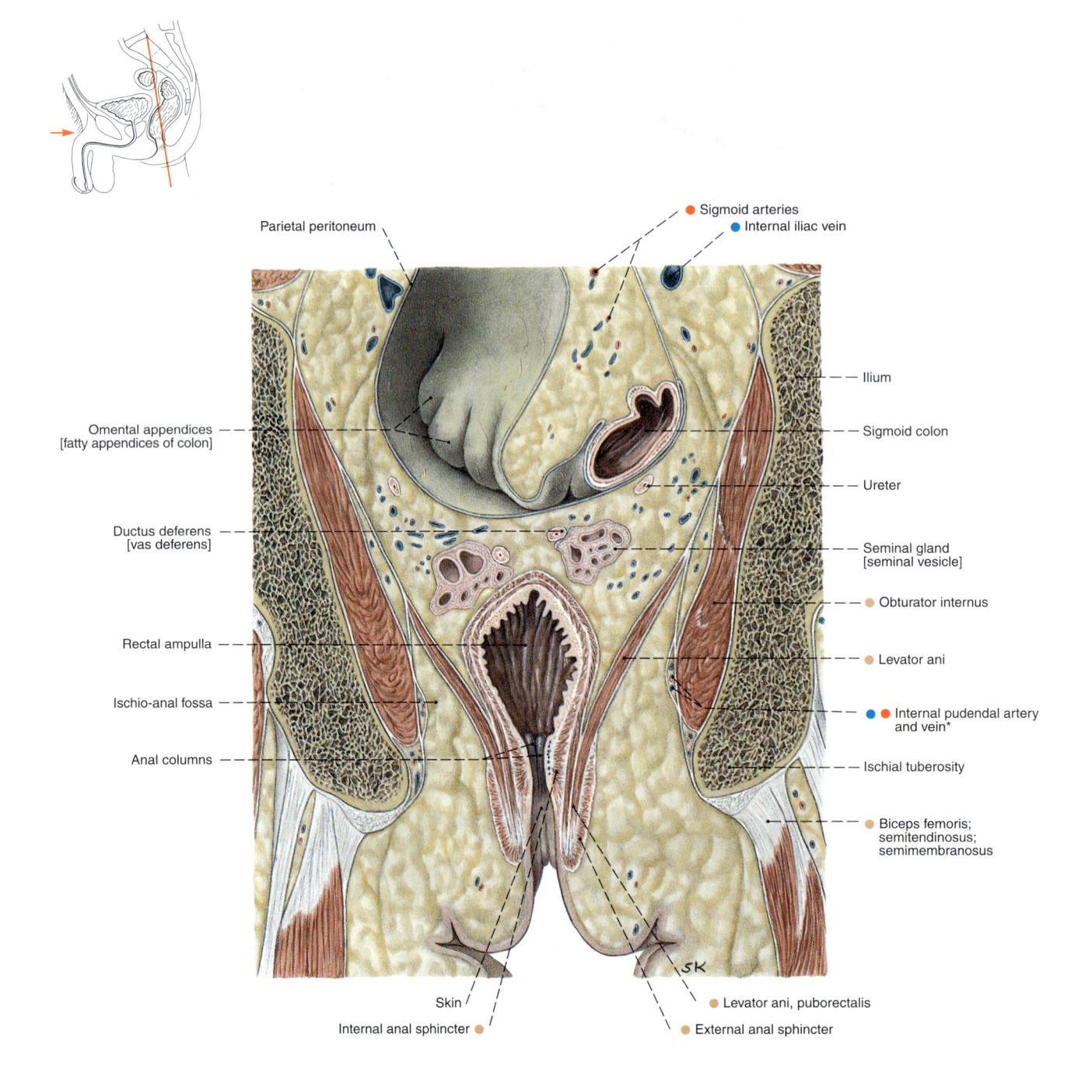

Fig. 1153 Male pelvis; frontal section through lesser pelvis [true pelvis]; ventral aspect.

* Clinically: ALCOCK's canal.

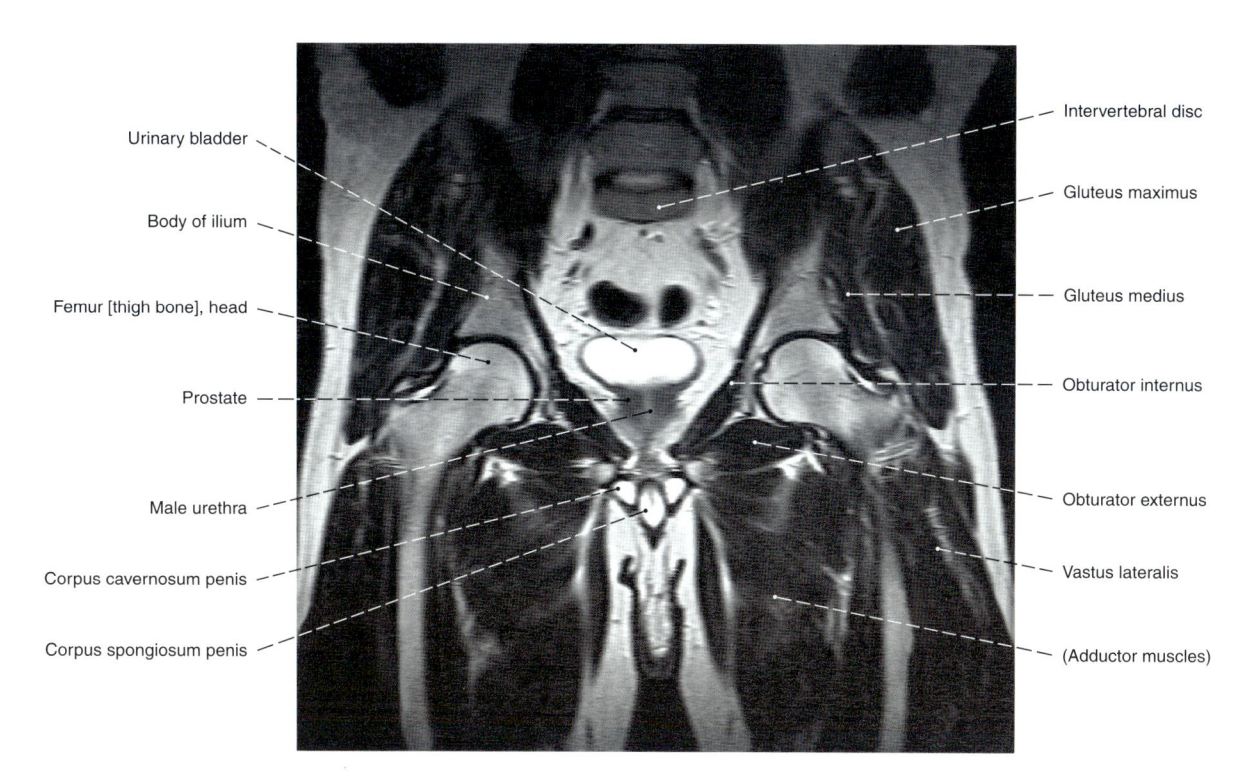

Fig. 1154 Male pelvis; magnetic resonance image; frontal section at level of hip joints; ventral aspect.

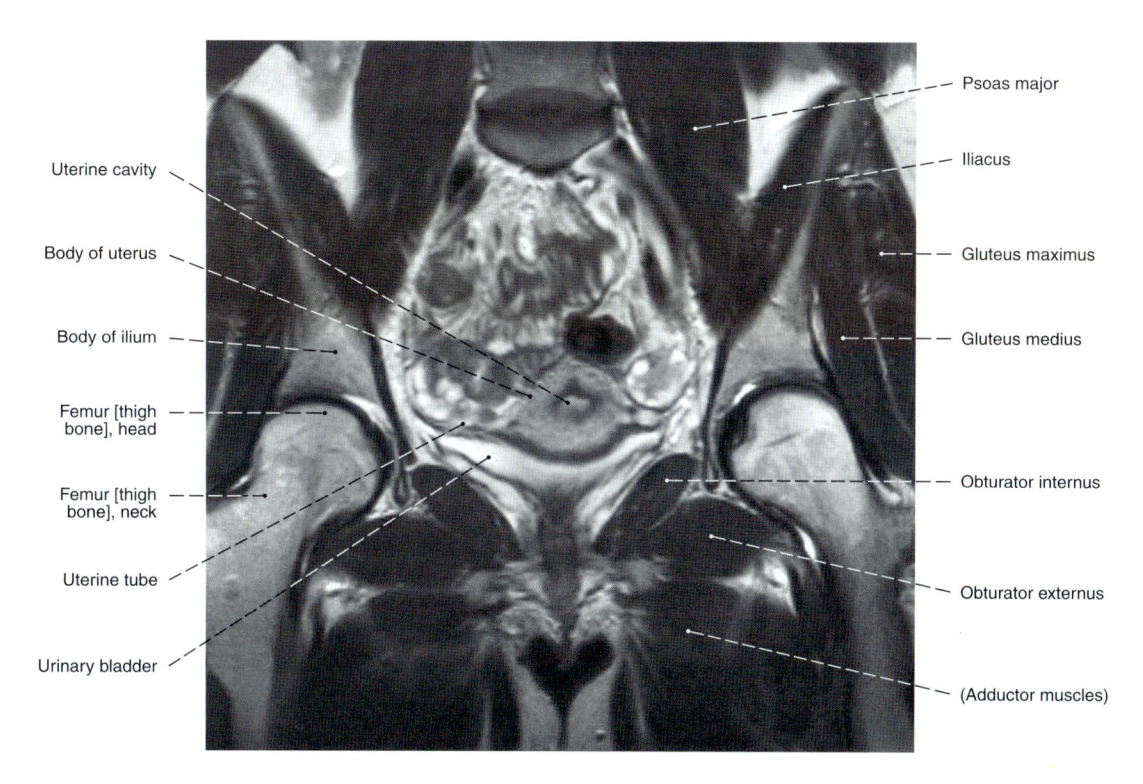

Fig. 1155 Female pelvis; magnetic resonance image; frontal section at level of hip joints; ventral aspect.

When the urinary bladder is empty, the uterus lies on top of the urinary bladder due to its anteflexion.

260 Pelvic viscera

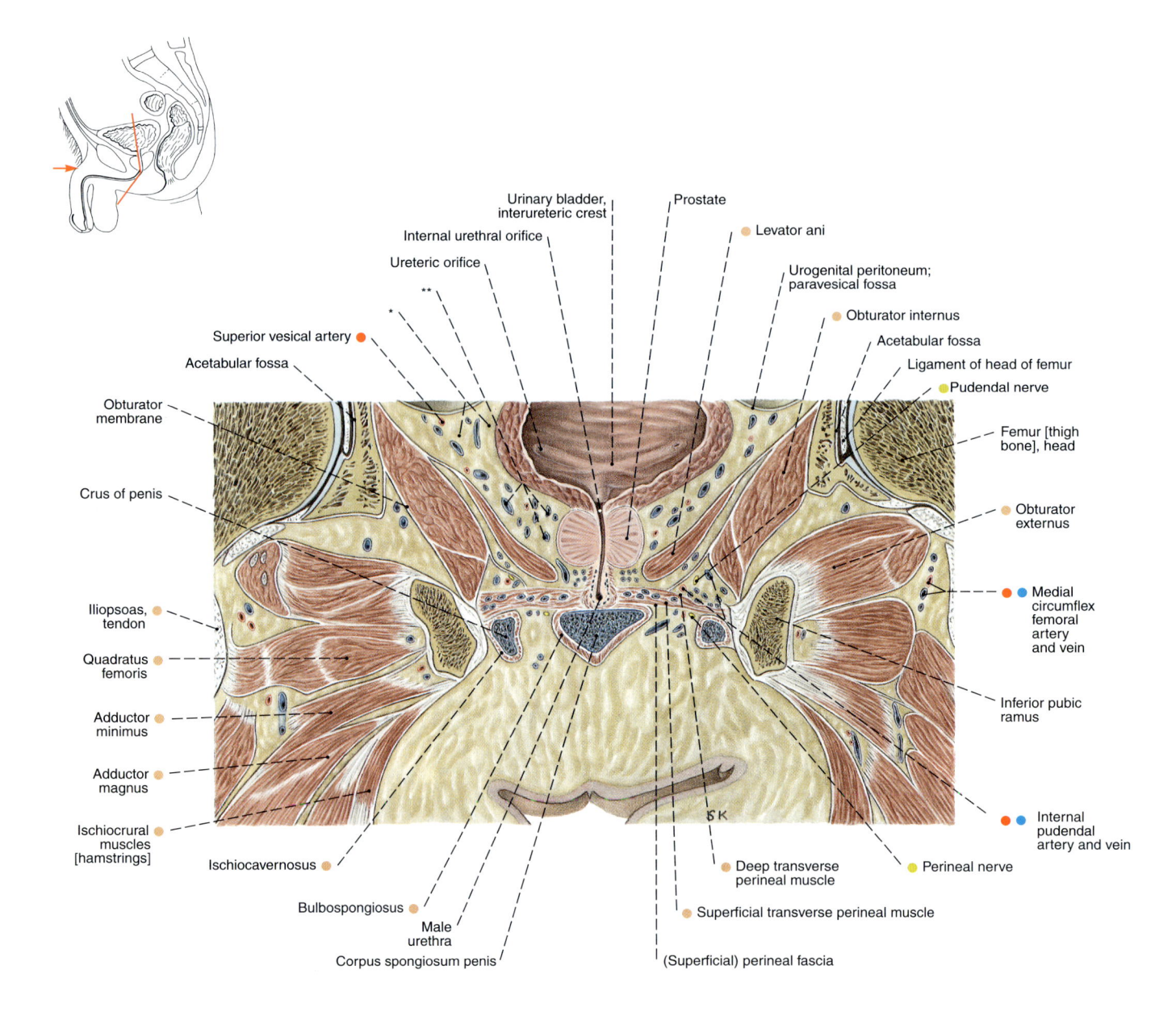

Fig. 1156 Male pelvis; oblique section through urinary bladder; ventral aspect.

* Clinically: paracystium.
** Clinically: prostatic venous plexus.

Pelvis **261**

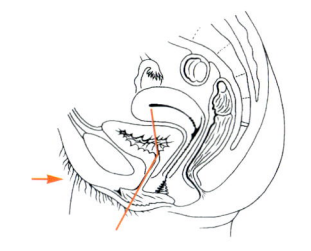

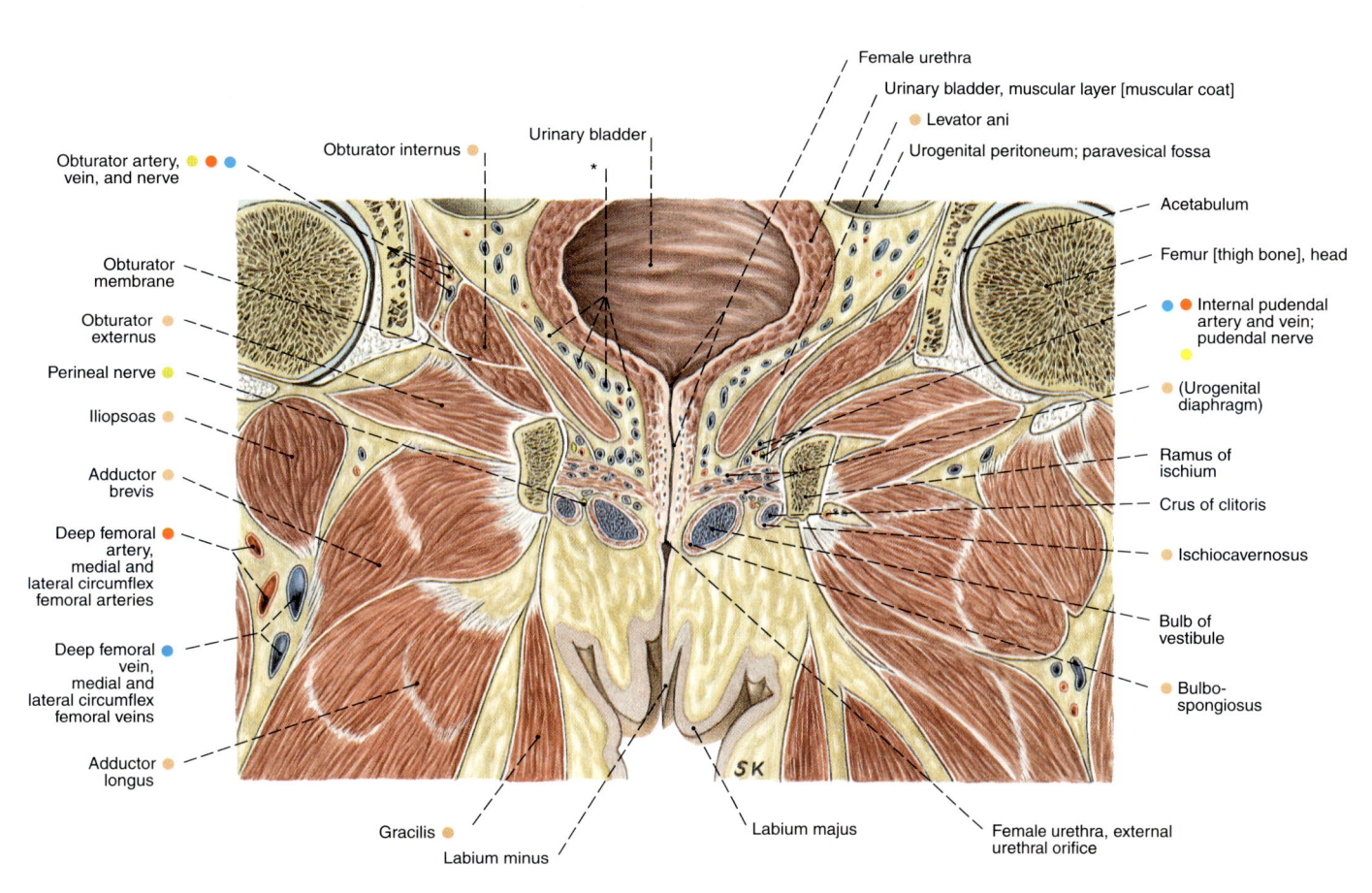

Fig. 1157 Female pelvis; oblique section through urinary bladder; ventral aspect.

* Clinically: paracystium with venous plexus.

262 Lower limb

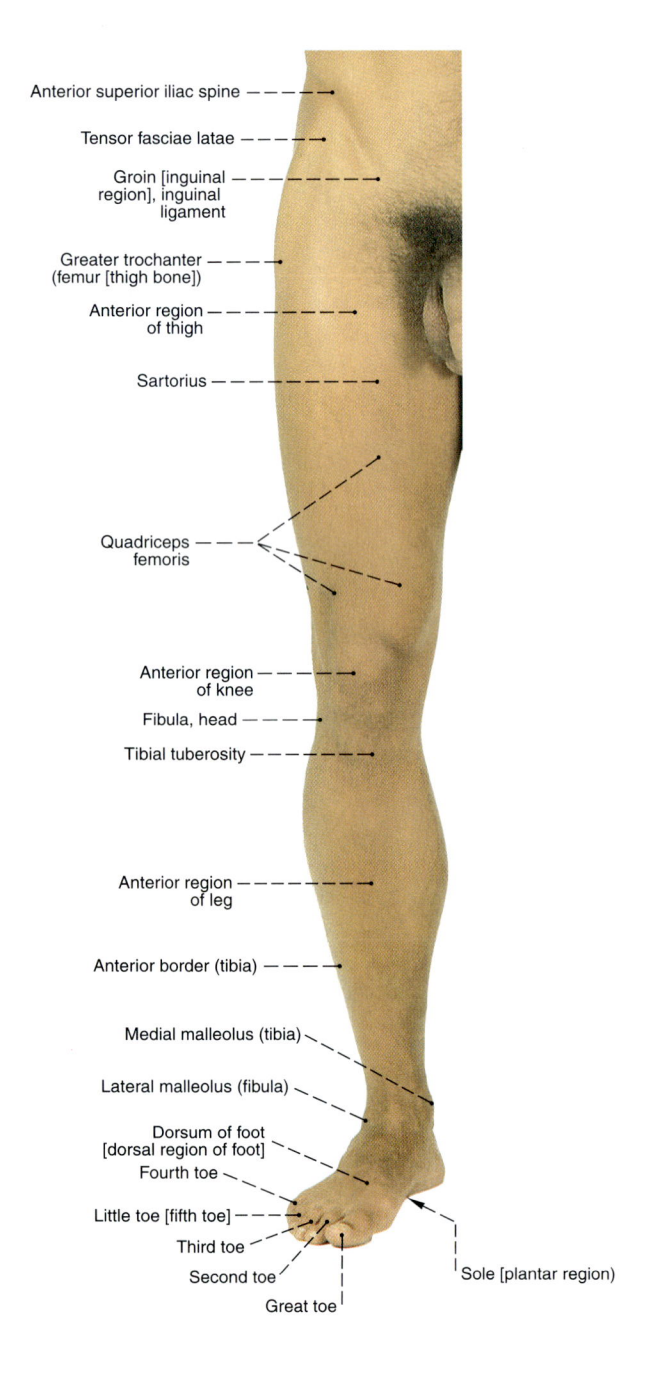

Fig. 1158 Right lower limb; surface anatomy; anterior aspect.

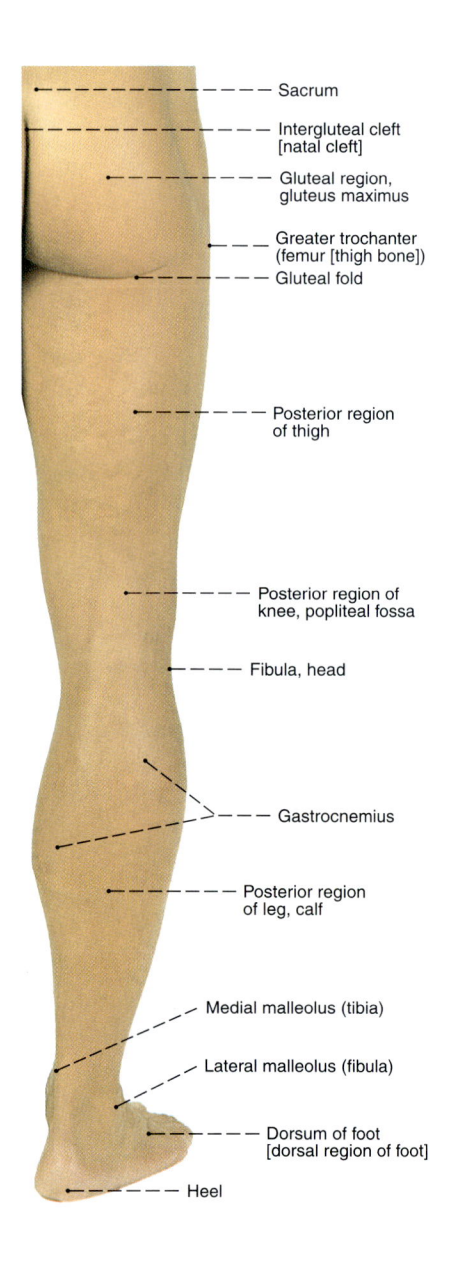

Fig. 1159 Right lower limb; surface anatomy; posterior aspect.

Pelvic girdle

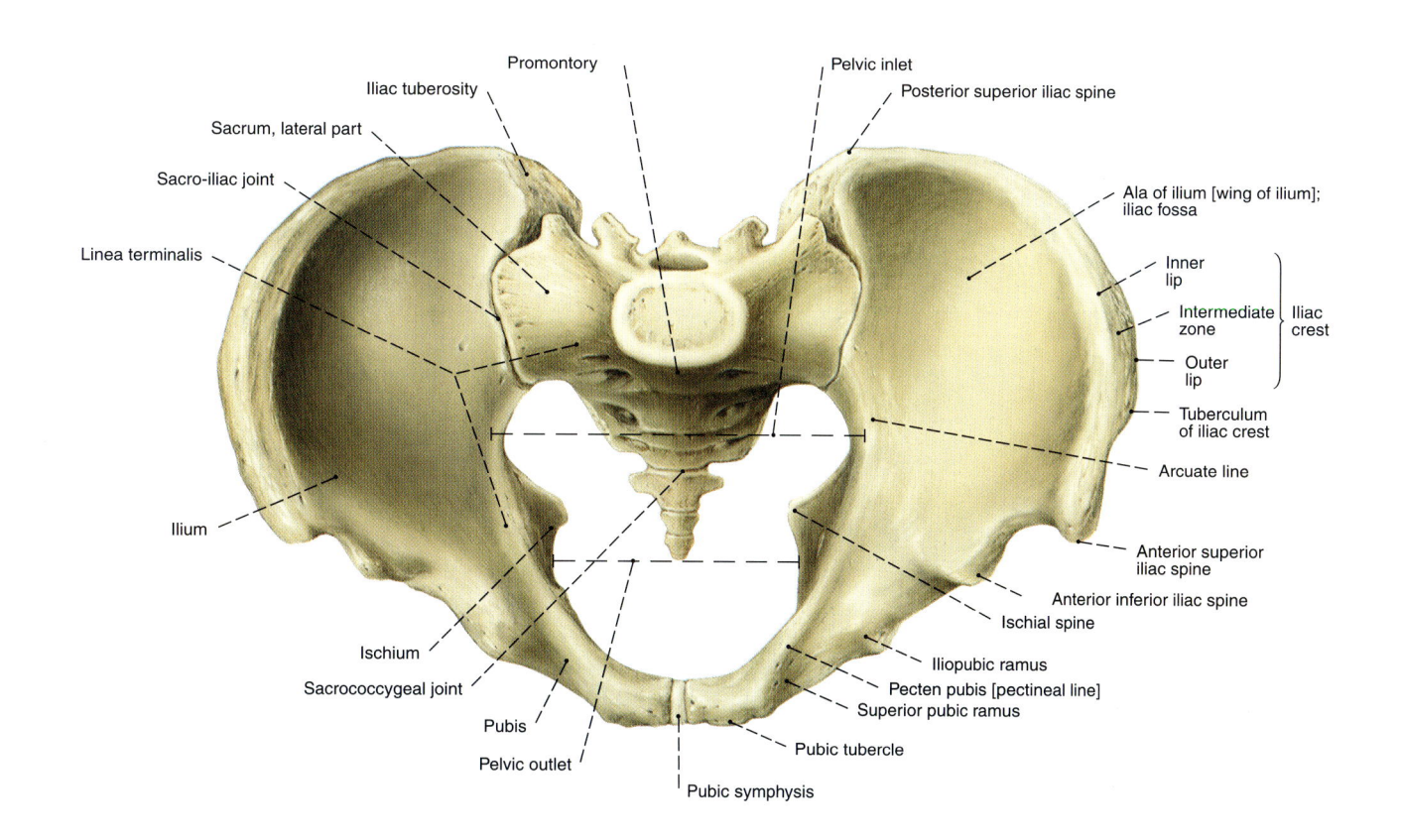

Fig. 1160 Sacrum and pelvic girdle; anterior superior aspect (40%).
The area cranial of the linea terminalis is called the greater pelvis [false pelvis]; the area caudal is called the lesser pelvis [true pelvis].

Joints of pelvic girdle

Name	Type	Movements
Pubic symphysis	Synchondrosis with interpubic disc [interpubic fibrocartilage]	
Sacro-iliac joint	Amphiarthrosis	
Anterior sacro-iliac ligaments Posterior sacro-iliac ligaments Interosseous sacro-iliac ligaments Sacrotuberous ligament Sacrospinal ligament Superior pubic ligament Inferior pubic ligament	Fibrous joints	Minimal translation and rotation during pelvic deformation caused by different loads

264　Lower limb

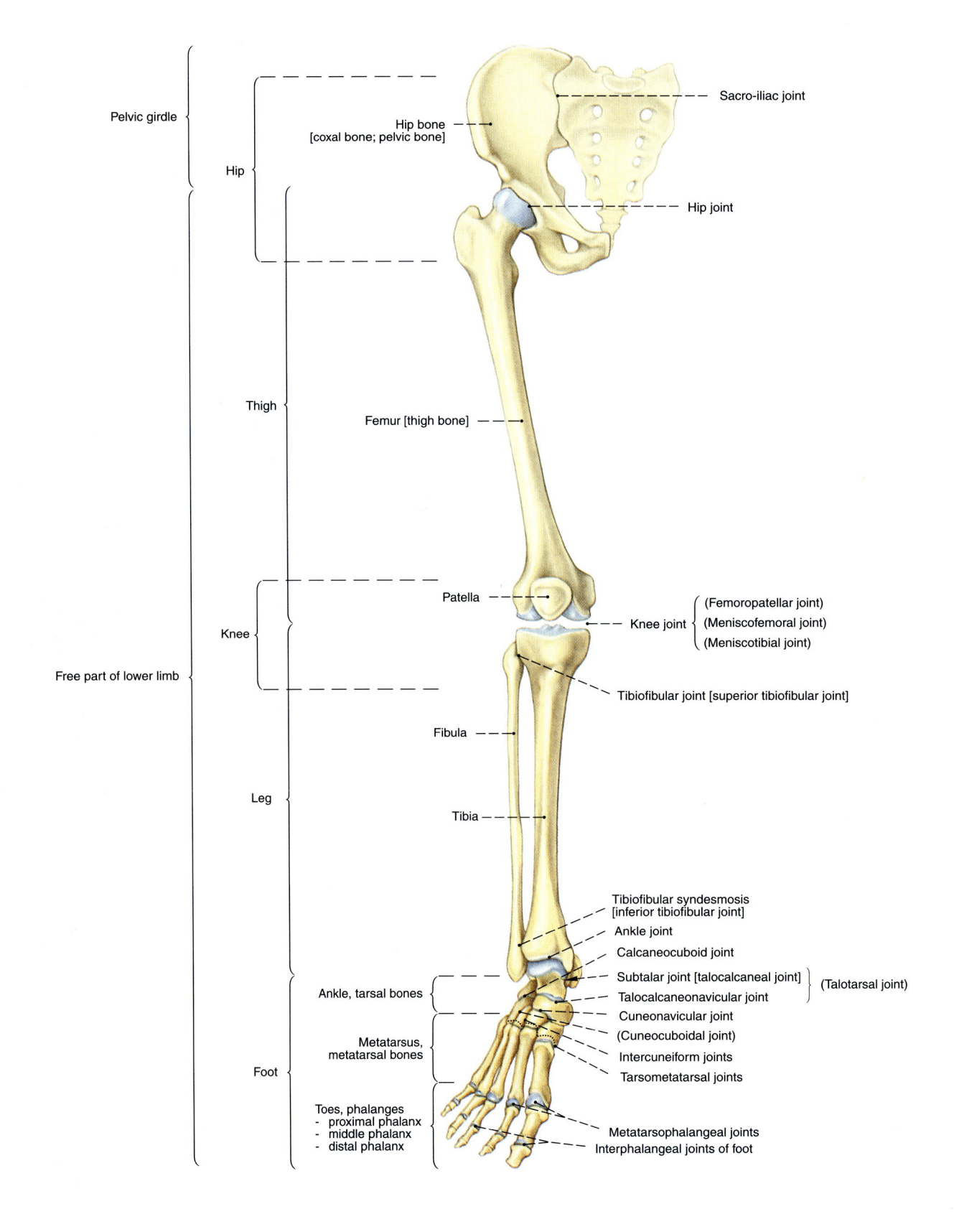

Fig. 1161　Right lower limb; diagram of skeleton and synovial joints; anterior aspect.

Joints of free lower limb (Fig. 1161)

Joint	Type	Movements
Hip joint	Ball-and-socket joint [spheroidal joint]	Flexion (anteversion), extension (retroversion), adduction, abduction, medial and lateral rotation
Knee joint	Pivot-hinge joint [trochoid joint and ginglymus]	Flexion, extension, medial and lateral rotation (only when knee is flexed)
Tibiofibular joint [superior tibiofibular joint]	Amphiarthrosis	Minimal translation in transverse and vertical directions, as well as minimal rotation
Tibiofibular syndesmosis [inferior tibiofibular joint]	Fibrous joint	Holds the malleoli together; in dorsiflexion of the ankle joint the malleoli drift somewhat apart
Ankle joint	Hinge joint [ginglymus]	Plantar flexion, dorsiflexion Supination (inversion), pronation (eversion)
Talotarsal joint a) Talocalcaneonavicular joint (anterior component) b) Subtalar joint [talocalcaneal joint] (posterior component)	Combined pivot-spherical joint	Little plantar and dorsiflexion and rotation; locks longitudinal arches of foot (key joint in talipes [flatfoot])
Transverse tarsal joint [CHOPART's joint] a) Talonavicular joint b) Calcaneocuboid joint	Amphiarthroses	Little movements causing deformation of foot during its adaptation to the floor (e.g. during walking)
Tarsal joints a) Cuneonavicular joint b) Intercuneiform joints c) Cuneocuboidal joint	Amphiarthroses	Little plantar and dorsiflexion and rotation of forefoot
Tarsometatarsal joints [LISFRANC's joint]	Amphiarthroses	Assist rotation of forefoot
Intermetatarsal joints	Amphiarthroses	
Metatarsophalangeal joints	Ball-and-socket joint [spheroidal joint], functionally limited	Flexion, extension of toes
Interphalangeal joints of foot	Hinge joints [ginglymi]	

Lower limb

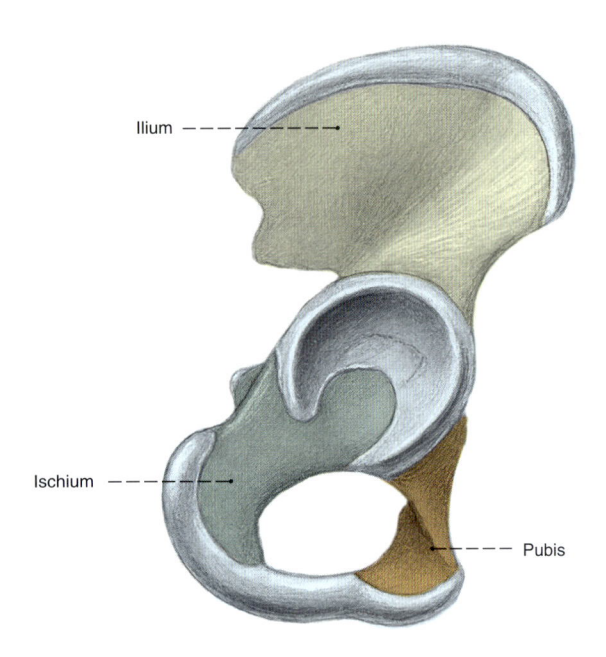

Fig. 1162 Right hip bone [coxal bone; pelvic bone]; extension of its three bony components in the newborn; lateral aspect (110%).

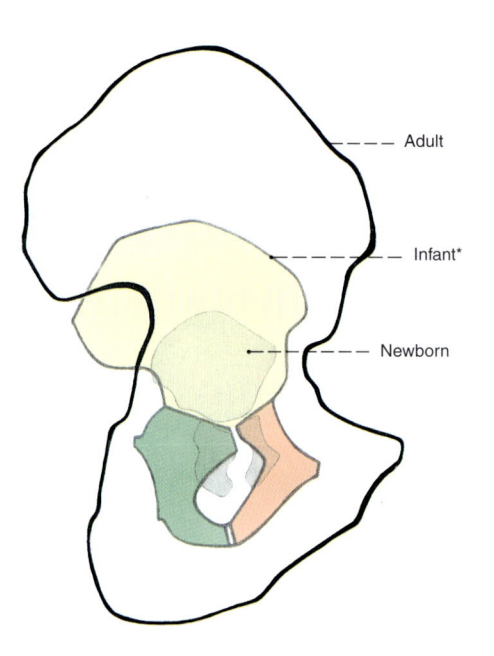

Fig. 1163 Right hip bone [coxal bone; pelvic bone]; extension of its three bony components at different ages; lateral aspect.

* Approximately 6 years of age.

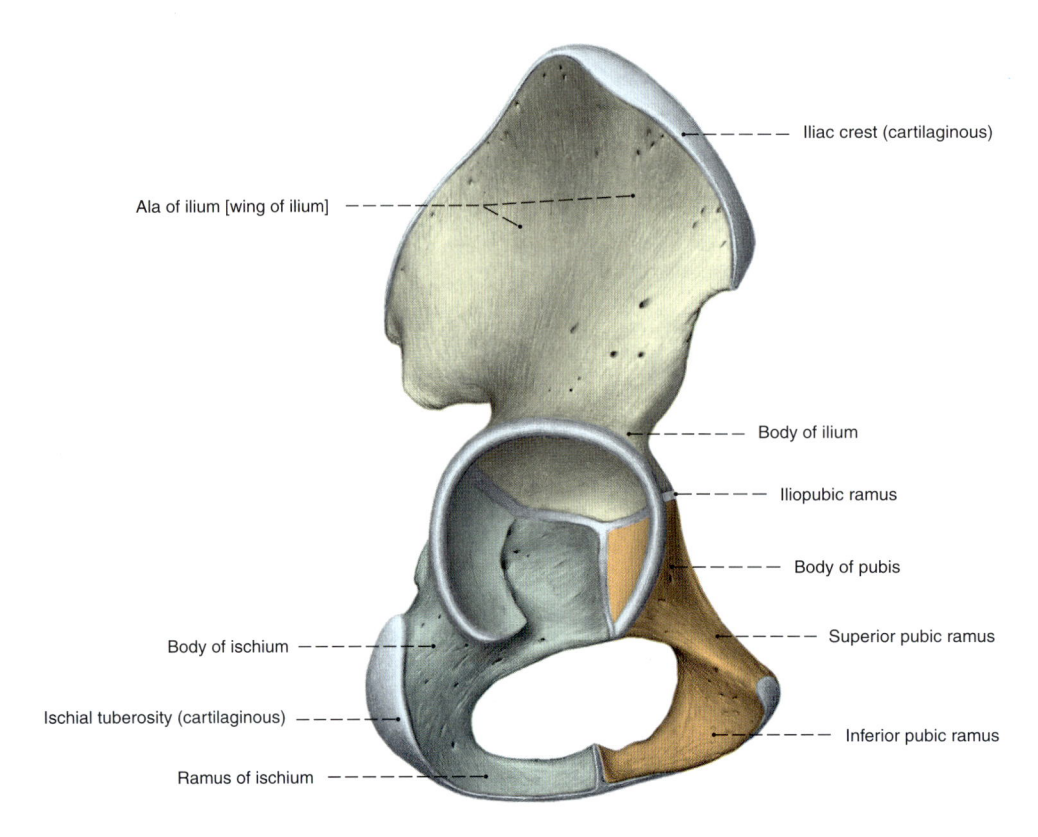

Fig. 1164 Right hip bone [coxal bone; pelvic bone]; developmental state at age of six; lateral aspect (90%). The three components of the hip bone [coxal bone; pelvic bone] are connected in the acetabulum by a Y-shaped cartilaginous joint, which ossifies at about 13–18 years of age.

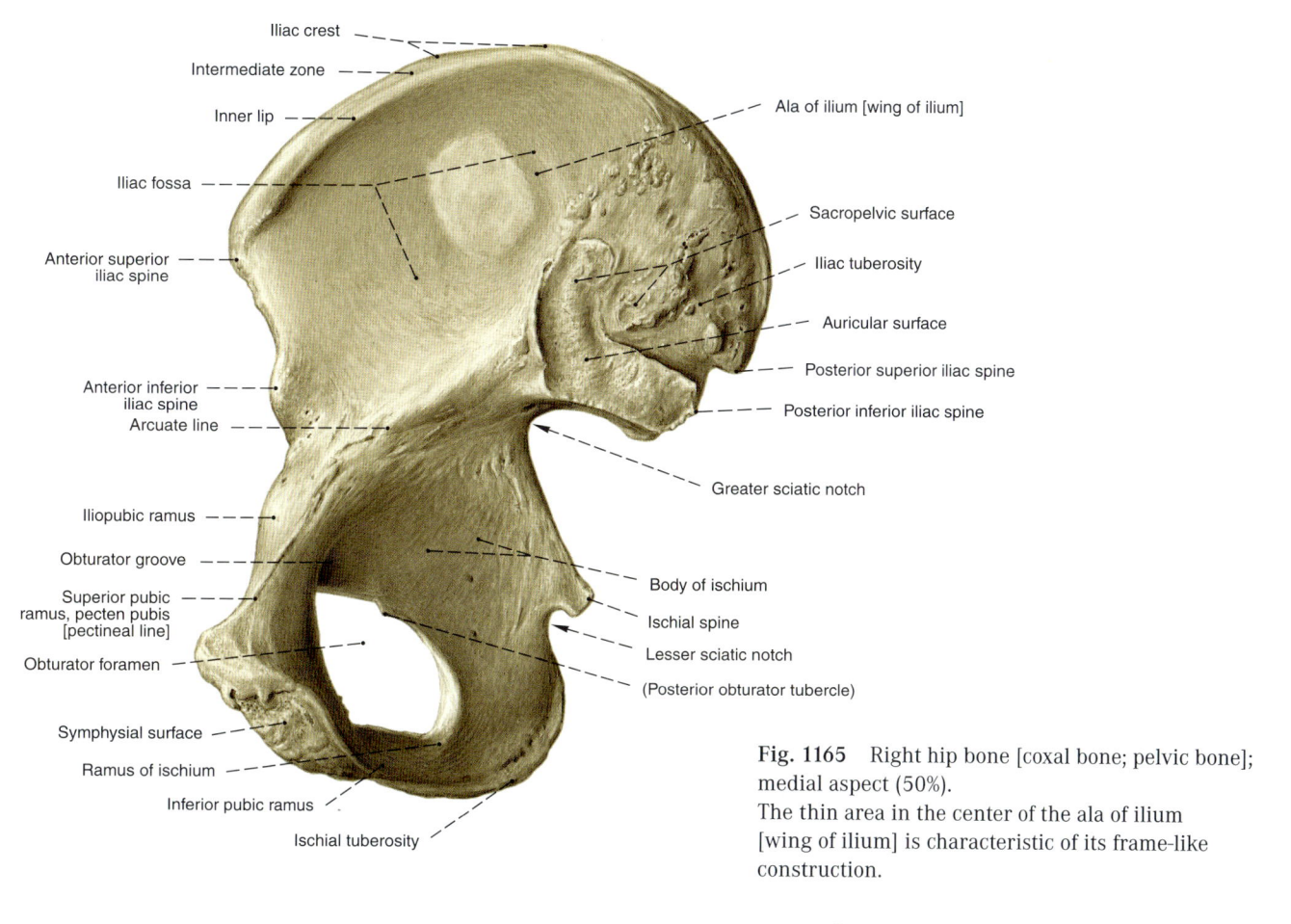

Hip bone [coxal bone, pelvic bone] 267

Fig. 1165 Right hip bone [coxal bone; pelvic bone]; medial aspect (50%).
The thin area in the center of the ala of ilium [wing of ilium] is characteristic of its frame-like construction.

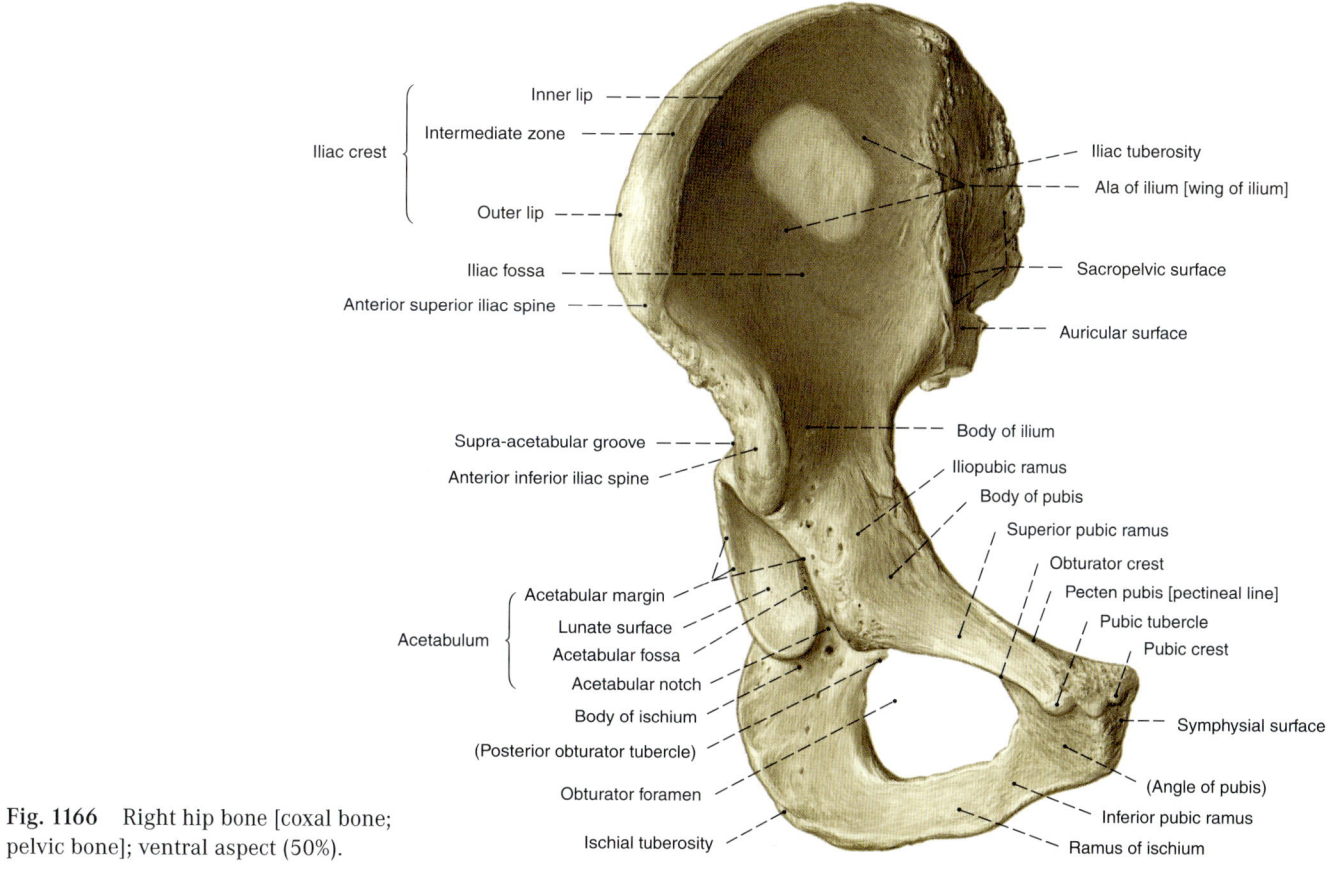

Fig. 1166 Right hip bone [coxal bone; pelvic bone]; ventral aspect (50%).

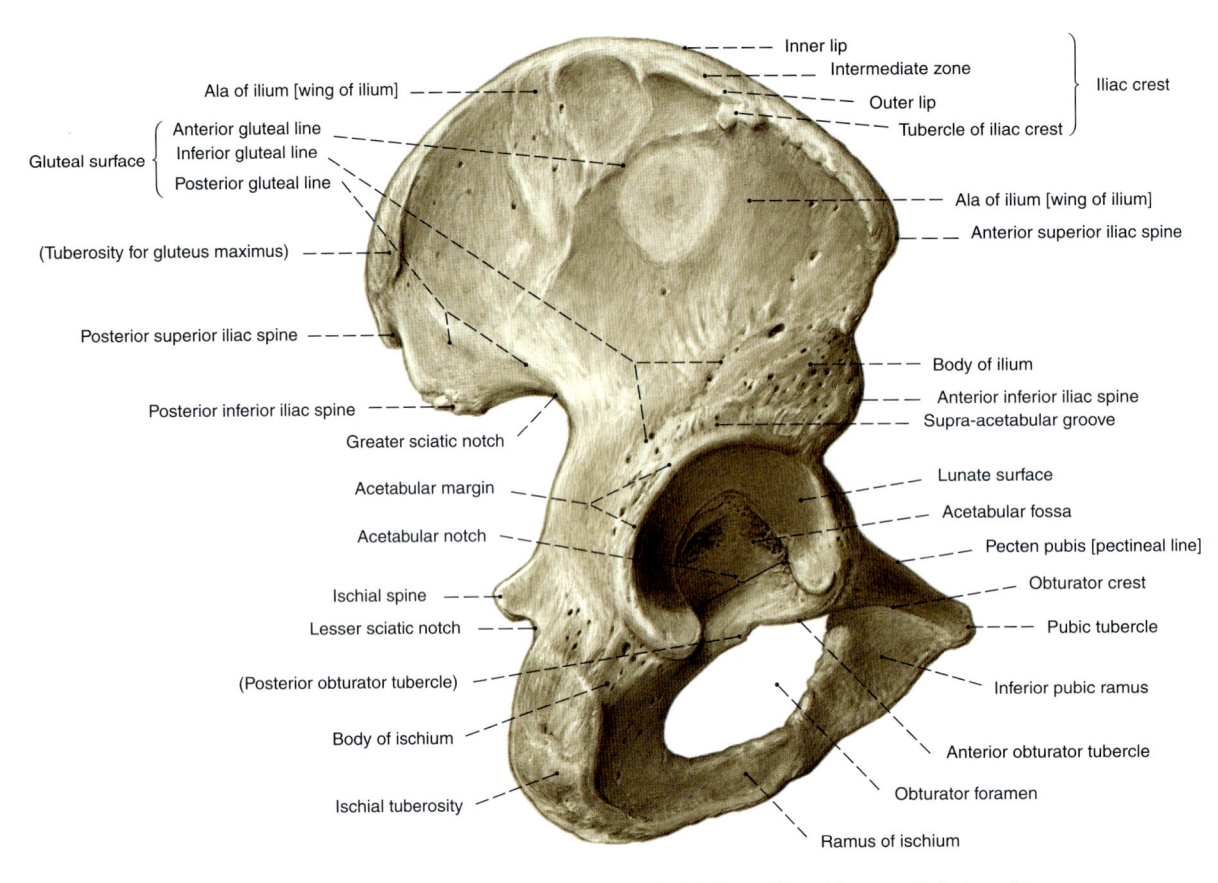

268 Lower limb

Fig. 1167 Right hip bone [coxal bone; pelvic bone]; lateral dorsal aspect (50%).

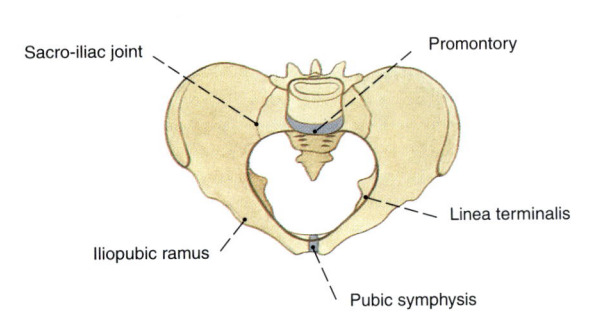

Fig. 1168 Pelvis; shape of pelvic inlet in the male pelvis; superior aspect.

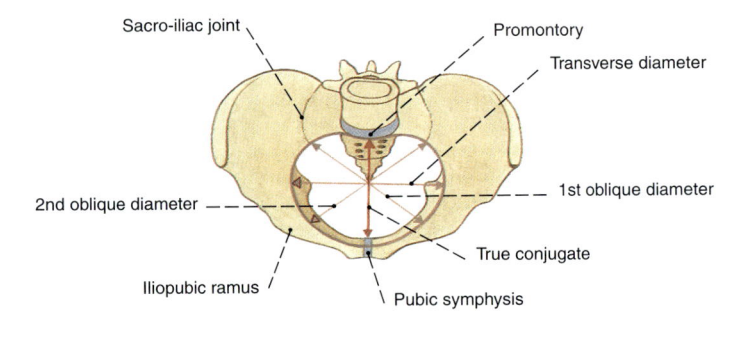

Fig. 1169 Pelvis; shape of pelvic inlet in the female pelvis; superior aspect.

Gender differences in the pelvis

Compared to the male pelvis, in which the pelvic inlet is clearly narrowed by the promontory, the female pelvis has a more rounded and oval-shaped pelvic inlet. The two inferior pubic rami form a right angle (subpubic angle) in the male and an arch (pubic arch) in the female. The alae [wings] of ilia are wider apart in the female pelvis. The widest diameter of the obturator foramina is in the transverse plane in the female and in the vertical plane in the male.

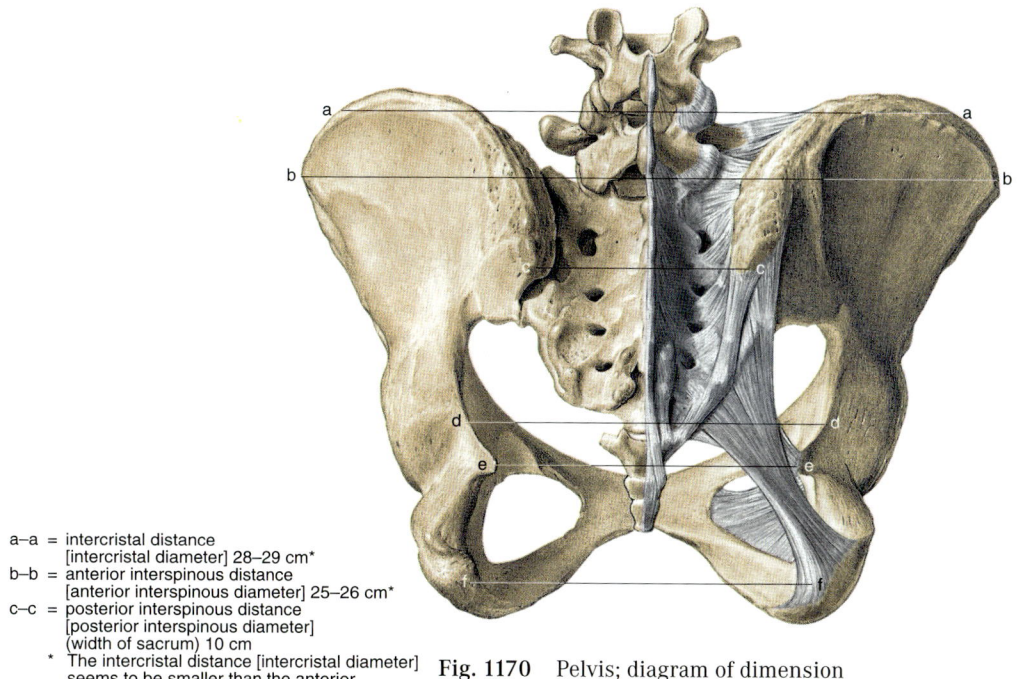

Pelvis 269

a–a = intercristal distance [intercristal diameter] 28–29 cm*
b–b = anterior interspinous distance [anterior interspinous diameter] 25–26 cm*
c–c = posterior interspinous distance [posterior interspinous diameter] (width of sacrum) 10 cm
  * The intercristal distance [intercristal diameter] seems to be smaller than the anterior interspinous distance [anterior interspinous diameter] due to the perspective.

Fig. 1170 Pelvis; diagram of dimension of the female pelvis; dorsal aspect.

d–d = transverse diameter of pelvic width (interacetabular line) 12–12.5 cm
e–e = transverse diameter of pelvic constriction (interspinous line) 10.5 cm
f–f = transverse diameter of pelvic outlet (tuberal diameter) 11–12 cm

k–k = axis of pelvis
a–b = clinically: anatomical conjugate
a–e = clinically: diagonal conjugate 12.5–13 cm
a–c = clinically: true conjugate 10.4–11 cm

Anterior superior iliac spine
Anterior inferior iliac spine
Linea terminalis
Pelvic inlet *

Greater sciatic notch
Sacrospinous ligament
Sacrotuberous ligament
Lesser sciatic notch
Pelvic outlet
Ischial tuberosity
Obturator foramen

h–d = clinically: sagittal diameter of pelvic width 12–12.5 cm
e–g = clinically: sagittal diameter of pelvic constriction 11–11.5 cm
e–f = clinically: sagittal diameter of pelvic outlet (pubococcygeal distance) 9–10 cm

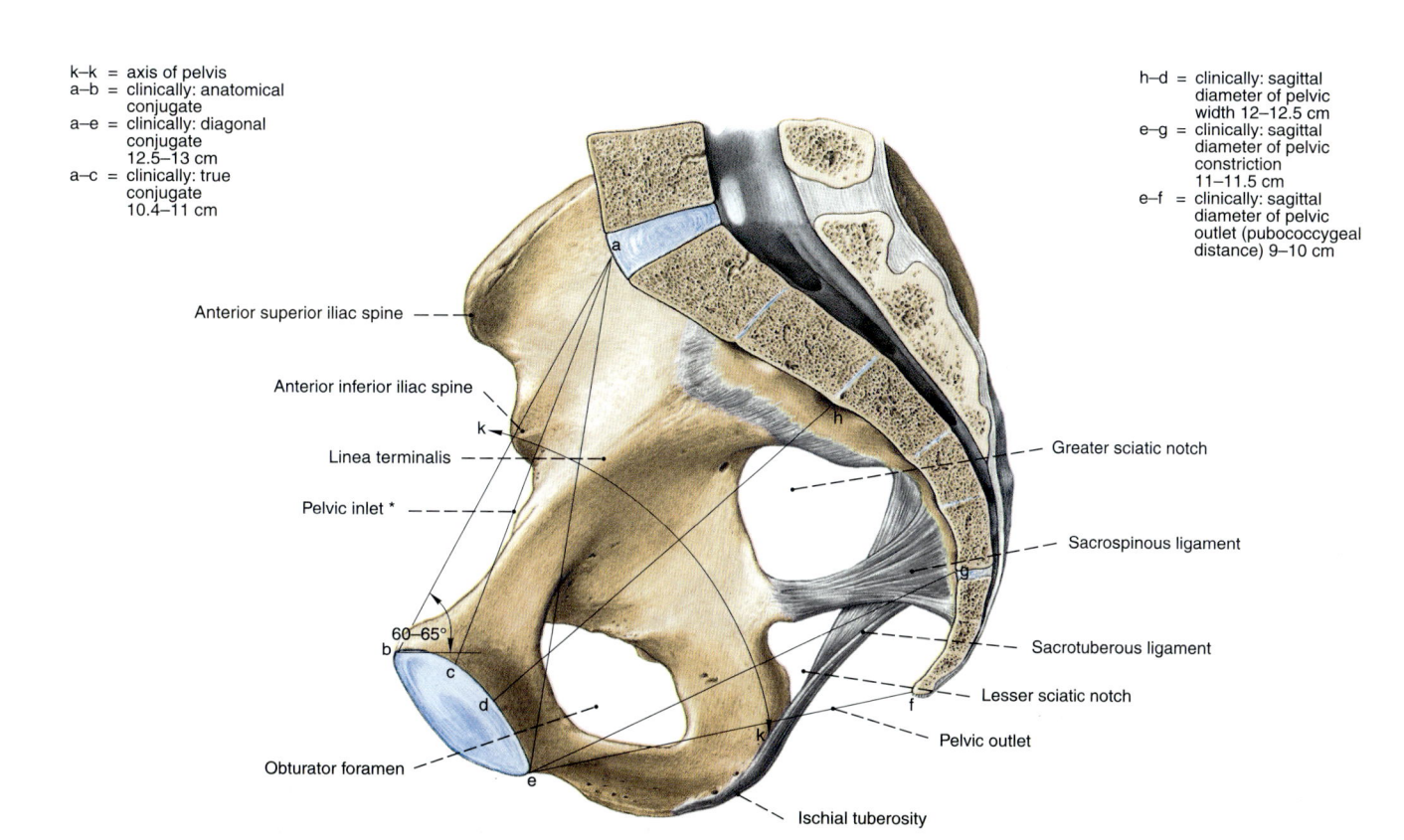

Fig. 1171 Pelvis; diagram of dimension of the female pelvis; median section; right medial aspect.

* The pelvic inlet is enclosed by the linea terminalis. Line a–c indicates the plan of the pelvic inlet. The pelvic outlet is enclosed by the coccyx, the ischial tuberosity, the ramus of ischium, and the inferior pelvic ramus on both sides.

270 *Lower limb*

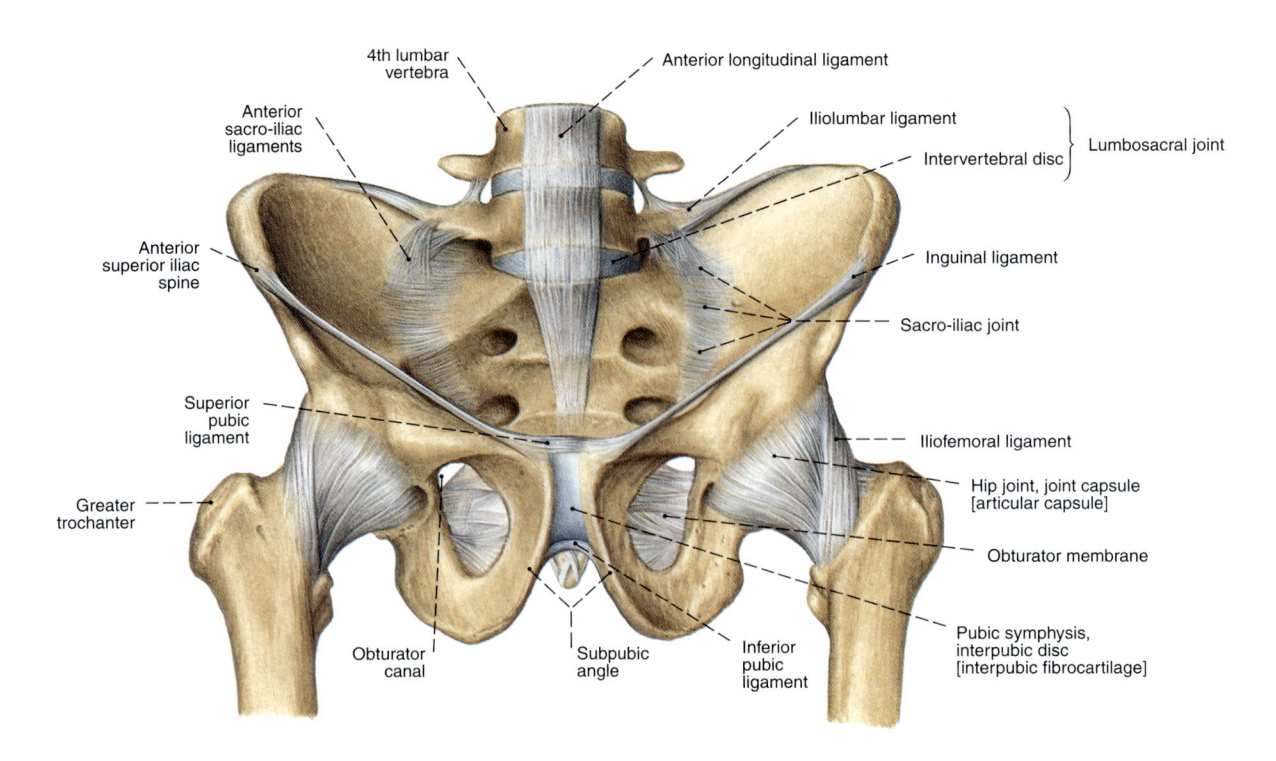

Fig. 1172 Joints of pelvic girdle and lumbosacral joint in the male; anterior inferior aspect (30%).

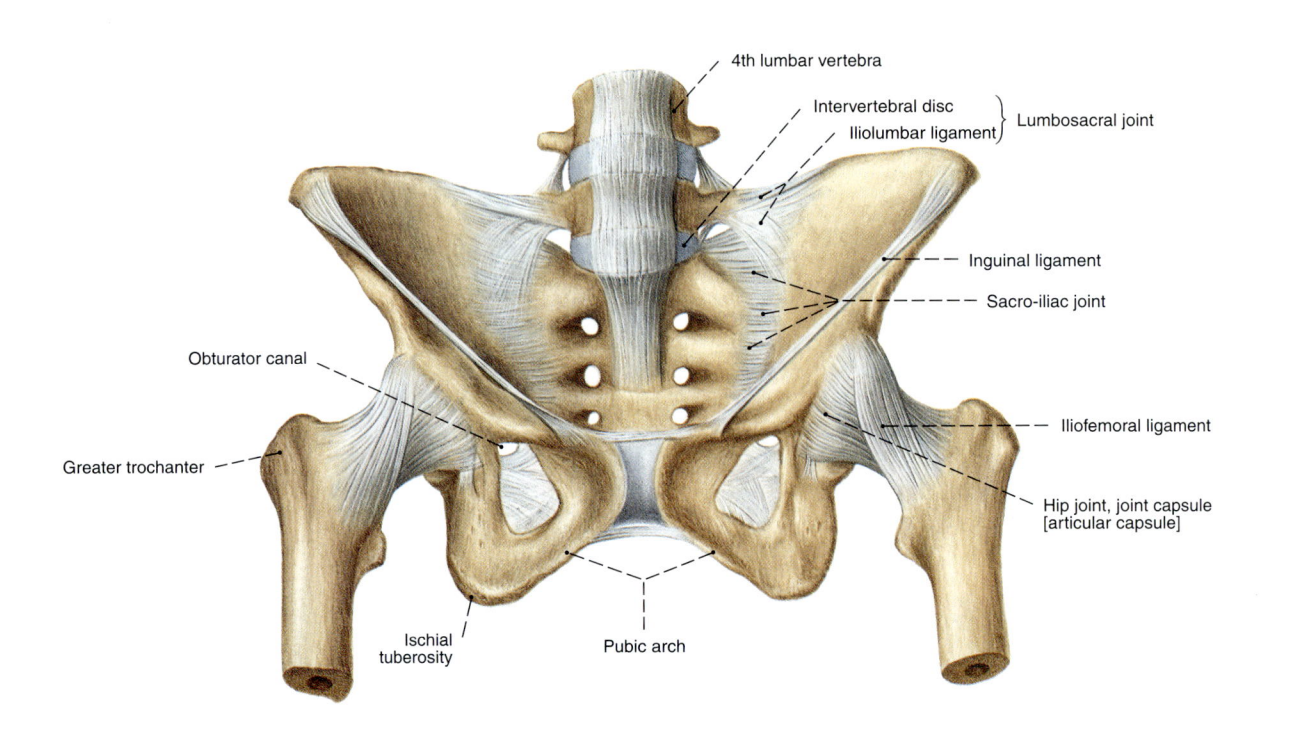

Fig. 1173 Joints of pelvic girdle and lumbosacral joint in the female; anterior inferior aspect (30%).

Pelvis 271

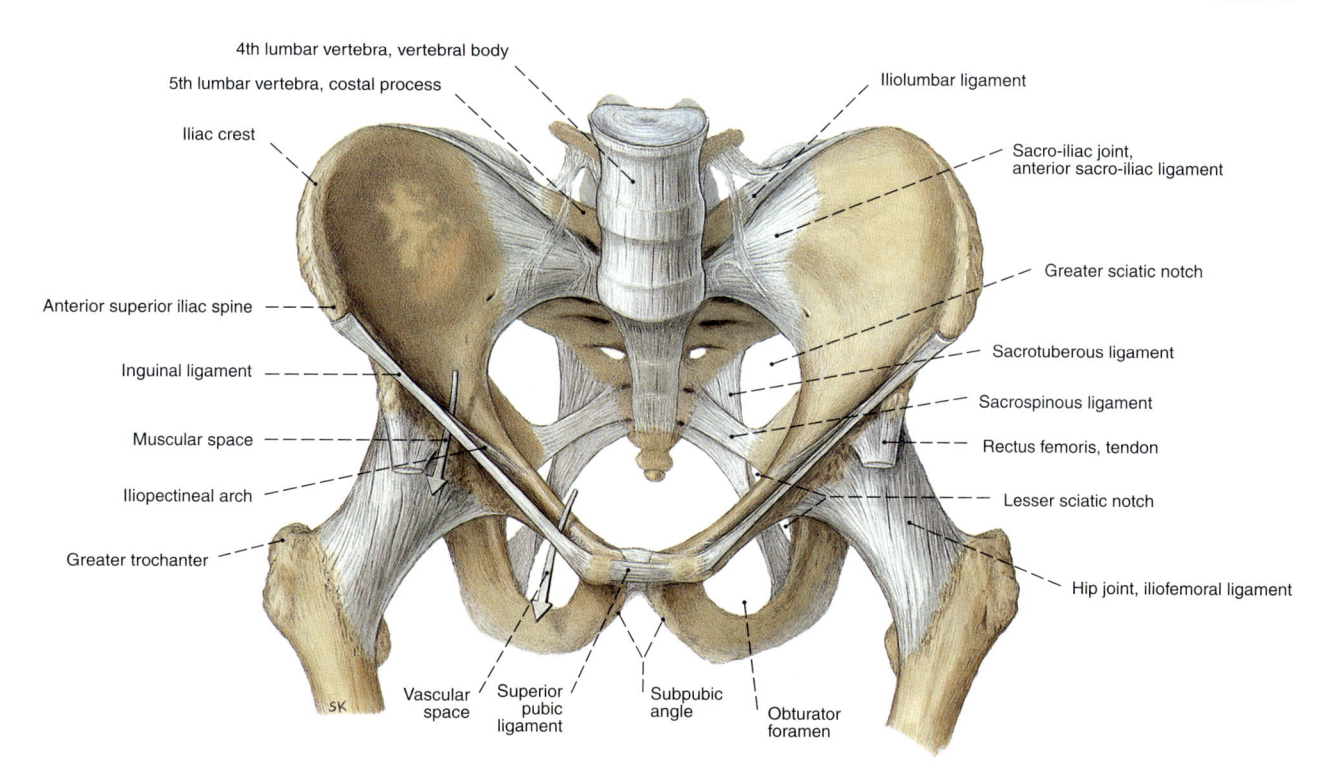

Fig. 1174 Joints of pelvic girdle and lumbosacral joint in the male; anterior superior aspect (30%).

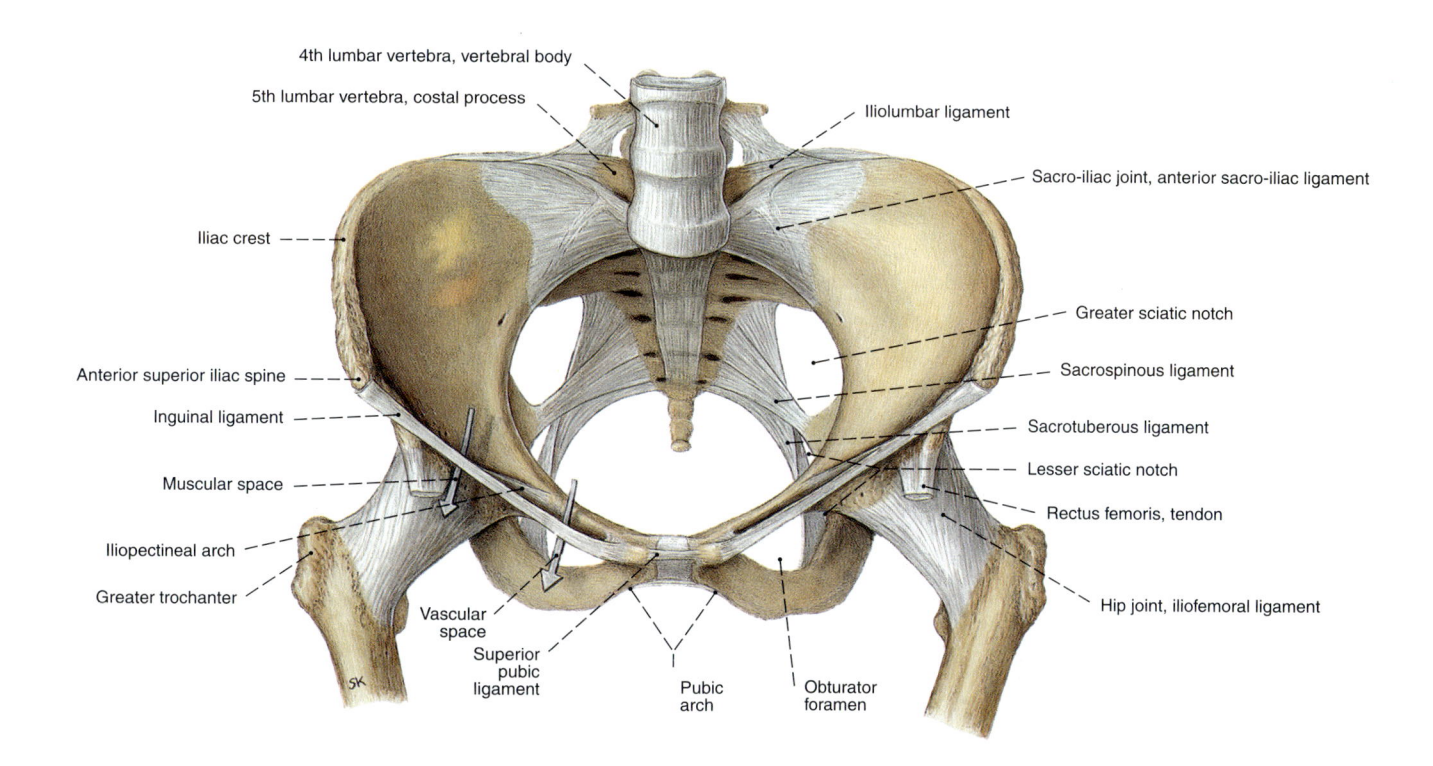

Fig. 1175 Joints of pelvic girdle and lumbosacral joint in the female; anterior superior aspect (30%).

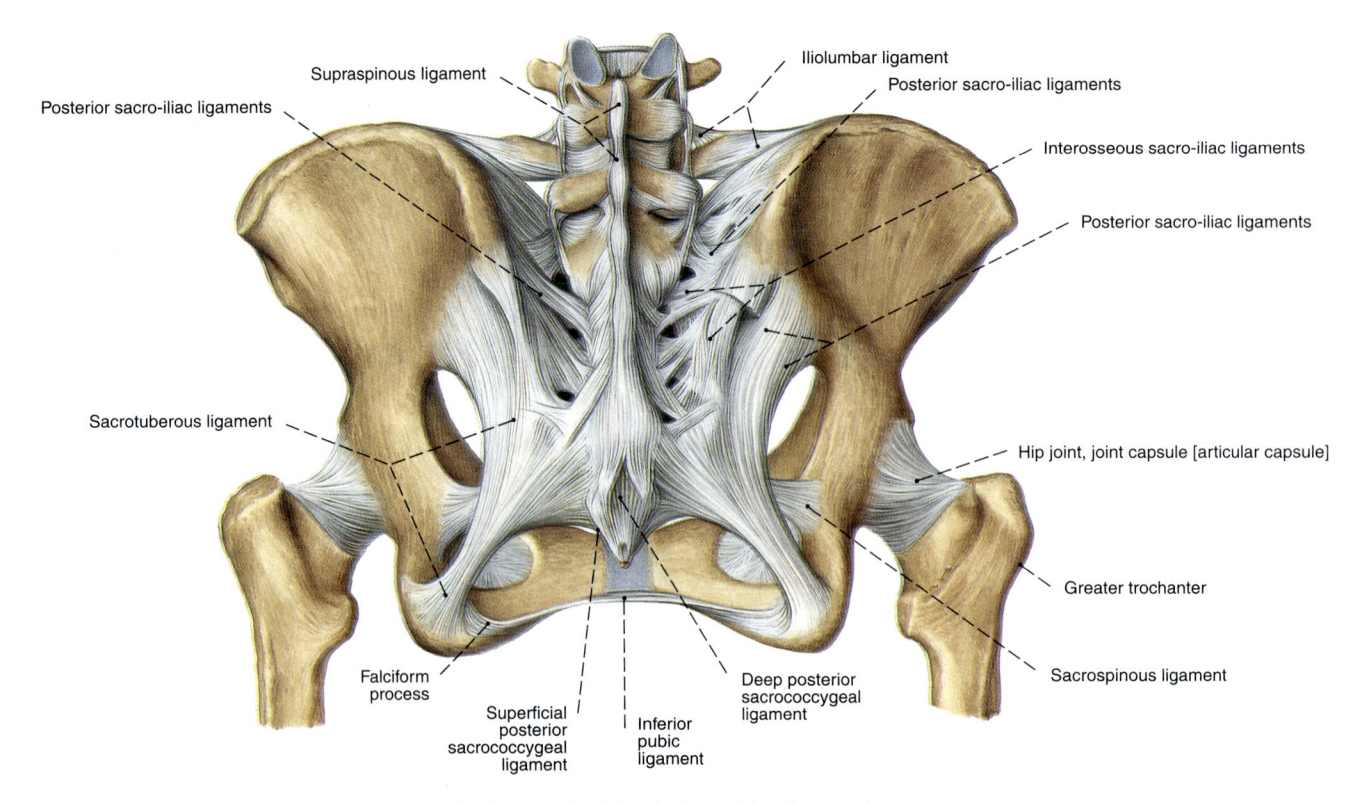

Fig. 1176 Joints of pelvic girdle and lumbosacral joint in the female; posterior aspect (30%).

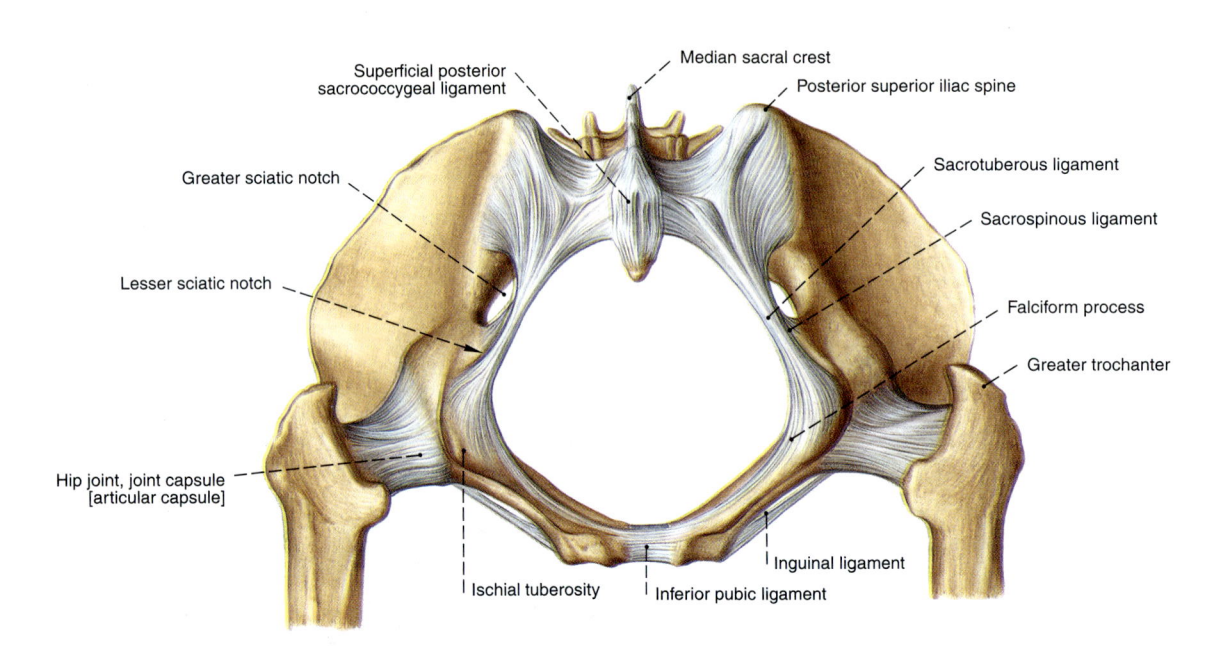

Fig. 1177 Joints of pelvic girdle in the female; inferior aspect (30%).

Pelvis 273

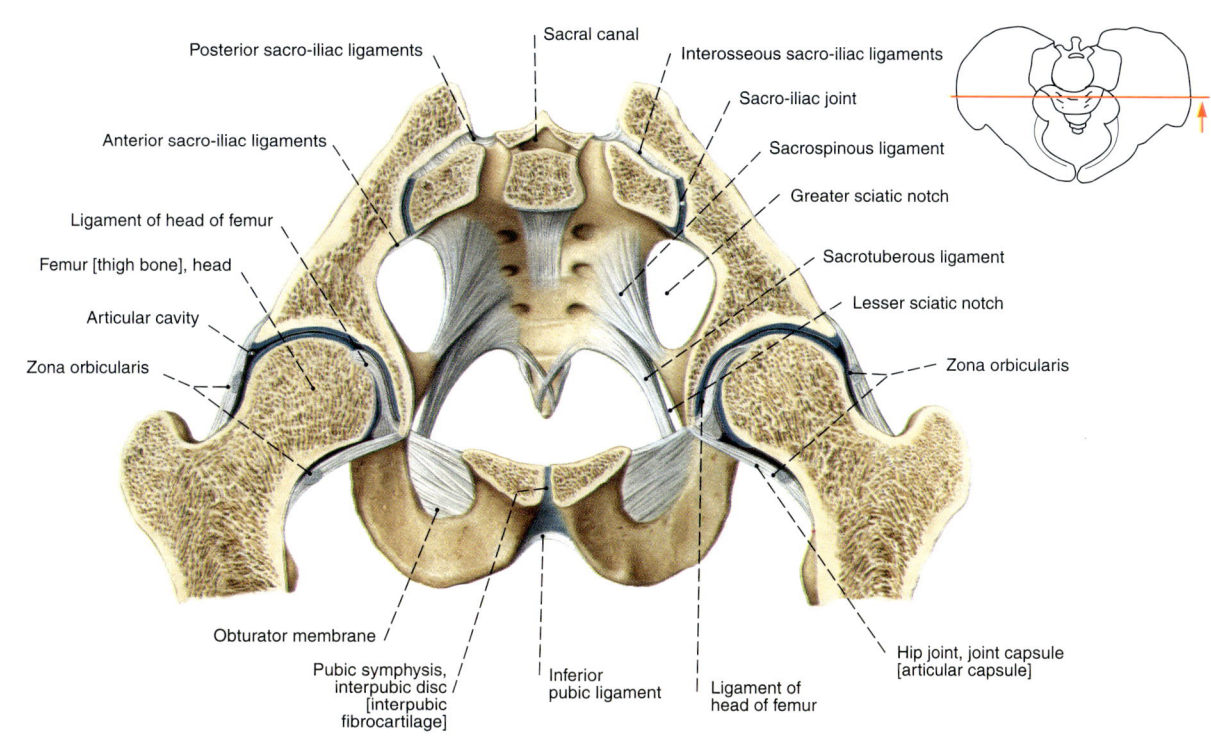

Fig. 1178 Joints of pelvic girdle in the female; frontal section at level of middle of acetabulum; anterior aspect (30%).

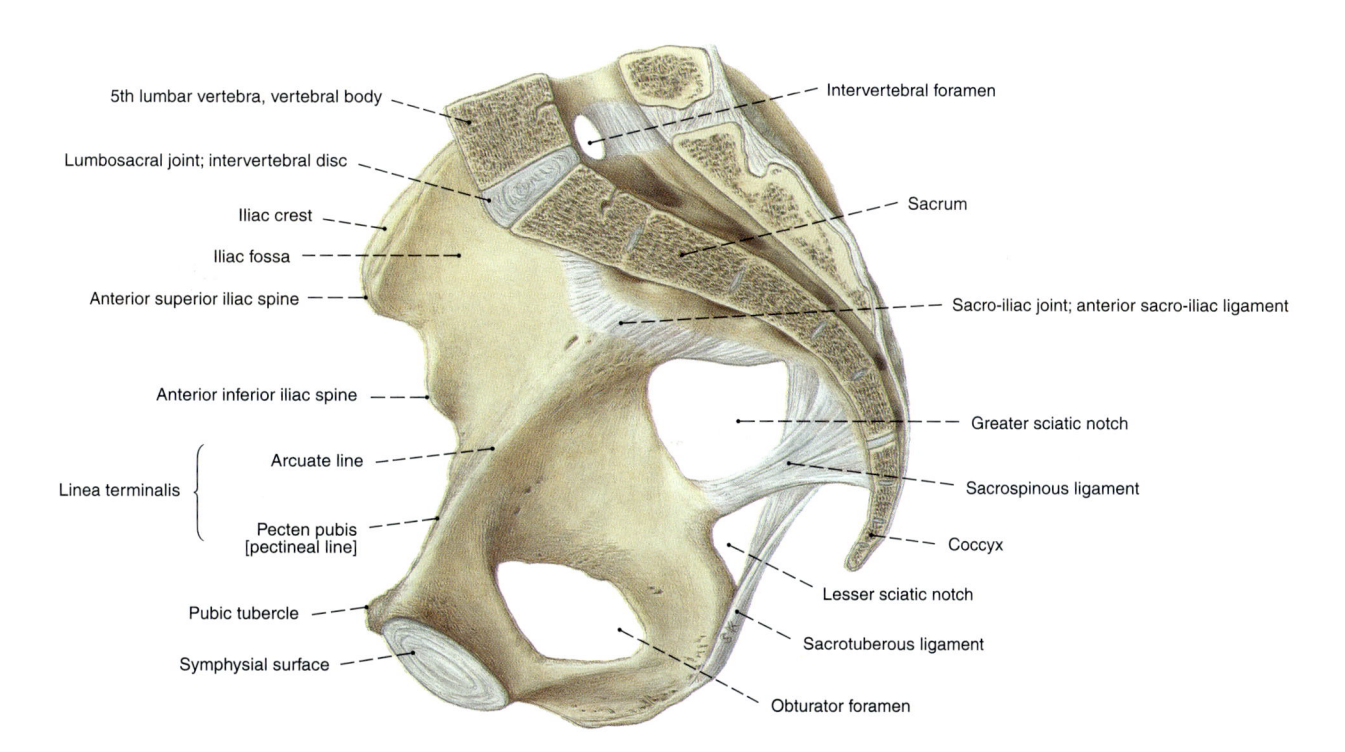

Fig. 1179 Joints of pelvic girdle and lumbosacral joint in the female; median section; medial aspect (35%). Normally, the anterior border of the lowest intervertebral disc forms the most ventral point of the posterior circumference of the pelvic inlet. In radiographs the most ventral point of the sacrum is called promontory.

274   Lower limb

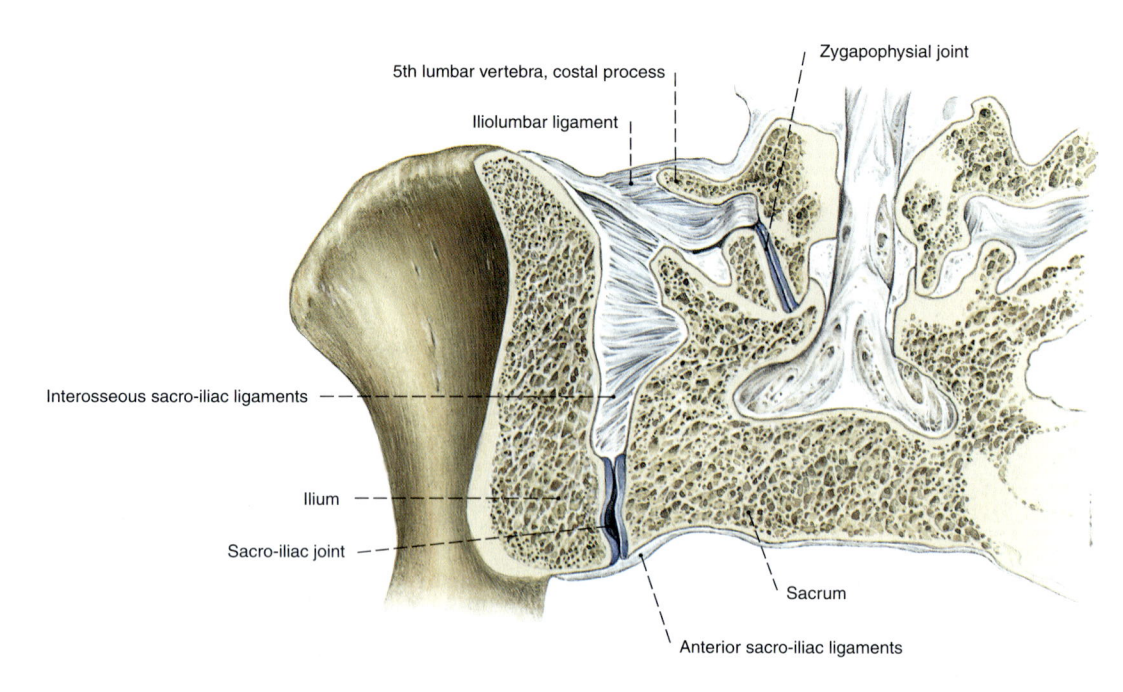

Fig. 1180   Left sacro-iliac joint; frontal section; anterior aspect (45%).

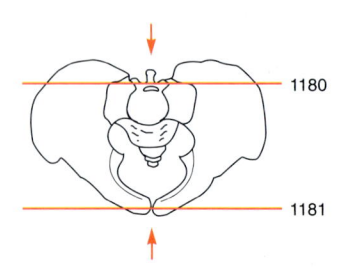

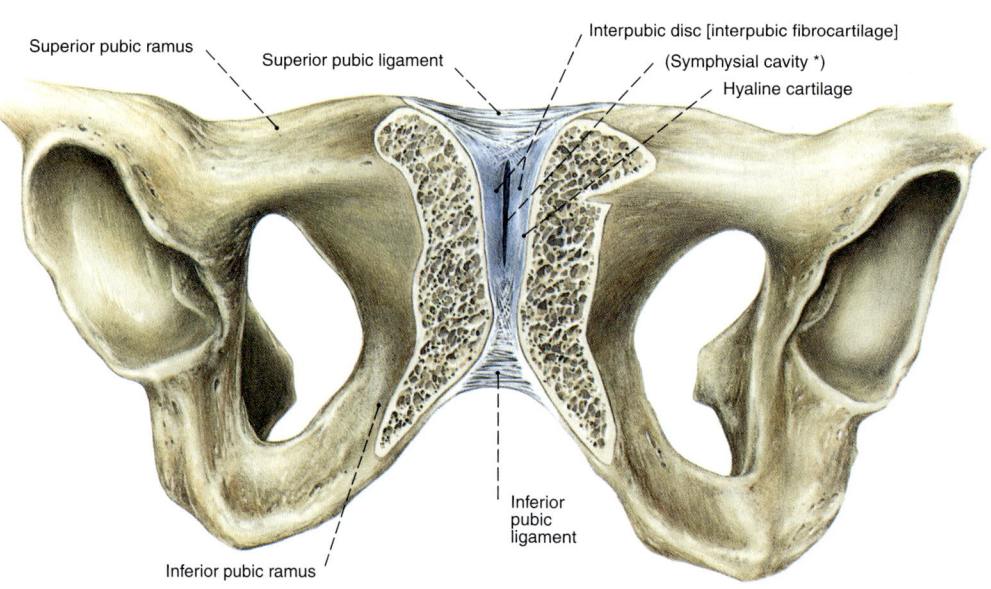

Fig. 1181   Pubic symphysis; oblique section in the direction of the longitudinal axis of the pubic symphysis, slightly tilted toward the frontal plane; inferior anterior aspect (60%). The interpubic disc [interpubic fibrocartilage] is made of fibrocartilage; only the symphysial surfaces are covered with hyaline cartilage. Starting in the 1st decade a longitudinal cleft can be observed (*).

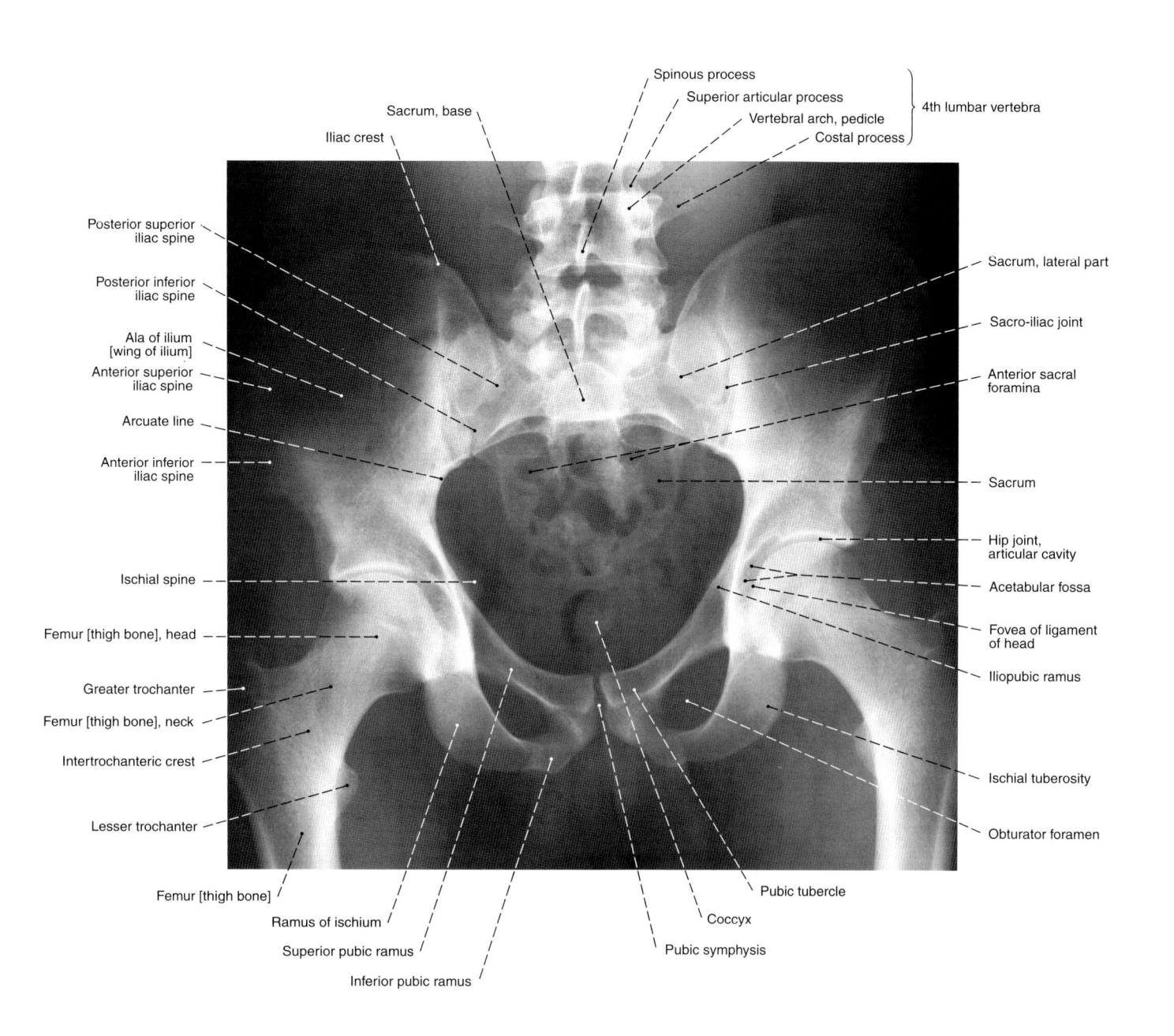

Fig. 1182 Male pelvis; AP radiograph in upright position; central beam directed onto 3rd sacral segment.

276 Lower limb

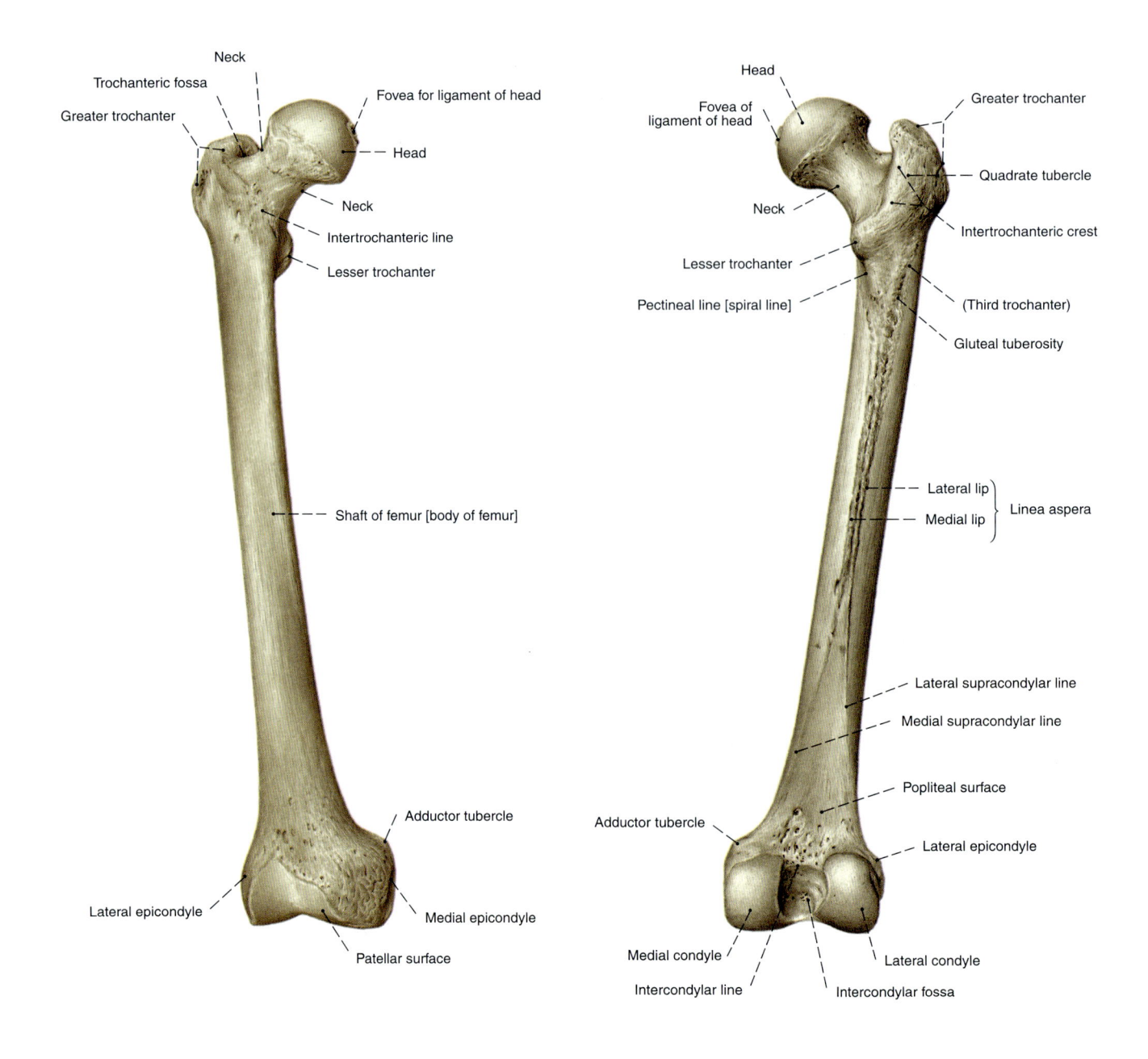

Fig. 1183 Right femur [thigh bone]; anterior aspect (30%).

Fig. 1184 Right femur [thigh bone]; posterior aspect (30%).

Femur [thigh bone]

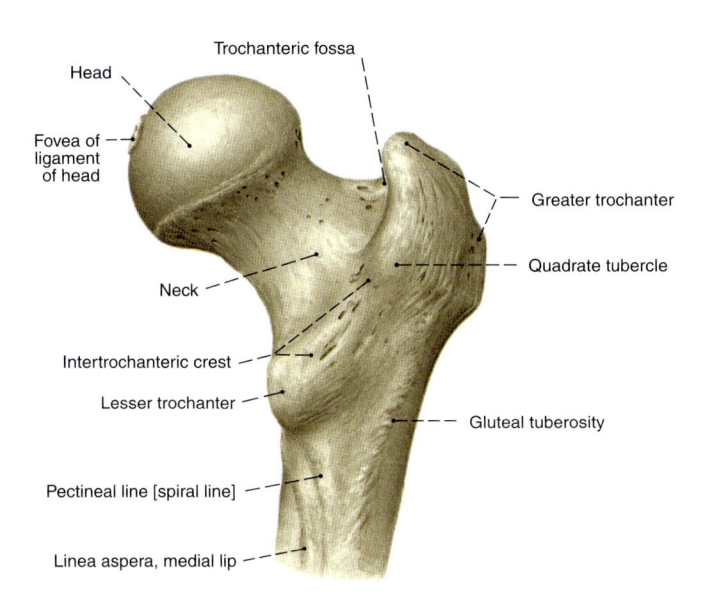

Fig. 1185 Right femur [thigh bone]; proximal extremity; posterior aspect (60%).

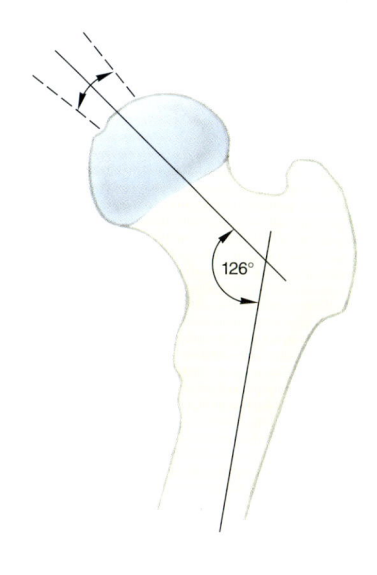

Fig. 1186 Right femur [thigh bone]; variability of angle of the neck; posterior aspect.
The angle of the neck is also known as angle of inclination or angle of depression. It is 150° in the newborn and approximately 126° in the adult.

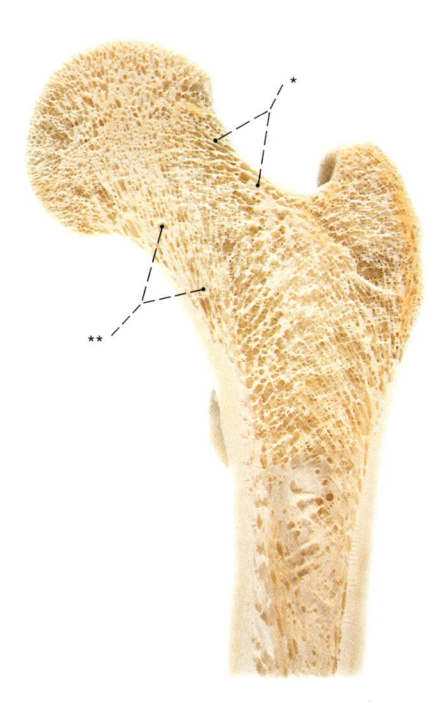

Fig. 1187 Femur [thigh bone]; structure of the spongy bone [trabecular bone] in large angle of inclination [angle of depression] (= coxa valga); section in the plane of the angle of anteversion [angle of declination] (60%). The lateral "tension bundle" (*) of the spongy bone [trabecular bone] is weakened; the medial "compression bundle" (**) is enlarged.

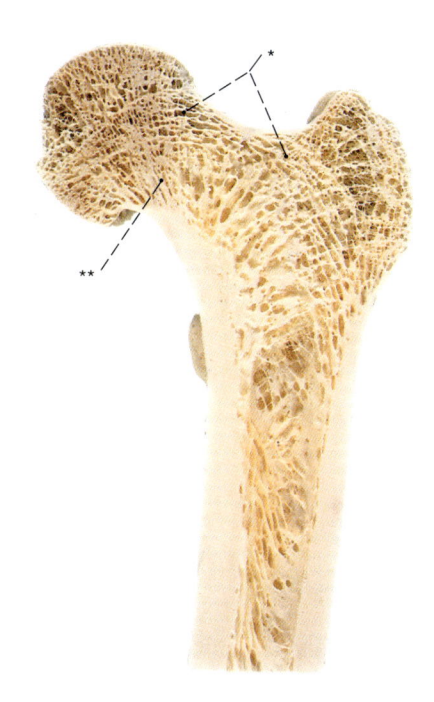

Fig. 1188 Femur [thigh bone]; structure of the spongy bone [trabecular bone] in small angle of inclination [angle of depression] (= coxa vara); section in the plane of the angle of anteversion [angle of declination] (60%). The lateral "tension bundle" (*) of the spongy bone [trabecular bone] is enlarged; the medial "compression bundle" (**) is weakened. Due to high-flexion stress the medial cortical bone of the neck is especially well developed.

Lower limb

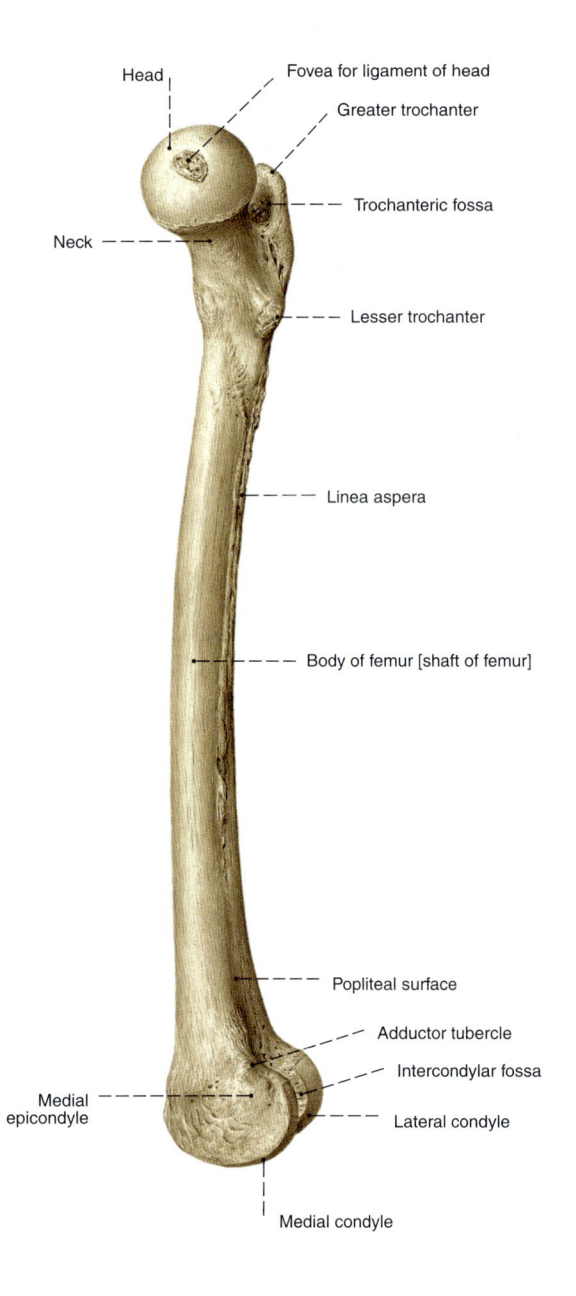

Fig. 1189 Right femur [thigh bone]; medial aspect (30%).

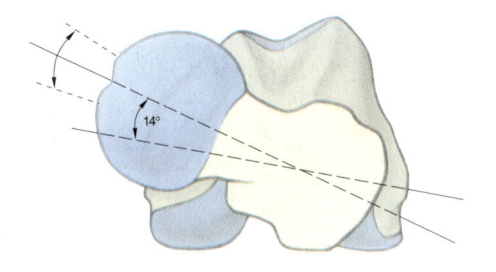

Fig. 1190 Right femur [thigh bone]; variability of angle of declination [angle of anteversion]; proximal and distal extremity projected over another; proximal aspect (70%). The angle of declination [angle of anteversion] is approximately 30° in the infant and approximately 14° in the adult.

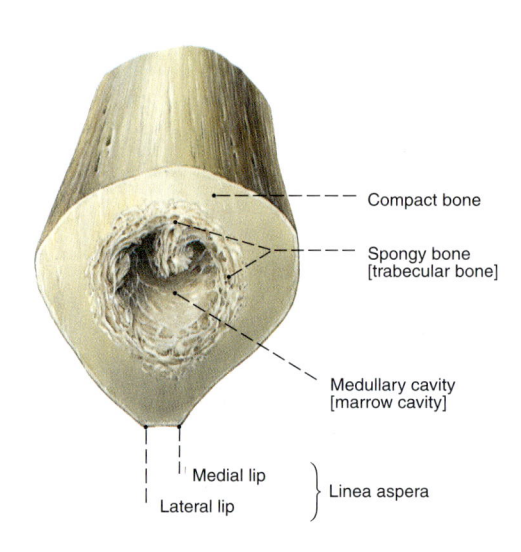

Fig. 1191 Right femur [thigh bone]; cross-section through middle of body of femur [shaft of femur]; distal aspect.

Pelvis and femur [thigh bone]

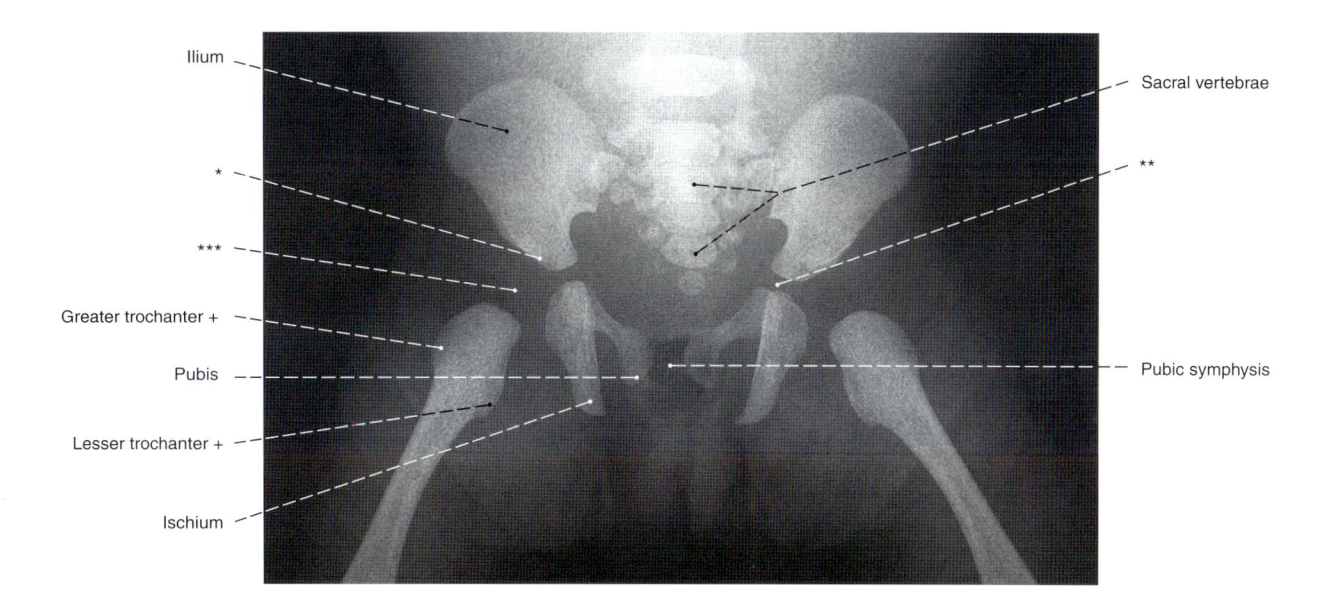

Fig. 1192 Pelvis and femur [thigh bone]; AP radiograph of a premature born female (fetus in the 8th month of pregnancy).

- * Bony roof of the acetabulum.
- ** Y-shaped epiphysial cartilage in acetabular fossa.
- *** The ossification center in the head of femur does not appear before the 3rd to 5th month of life.
- + Both trochanters are only bony projection of the diaphysis at this age.

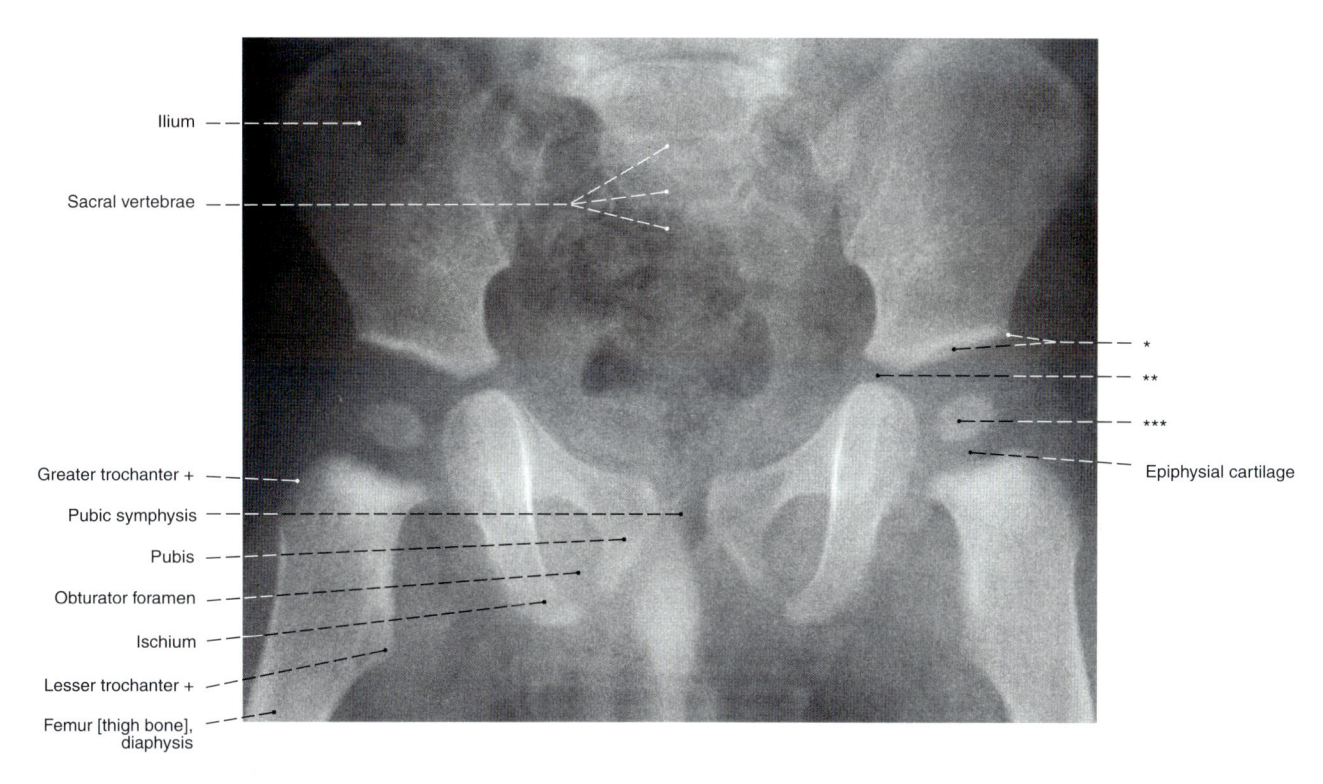

Fig. 1193 Pelvis and femur; AP radiograph of a 12-month-old boy.

- * Bony roof of the acetabulum.
- ** Y-shaped epiphysial cartilage in acetabular fossa.
- *** Ossification center in the head of femur.
- + Both trochanters are only bony projection of the diaphysis at this age.

Lower limb

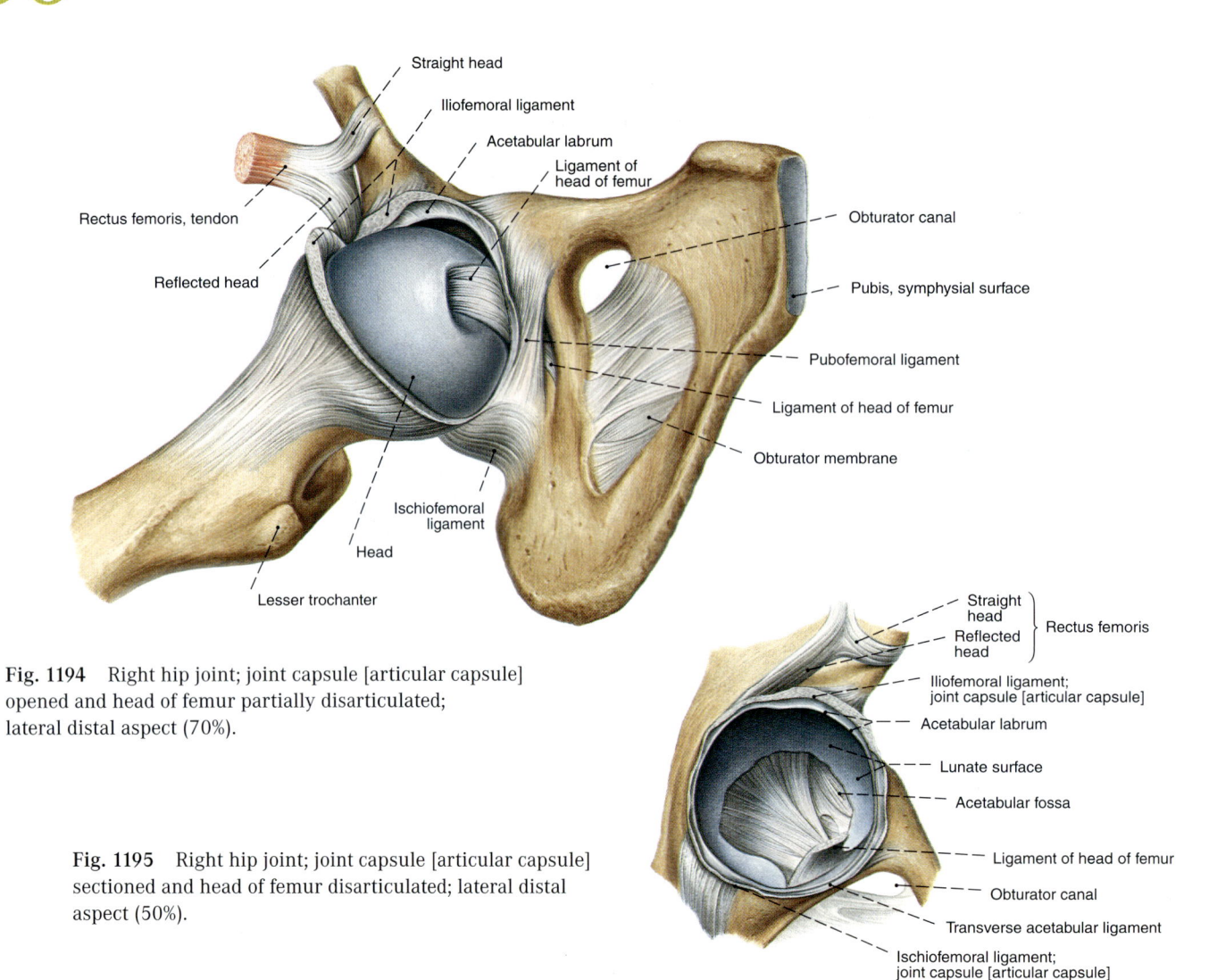

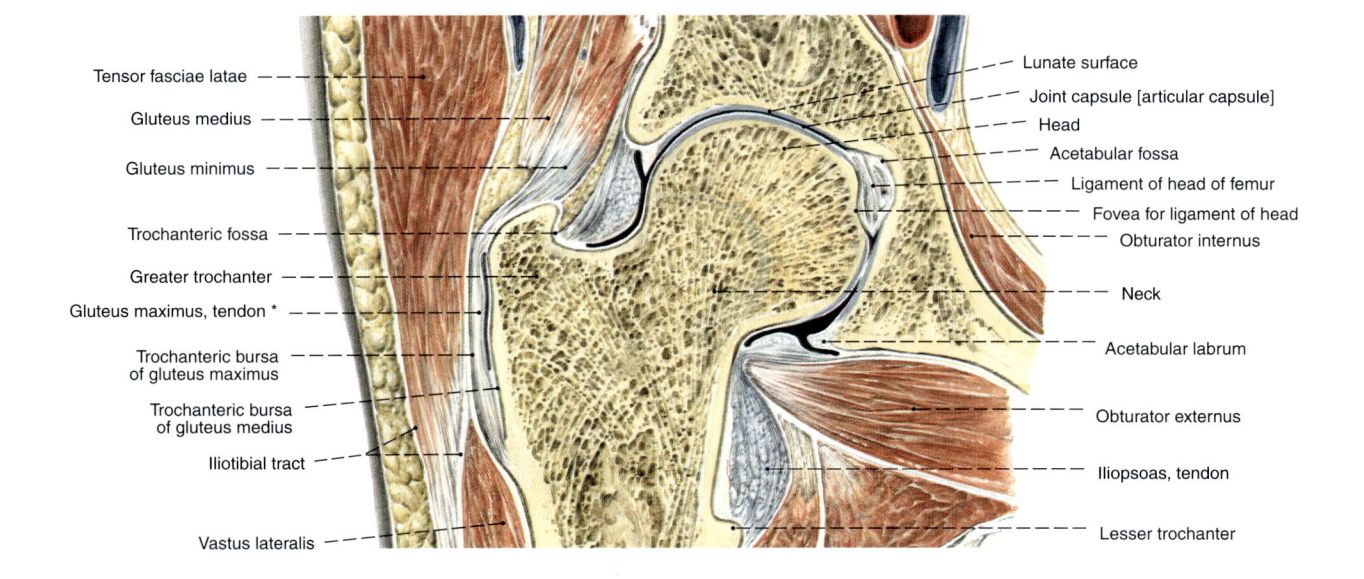

Fig. 1194 Right hip joint; joint capsule [articular capsule] opened and head of femur partially disarticulated; lateral distal aspect (70%).

Fig. 1195 Right hip joint; joint capsule [articular capsule] sectioned and head of femur disarticulated; lateral distal aspect (50%).

Fig. 1196 Right hip joint; vertical section in plane of angle of declination [angel of anteversion]; anterior aspect (65%).

* Merges into iliotibial tract.

Hip joint 281

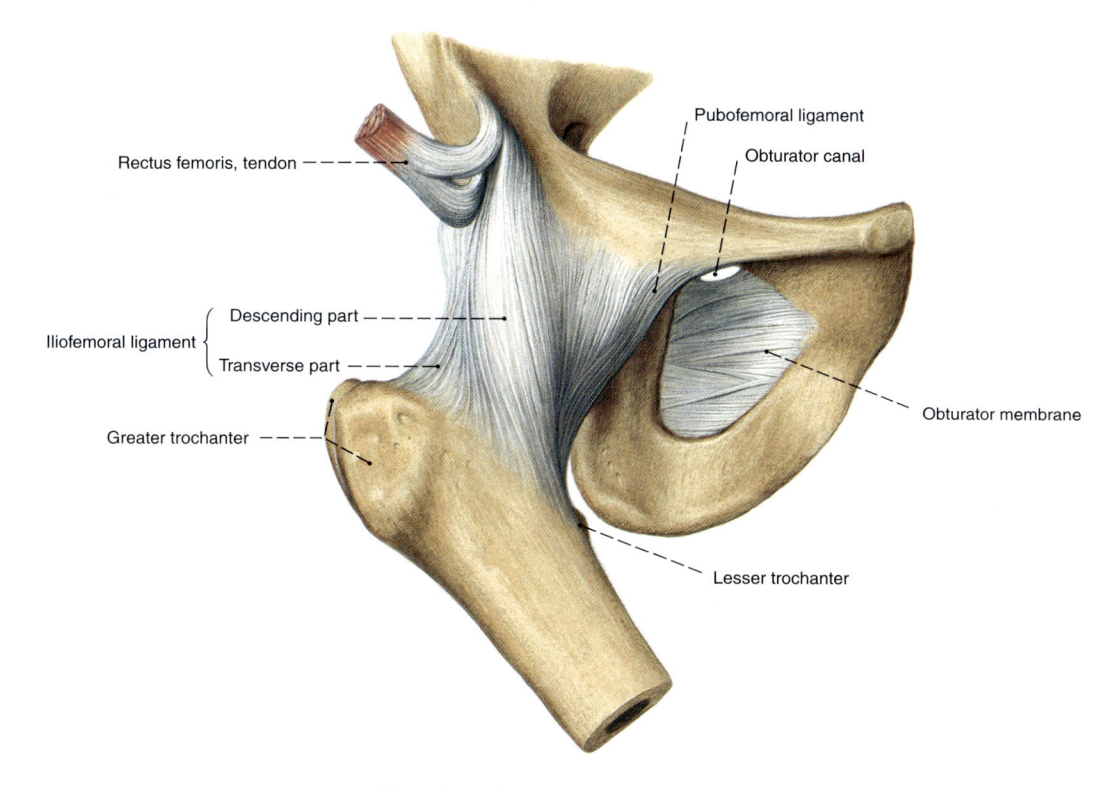

Fig. 1197 Right hip joint; anterior distal aspect (50%).

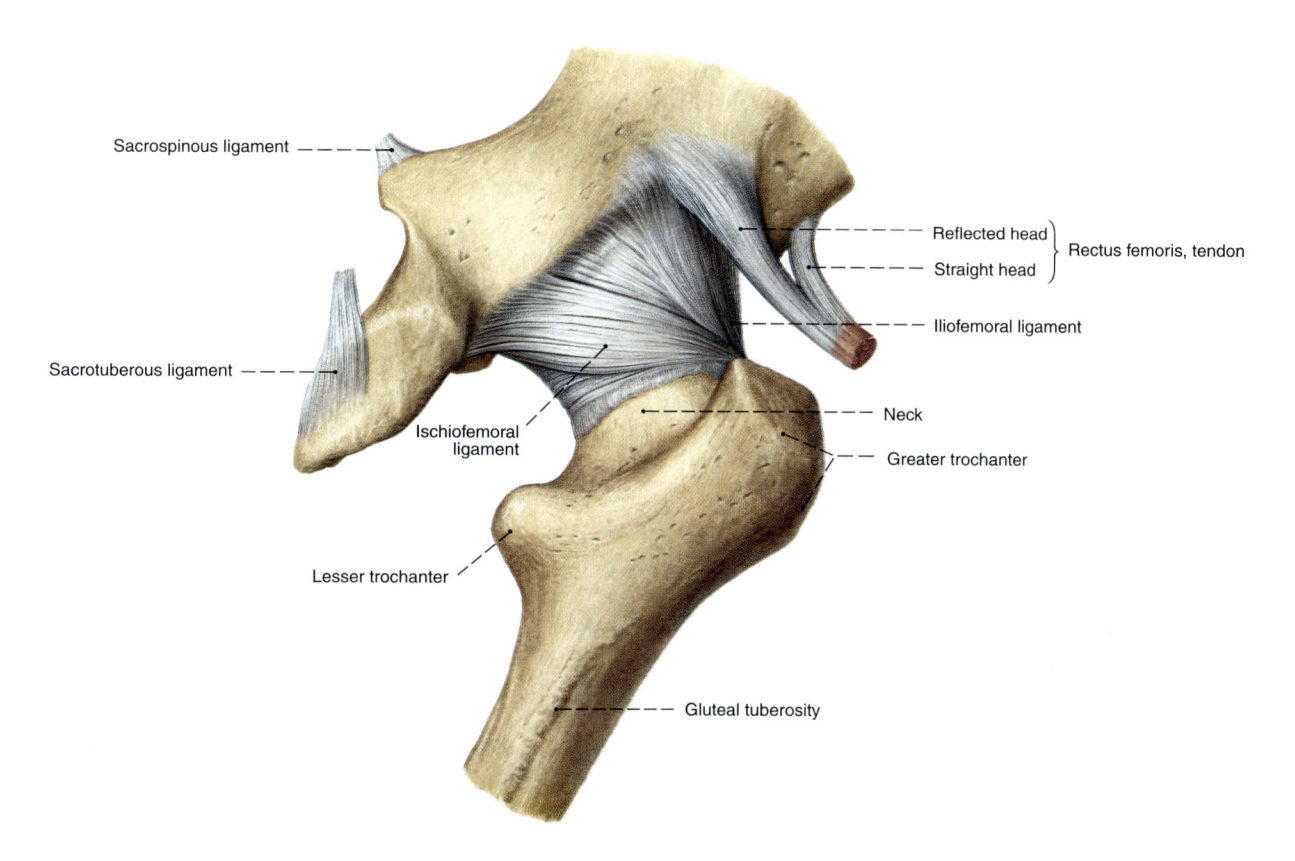

Fig. 1198 Right hip joint; posterior aspect (50%).

Lower limb

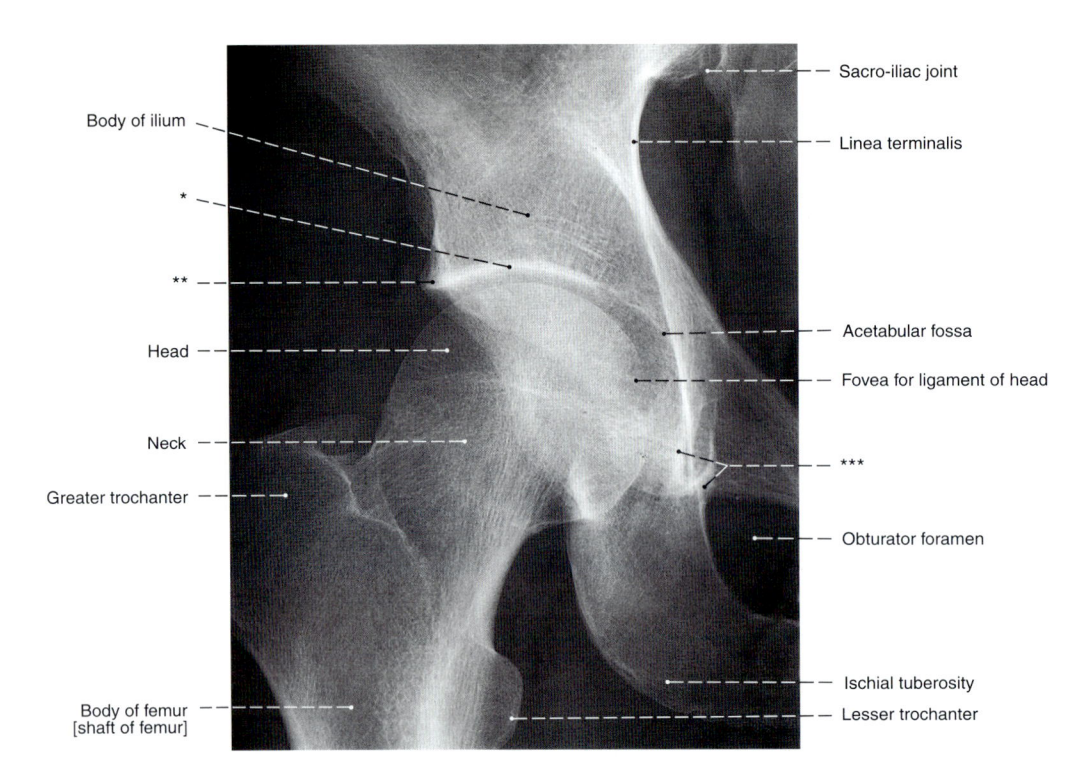

Fig. 1199 Hip joint; AP radiograph in upright position, standing on both legs.

* Clinically: roof of acetabulum = tangential projection of lunate surface.
** Clinically: edge of roof of acetabulum = outermost part of acetabulum.
*** Clinically: KÖHLER'S teardrop = projection of acetabular fossa.

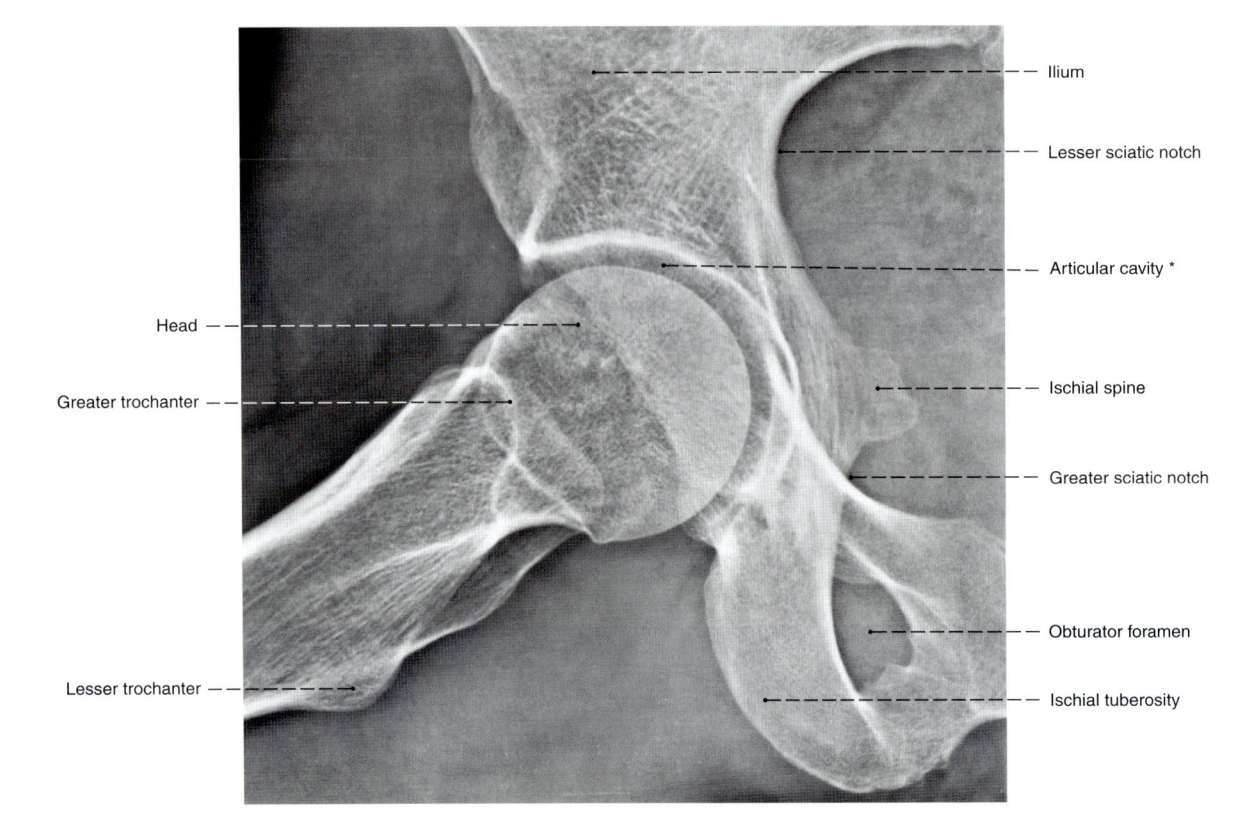

Fig. 1200 Hip joint; AP radiograph in supine position and abduction and flexion of the thigh (so-called LAUENSTEIN projection).

* Due to little absorption of X-rays by cartilage, the articular cavity seems to be abnormally wide in radiographs.

Femur [thigh bone] 283

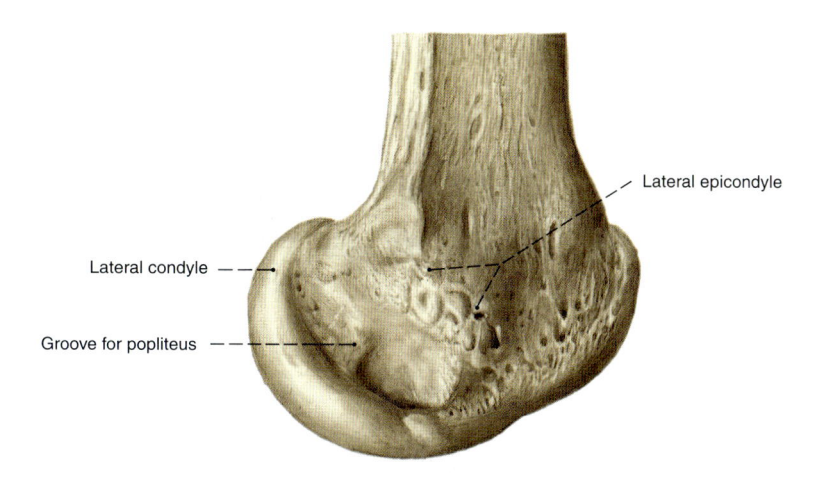

Fig. 1201 Right femur [thigh bone]; distal extremity; lateral aspect (80%).

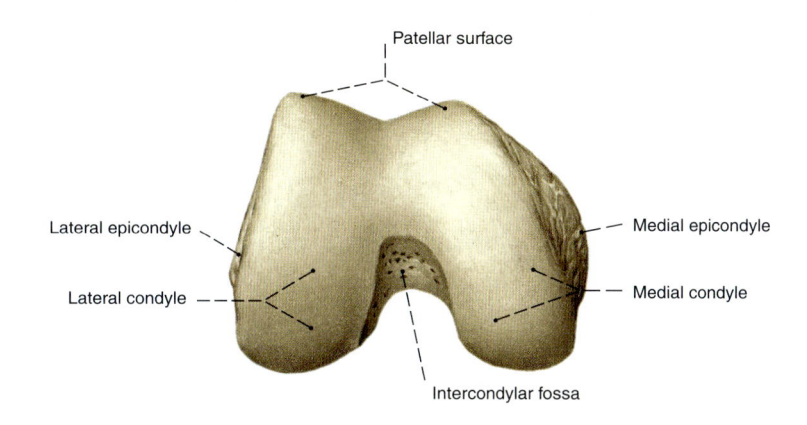

Fig. 1202 Right femur [thigh bone]; distal extremity; distal aspect (50%).

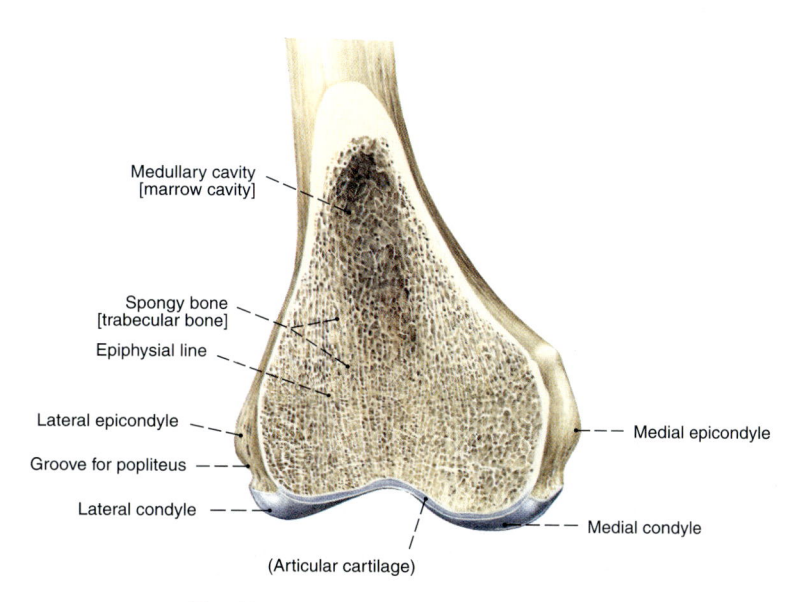

Fig. 1203 Right femur [thigh bone]; frontal section through distal extremity; anterior aspect (50%).

Lower limb

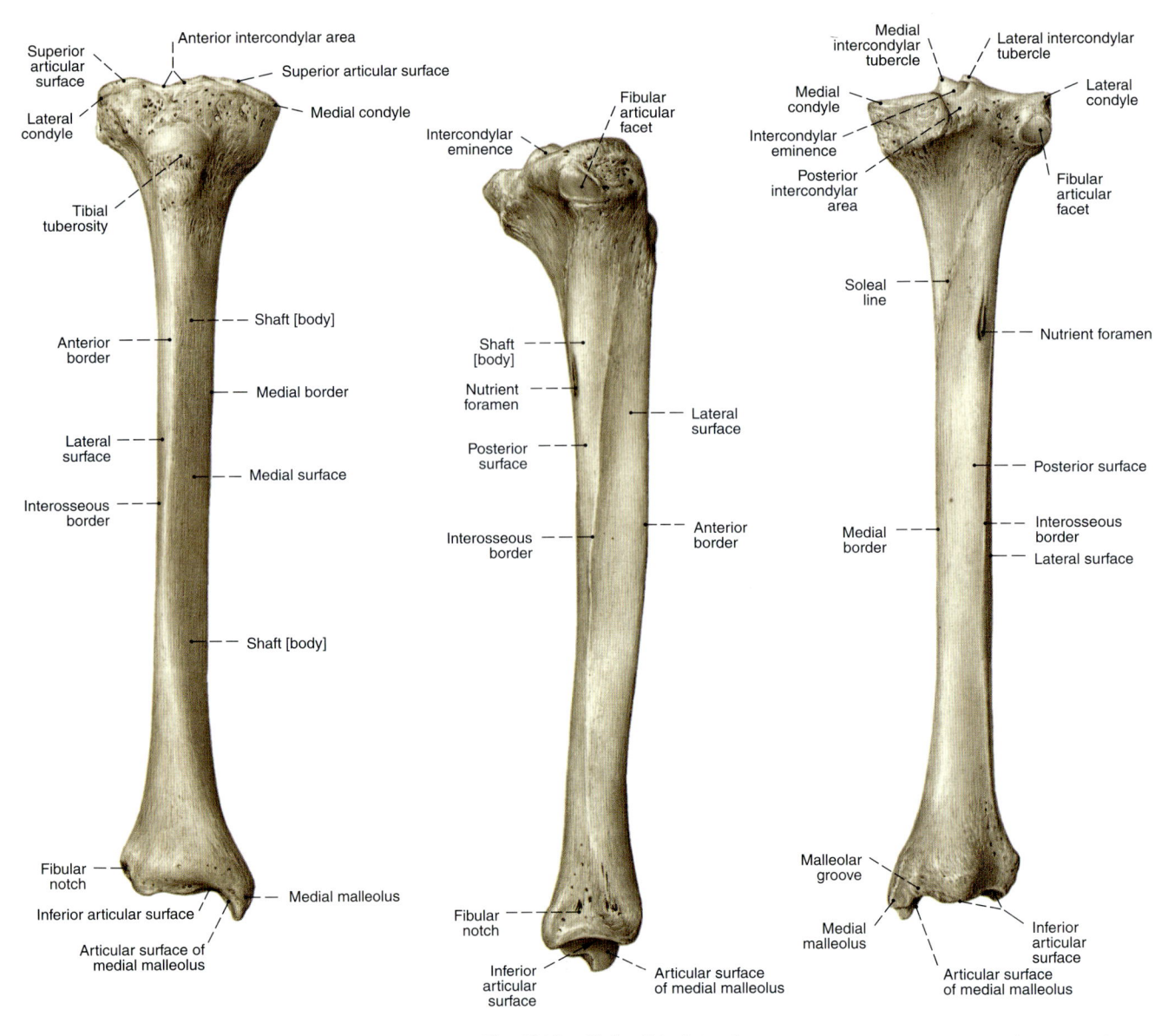

Fig. 1204 Right tibia; anterior aspect (35%).

Fig. 1205 Right tibia; lateral aspect (35%).

Fig. 1206 Right tibia; posterior aspect (35%).

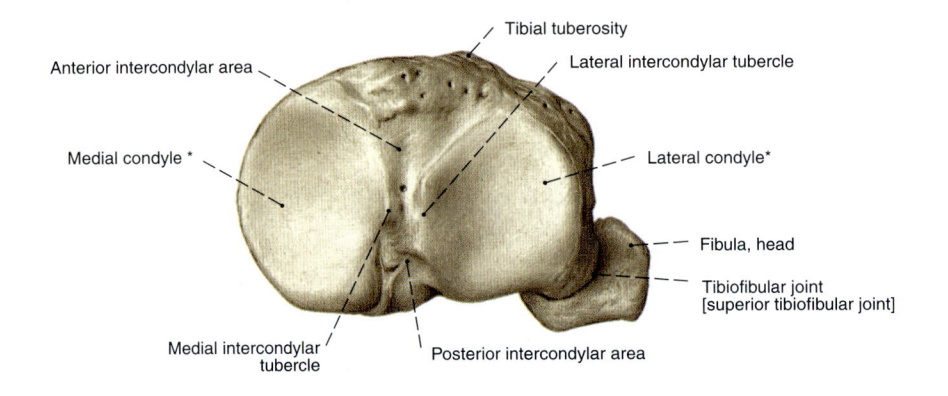

Fig. 1207 Right tibia and fibula; proximal aspect (70%).

* The articular surfaces of both condyles are together called the superior articular surface.

Tibia and fibula 285

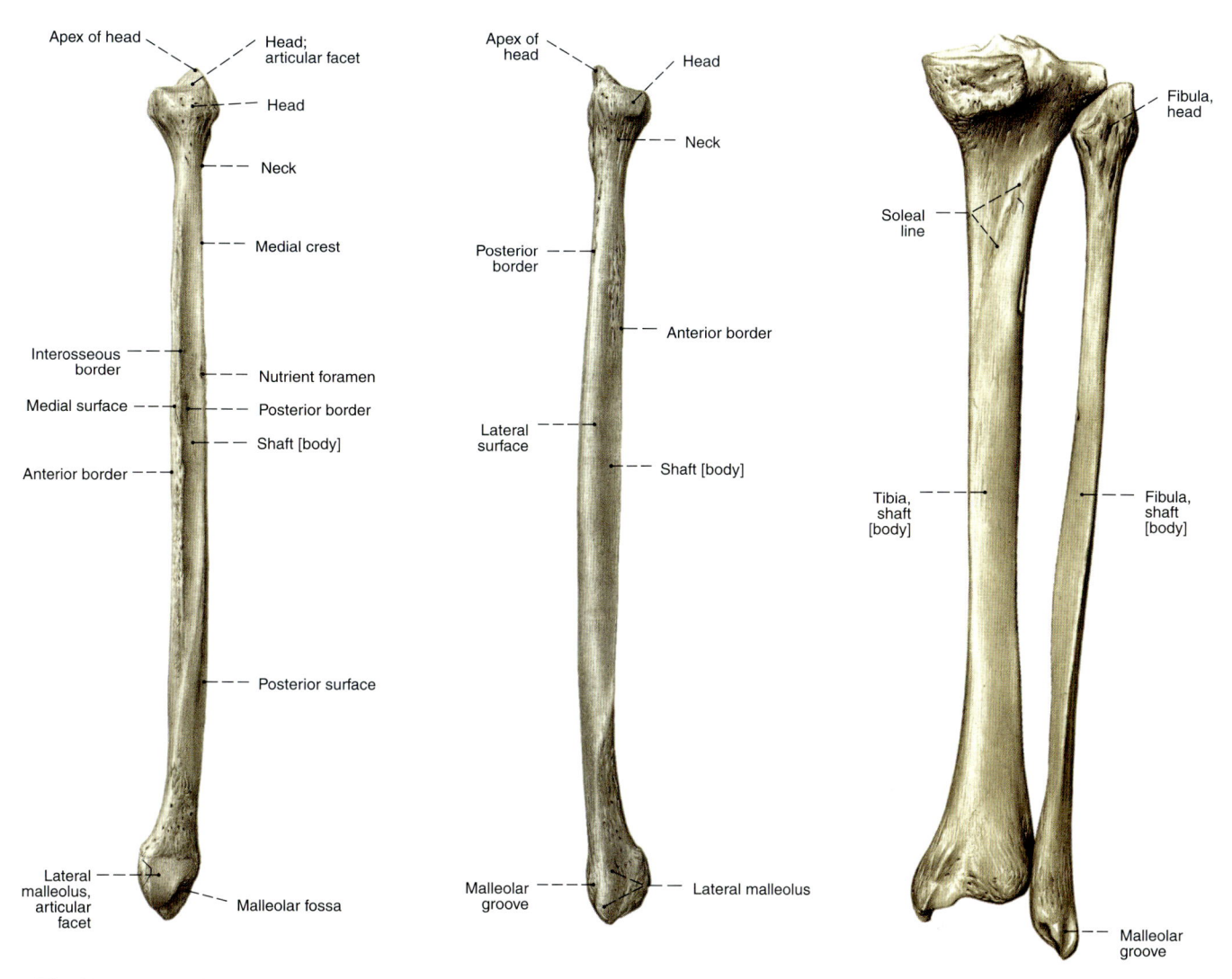

Fig. 1208 Right fibula; medial aspect (35%).

Fig. 1209 Right fibula; lateral aspect (35%).

Fig. 1210 Right tibia and fibula; posterior aspect (35%).

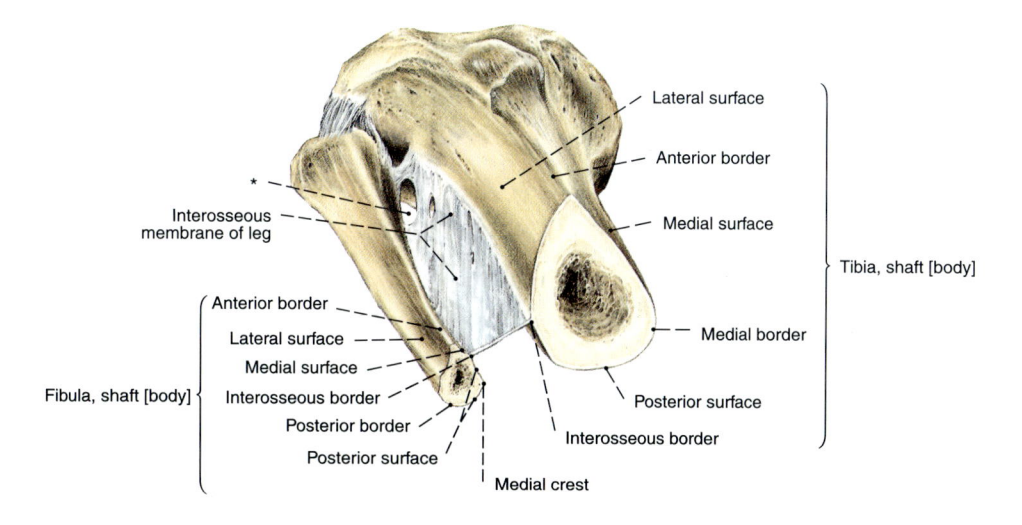

Fig. 1211 Right tibia and fibula; cross-section with interosseous membrane of leg; distal aspect (60%).
* Opening for passage of anterior tibial artery.

286 Lower limb

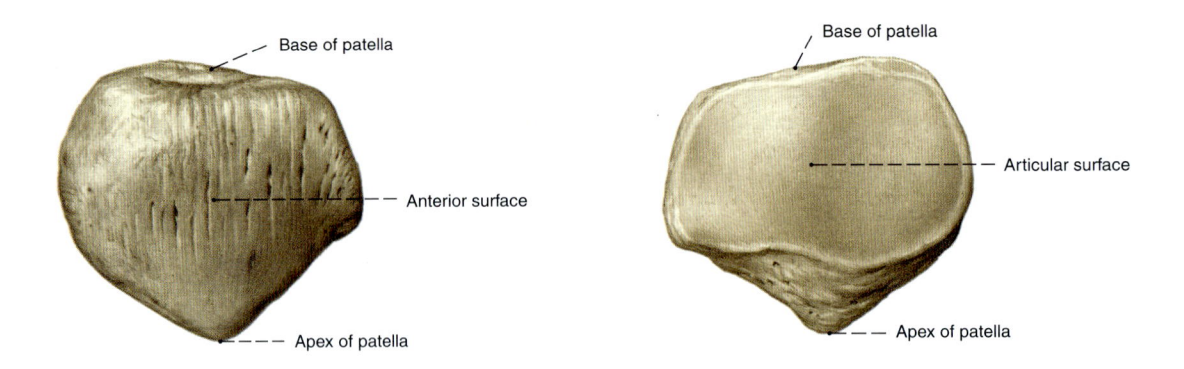

Fig. 1212 Right patella; anterior aspect (80%).

Fig. 1213 Right patella; posterior aspect (80%).

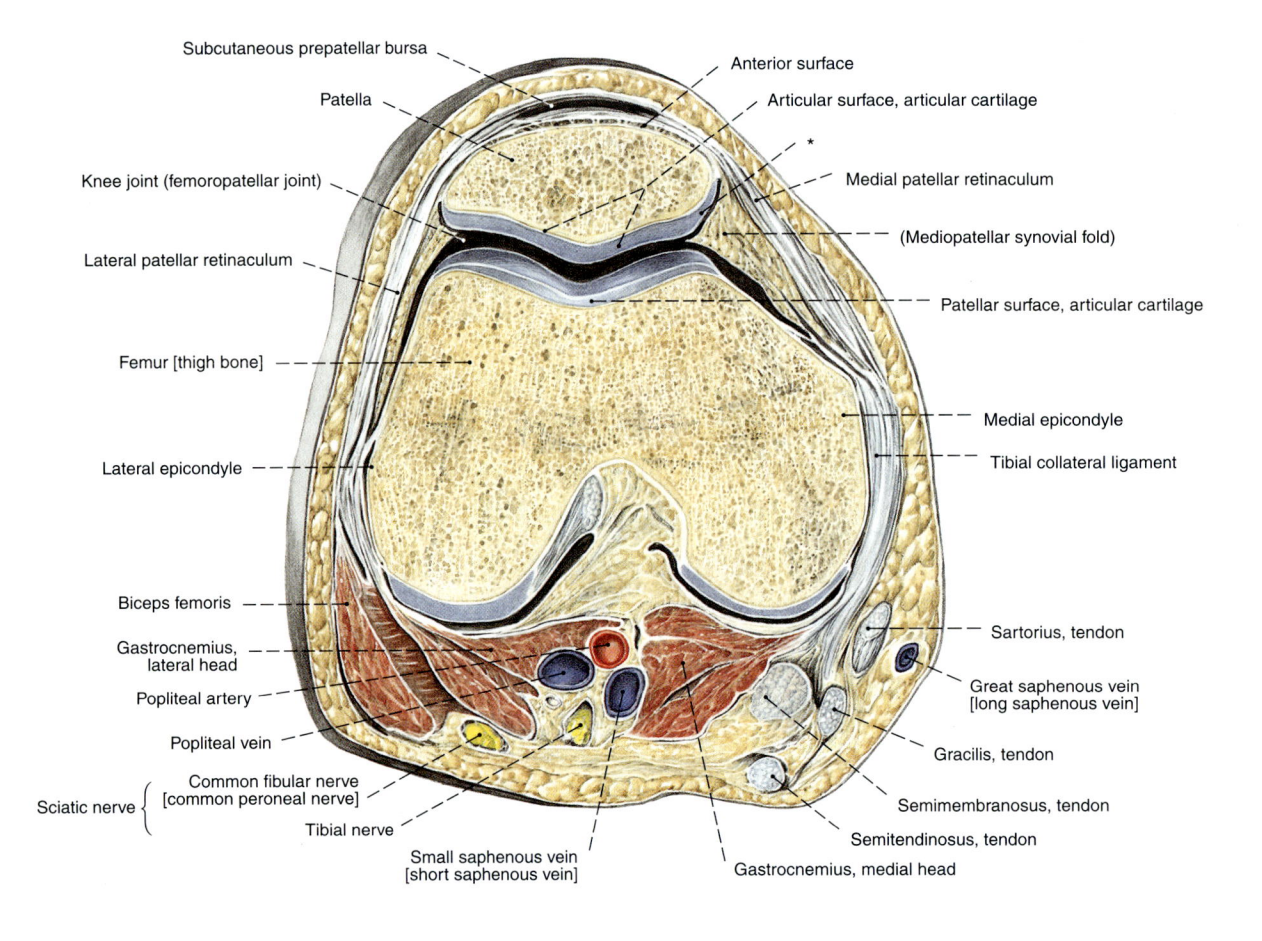

Fig. 1214 Right patella and femur [thigh bone]; cross-section through knee joint at level of middle of femoropatellar joint in extension; distal aspect (70%).
* Medial border facet.

Knee joint 287

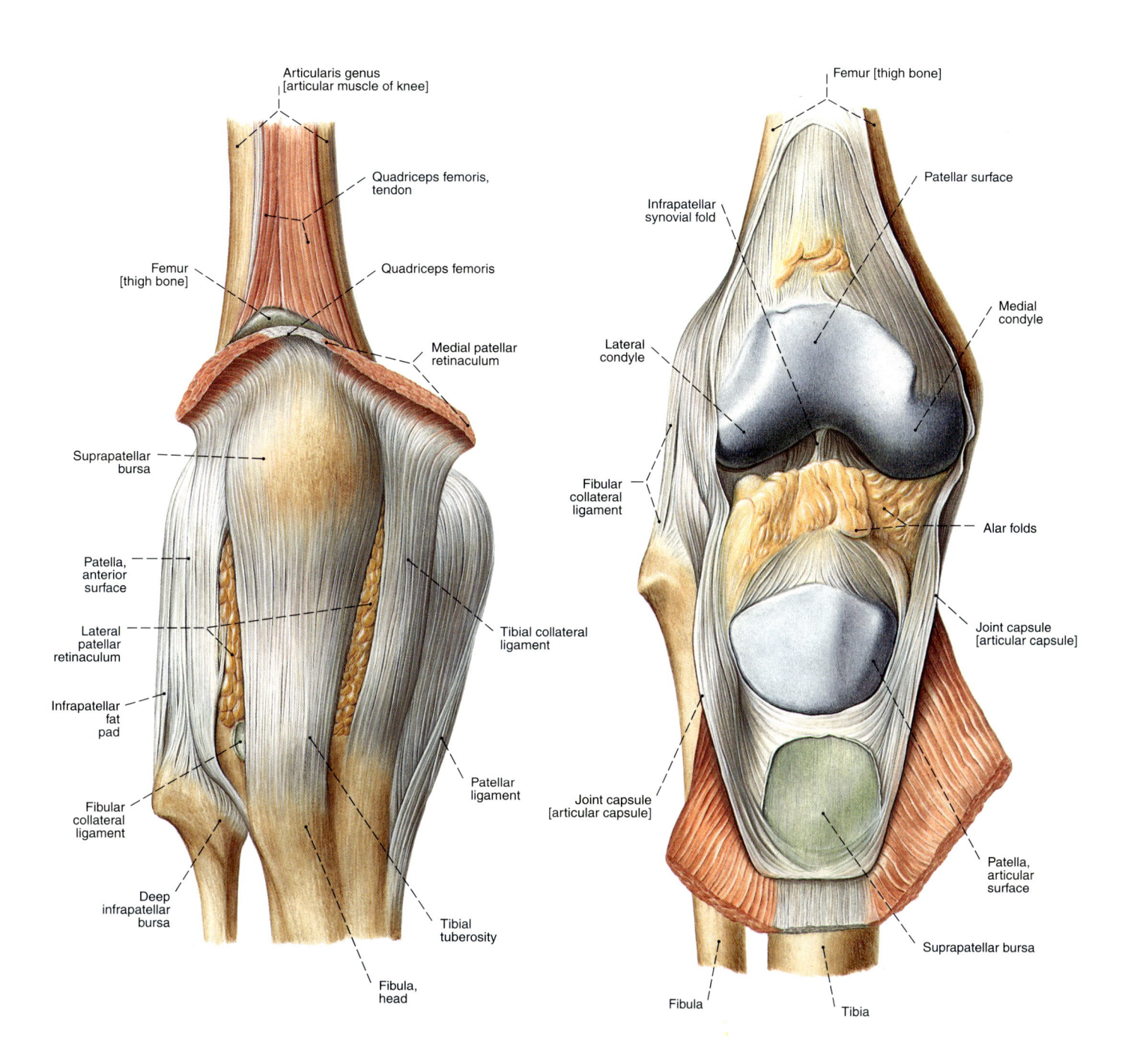

Fig. 1215 Right knee joint with intact joint capsule [articular capsule]; anterior aspect [65%].

Fig. 1216 Right knee joint; quadriceps sectioned and anterior part of joint capsule [articular capsule] reflected distally; suprapatellar bursa opened; anterior aspect [65%].

288 Lower limb

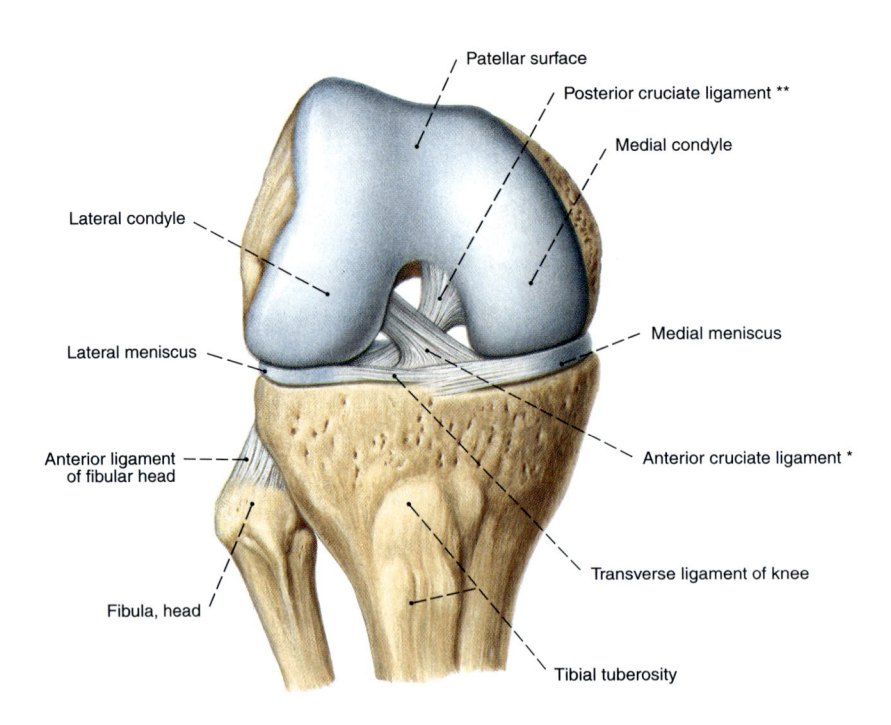

Fig. 1217 Right knee joint in 90° flexion; joint capsule [articular capsule] and collateral ligaments removed; anterior aspect [65%].
* Clinically: ACL.
** Clinically: PCL.

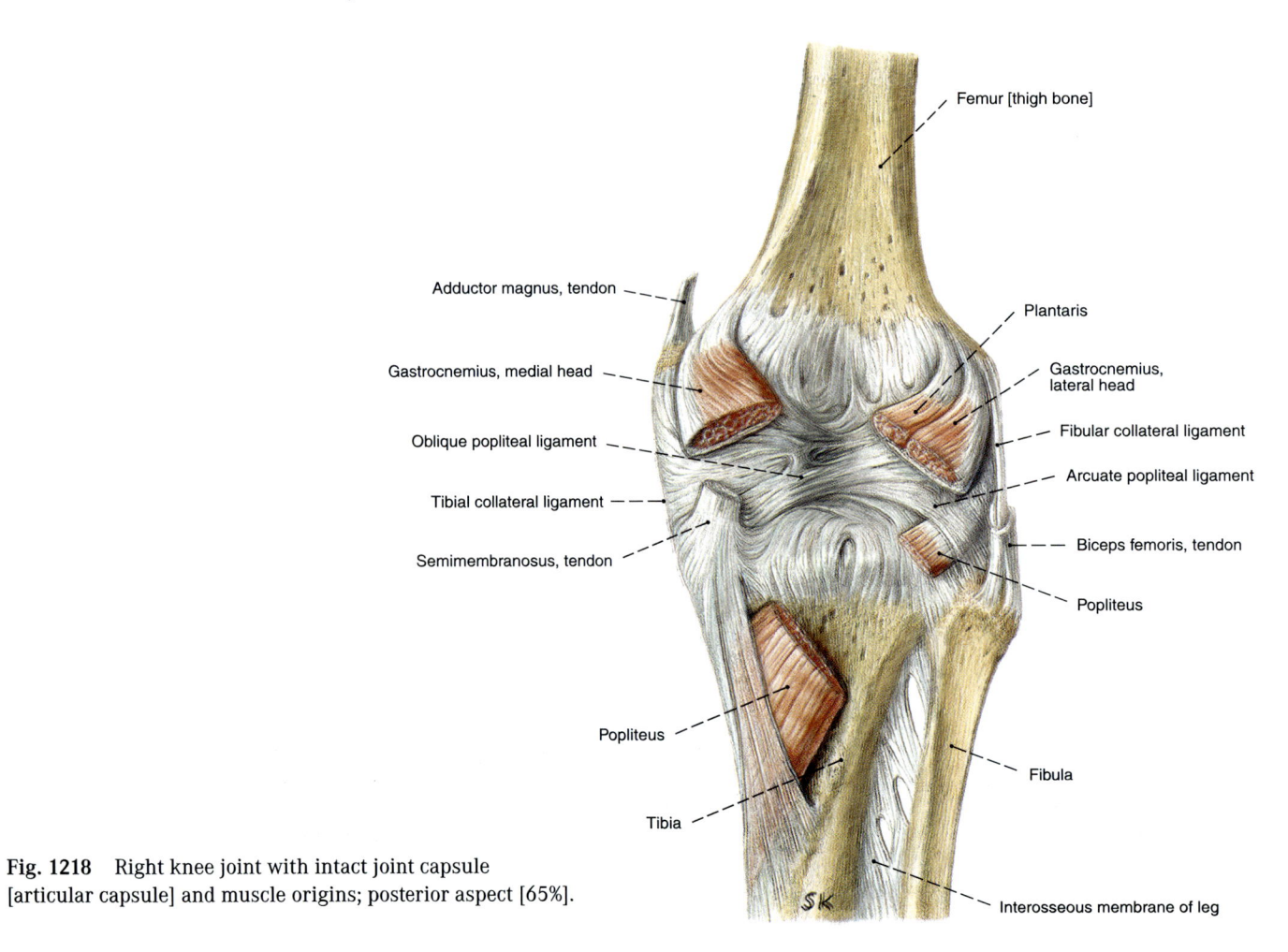

Fig. 1218 Right knee joint with intact joint capsule [articular capsule] and muscle origins; posterior aspect [65%].

Knee joint

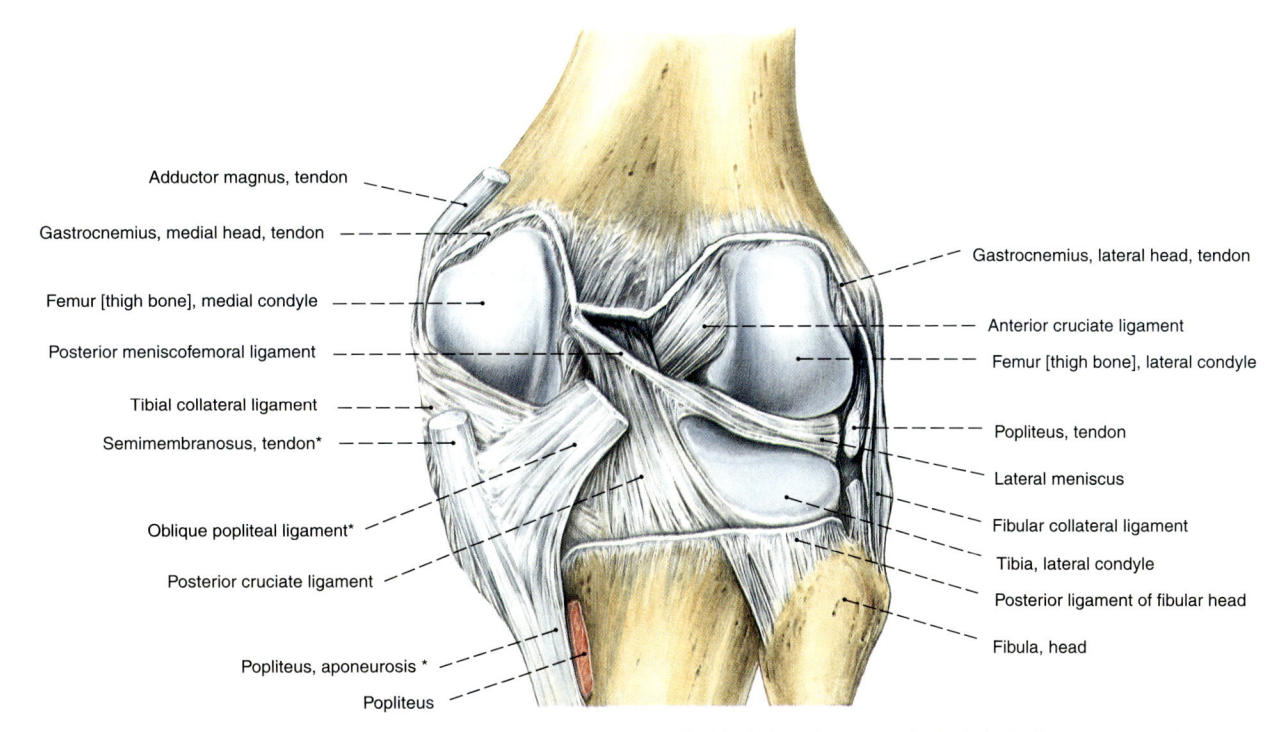

Fig. 1219 Right knee joint; cruciate ligaments and menisci exposed; posterior aspect (65%).

* Besides its bony insertion at the medial side of the tibia, below the medial condyle, the tendon of the semimembranosus also ends with the oblique popliteal ligament and an aponeurosis that covers the origin of the popliteus muscle.

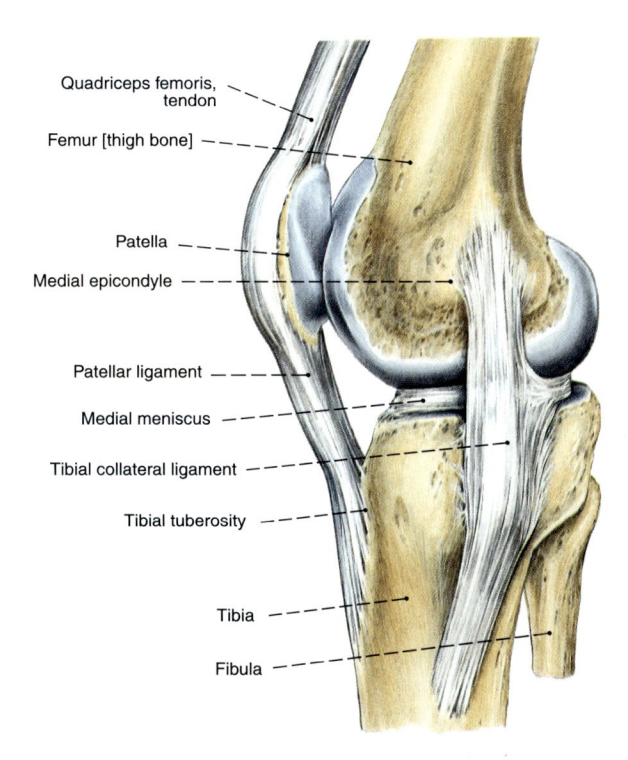

Fig. 1220 Right knee joint; arrangement of fibers of tibial collateral ligament in extension; medial aspect (60%).
Only the posterior fibers of the tibial collateral ligament are attached to the medial meniscus.

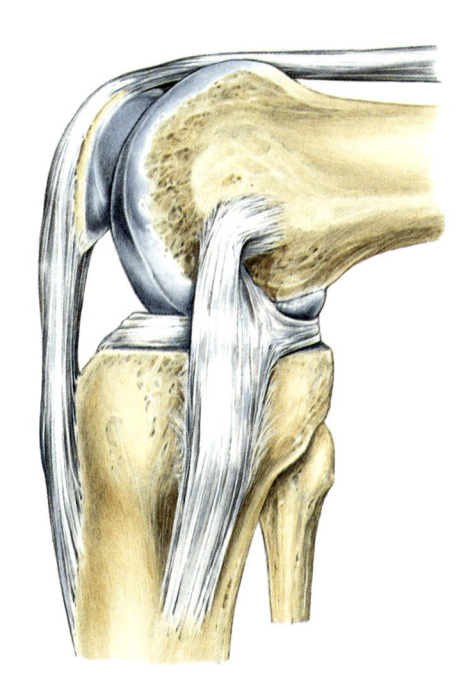

Fig. 1221 Right knee joint; arrangement of fibers of tibial collateral ligament in flexion; medial aspect (60%).
During flexion the posterior and proximal fibers of the tibial collateral ligament become twisted, which stabilizes the medial meniscus.

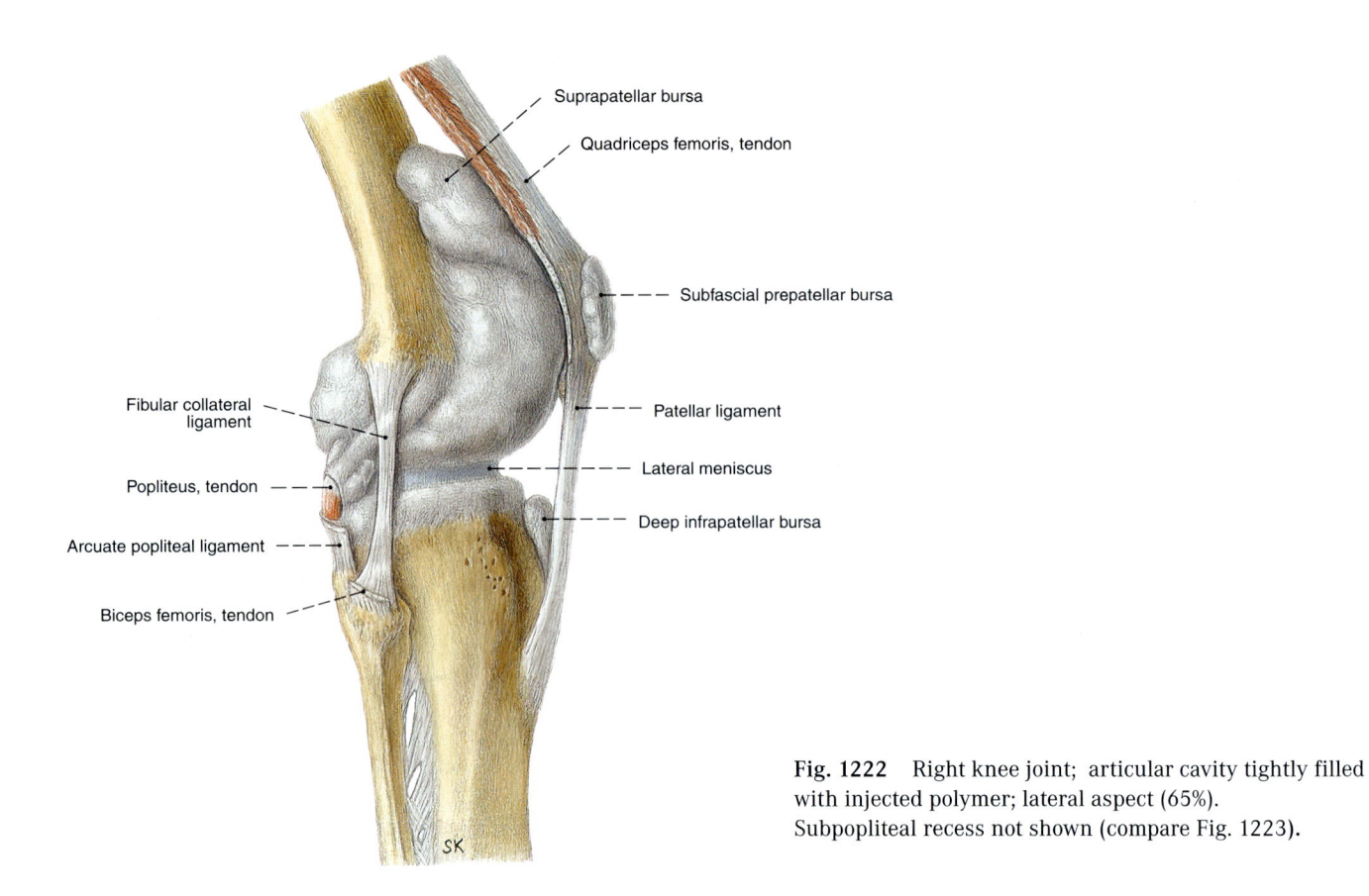

Fig. 1222 Right knee joint; articular cavity tightly filled with injected polymer; lateral aspect (65%). Subpopliteal recess not shown (compare Fig. 1223).

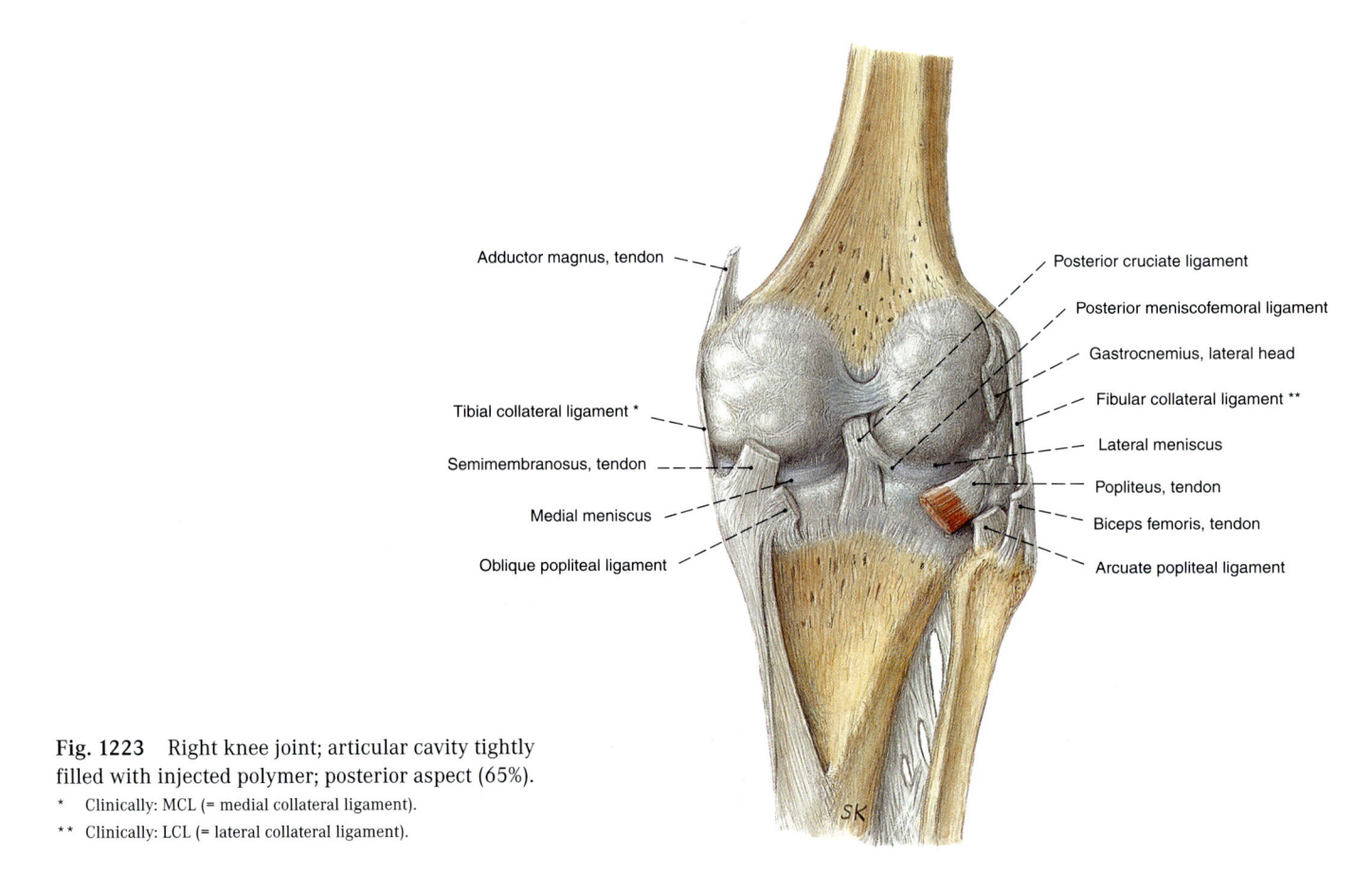

Fig. 1223 Right knee joint; articular cavity tightly filled with injected polymer; posterior aspect (65%).
 * Clinically: MCL (= medial collateral ligament).
 ** Clinically: LCL (= lateral collateral ligament).

Knee joint

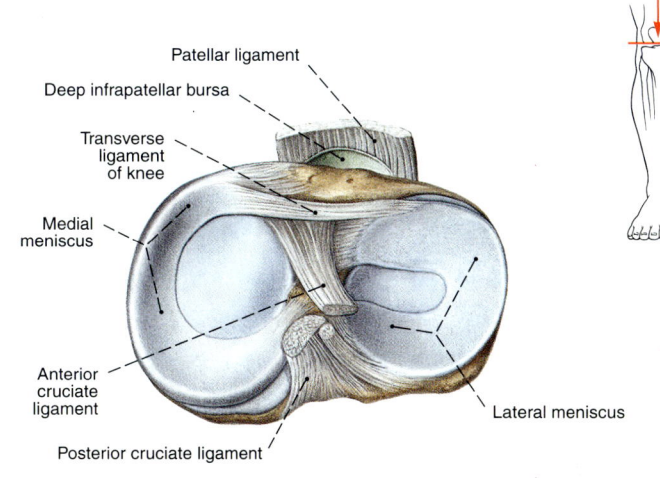

Fig. 1224 Right knee joint; menisci after transverse section of joint capsule [articular capsule], cruciate and collateral ligaments; proximal aspect (65%).

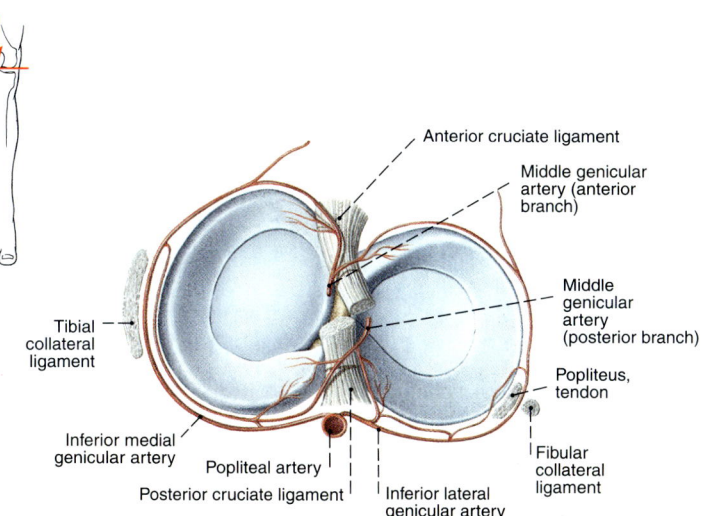

Fig. 1225 Right knee joint; arterial supply of menisci after transverse section of joint capsule [articular capsule], cruciate and collateral ligaments; proximal aspect (65%).

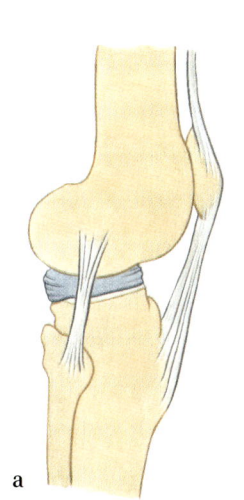

Fig. 1226 a, b Right knee joint; displacement of menisci during movement; lateral aspect.

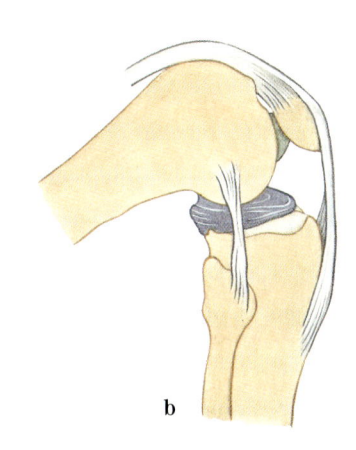

a In extension
b In flexion

Fig. 1227 Right knee joint; displacement of menisci during flexion; proximal aspect.
During flexion both menisci are displaced posteriorly over the borders of the condyles of the tibia. The lower risk of injury of the lateral meniscus is explained by its greater mobility.

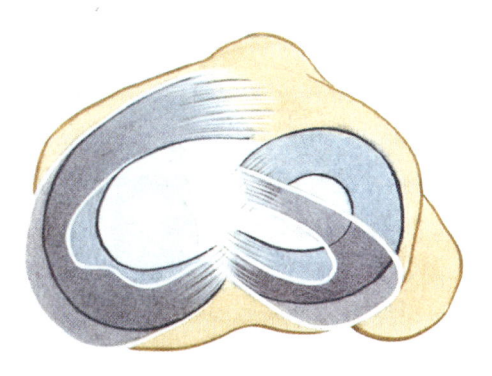

Components of knee joints

The complex arrangement of three articulating bones and the partial transverse separation by the menisci results in a functional division of the knee joint into three component: the femoropatellar joint, the meniscofemoral joint, and the meniscotibial joint. The menisci act as transportable articular surfaces and enable a better transmission of pressure to the condyles of tibia.

292 Lower limb

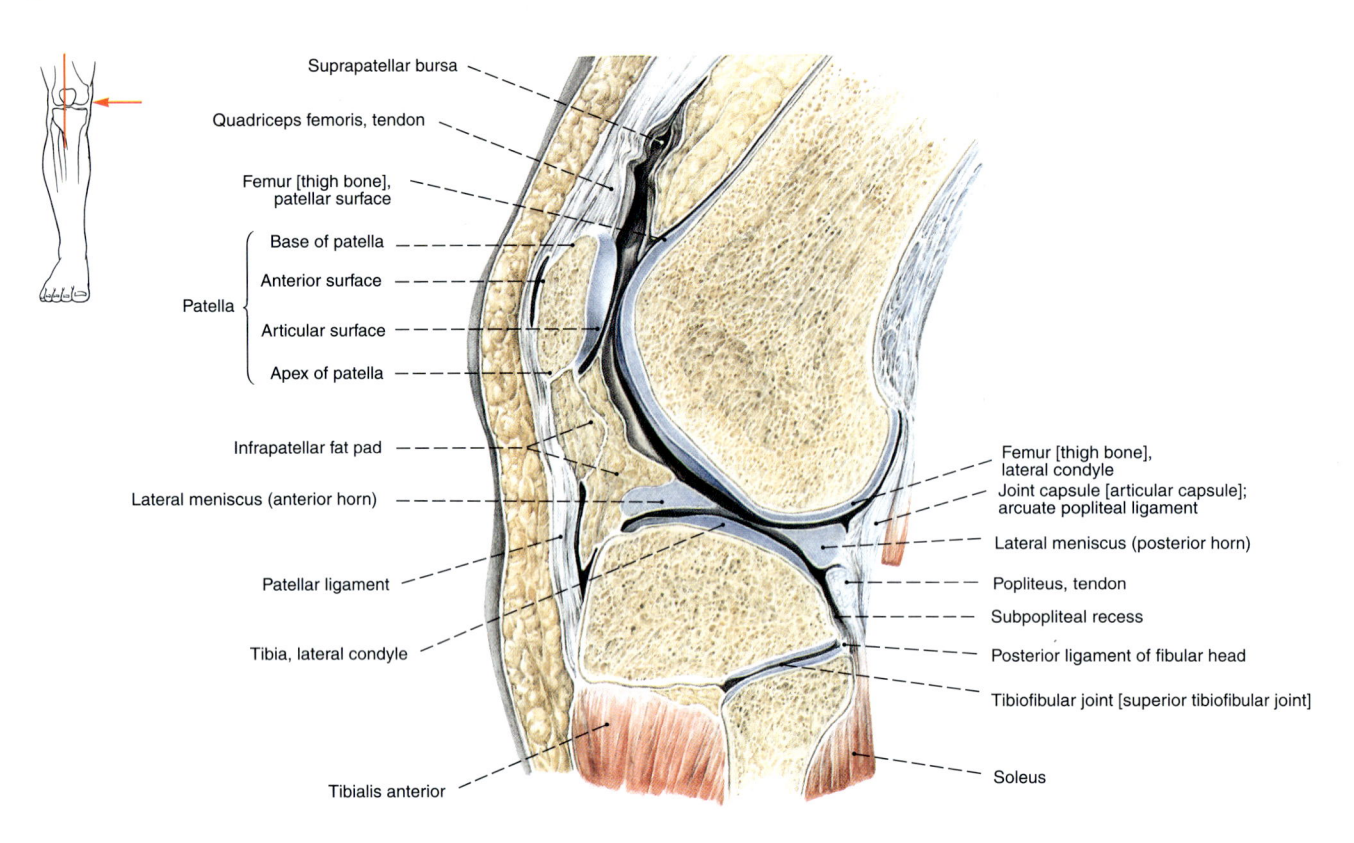

Fig. 1228 Right knee joint; sagittal section though lateral part of joint; lateral aspect [65%].

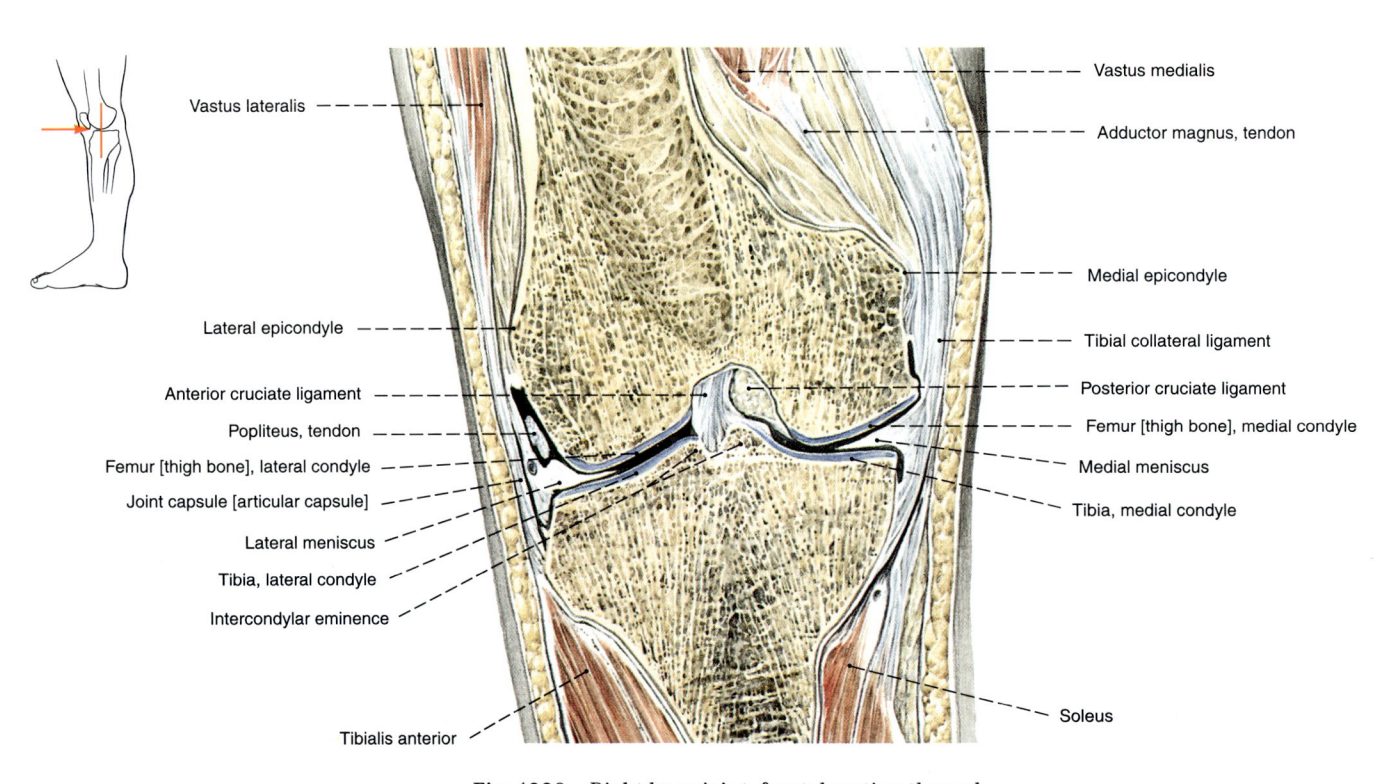

Fig. 1229 Right knee joint; frontal section through middle of joint; anterior aspect [65%].

Knee joint 293

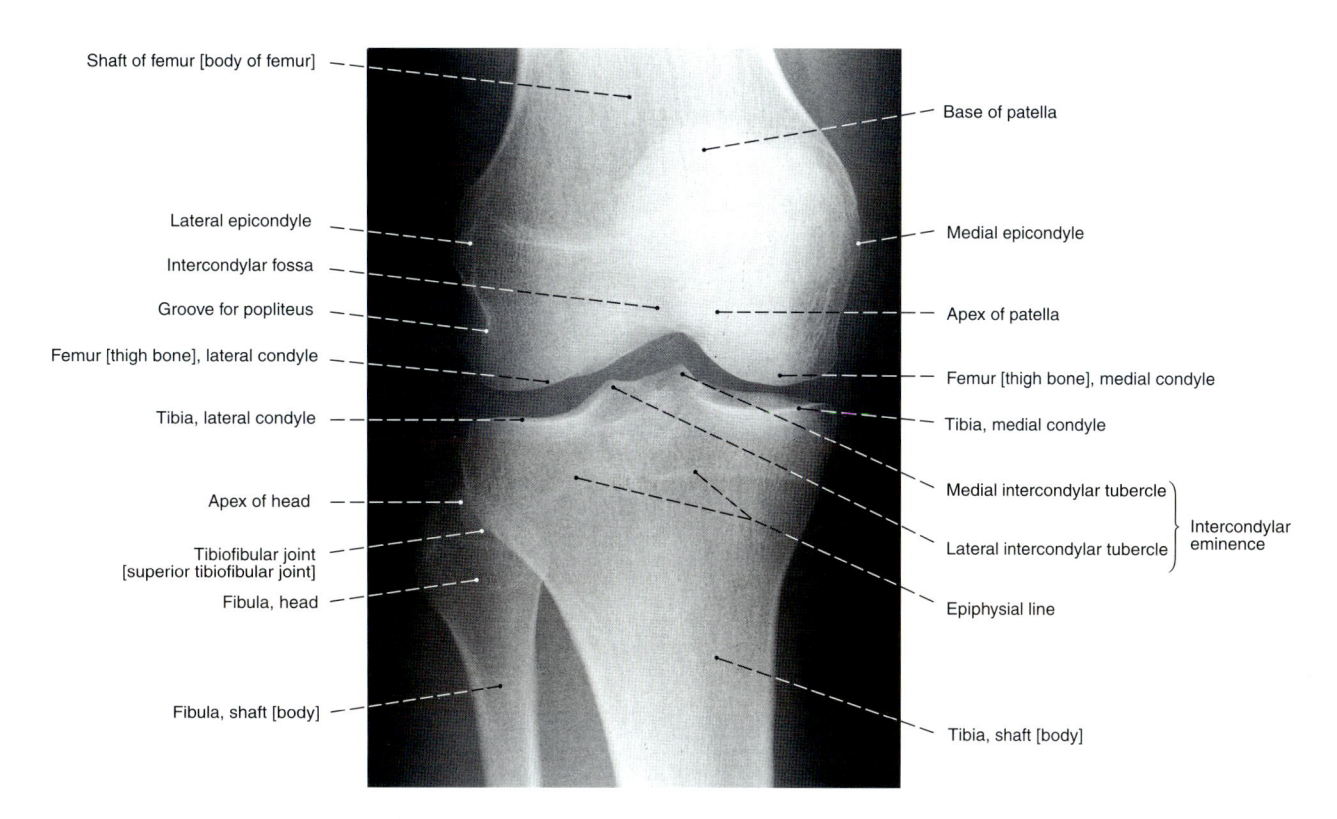

Fig. 1230 Knee joint; AP radiograph in supine position; central beam directed onto middle of joint.

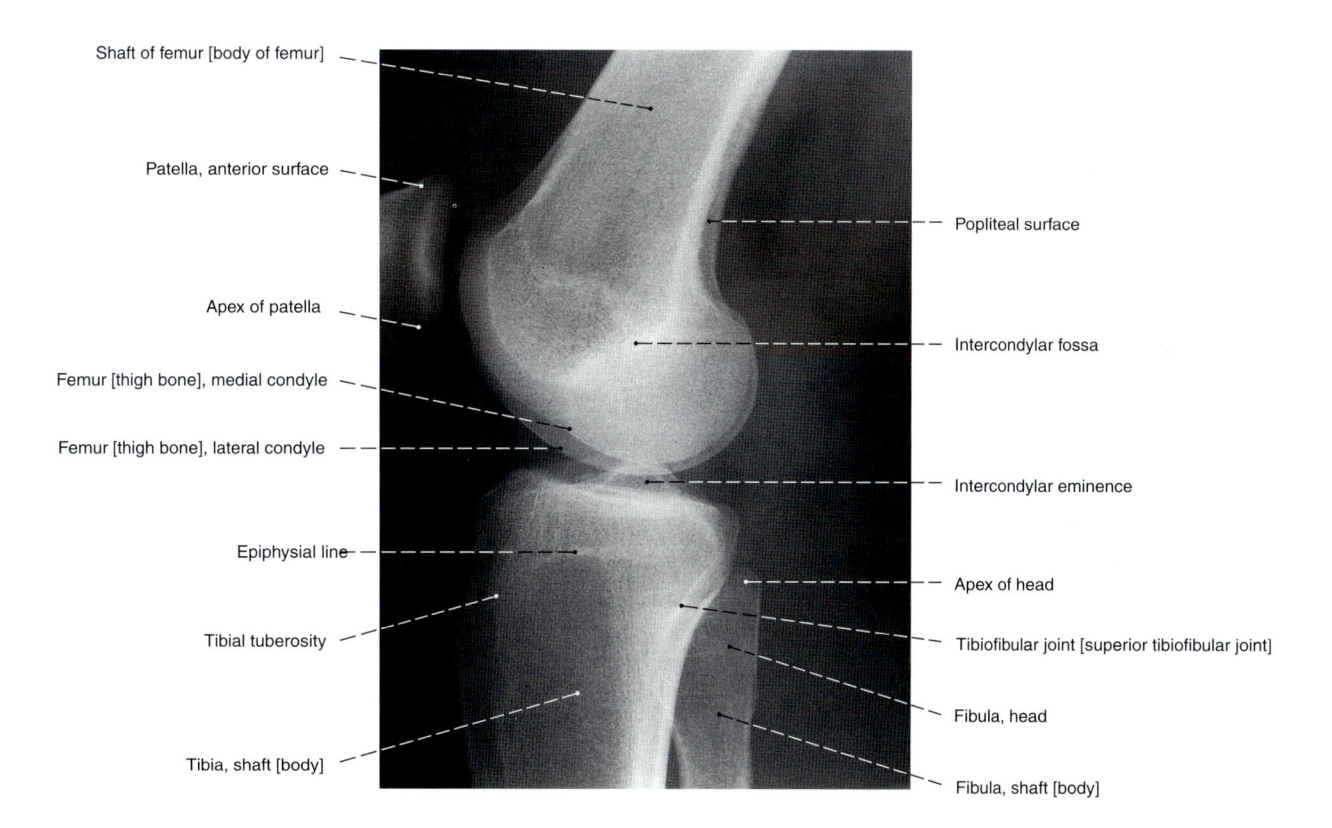

Fig. 1231 Knee joint; lateral radiograph in supine position; central beam directed onto middle of joint.

294　Lower limb

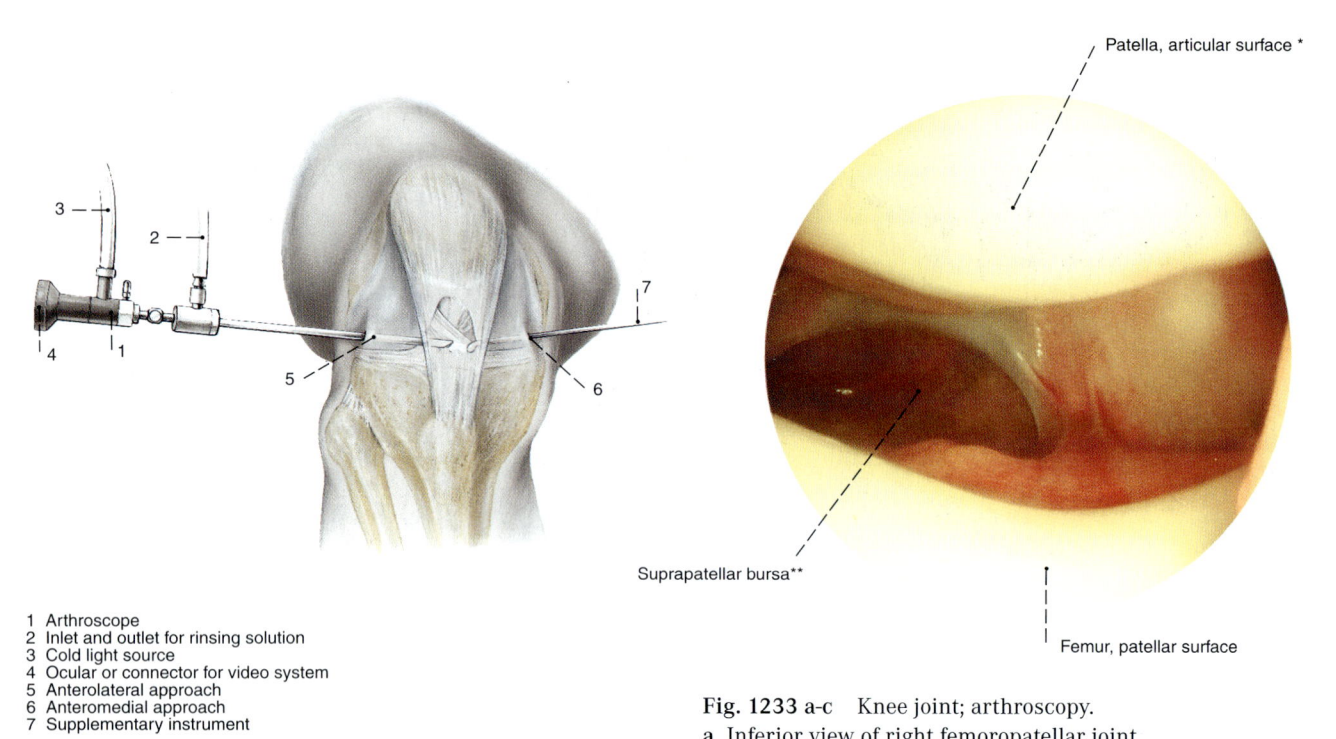

1 Arthroscope
2 Inlet and outlet for rinsing solution
3 Cold light source
4 Ocular or connector for video system
5 Anterolateral approach
6 Anteromedial approach
7 Supplementary instrument

Fig. 1232　Arthroscopic approaches.

Fig. 1233 a-c　Knee joint; arthroscopy.
a Inferior view of right femoropatellar joint
* Patellar roof ridge: roof ridge between medial and lateral articular surface.
** Clinically: suprapatellar recess.

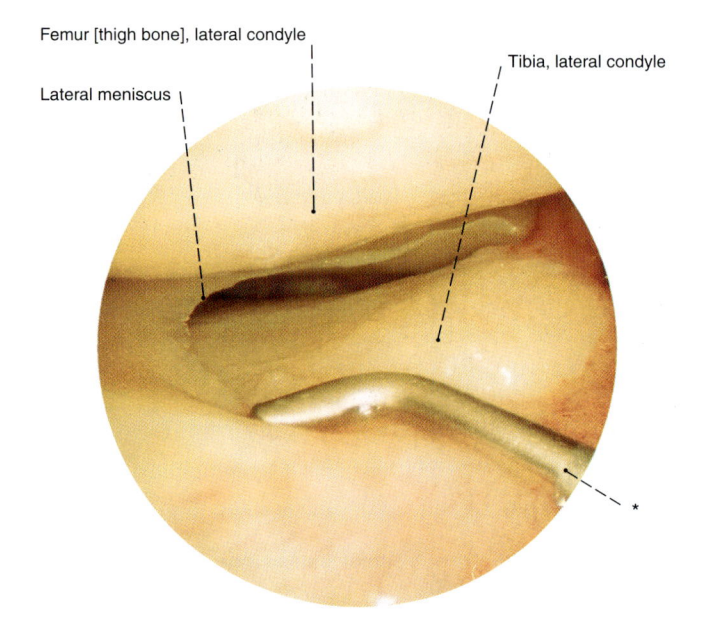

b Medial view of free medial border of right lateral meniscus. The anterior part of the meniscus is depressed by a probing hook (*).

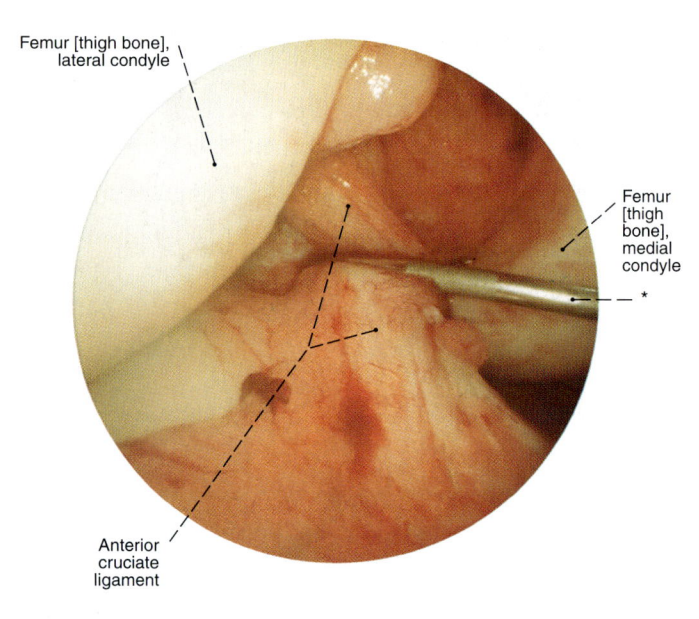

c Anterolateral view of distal part of right anterior cruciate ligament.
The ligament is covered with a rich-vascular synovial membrane [synovial layer]; it is retracted medially by a probing hook (*).

Knee joint

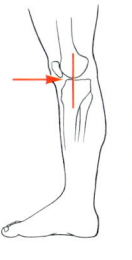

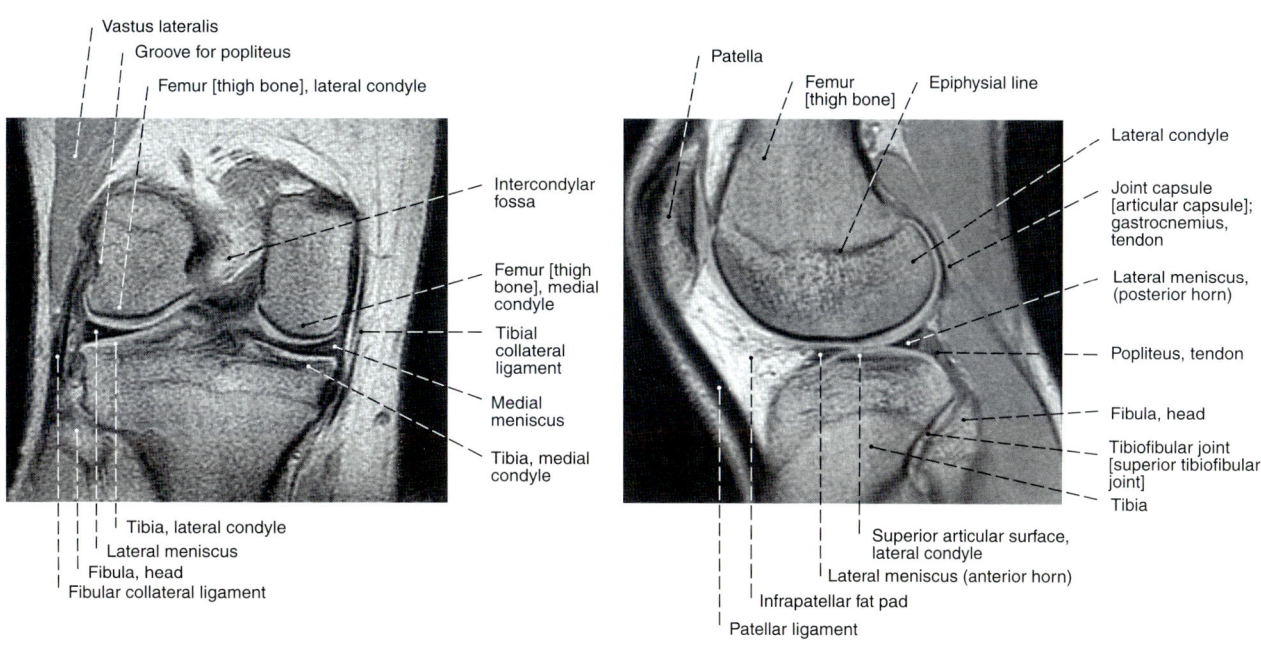

Fig. 1234 Knee joint; magnetic resonance image; frontal section through middle of intercondylar eminence; knee in extension. Compact bone is visualized in black using this MRI technique.

Fig. 1235 Knee joint; magnetic resonance image; sagittal section through lateral part of joint; knee in extension.

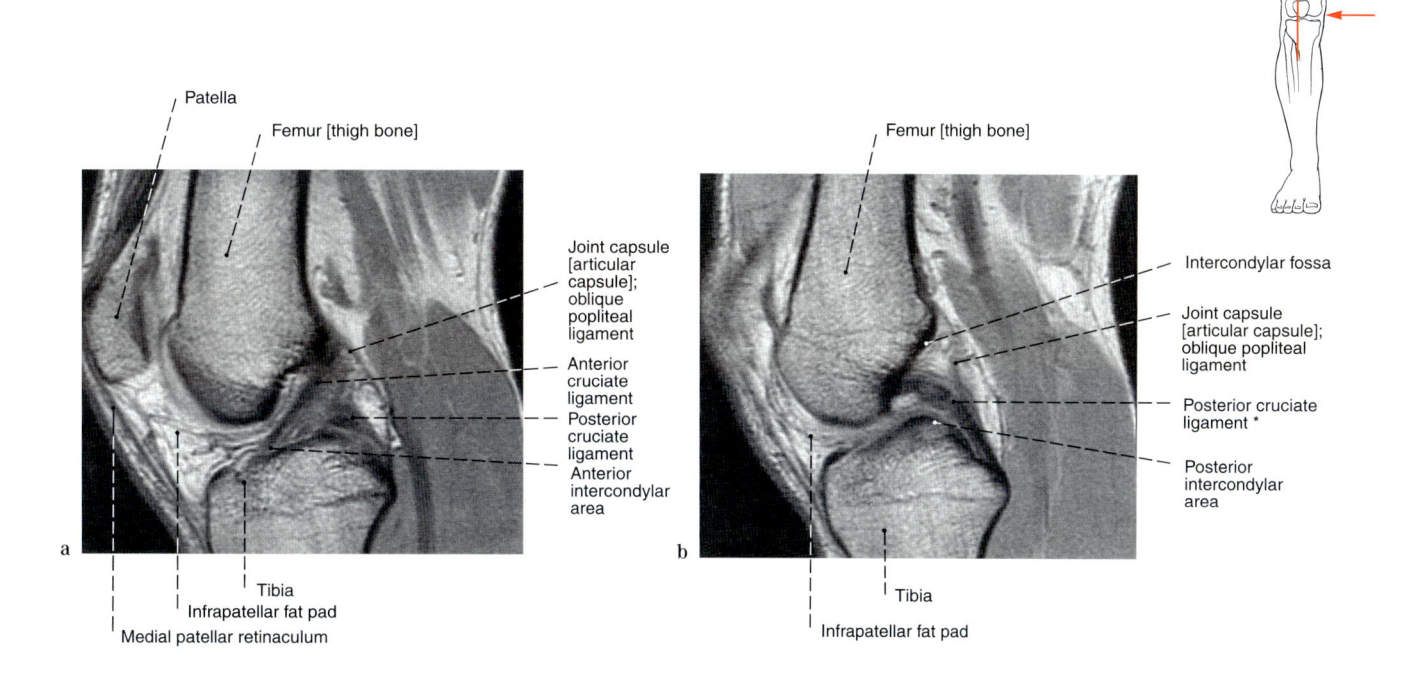

Fig. 1236 a, b Knee joint; magnetic resonance image; sagittal sections; knee in extension.

   a Anterior cruciate ligament
   b Posterior cruciate ligament

* The inhomogeneity is caused by oblique sections of the fiber bundles.

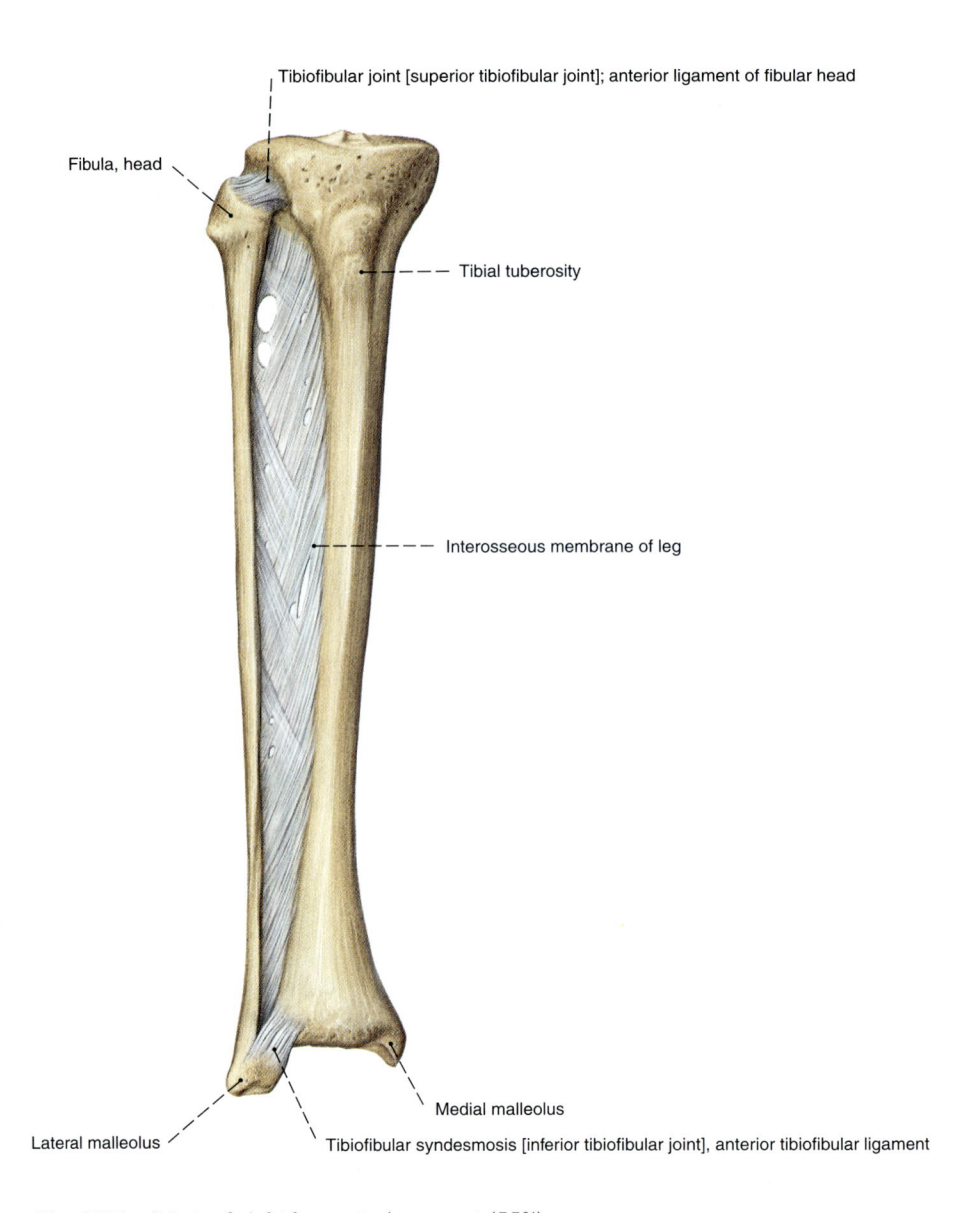

Fig. 1237 Joints of right leg; anterior aspect (55%).

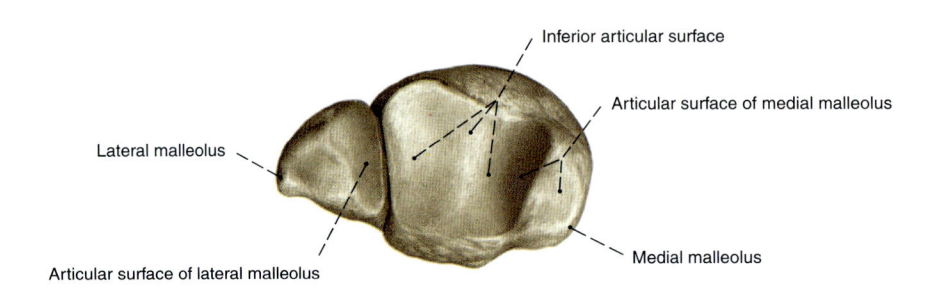

Fig. 1238 Right tibia and fibula; distal aspect (55%).

Bones of foot **297**

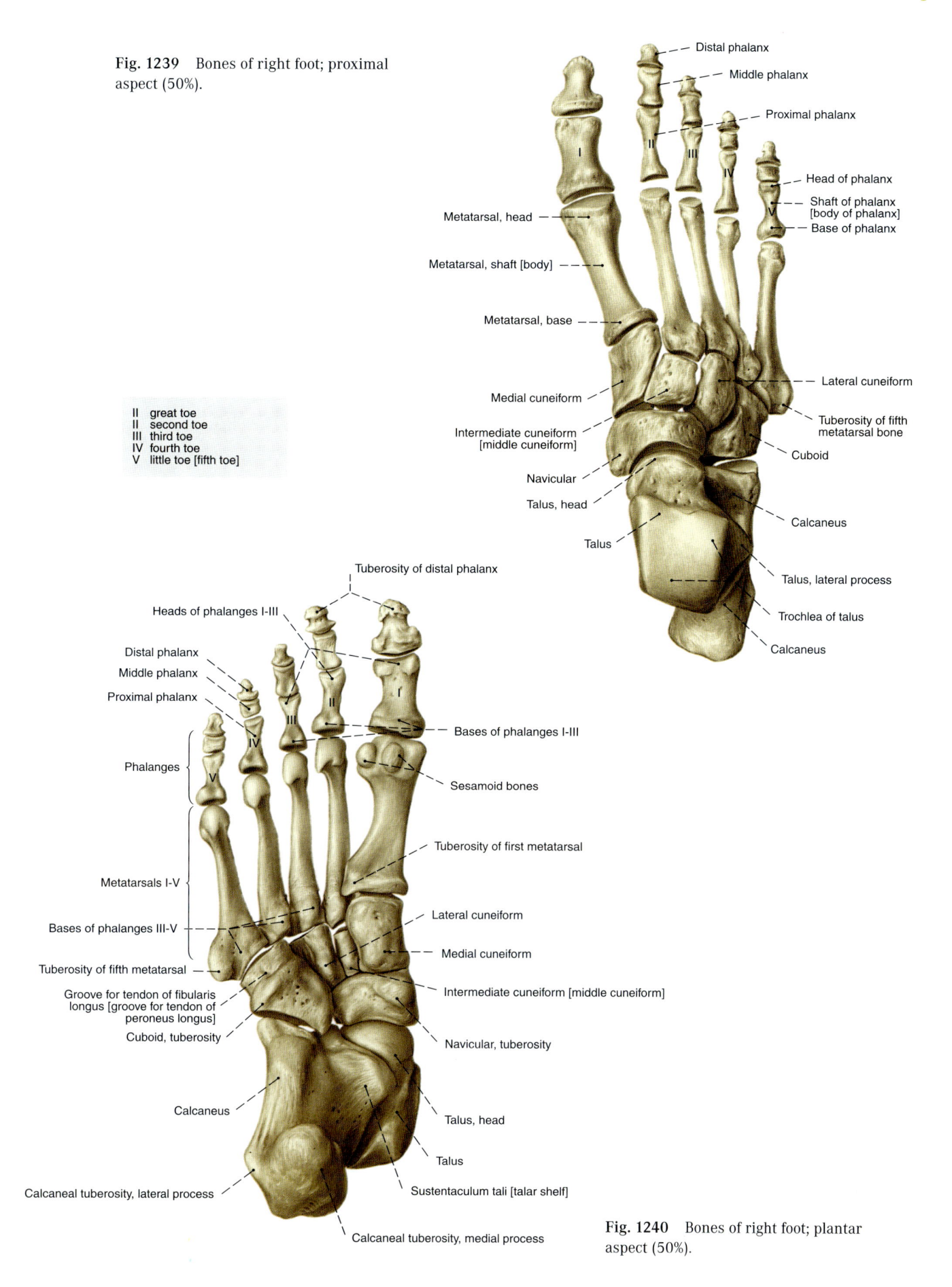

Fig. 1239 Bones of right foot; proximal aspect (50%).

- I great toe
- II second toe
- III third toe
- IV fourth toe
- V little toe [fifth toe]

Labels (Fig. 1239): Distal phalanx; Middle phalanx; Proximal phalanx; Head of phalanx; Shaft of phalanx [body of phalanx]; Base of phalanx; Metatarsal, head; Metatarsal, shaft [body]; Metatarsal, base; Lateral cuneiform; Medial cuneiform; Tuberosity of fifth metatarsal bone; Intermediate cuneiform [middle cuneiform]; Cuboid; Navicular; Talus, head; Calcaneus; Talus; Talus, lateral process; Trochlea of talus; Calcaneus.

Fig. 1240 Bones of right foot; plantar aspect (50%).

Labels (Fig. 1240): Tuberosity of distal phalanx; Heads of phalanges I–III; Distal phalanx; Middle phalanx; Proximal phalanx; Phalanges; Bases of phalanges I–III; Sesamoid bones; Metatarsals I–V; Tuberosity of first metatarsal; Bases of phalanges III–V; Lateral cuneiform; Medial cuneiform; Tuberosity of fifth metatarsal; Intermediate cuneiform [middle cuneiform]; Groove for tendon of fibularis longus [groove for tendon of peroneus longus]; Cuboid, tuberosity; Navicular, tuberosity; Calcaneus; Talus, head; Talus; Calcaneal tuberosity, lateral process; Sustentaculum tali [talar shelf]; Calcaneal tuberosity, medial process.

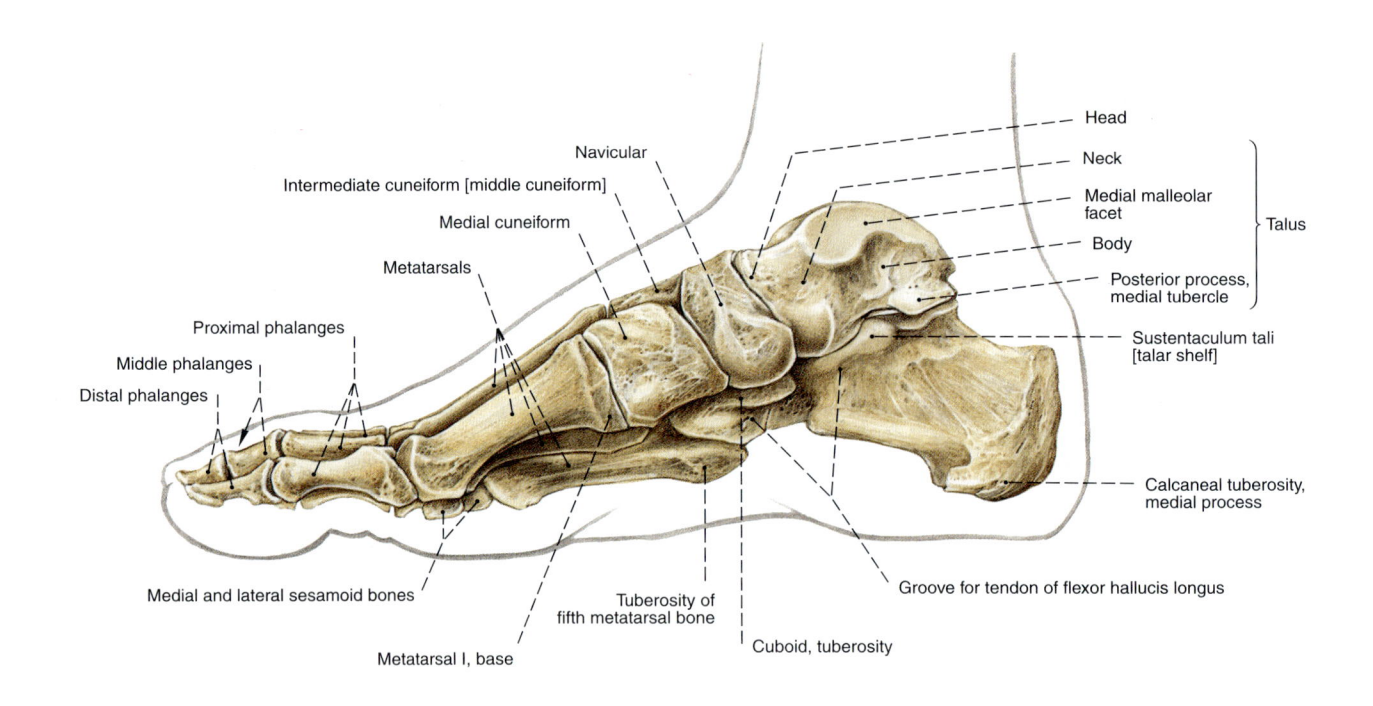

Fig. 1241 Bones of right foot; medial aspect (45%).

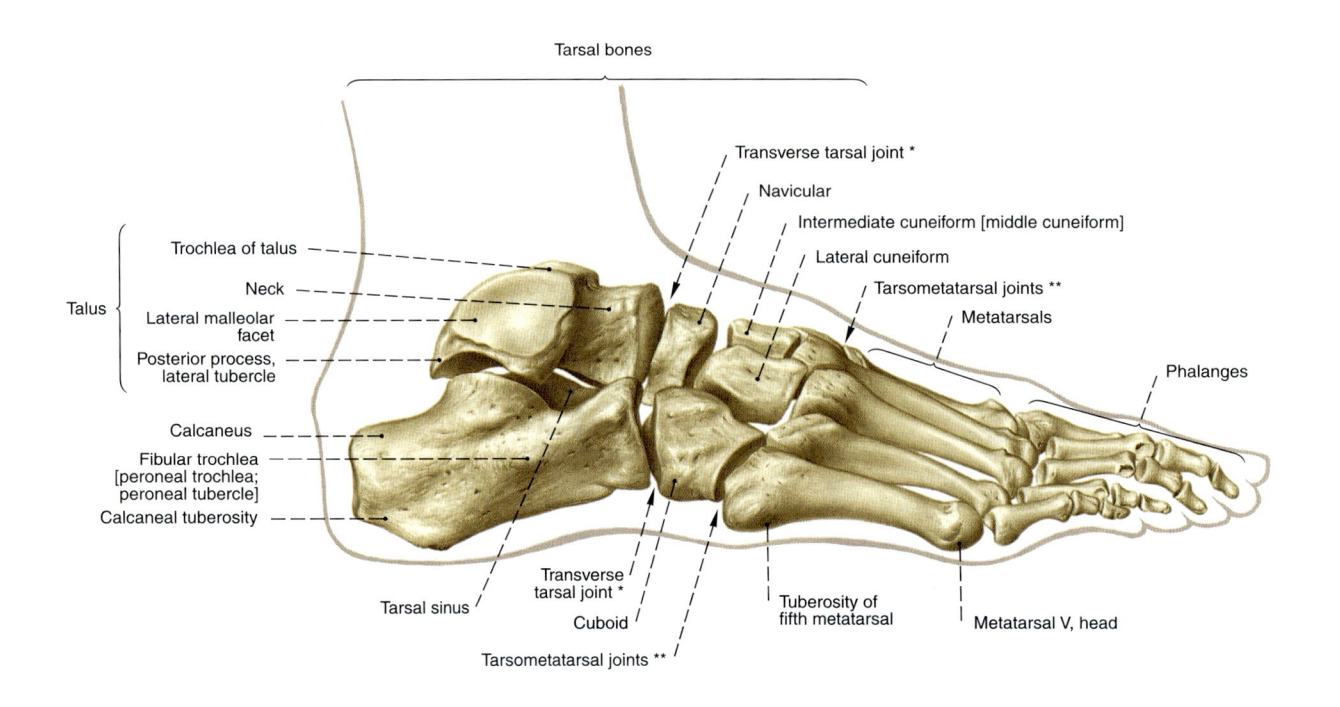

Fig. 1242 Bones of right foot; lateral aspect (45%).
* Also: CHOPART's joint.
** Also: LISFRANC's joint.

Talus and calcaneus

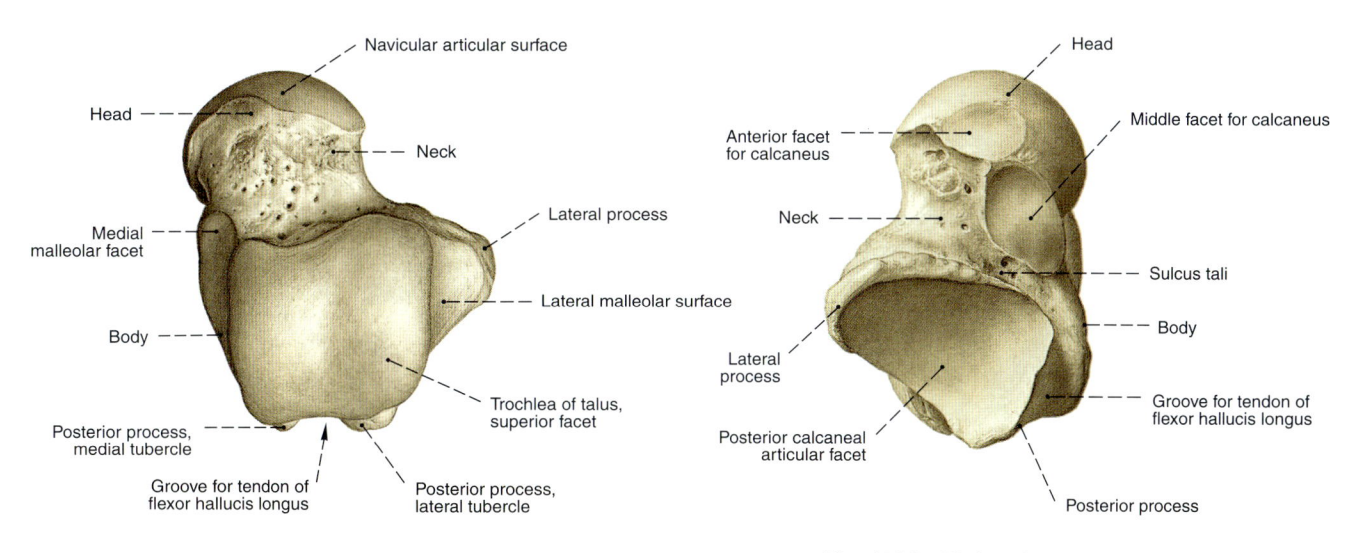

Fig. 1243 Right talus; proximal aspect (85%).

Fig. 1244 Right talus; plantar aspect (85%).

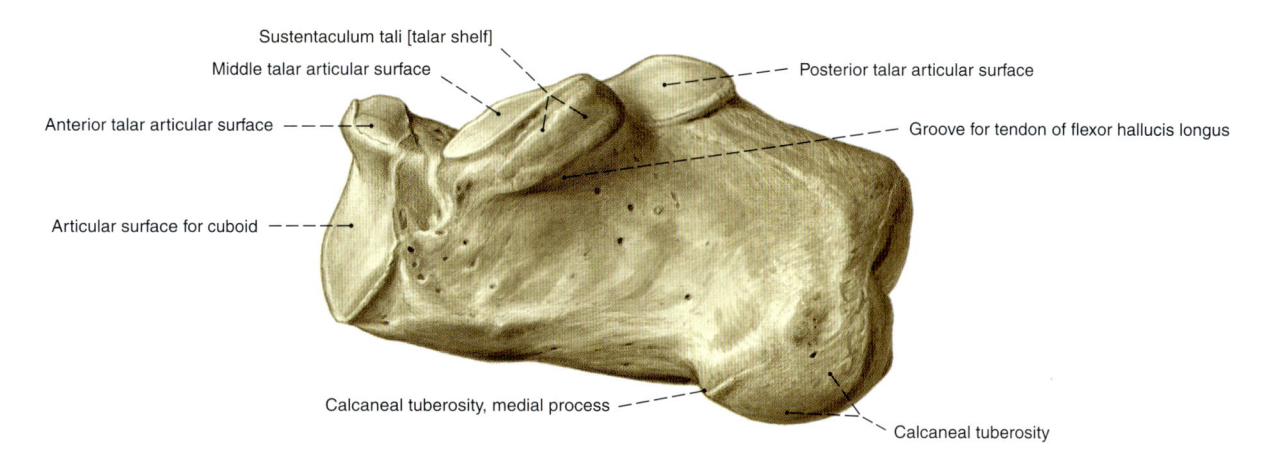

Fig. 1245 Right calcaneus; medial aspect (90%).

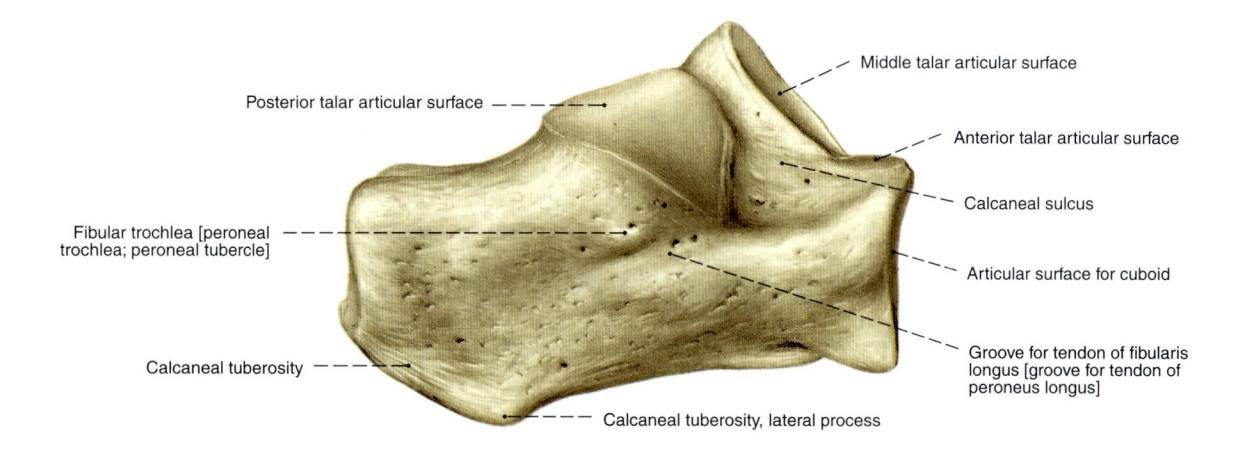

Fig. 1246 Right calcaneus; lateral aspect (90%).

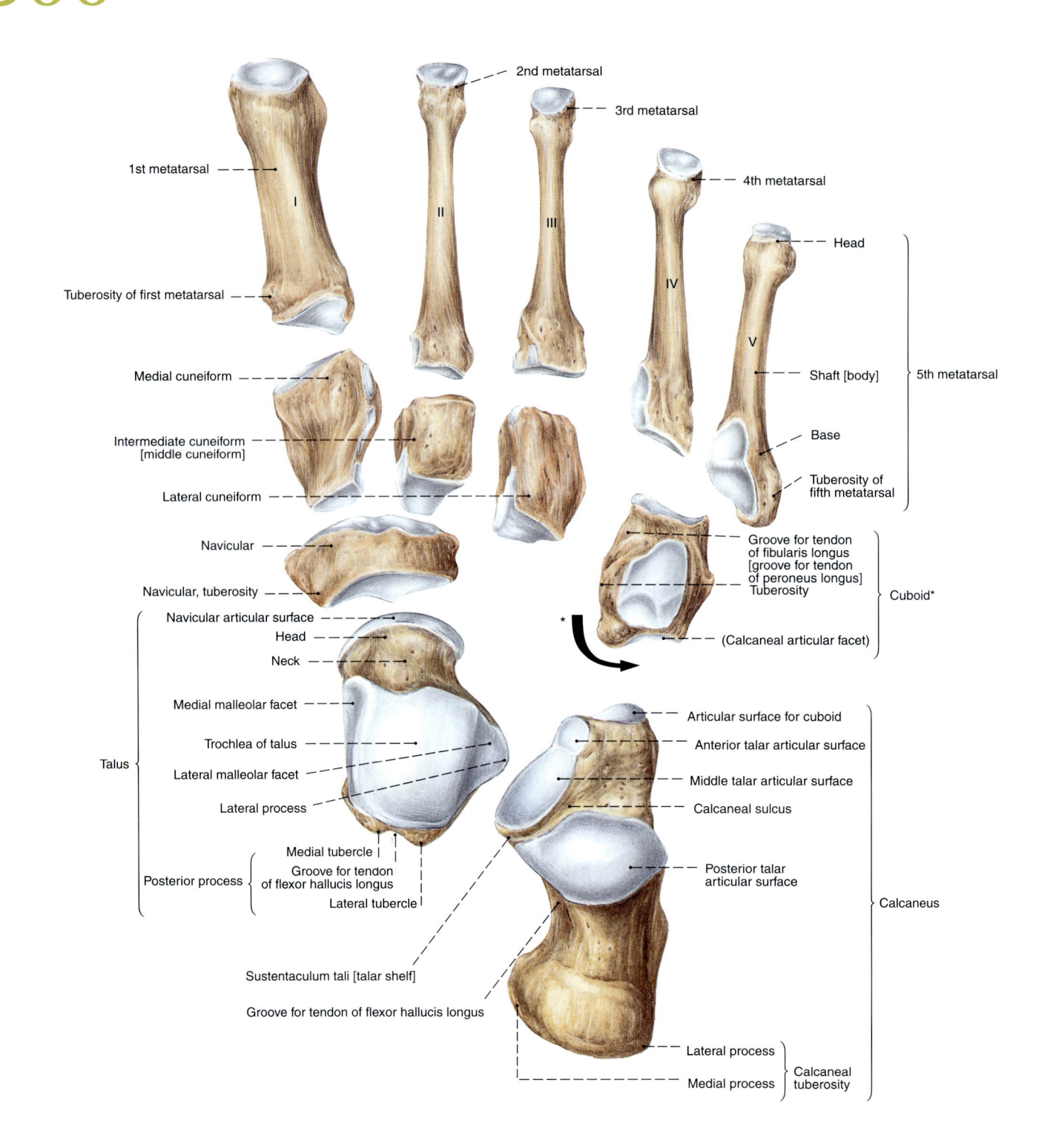

Fig. 1247 Tarsal bones and metatarsals of right foot; distances between bones increased for didactic reasons; proximal aspect (80%).

* The cuboid is shown from the medial aspect.

Bones of foot

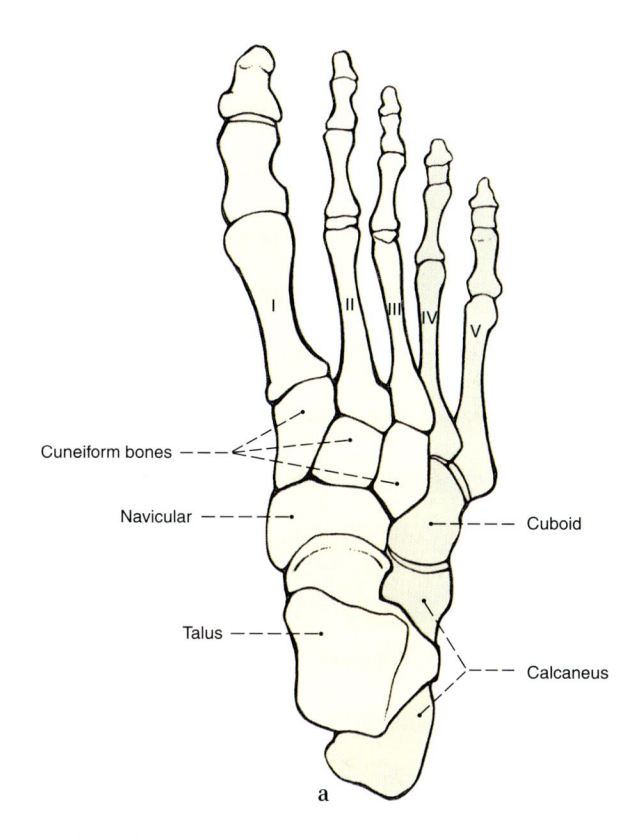

Fig. 1248 a, b Bones of right foot; arrangement of bones.
a Proximal aspect
b Plantar aspect

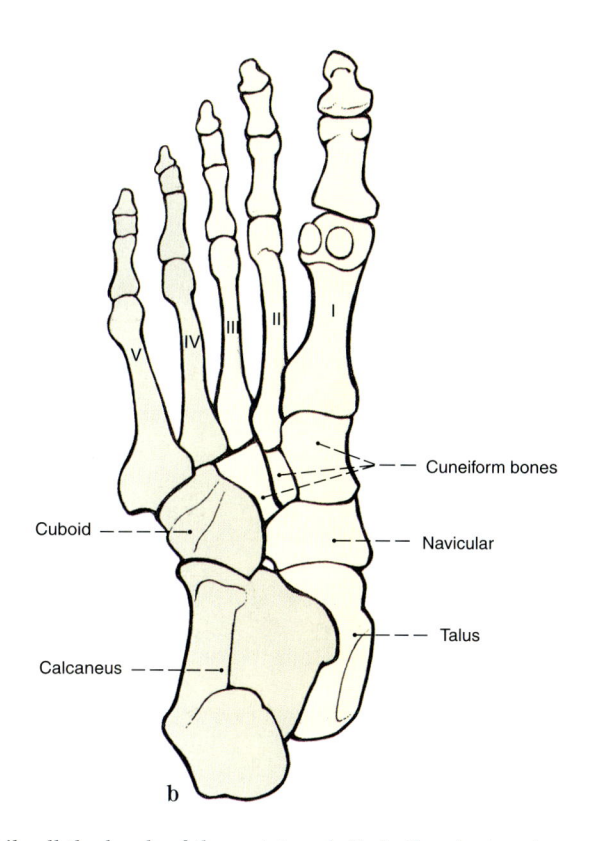

While all the heads of the metatarsals lie in the plantar plane, the cuneiform bones, the navicular, and the talus lie more and more dorsally above the lateral skeletal parts, so that the talus lies over the calcaneus. Thus, the longitudinal arch is formed on the medial side.

The wedge-shaped cross-section of the cuneiform bones and the bases of the metatarsals create the formation of the transverse arch.

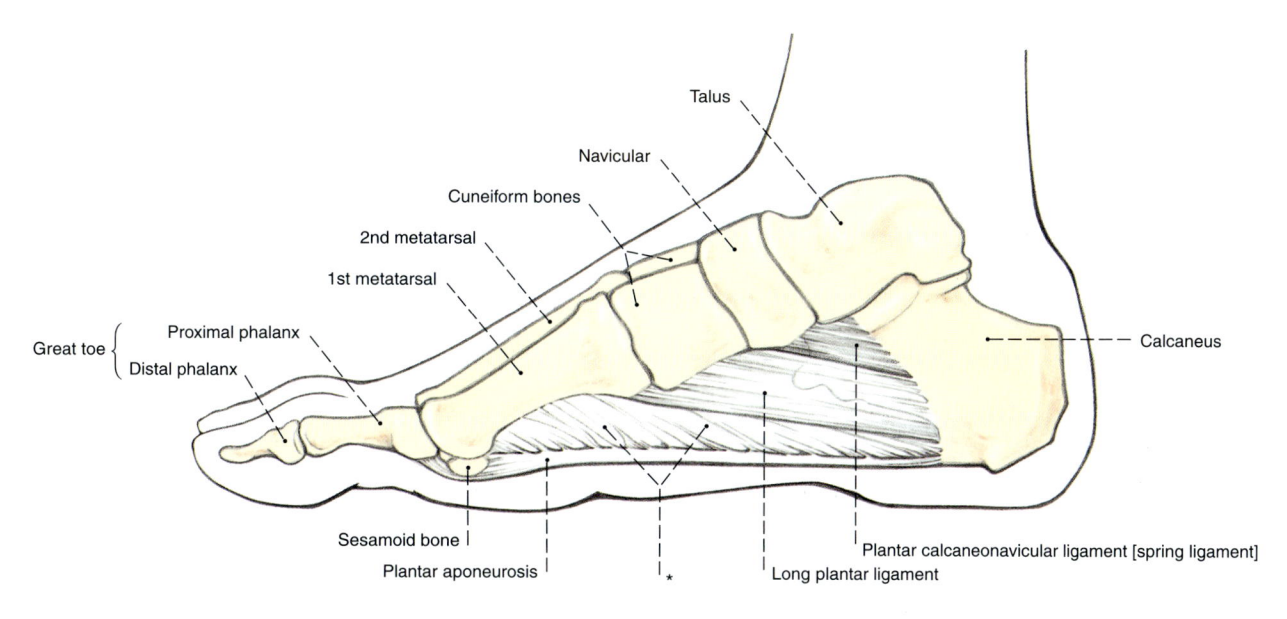

Fig. 1249 Bracing of the medial longitudinal arch of the right foot; medial aspect.
*Medial intermuscular septum.

The shown longitudinal ligamentous structures brace the longitudinal arch passively. These ligaments are supported by the short muscles of the foot.

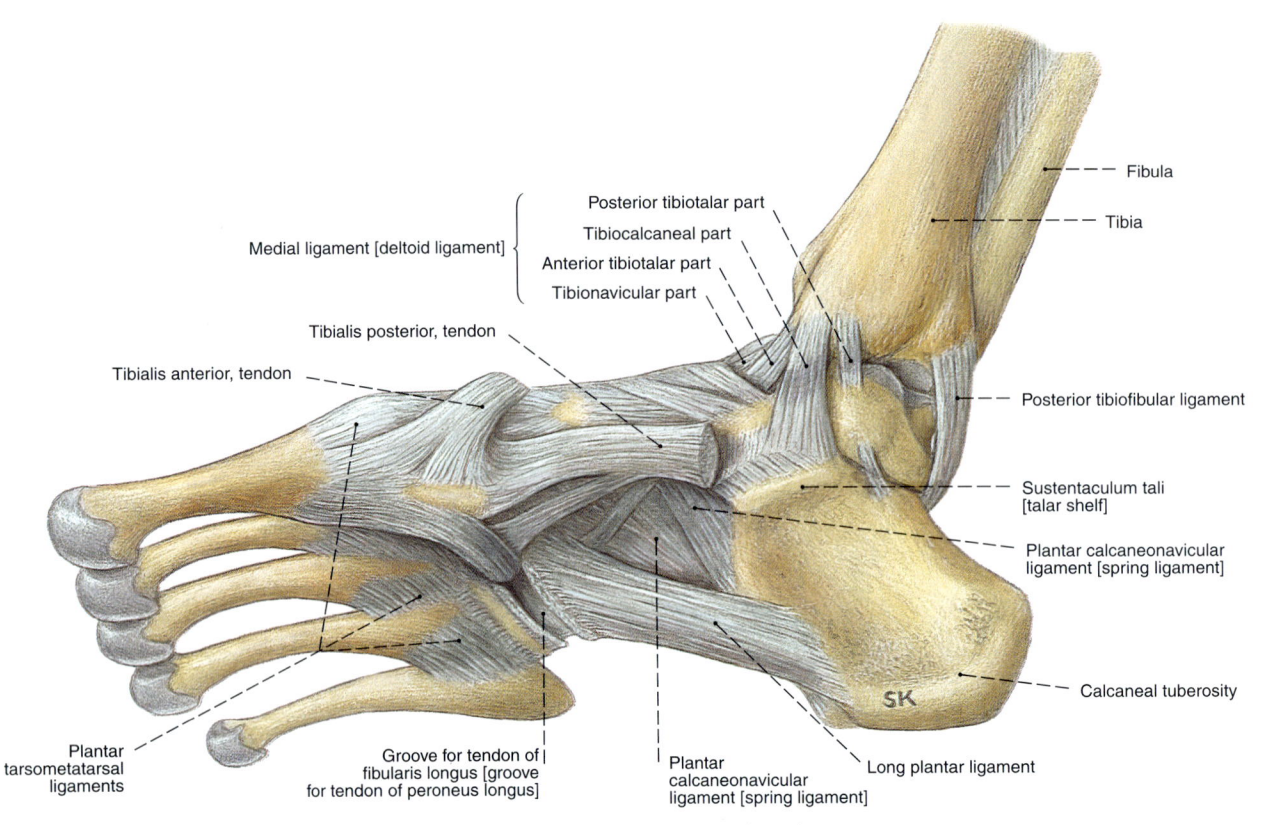

Fig. 1250 Joints of right foot; ligaments and tendons of tarsus and ankle joint; medial aspect (70%).

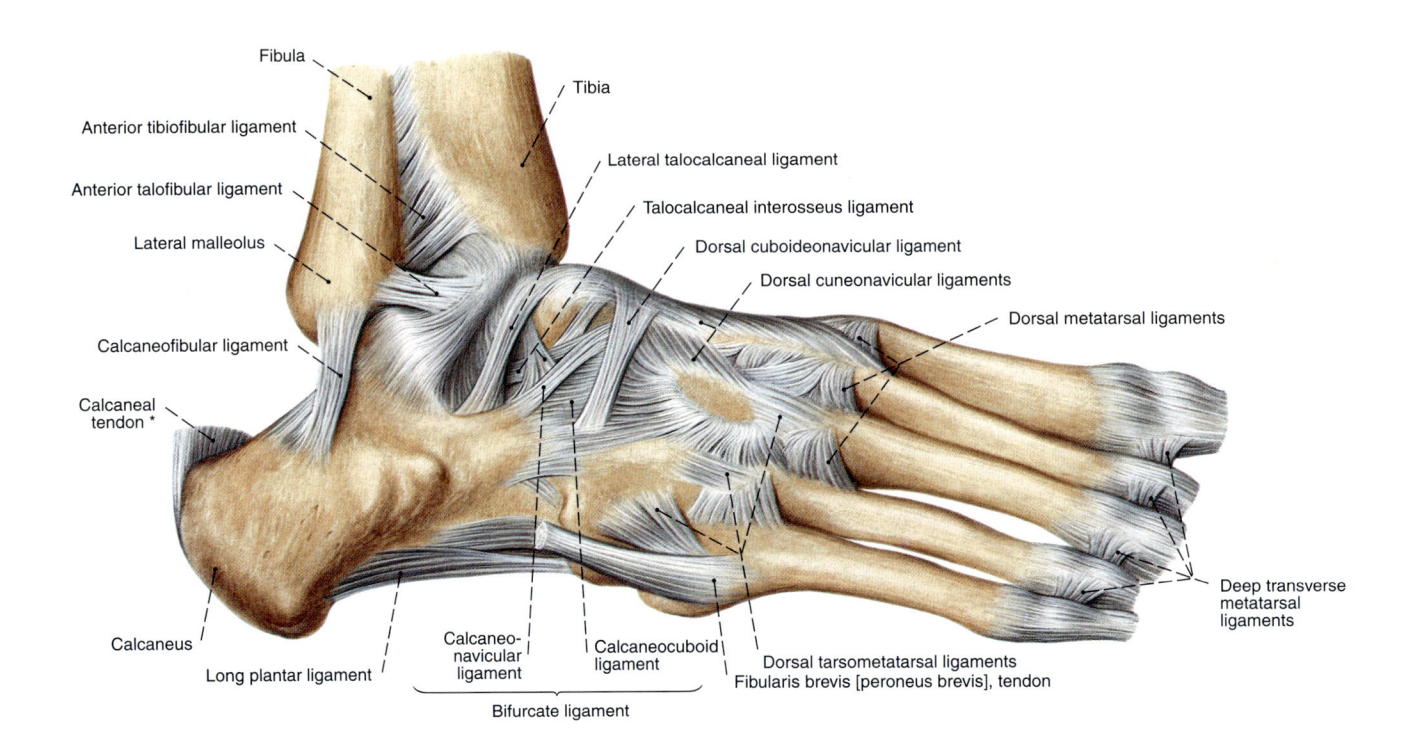

Fig. 1251 Joints of right foot; ligaments and tendons of tarsus and metatarsus; lateral aspect (70%).
*Also ACHILLES tendon.

Joints of foot 303

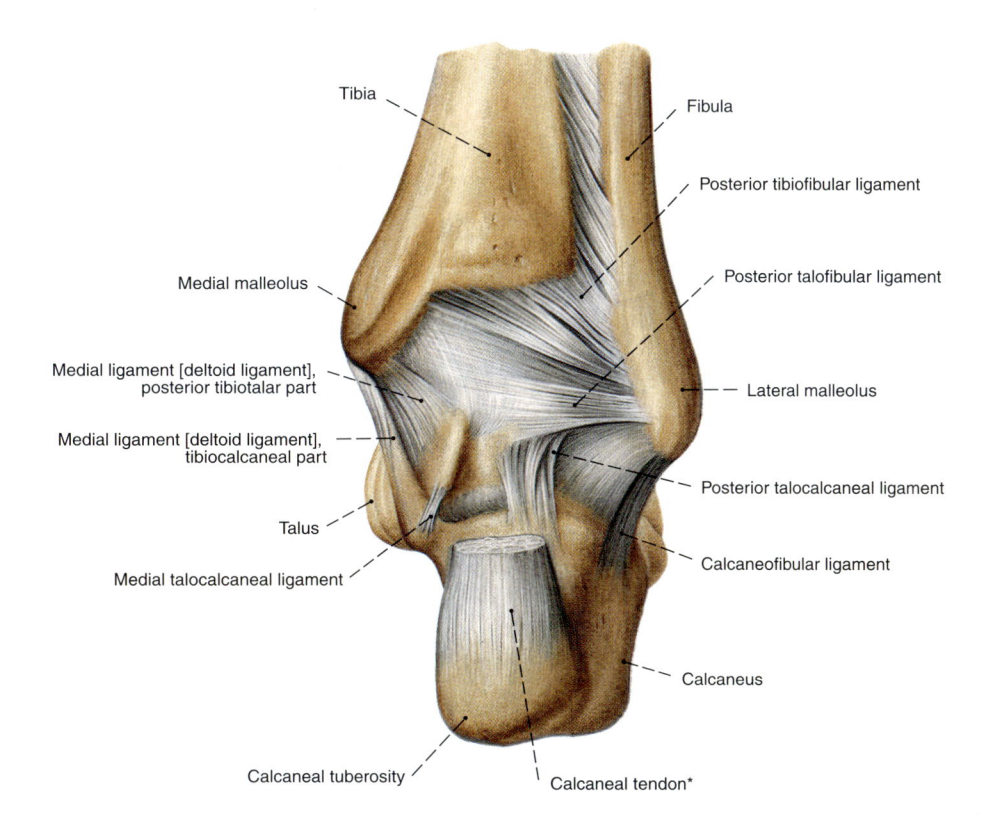

Fig. 1252 Joints of right foot; ligaments and tendons of tarsus; posterior aspect (70%).
*Also ACHILLES tendon.

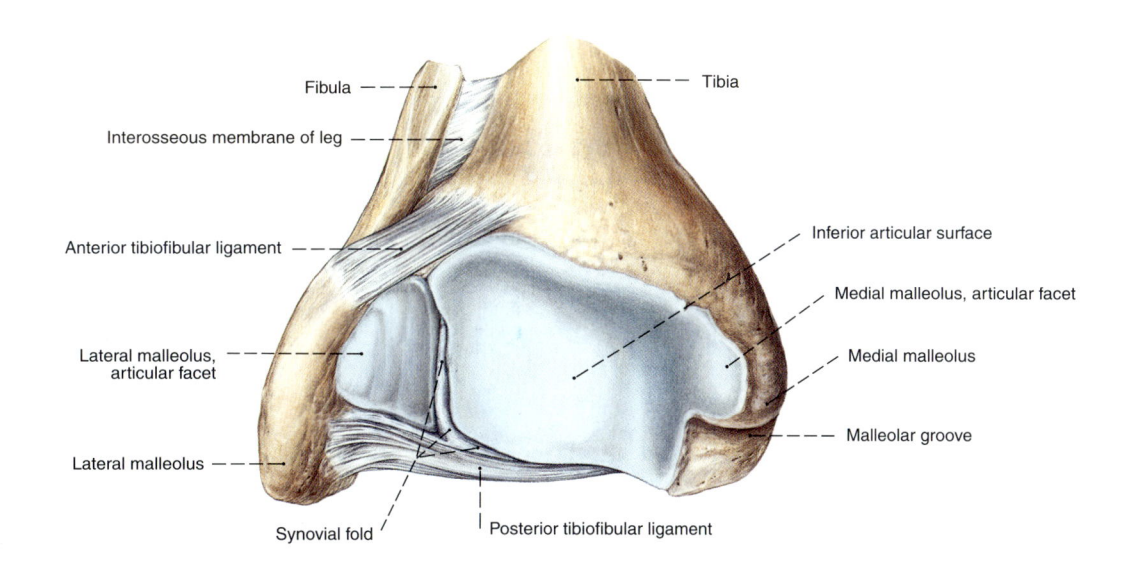

Fig. 1253 Right ankle joint; proximal articular surfaces; distal aspect (120%).

Lower limb

Fig. 1254 Joints of right foot; plantar aspect (55%).
* The long plantar ligament closes the groove, creating a canal for tendon of fibularis [peroneus] longus.

Fig. 1255 Joints of right foot; ligaments and tendons of tarsus and metatarsus; plantar aspect (55%).

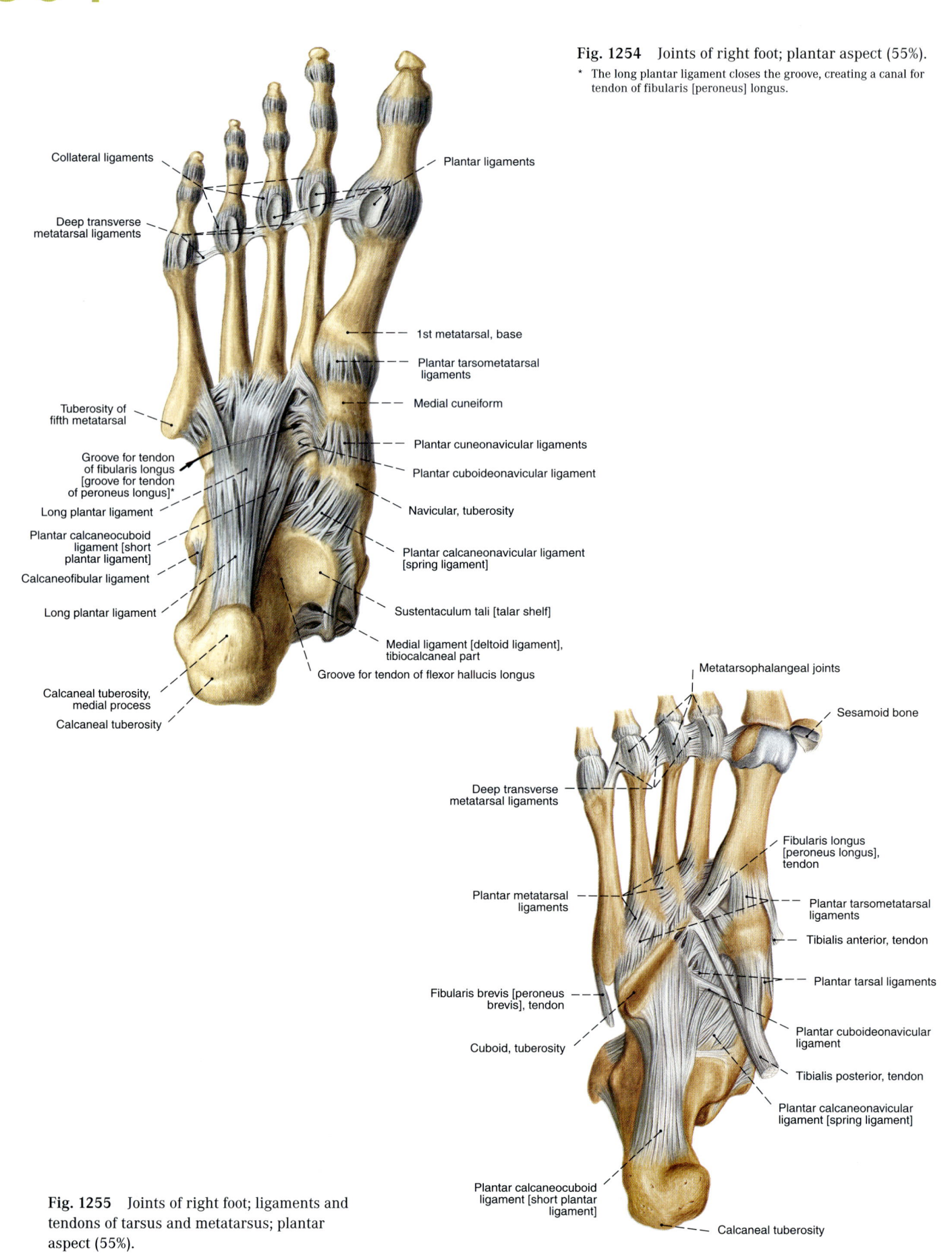

Joints of foot 305

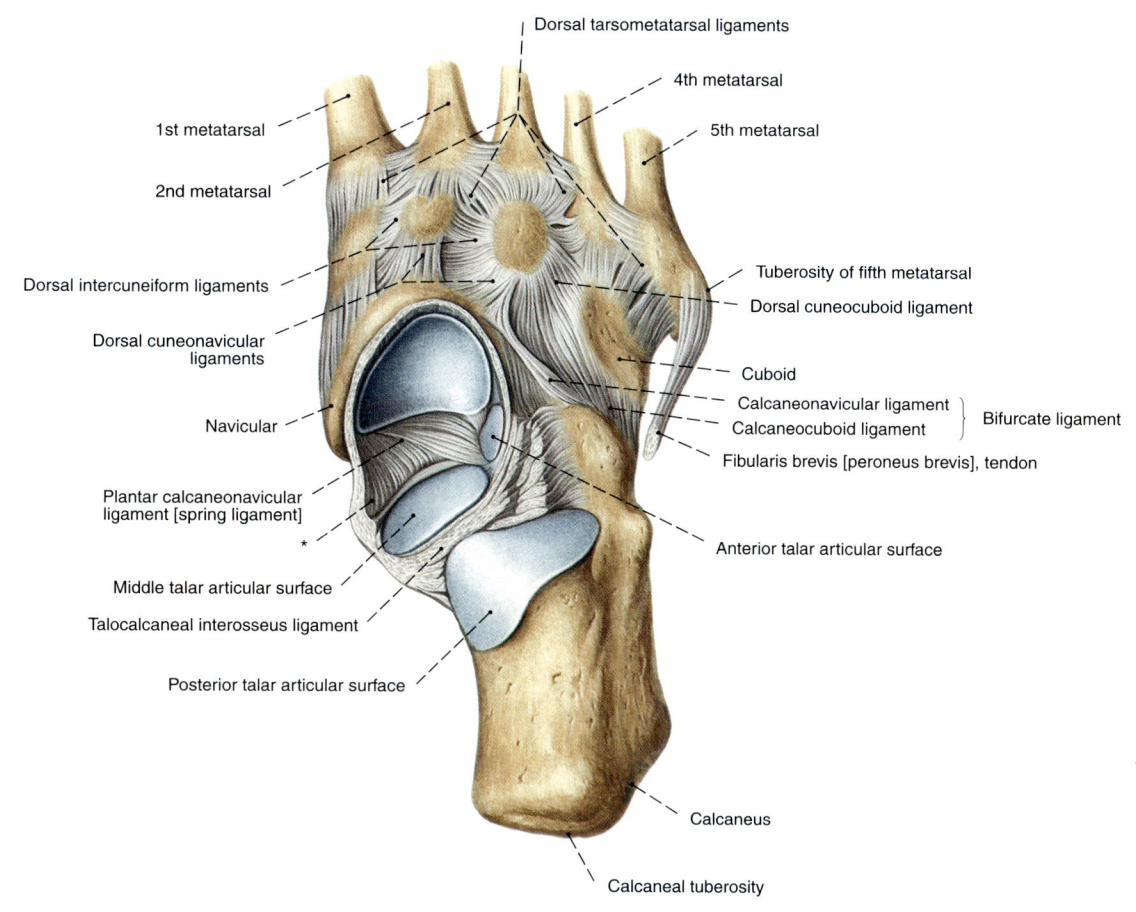

Fig. 1256 Joints of right foot; subtalar [talocalcaneal] and talocalcaneonavicular joints disarticulated; proximal aspect (70%).
* See Fig. 1257.

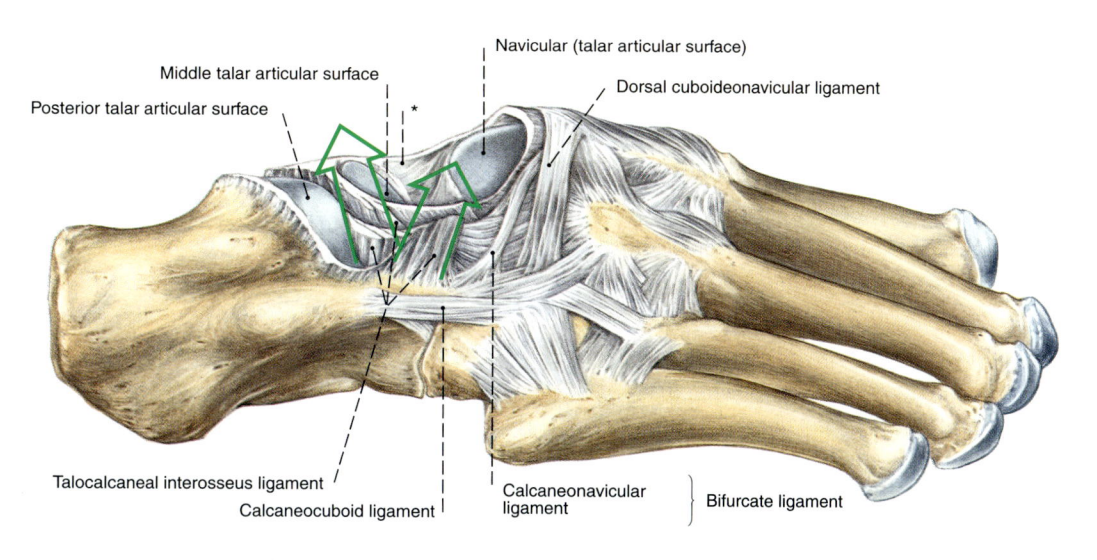

Fig. 1257 Subtalar [talocalcaneal] and talocalcaneonavicular joints of right foot; talus and lateral ligaments removed; lateral aspect (70%).
The two arrows indicate the torsion of the talocalcaneal interosseus ligament.

* Sheet of dense connective tissue between the plantar calcaneonavicular ligament [spring ligament] and the tibionavicular part of the medial ligament [deltoid ligament] that opposes the medially directed shearing force of the head of talus.
Weakening of this sheet causes flattening of the medial longitudinal arch (flatfoot; splayfoot; talipes planus).

306　Lower limb

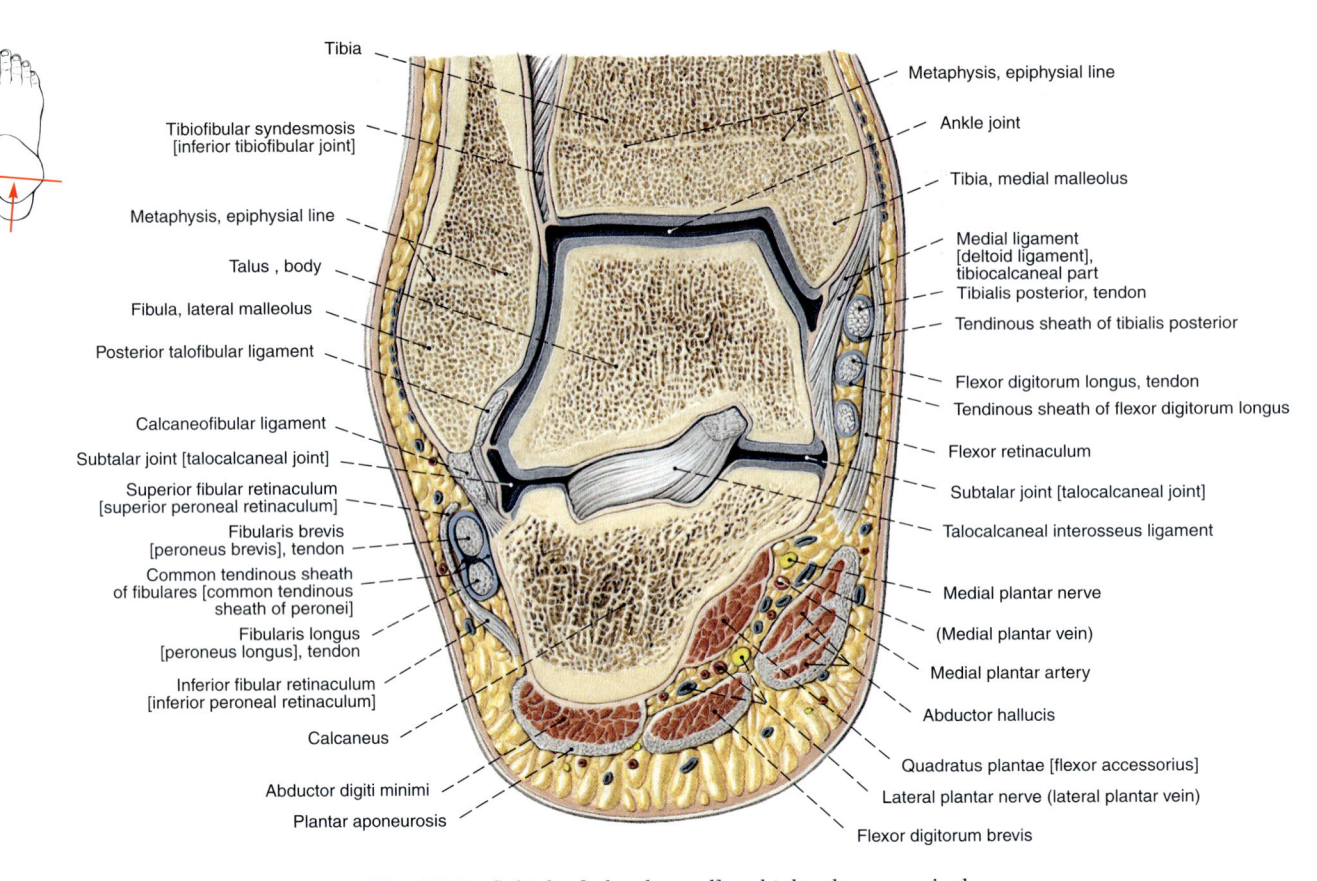

Fig. 1258　Subtalar [talocalcaneal] and talocalcaneonavicular joints of right foot; frontal section through malleoli distal aspect (90%).
* See Fig. 1257.

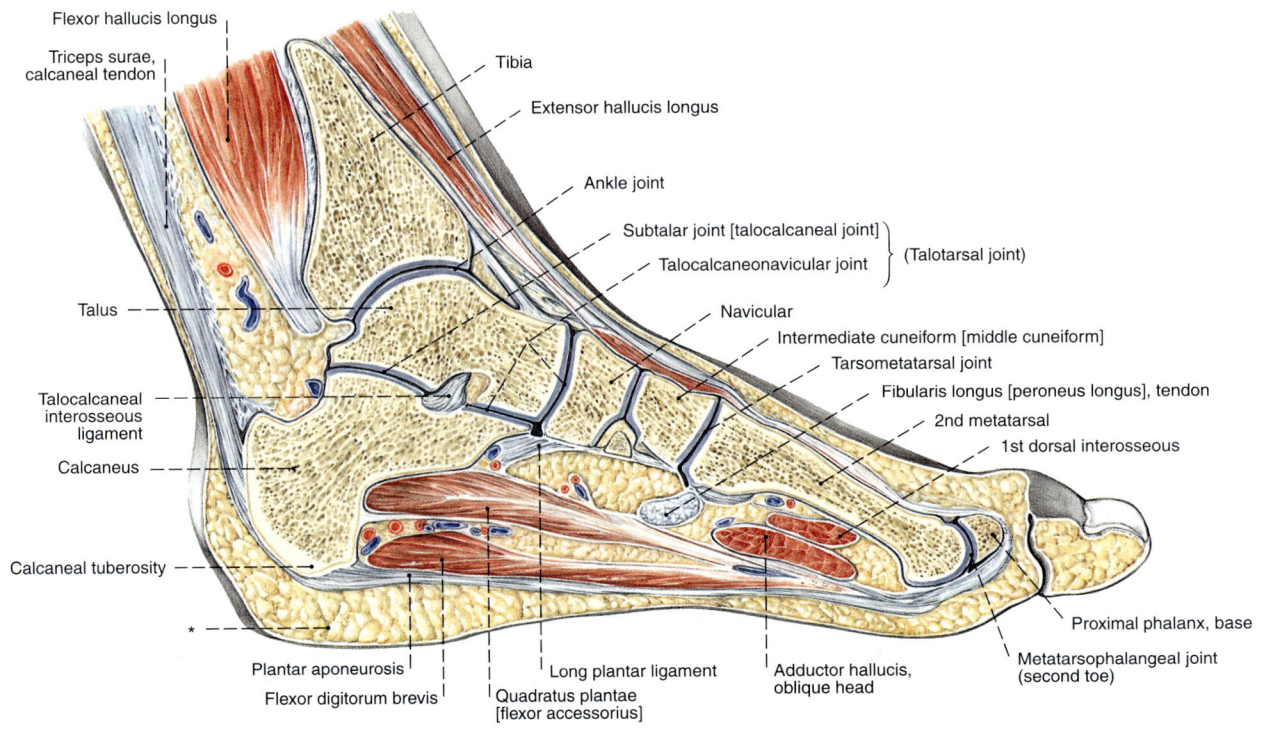

Fig. 1259　Subtalar [talocalcaneal] and talocalcaneonavicular joints of right foot; sagittal section through middle of trochlea of talus; lateral aspect (50%).

* Calcaneal fat pad.

Subtalar [talocalcaneal] and talocalcaneonavicular joints

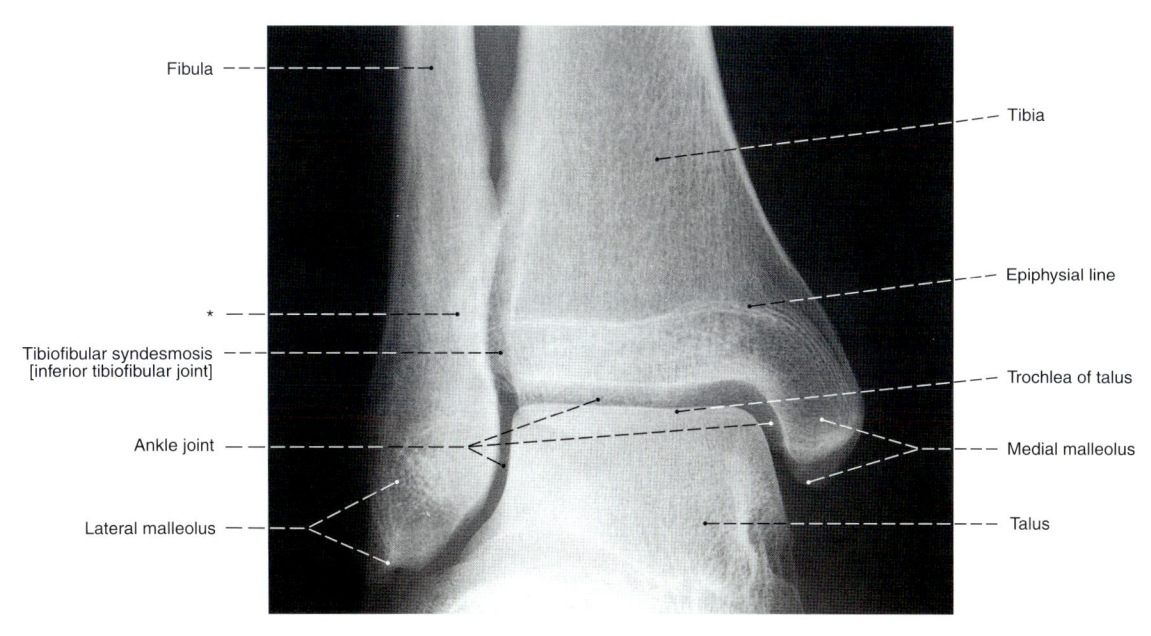

Fig. 1260 Ankle and talocalcaneonavicular joints; AP radiograph in supine position; central beam directed tangential to the trochlea of talus.

* Clinically the posterior border of the fibular notch is also called third malleolus.

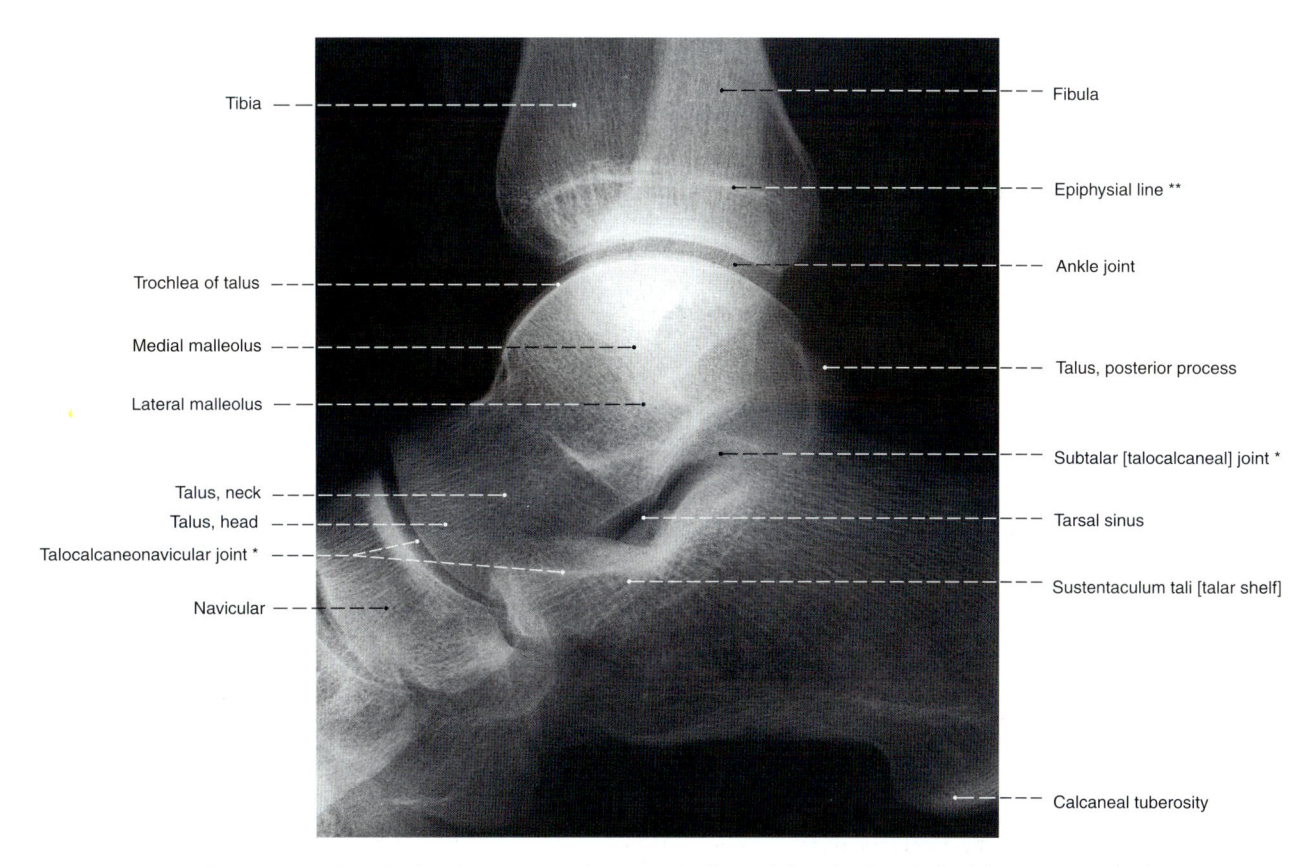

Fig. 1261 Subtalar [talocalcaneal] and talocalcaneonavicular joints; lateral radiograph in supine position; central beam directed onto the top of the trochlea of talus.

* Due to their torsion the articular clefts are not viewed orthogonally.
** Superposition of epiphysial lines of tibia and fibula.

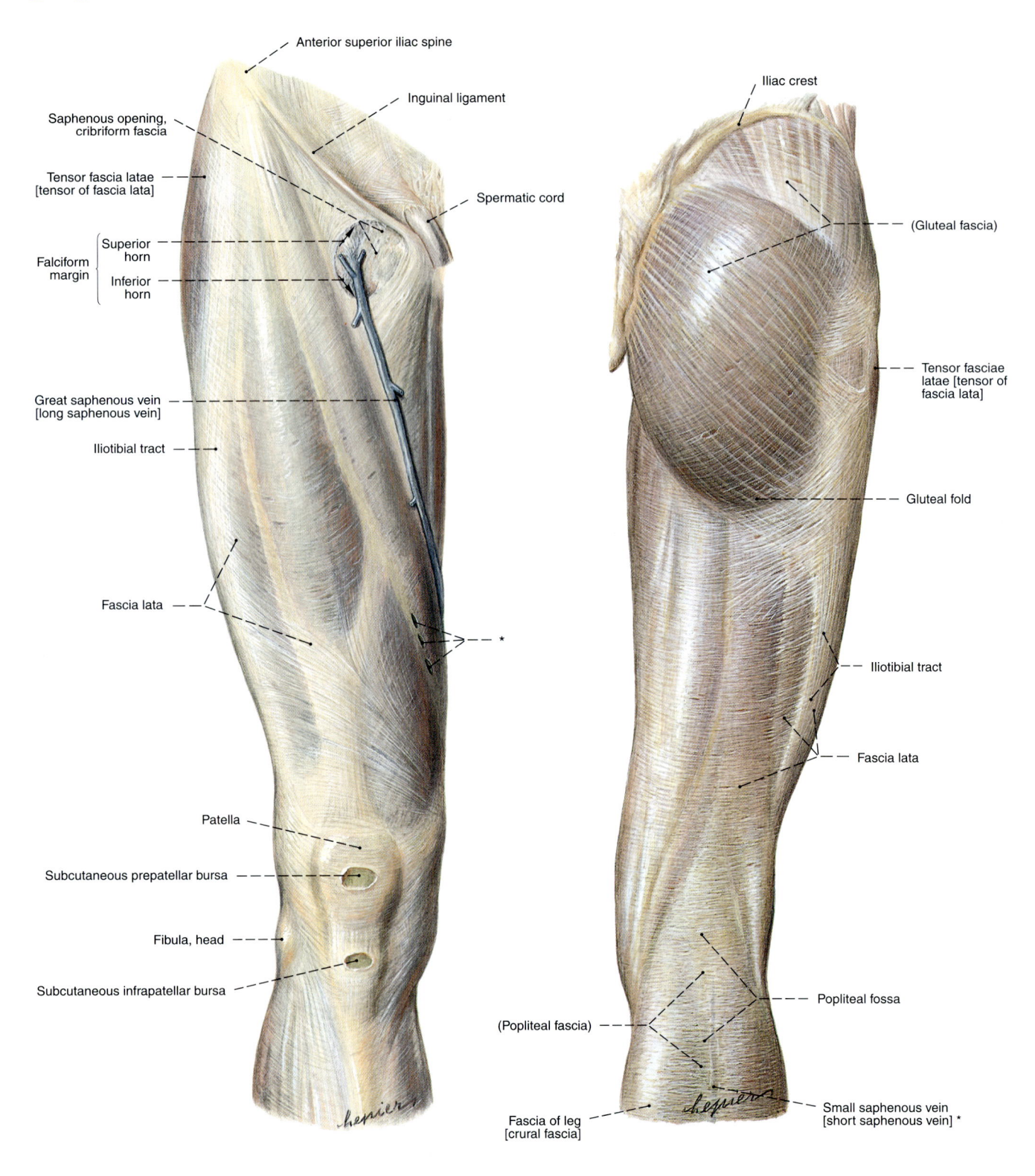

Fig. 1262 Fascia lata of right thigh; anterior aspect.
The transition zone between the aponeurosis of the external oblique and the fascia lata is called inguinal ligament. This ligament is attached laterally to the anterior superior iliac spine and medially to the pubic tubercle.

* Openings for perforating veins (DODD's veins).

Fig. 1263 Fascia lata of right thigh; posterior aspect.

* Sub- or intrafascial course of small saphenous vein [short saphenous vein].

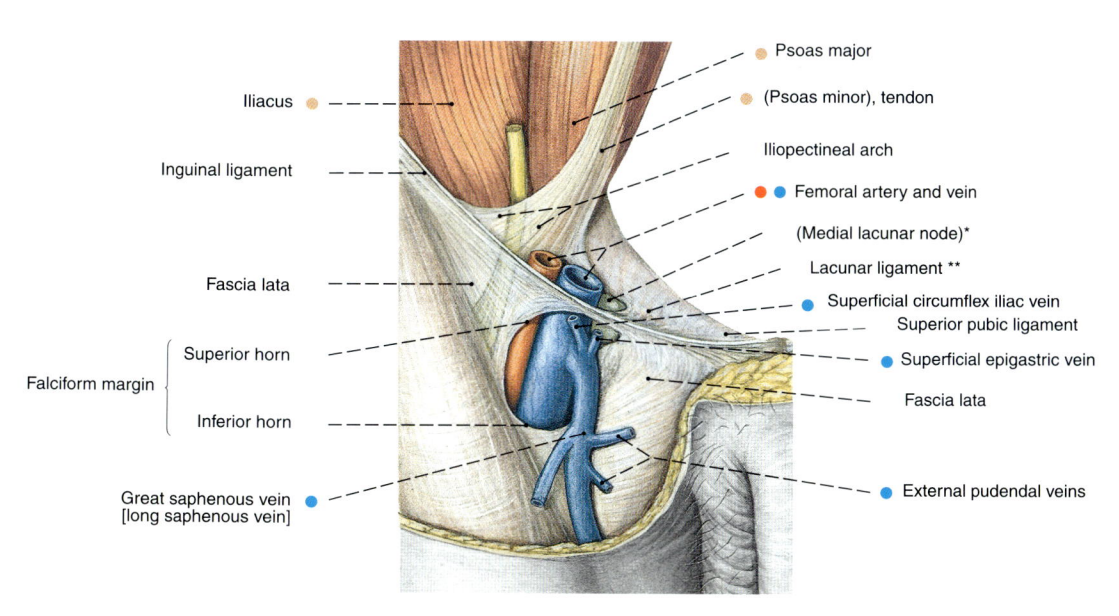

Saphenous opening, muscular and vascular spaces

Fig. 1264 Right saphenous opening and vascular space; anterior abdominal wall, contents of abdomen, iliac fascia, and femoral septum (CLOQUET's septum) removed; anterior aspect.

* Also: ROSNEMUELLER'S gland [node].
** Also: GIMBERNAT's ligament.

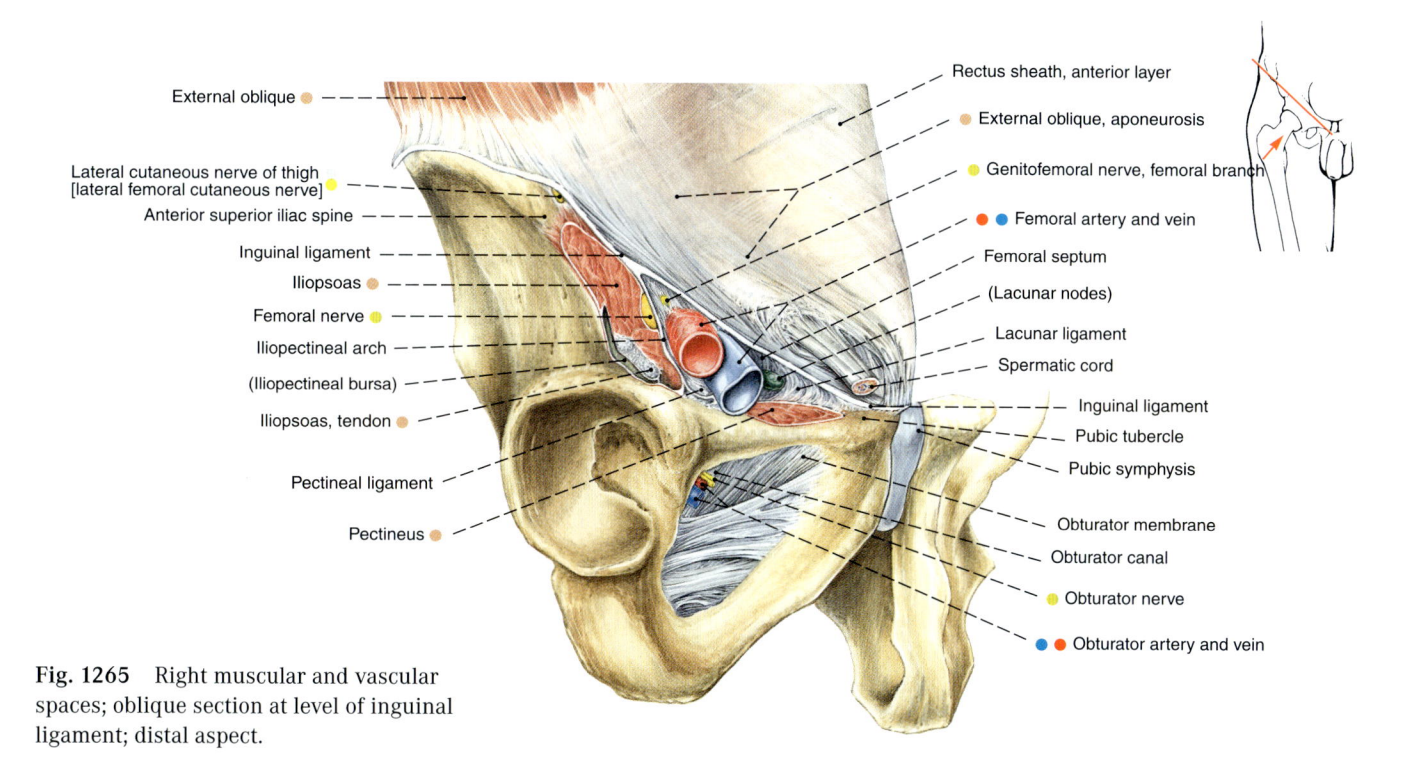

Fig. 1265 Right muscular and vascular spaces; oblique section at level of inguinal ligament; distal aspect.

Muscular and vascular spaces of the groin [inguinal region]

The space beneath the inguinal ligament is divided into two passage spaces by the iliopectineal arch. Lateral to this arch lies the muscular space, medial the vascular space. Through the muscular space pass the iliopsoas, the lateral cutaneous nerve of thigh [lateral femoral cutaneous nerve], and the femoral nerve to reach the thigh. In the vascular space are the femoral artery and vein, the femoral branch of genitofemoral nerve, and the lacunar nodes (lateral, medial, and intermediate), as well as lymphatic vessels. The space between the femoral vein (lateral), the sharp-edged lacunar ligament (medial), the inguinal ligament (ventral), and the pectineal ligament (dorsal) is filled with loose connective tissue, the femoral septum (CLOQUETS' s septum) and is also called femoral ring or femoral canal.

Here a femoral hernia may develop; the femoral ring then becomes the inner and the saphenous opening the outer opening of the hernia.

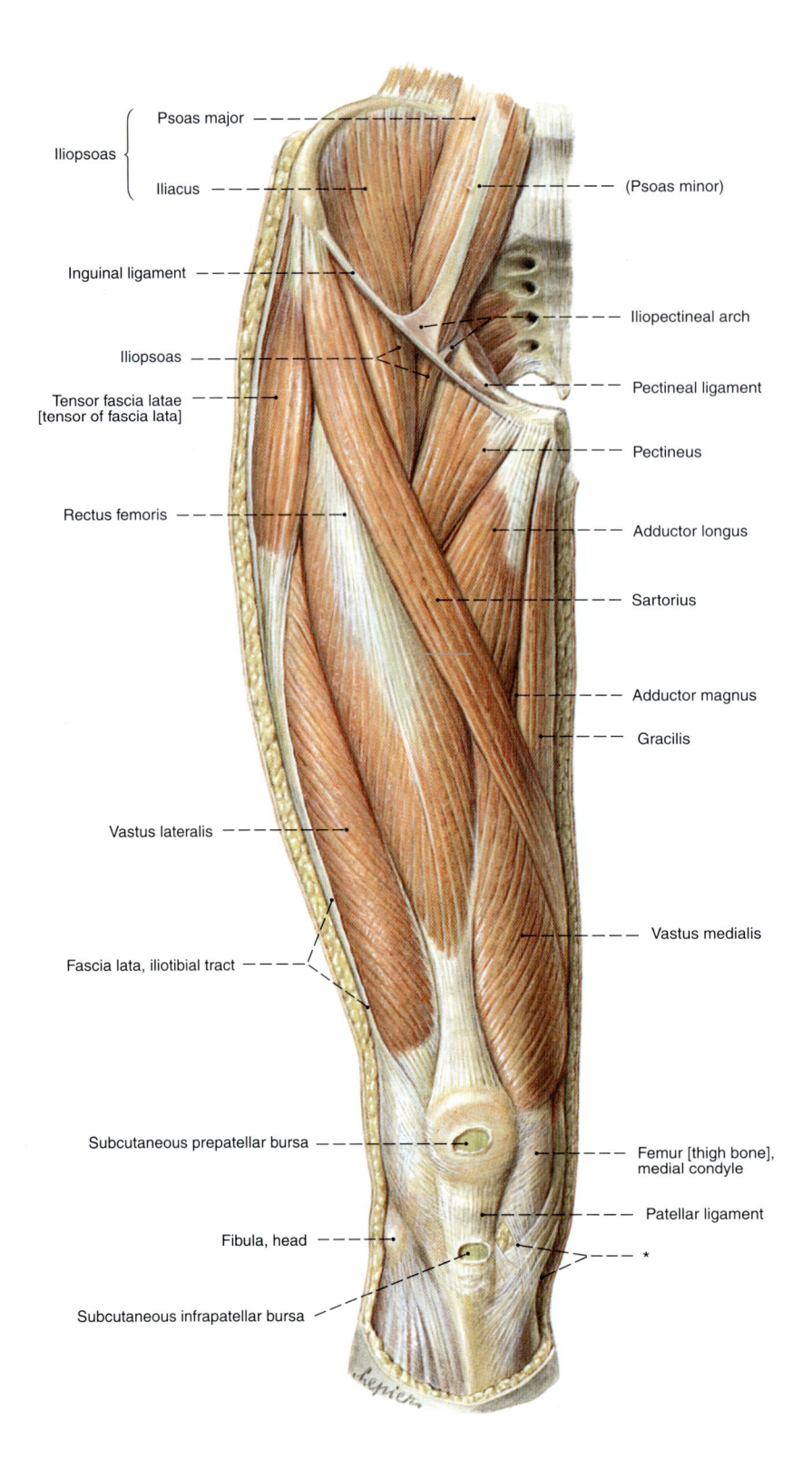

Fig. 1266 Muscles of right thigh and hip; fascia lata except iliotibial tract removed; anterior aspect.

* Common insertion of sartorius, gracilis, and semitendinosus beneath the medial condyle of tibia (formerly superficial pes anserinus).

Muscles of thigh 311

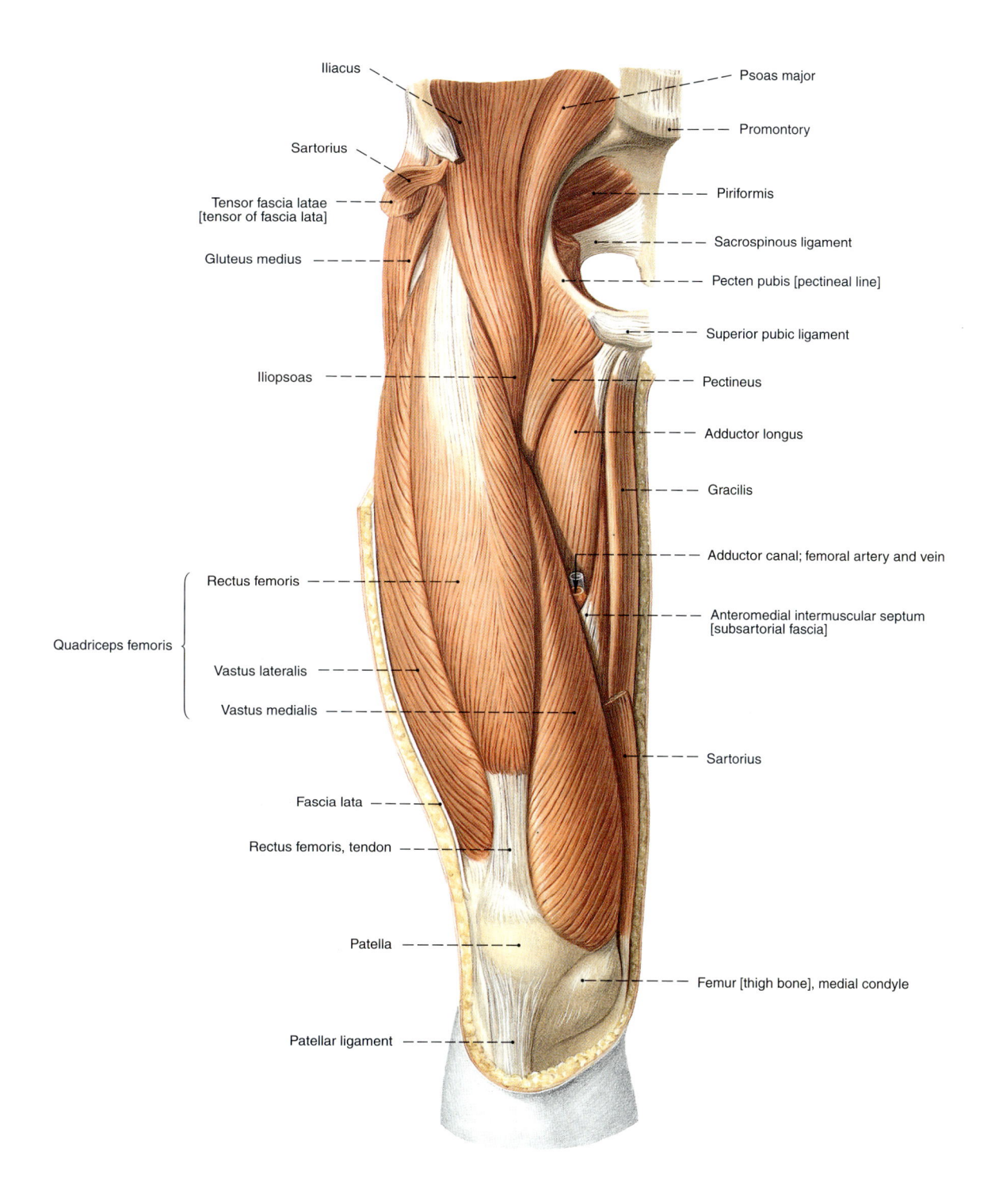

Fig. 1267 Muscles of right thigh and hip; fascia lata, tensor fasciae latae [tensor of fascia lata], and sartorius removed; anterior aspect.

312 Lower limb

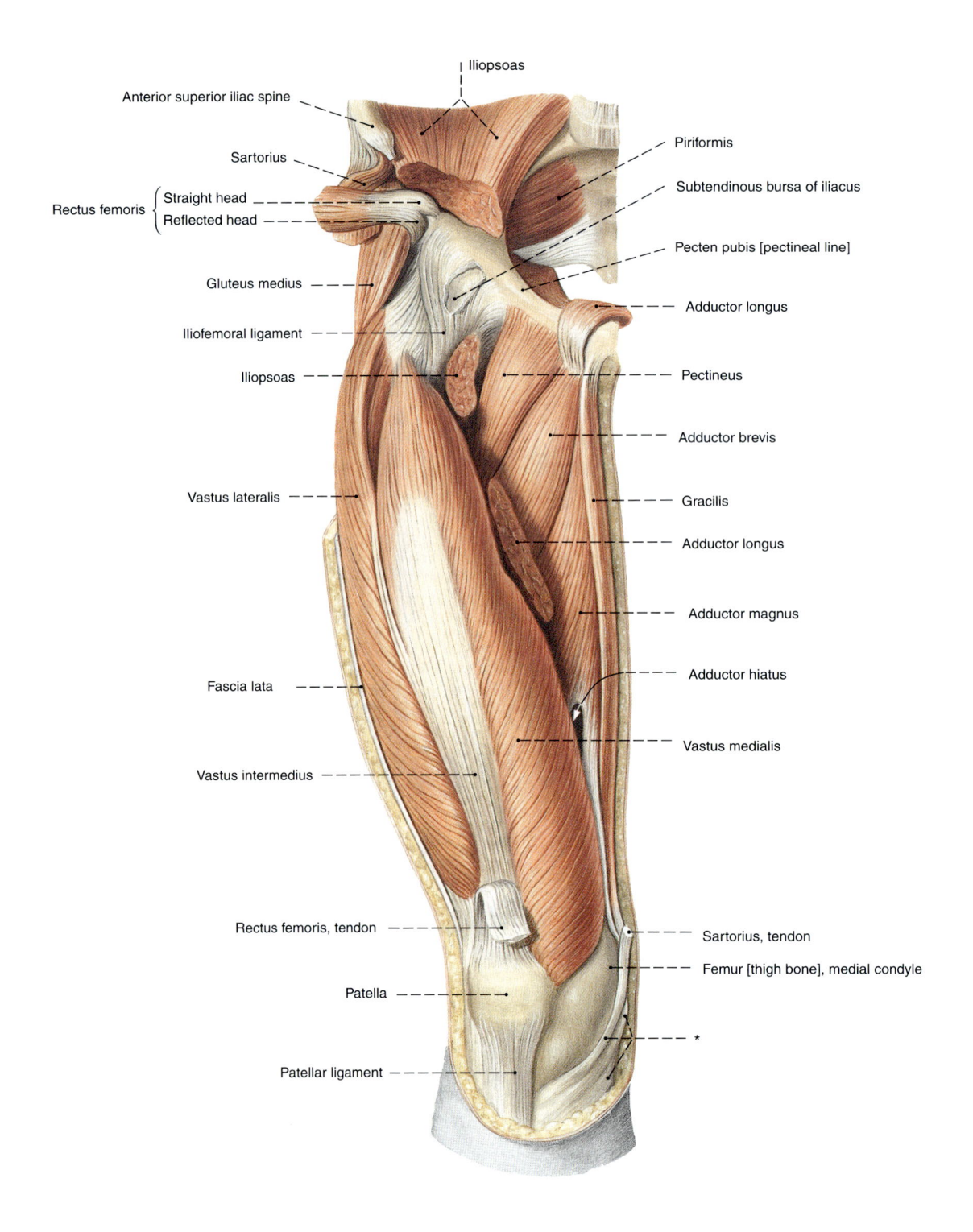

Fig. 1268   Muscles of right thigh and hip; deep layer after removal of sartorius, rectus femoris, and adductor longus as well as partial removal of iliopsoas in the region of the joint; anterior and lateral wall of adductor canal and anteromedial intermuscular septum [subsartorial fascia] removed to expose adductor hiatus; anterior aspect.

* Common insertion of sartorius, gracilis, and semitendinosus beneath the medial condyle of tibia.
** Origin of rectus femoris reflected laterally.

Muscle of thigh

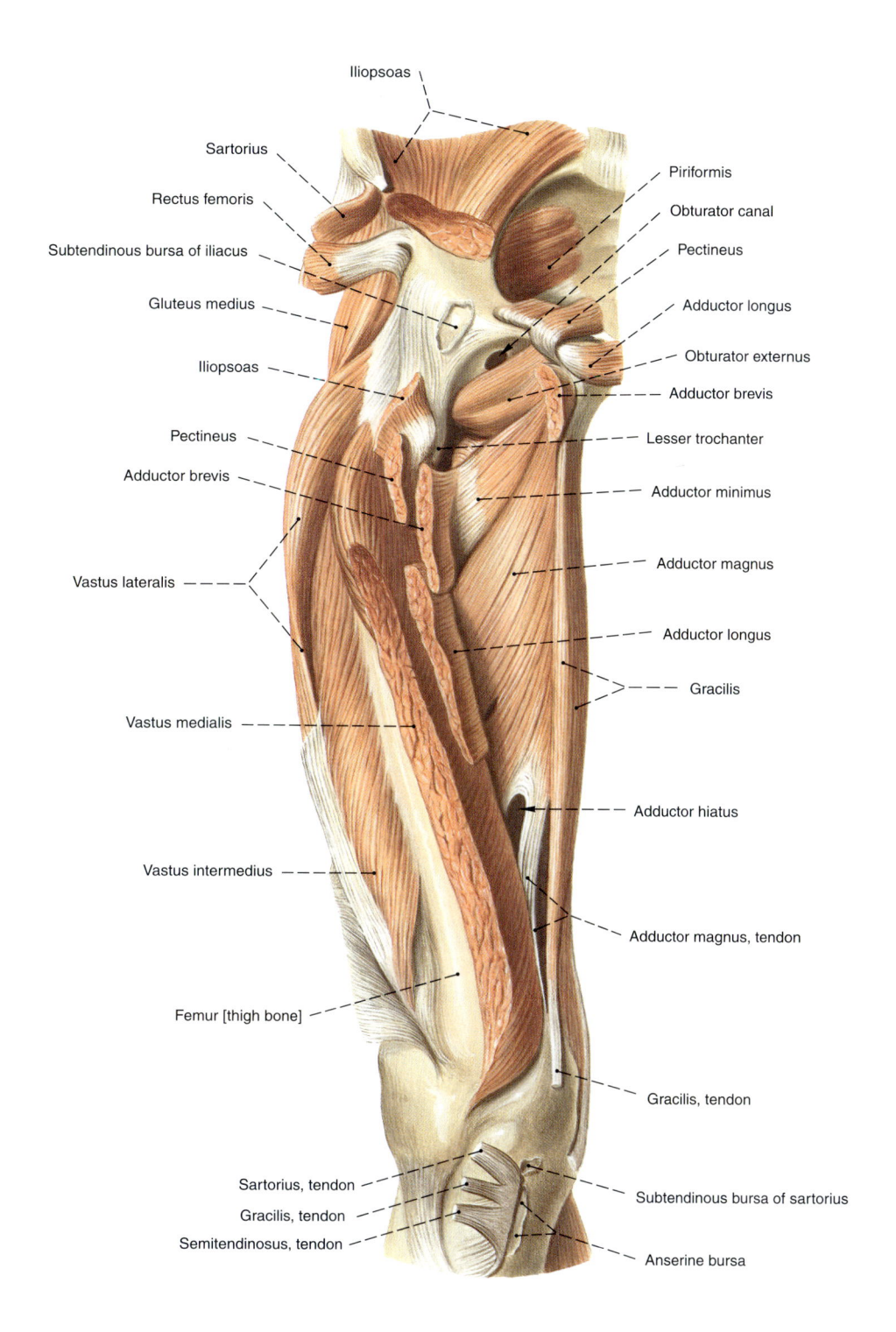

Fig. 1269　Muscles of right thigh and hip; superficial muscles extensively and also several deep muscle removed; anterior and lateral wall of adductor canal removed; anterior aspect.

Lower limb

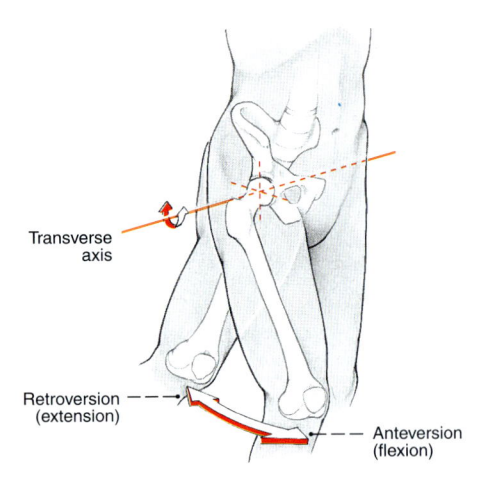

Fig. 1270 Hip joint; movement in the sagittal plane.

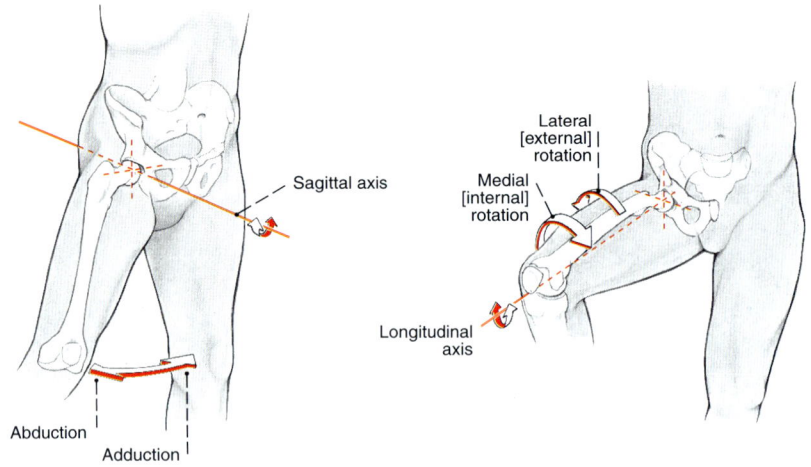

Fig. 1271 Hip joint; movement in the frontal plane.

Fig. 1272 Hip joint; movement in the transverse plane.

Ventral muscles of hip (Figs. 1266-1268, 1285)

This group comprises only the iliacus and psoas major, which assemble the iliopsoas. The iliopsoas is the only muscle passing only the hip joint anteriorly. The other muscles ventral to the hip joint also pass the knee joint and, thus, are explained with the muscles of the thigh.

Muscle *Innervation*	Origin	Insertion	Function
1. **Iliacus** *Muscular branches (lumbar plexus)*	Iliac fossa and anterior inferior iliac spine, anterior part of joint capsule of hip joint	Lesser trochanter and adjacent area of medial lip of linea aspera	
2. **Psoas major** *Muscular branches (lumbar plexus)*	**Superficial part:** vertebral bodies of 12th thoracic-4th lumbar vertebrae (lateral surfaces), intervertebral discs **Deep part:** costal processes of 1st-4th lumbar vertebrae	Lesser trochanter	**Lumbar vertebral column:** Lateral flexion, extension (increases lumbar lordosis)
3. **Psoas minor** *Muscular branches (lumbar plexus)* (inconstant muscle)	Vertebral bodies of 12th thoracic and 1st lumbar vertebrae (lateral surfaces)	Fascia of iliopsoas, iliopectineal arch (frequently via along flat tendon)	**Hip joint :** Flexion, medial rotation (lateral rotation when gluteal muscles contract simultaneously)

Ventral muscles of thigh (Figs. 1266, 1267, 1285)

Sartorius spirals from proximal lateral across the thigh toward its distal medial insertion. The short muscle belly of tensor fascia latae lies most lateral, embedded in the fascia lata, that blends with the iliotibial tract. The majority of the ventral muscles of thigh is made by the quadriceps femoris.

Muscle *Innervation*	Origin	Insertion	Function
1. **Quadriceps femoris** *Femoral nerve (lumbar plexus)* Rectus femoris acts on two joints Vastus medialis, lateralis, and intermedius acts on one joint	**Rectus femoris, straight head:** anterior inferior iliac spine **Rectus femoris, reflected head:** superior border of acetabulum **Vastus medialis:** medial lip of linea aspera (lower 2/3)	Patella (proximal and lateral borders), tibial tuberosity (via patellar ligament), proximal extremity of tibia (regions lateral and medial to tibial tuberosity, via patellar retinacula)	**Hip joint** (rectus femoris only): flexion **Knee joint:** extension

Muscle *Innervation*	Origin	Insertion	Function
	Vastus lateralis: greater trochanter (distal circumference), lateral lip of linea aspera **Vastus intermedius:** anterior surface of femur (upper 2/3) **Articularis genus [articular muscle of knee]:** anterior surface of femur (distal 1/3)		
2. Sartorius *Femoral nerve (lumbar plexus)*	Anterior superior iliac spine	Tibial tuberosity (medial facet)	**Hip joint:** Flexion, lateral rotation, abduction **Knee joint:** Flexion, medial rotation
3. Tensor fasciae latae [tensor of fascia lata] *Superior gluteal nerve (sacral plexus)*	Anterior superior iliac spine	Lateral surface of tibia (via iliotibial tract beneath lateral condyle)	**Hip joint:** Flexion, abduction, medial rotation **Knee joint:** Stabilization in extended position

Medial muscles of thigh (Figs. 1266, 1268, 1269, 1285, 1286)

The medial group of muscles of thigh are also known as the adductor compartment due to their main function. They form the triangular medial compartment of thigh. Most medial lies gracilis. From proximal to distal pectineus is followed by adductor brevis, adductor longus, and adductor magnus. Obturator externus lies deep to pectineus and close to the inferior circumference of the femoral neck.

Muscle *Innervation*	Origin	Insertion	Function
1. Gracilis *Obturator nerve (lumbar plexus)*	Inferior pubic ramus (medial border, near symphysis)	Proximal extremity of tibia (medial to tibial tuberosity)	**Hip joint:** Adduction, flexion, lateral rotation **Knee joint:** Flexion, medial rotation
2. Pectineus *Femoral and obturator nerves (lumbar plexus)*	Pecten pubis [pectineal line]	Pectineal line [spiral line] of femur [thigh bone]	**Hip joint:** Adduction, flexion, lateral rotation
3. Adductor brevis *Obturator nerve (lumbar plexus)*	Inferior pubic ramus (closer to obturator foramen compared to adductor longus)	Medial lip of linea aspera (proximal 1/3)	**Hip joint:** Adduction, flexion, lateral rotation
4. Adductor longus *Obturator nerve (lumbar plexus)*	Pubis (beneath pubic crest up to symphysis)	Medial lip of linea aspera (middle 1/3)	**Hip joint:** Adduction, flexion, lateral rotation (most anterior fibers rotate medially)
5. Adductor magnus *Obturator nerve (lumbar plexus) and sciatic nerve (tibial part-sacral plexus)* The adductor minimus is a proximal part of adductor magnus	Inferior pubic ramus and ramus of ischium (medial border)	Medial lip of linea aspera (proximal 2/3), gluteal tuberosity, adductor tubercle (adductor hiatus between both insertions)	**Hip joint:** Adduction, lateral rotation, flexion (anterior part), extension (posterior part)
6. Obturator externus *Obturator nerve (lumbar plexus)*	Circumference of obturator foramen (lateral surface), obturator membrane	Trochanteric fossa	**Hip joint:** Lateral rotation, adduction, flexion

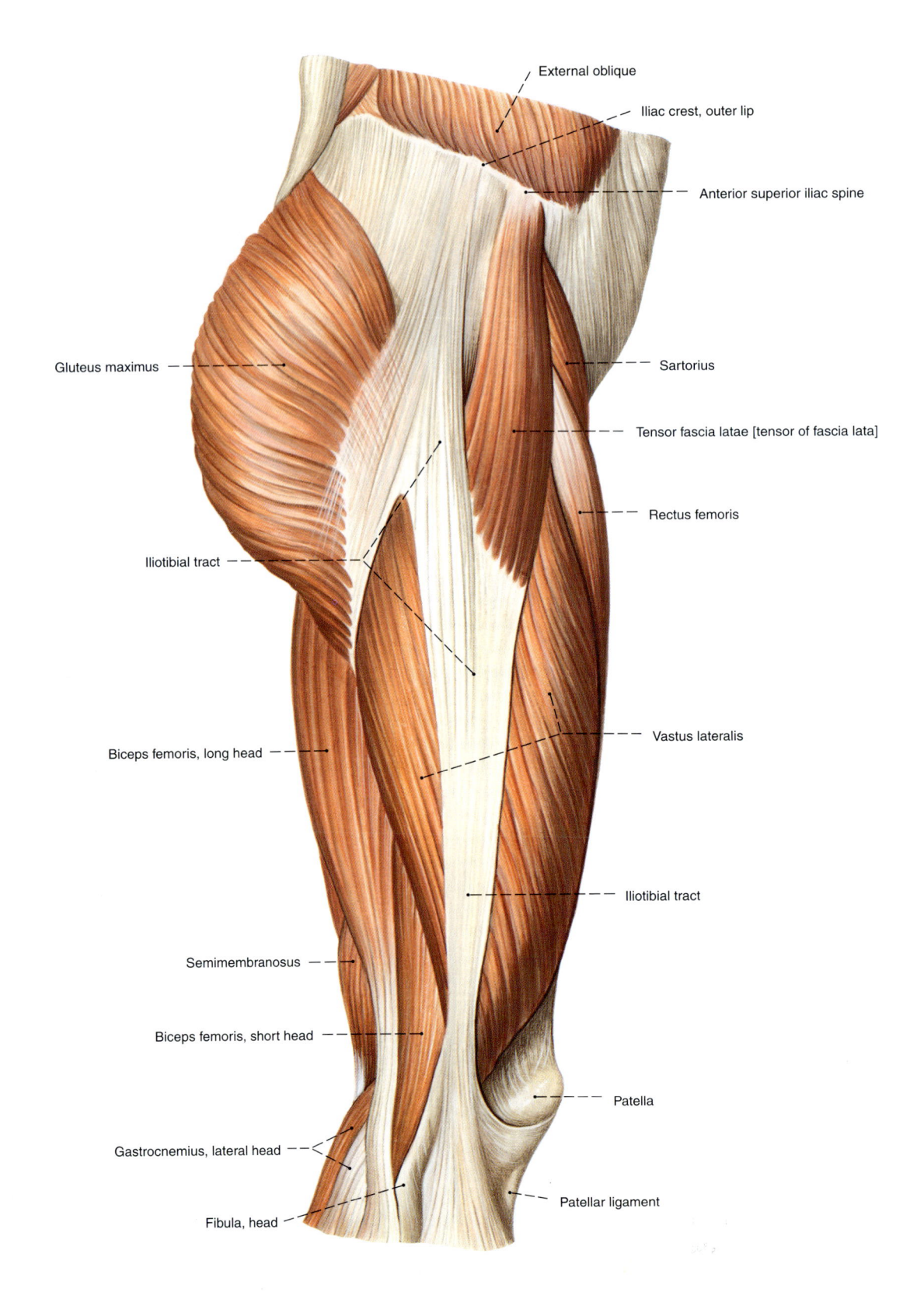

Fig. 1273 Muscles of right thigh and hip; fascia lata removed except for iliotibial tract; lateral aspect.

Muscles of thigh and hip 317

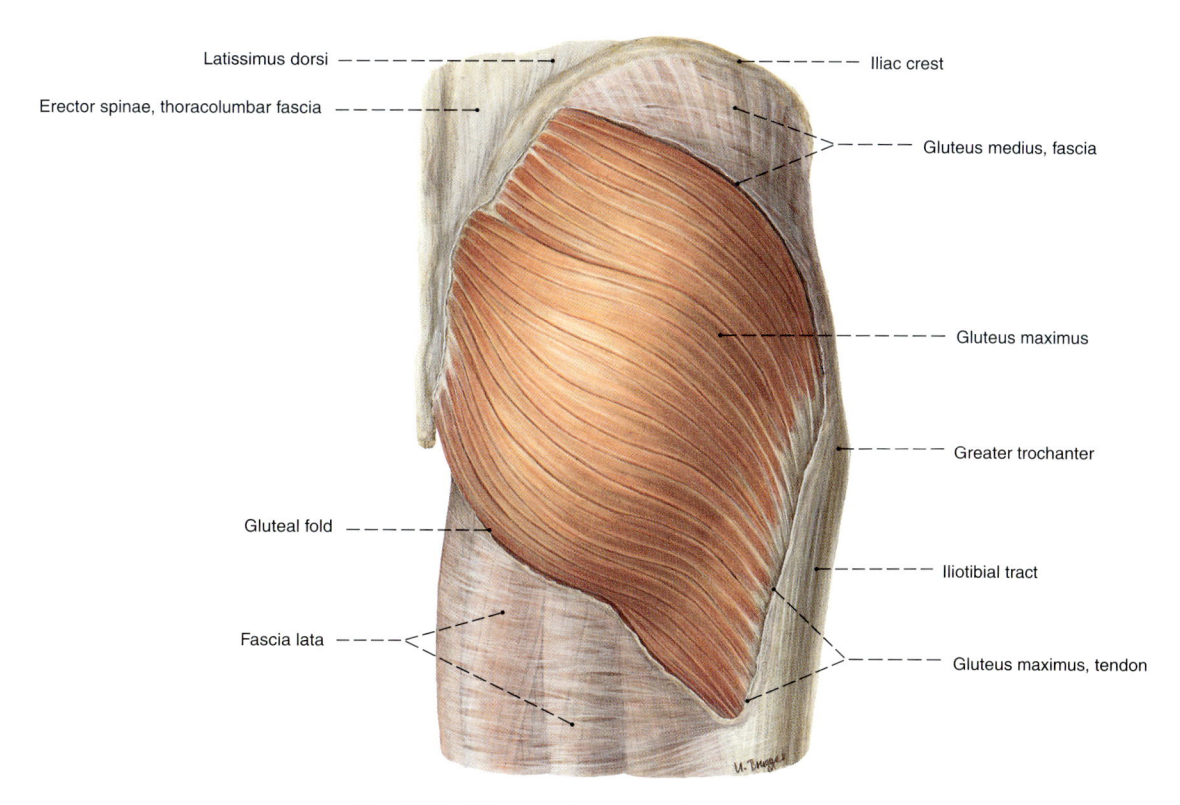

Fig. 1274 Muscles of right thigh and hip; superficial muscles after removal of fascia of gluteus maximus; dorsal aspect.

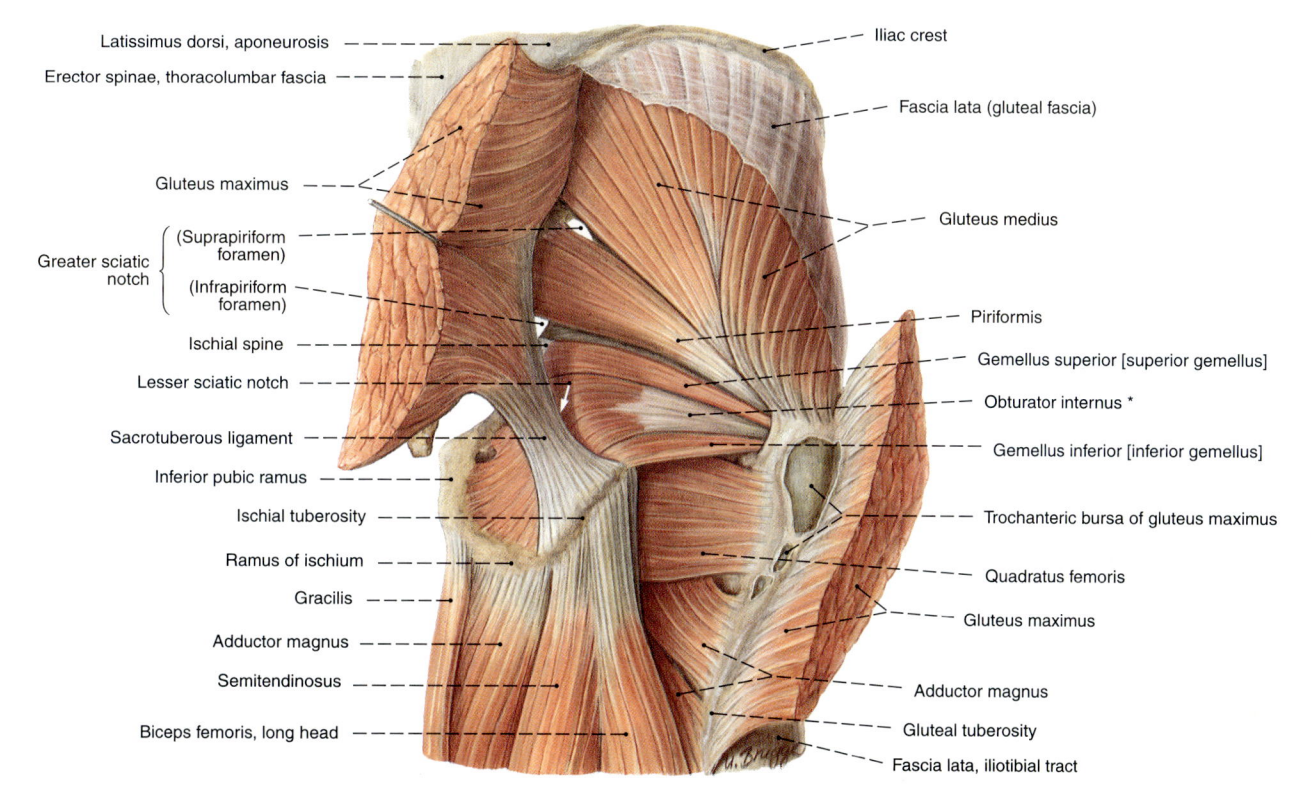

Fig. 1275 Muscles of right thigh and hip; deep muscles after sectioning of gluteus maximus; dorsal aspect.

*The part of obturator internus between the lesser sciatic notch and its insertion is frequently made only of tendinous bands.

318 Lower limb

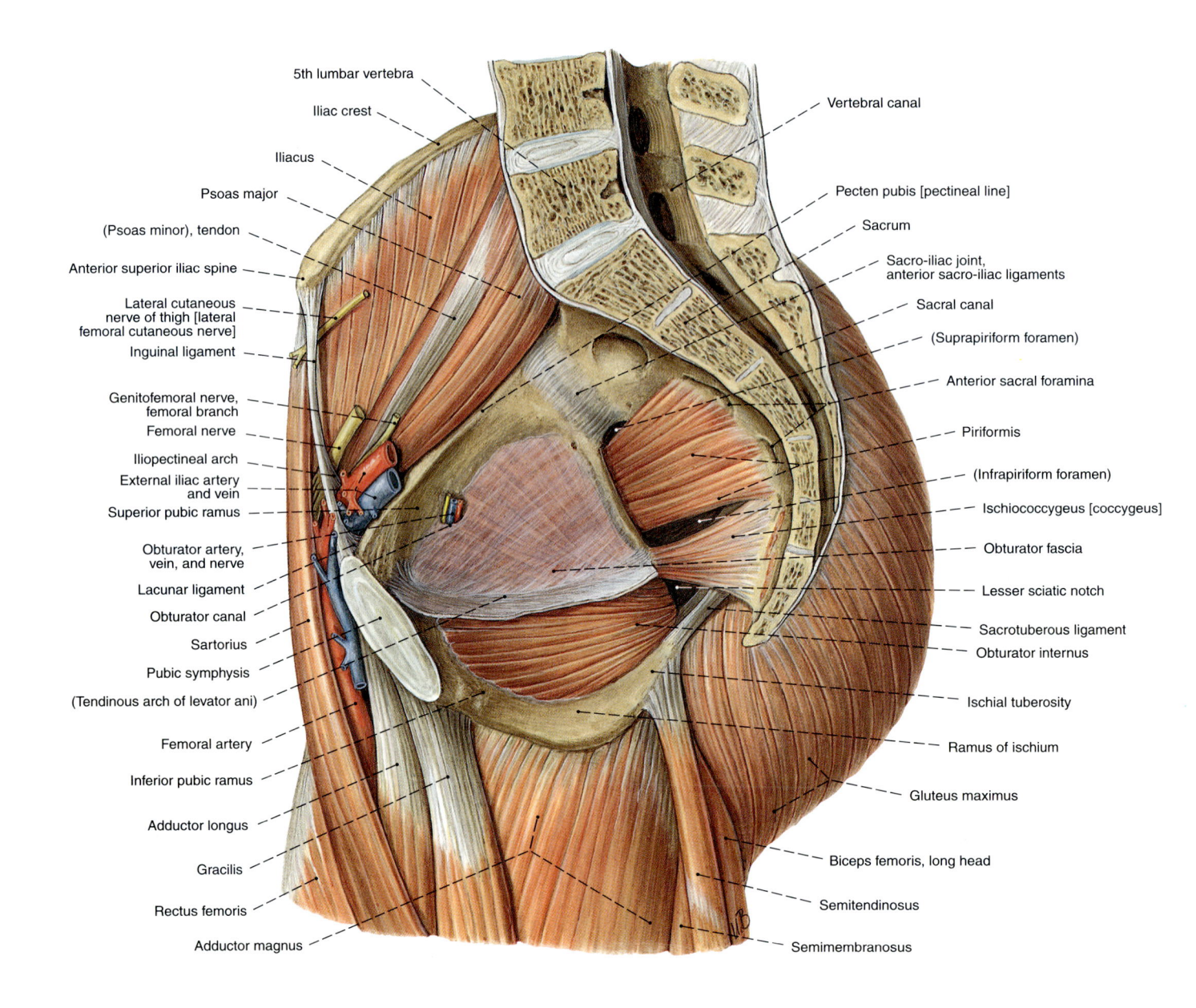

Fig. 1276 Muscles of right thigh and hip; pelvis and lumbar vertebral column sectioned in the median plane; medial aspect.

Muscles of thigh and hip 319

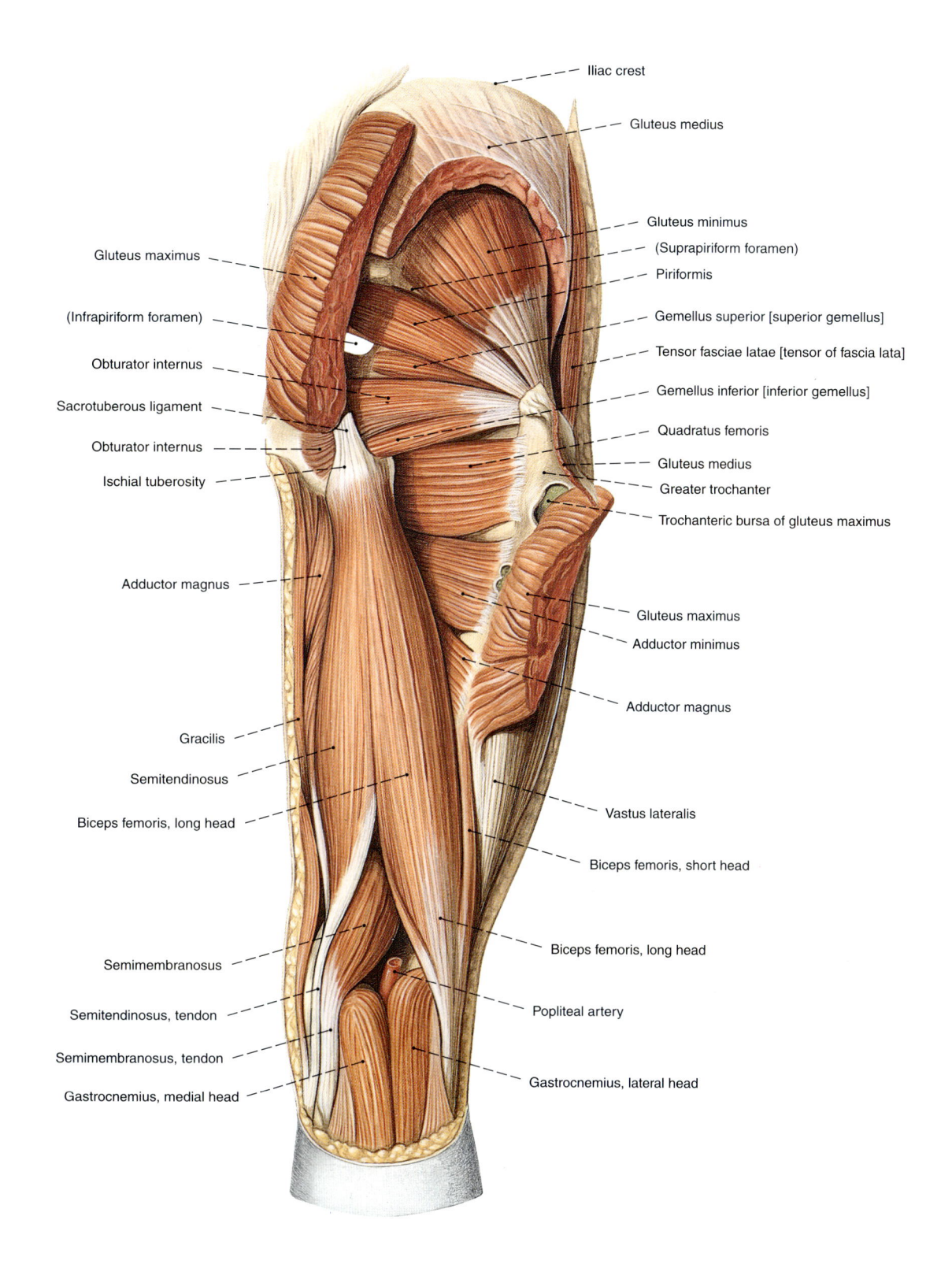

Fig. 1277 Muscles of right thigh and hip; gluteus maximus and medius partially removed; posterior aspect.

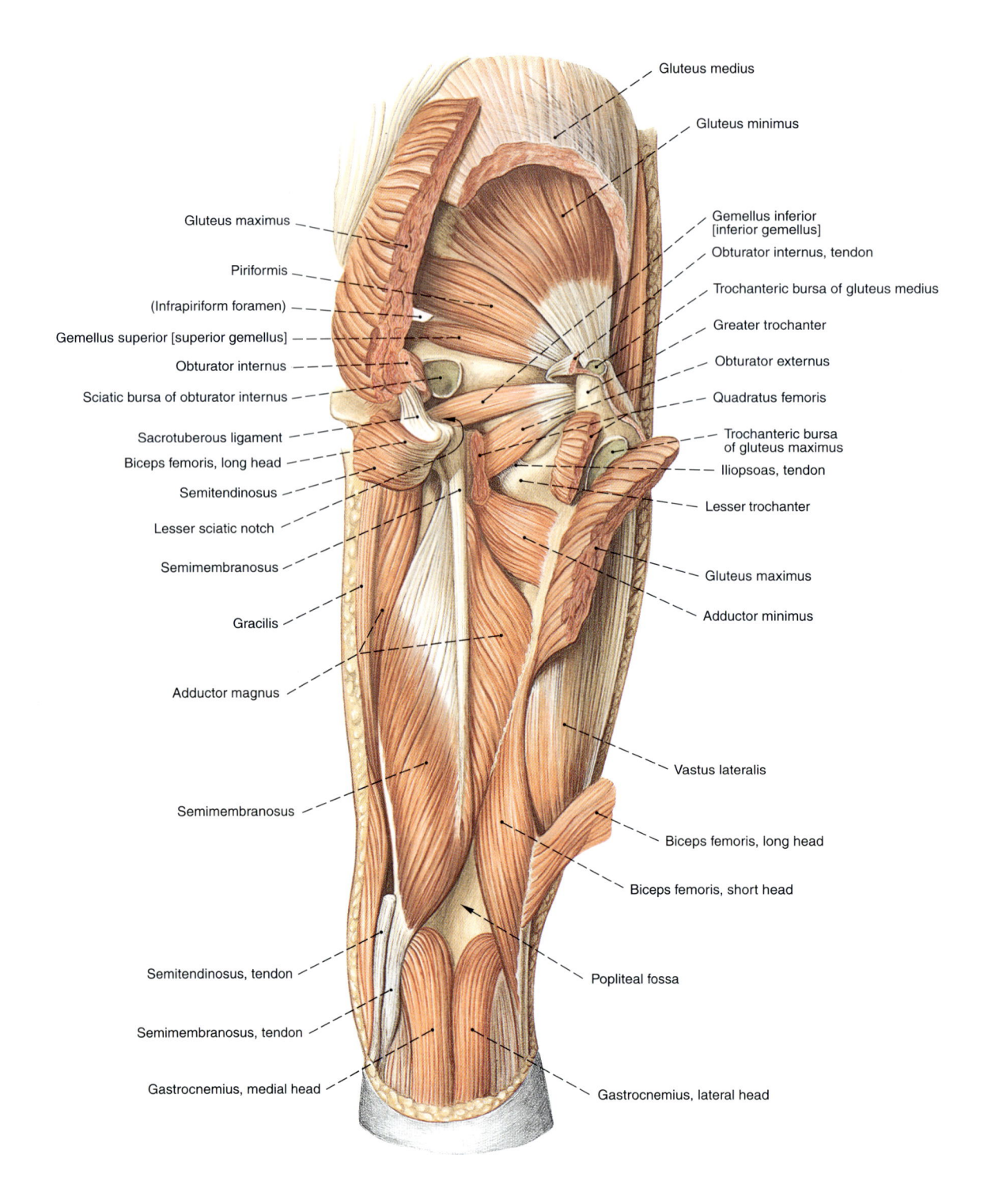

Fig. 1278 Muscles of right thigh and hip; deep layer after extensive removal of superficial gluteal and ischiocrural muscles [hamstrings]; posterior aspect.

Dorsal muscles of hip (Figs. 1274, 1275, 1277, 1285, 1286)

The gluteus maximus is the most superficial muscle of the gluteal region and covers almost entirely the other muscles of this group. The most ventral superior part of gluteus medius, which covers the gluteus minimus, is not covered by the gluteus maximus. Caudally, the deep muscles follow: piriformis, gemellus superior [superior gemellus], obturator internus, gemellus inferior [inferior gemellus], and quadratus femoris.

Muscle *Innervation*	Origin	Insertion	Function
1. Gluteus maximus *Inferior gluteal nerve [sacral plexus]*	Gluteal surface of ala of ilium [wing of ilium] (dorsal to posterior gluteal line), posterior surface of sacrum, thoracolumbar fascia, sacrotuberous ligament	**Cranial part:** tibia beneath lateral condyle (via iliotibial tract). Between greater trochanter and iliotibial tract lies the trochanteric bursa of gluteus maximus **Caudal part:** gluteal tuberosity, lateral femoral intermuscular septum	**Hip joint:** cranial part: extension, lateral rotation, abduction caudal part: extension, lateral rotation, adduction **Knee joint** (via iliotibial tract): extension
2. Gluteus medius *Superior gluteal nerve [sacral plexus]*	Gluteal surface of ala of ilium [wing of ilium] (between anterior and posterior gluteal lines)	Greater trochanter (tip and lateral border)	**Hip joint:** Ventral part: abduction, flexion, medial rotation Dorsal part: abduction, extension, lateral rotation
3. Gluteus minimus *Superior gluteal nerve [sacral plexus]*	Gluteal surface of ala of ilium [wing of ilium] (between anterior and inferior gluteal lines)	Greater trochanter (tip and lateral border)	**Hip joint:** Ventral part: abduction, flexion, medial rotation Dorsal part: abduction, extension, lateral rotation
4. Piriformis *Sciatic nerve and/ or nerve to piriformis [sacral plexus]*	Pelvic surface of sacrum (lateral to anterior sacral foramina of 3rd and 4th sacral vertebrae), greater sciatic notch (close to sacrum)	Greater trochanter (medial of tip)	**Hip joint:** Lateral rotation, extension, adduction
5. Obturator internus *Nerve to obturator internus and muscular branches [sacral plexus]*	Circumference of obturator foramen (medial surface)	Trochanteric fossa	
6. Gemellus superior [superior gemellus] *Nerve to obturator internus and muscular branches [sacral plexus]*	Ischial spine	Trochanteric fossa	
7. Gemellus inferior [inferior gemellus] *Nerve to obturator internus and muscular branches [sacral plexus]*	Ischial tuberosity	Trochanteric fossa	**Hip joint:** Lateral rotation, adduction, extension
8. Quadratus femoris *Nerve to quadratus femoris [sacral plexus]*	Ischial tuberosity (lateral border)	Intertrochanteric crest	

Posterior muscles of thigh (Figs. 1277, 1286)

The posterior muscles of thigh comprise the biceps femoris, semitendinosus, and semimembranosus from lateral to medial.

Muscle *Innervation*	Origin	Insertion	Function
1. Biceps femoris Long head: *Sciatic nerve, tibial part [sacral plexus]* Short head: *Sciatic nerve, fibular part [sacral plexus]* Long head acts at two joints; short head acts at one joint	**Long head:** ischial tuberosity (common head with semitendinosus) **Short head:** lateral lip of linea aspera (middle 1/3)	Head of fibula (embraces fibular collateral ligament) Blends with crural fascia [fascia of leg]	**Hip joint:** Extension, adduction, lateral rotation **Knee joint:** Flexion, lateral rotation
2. Semitendinosus *Sciatic nerve, tibial part [sacral plexus]*	Ischial tuberosity (common head with long head of biceps femoris)	Tibial tuberosity (medial surface)	**Hip joint:** Extension, adduction, lateral rotation **Knee joint:** Flexion, medial rotation
3. Semimembranosus *Sciatic nerve, tibial part [sacral plexus]*	Ischial tuberosity	Proximal extremity of fibula (beneath medial condyle)	**Hip joint:** Extension, adduction, lateral rotation **Knee joint:** Flexion, medial rotation

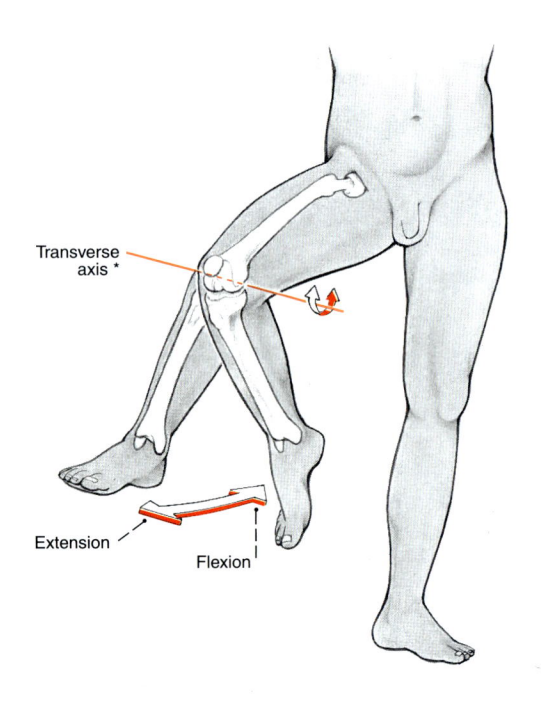

Fig. 1279 Knee joint; movement in the sagittal plane.

* Due to the inhomogeneous curvature of the condyles of femur [thigh bone] the position of this axis changes during movement (instantaneous axis).

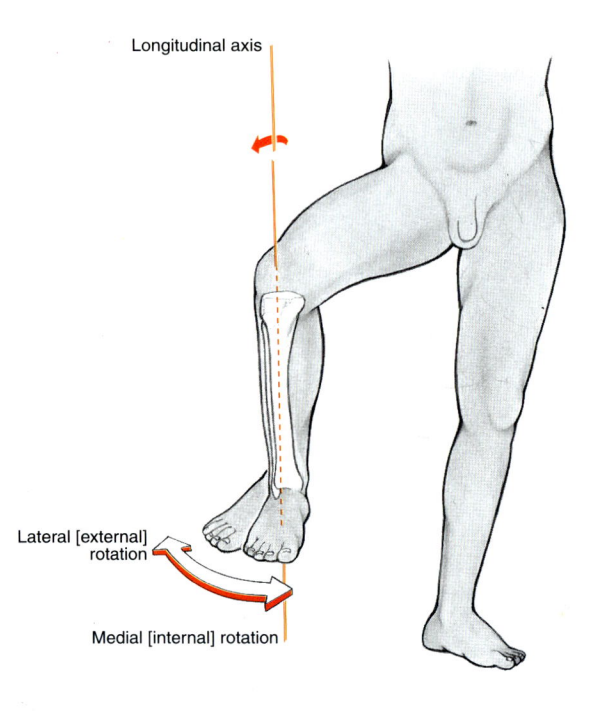

Fig. 1280 Knee joint; movement in the transverse plane.

Mechanics of hip and knee joints 323

S_4	center of gravity of 4/6 parts of body weight
F_{S4}	load of parts of body weight effective in the hip joints
R_Z	resulting force in each hip joint in two-legged standing
S_6	center of gravity of 5/6 parts of body weight
F_{S5}	load of parts of body weight effective in the hip joints
R_E	resulting force in each hip joint in one-legged standing
F_{Ab}	force of abductors
l_1	lever arm of F_{S5}
l_2	lever arm of F_{Ab}
*	Centroidal axis.
**	Angle of inclination [depression] of neck (approx. 125°).

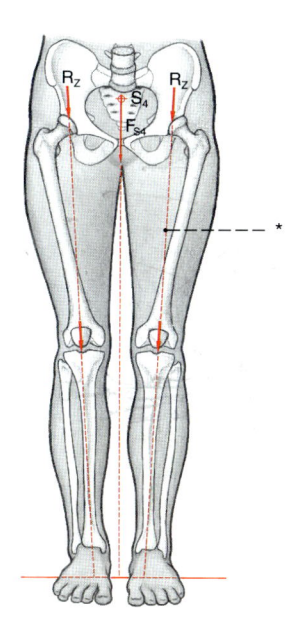

Fig. 1281 Load on hip joints in two-legged standing.

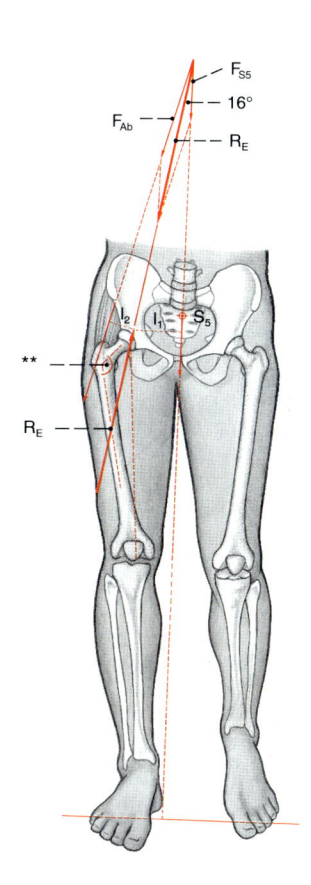

Fig. 1282 Unilateral load on hip joint in the stance phase.

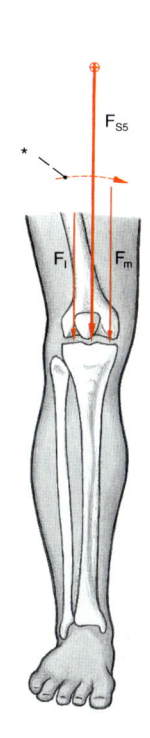

F_l	partial force effective in lateral compartment
F_m	partial force effective in medial compartment
F_{S5}	load of approx. 5/6 parts of body weight effective in the knee joints

Fig. 1283 Load on knee joint in the frontal plane.

F_{Qu}	force of quadriceps femoris
F_{Lig}	force of patellar ligament
R_{FP}	resulting force in femoropatellar joint
R_{FT}	resulting force in femorotibial joint

l_1	lever arm of 5/6 parts of body weight effective in this position
l_2	lever arm of patellar ligament
*	Torque of body

Fig. 1284 a, b Load on knee joint in the sagittal plane.
a Femorotibial joint   **b** Femoropatellar joint

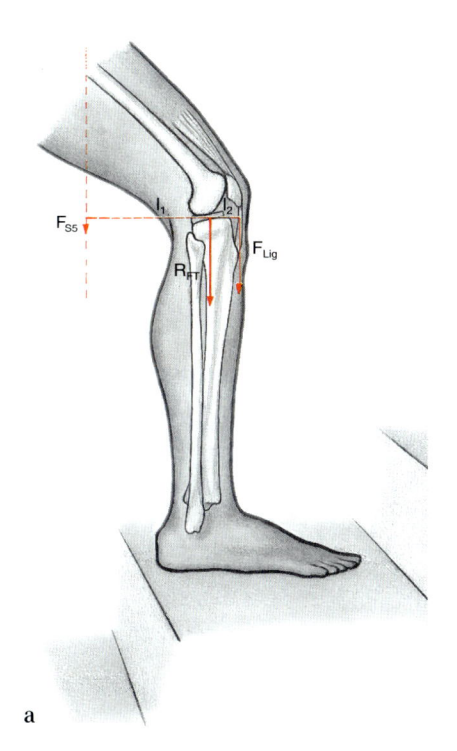

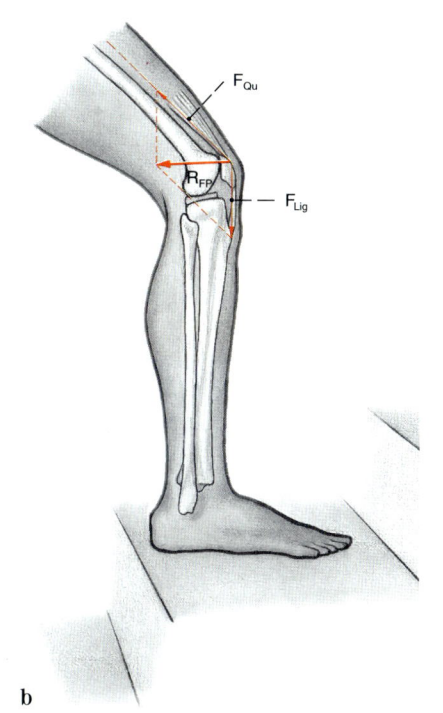

324 Lower limb

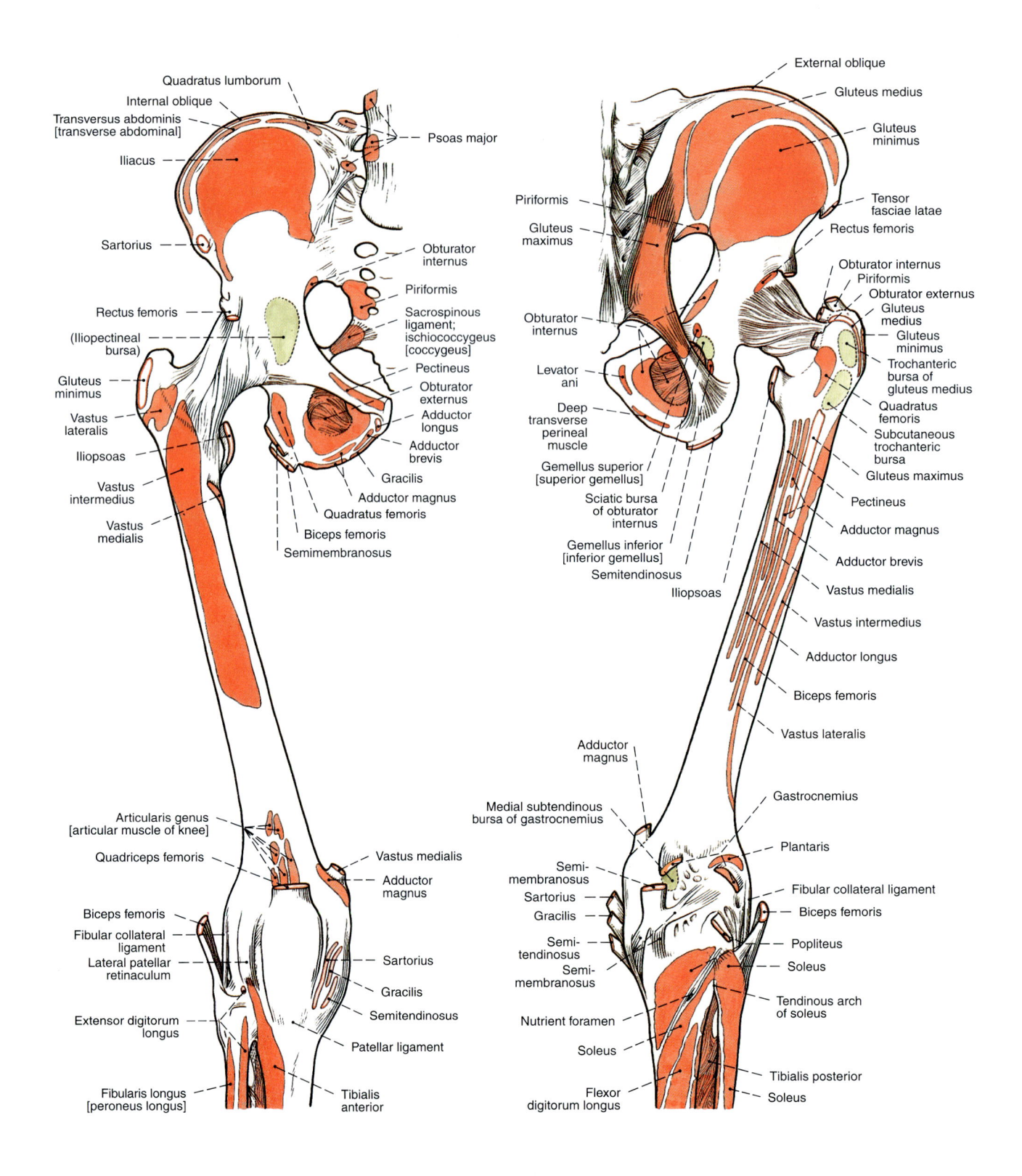

Fig. 1285 Muscle origins and insertions on the lower lumbar vertebrae, right pelvic girdle, femur [thigh bone], and proximal extremities of bones of right leg; anterior aspect.

Fig. 1286 Muscle origins and insertions of lower lumbar vertebrae, right pelvic girdle, femur [thigh bone], and proximal extremities of bones of right leg; posterior aspect.

Fasciae of knee and leg 325

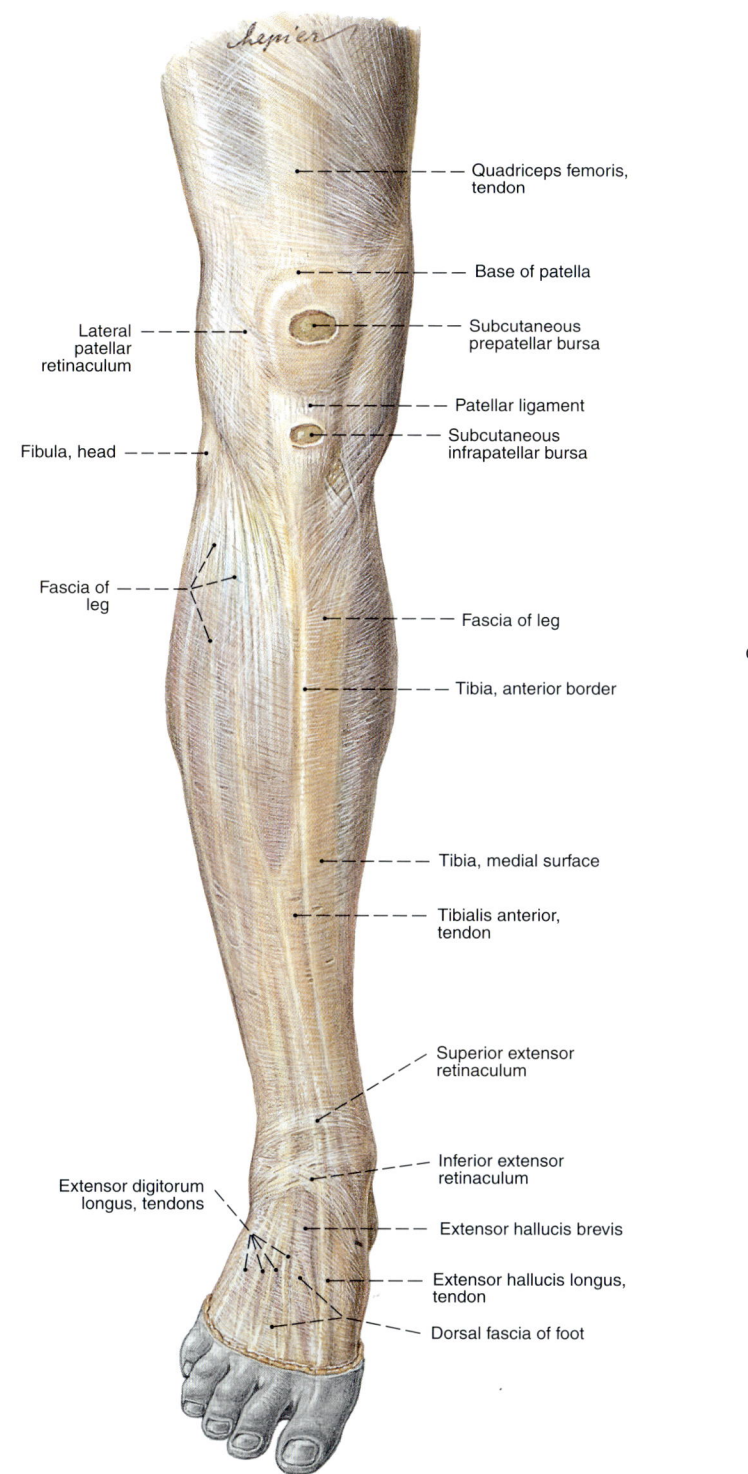

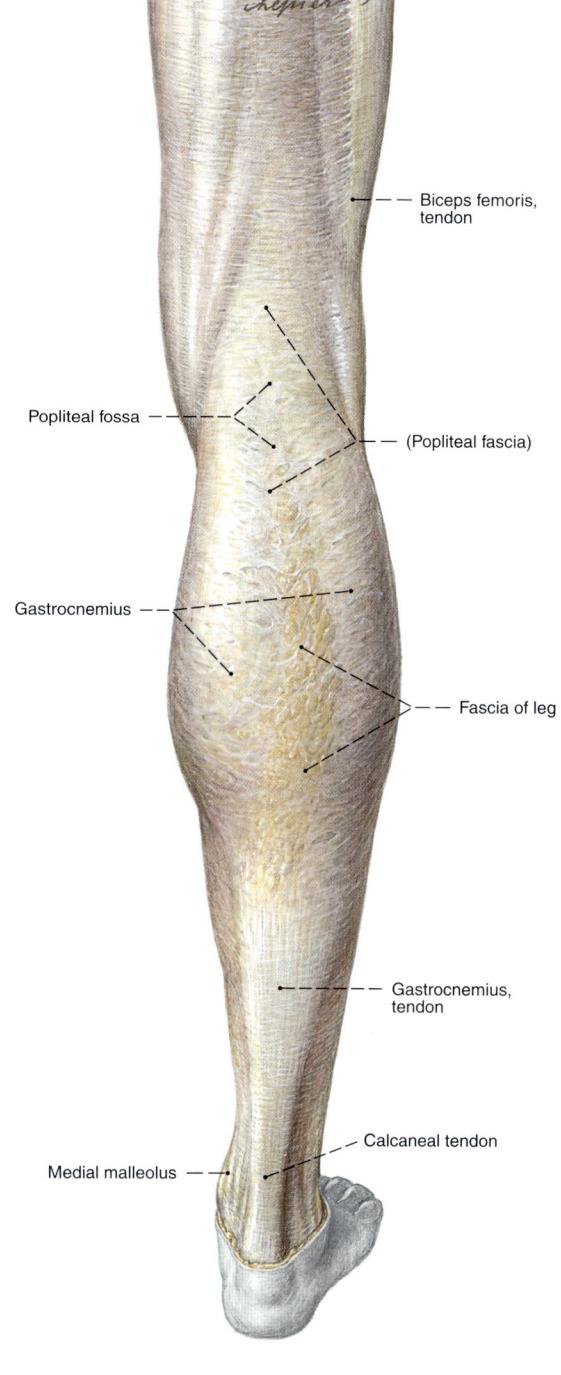

Fig. 1287 Fasciae of right knee and leg; anterior aspect.

Fig. 1288 Fasciae of right knee and leg; posterior aspect.

Lower limb

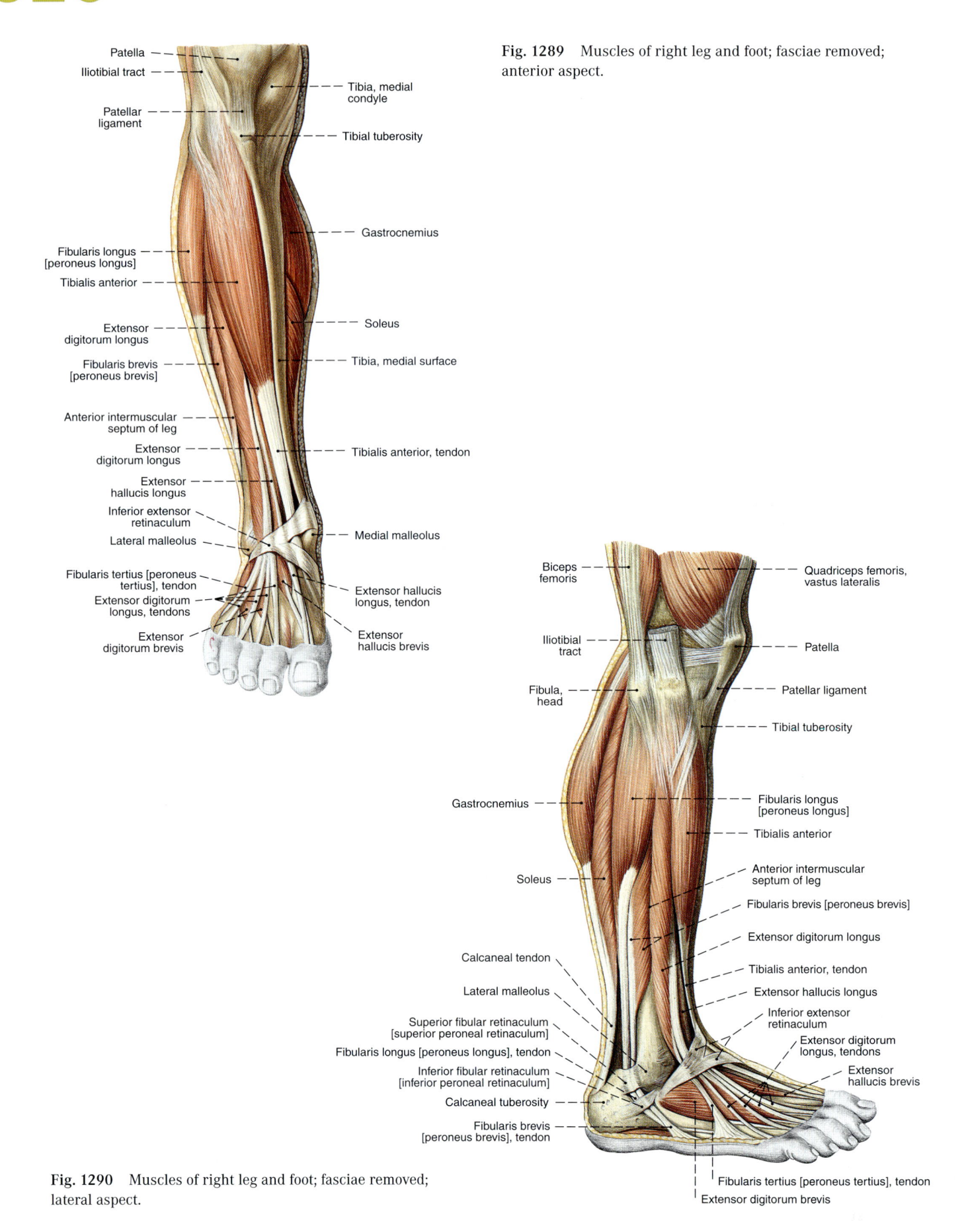

Fig. 1289 Muscles of right leg and foot; fasciae removed; anterior aspect.

Fig. 1290 Muscles of right leg and foot; fasciae removed; lateral aspect.

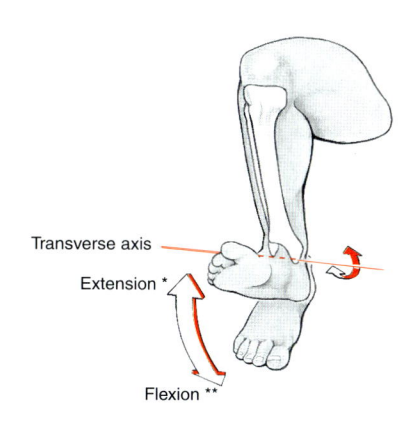

Muscles of leg 327

Fig. 1291 Ankle joint; movement in the sagittal plane.
  Flexion and extension are the main movements of the ankle joint.
  To avoid misunderstanding, flexion** is also known as plantar flexion and extension* is also known as dorsiflexion.

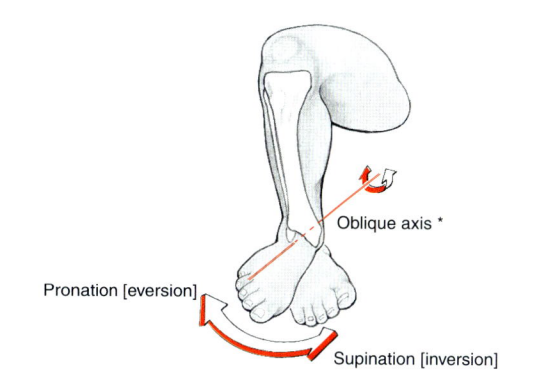

Fig. 1292 Ankle joint; rotation movements.
Starting from maximal plantar flexion, pronation is also known as lateral abduction and supination is also known as medial abduction.
* This axis courses from the medial side of the neck of talus posteriorly beneath the lateral process of the calcaneal tuberosity. It is slightly more exaggerated than shown in this figure for didactic reasons (see Fig. 1310).

Ventral muscles of leg (Figs. 1289, 1300, 1308, 1310)

Most superficially and medially, tibialis anterior bulges the fascia of leg. Medially follows extensor digitorum longus, which laterally frequently ends in fibularis [peroneus] tertius. The deepest muscle is the extensor hallucis longus.

Muscle *Innervation*	Origin	Insertion	Function
1. **Tibialis anterior** *Deep fibular [peroneal] nerve (sciatic nerve)*	Proximal extremity of tibia (beneath lateral condyle), lateral surface of tibia [upper 2/3], interosseous membrane of leg, fascia of leg	Base of 1st metatarsal (medial border), medial cuneiform (plantar surface)	**Ankle joint:** Dorsiflexion **Talotarsal joint:** Supination
2. **Extensor hallucis longus** *Deep fibular [peroneal] nerve (sciatic nerve)*	Medial surface of fibula (distal 2/3), interosseous membrane of leg, fascia of leg	Base of distal phalanx of great toe, proximal phalanx	**Ankle joint:** Dorsiflexion **Talotarsal joint:** Supination **Joints of great toe:** Extension
3. **Extensor digitorum longus** *Deep fibular [peroneal] nerve (sciatic nerve)*	Proximal extremity of tibia (beneath lateral condyle), anterior border of fibula, interosseous membrane of leg, anterior intermuscular septum of leg, fascia of leg	Extensor expansion of 2nd–5th toes	**Ankle joint:** Dorsiflexion **Talotarsal joint:** Pronation **Joints of toes:** Extension
4. **Fibularis [peroneus] longus** *Deep fibular [peroneal] nerve (sciatic nerve) (variable)*	Limb of extensor digitorum longus	Base of 5th metatarsal	

328 Lower limb

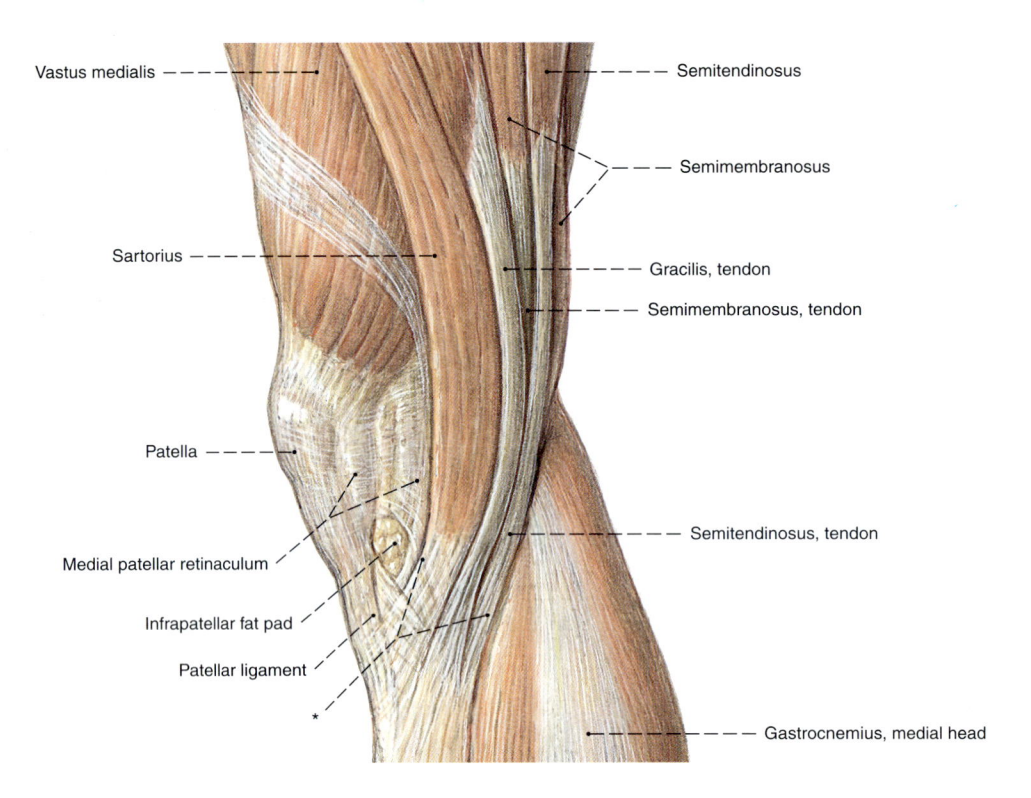

Fig. 1293 Muscles in the region of the right knee joint; fasciae removed; medial aspect.

* Common insertion of sartorius, gracilis, and semitendinosus beneath the medial condyle of tibia (formerly superficial pes anserinus).

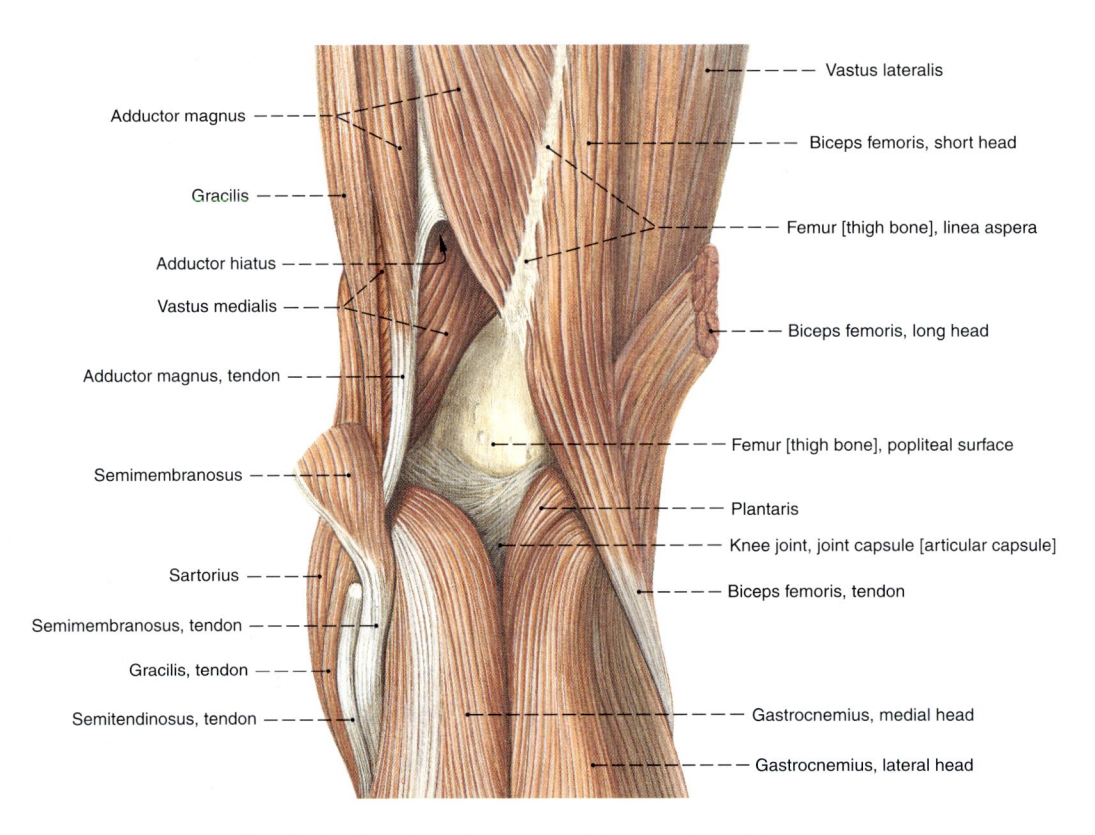

Fig. 1294 Muscles in the region of the right knee joint; fasciae and ischiocrural muscles [hamstrings] extensively removed; posterior aspect.

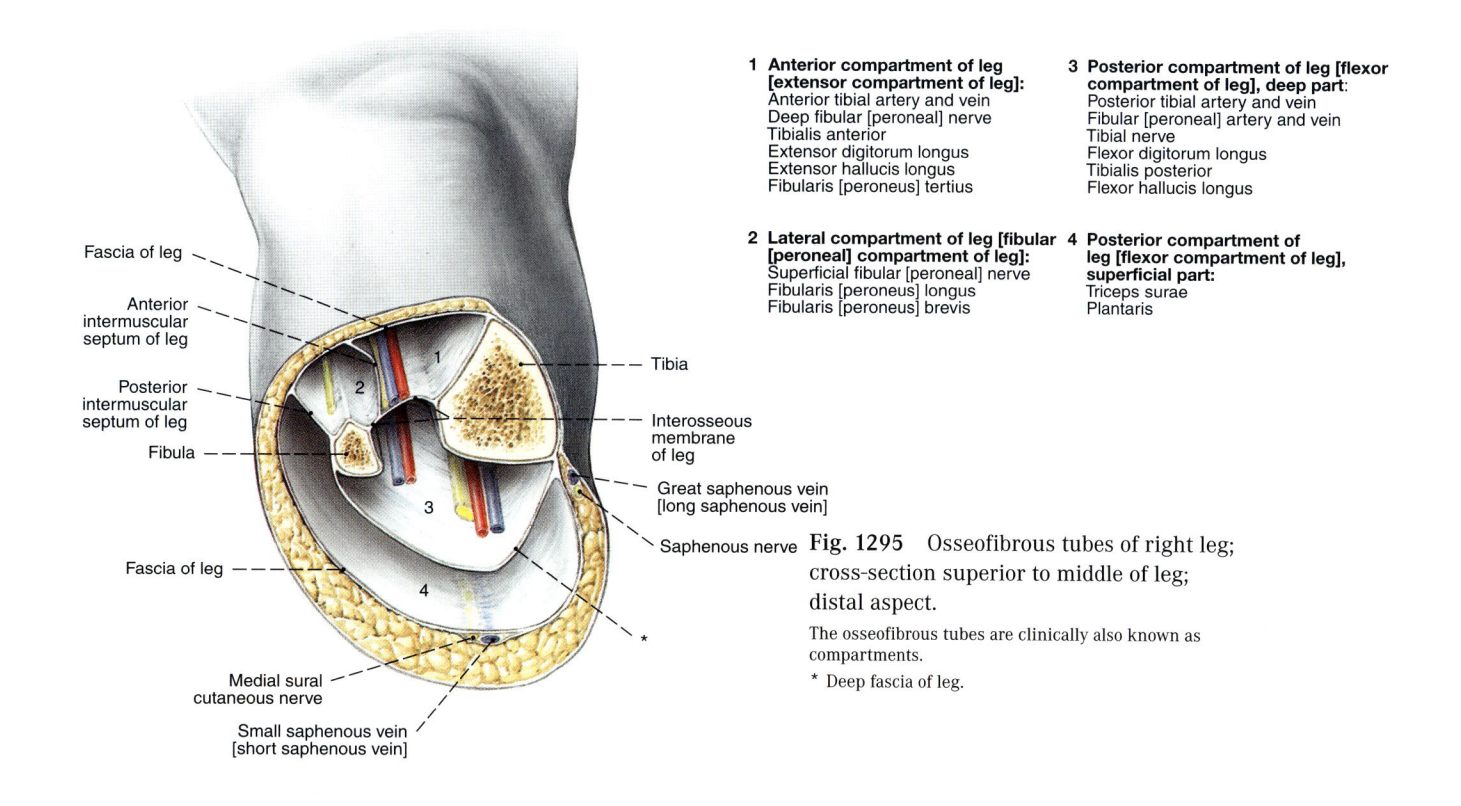

Muscles of leg

1 Anterior compartment of leg [extensor compartment of leg]:
Anterior tibial artery and vein
Deep fibular [peroneal] nerve
Tibialis anterior
Extensor digitorum longus
Extensor hallucis longus
Fibularis [peroneus] tertius

2 Lateral compartment of leg [fibular [peroneal] compartment of leg]:
Superficial fibular [peroneal] nerve
Fibularis [peroneus] longus
Fibularis [peroneus] brevis

3 Posterior compartment of leg [flexor compartment of leg], deep part:
Posterior tibial artery and vein
Fibular [peroneal] artery and vein
Tibial nerve
Flexor digitorum longus
Tibialis posterior
Flexor hallucis longus

4 Posterior compartment of leg [flexor compartment of leg], superficial part:
Triceps surae
Plantaris

Fig. 1295 Osseofibrous tubes of right leg; cross-section superior to middle of leg; distal aspect.

The osseofibrous tubes are clinically also known as compartments.

* Deep fascia of leg.

The strong fascia of leg and the equally strong intermuscular septa of leg together with the interosseous membrane and the bones of leg form osseofibrous tubes that are also known as compartments. Anterior, lateral, superficial posterior, and deep posterior compartments can be differentiated. In addition to a girding function to decrease flexion forces on the bones of leg, they increase pressure during muscle action. When the venous valves are intact they essentially support venous drainage. When physiologic pressure equilibrium is disturbed, e.g. due to effusion of blood, compression of nerves and blood vessels within the osseofibrous tube may cause the so-called compartment syndrome.

Lateral muscles of leg (Fig. 1290)

Lateral superficial lies the fibularis [peroneus] longus, beneath it the fibularis [peroneus] brevis.

Muscle *Innervation*	Origin	Insertion	Function*
1. Fibularis [peroneus] longus *Superficial fibular [peroneal] nerve (sciatic nerve)*	Head of fibula, lateral surface and posterior border of fibula (proximal 2/3), anterior and posterior intermuscular septa of leg, fascia of leg	Tuberosity of 1st metatarsal, intermediate [middle] cuneiform (plantar surface)	**Ankle joint:** Plantar flexion **Talotarsal joint:** Pronation
2. Fibularis [peroneus] brevis *Superficial fibular [peroneal] nerve (sciatic nerve)*	Lateral surface and anterior border of fibula (distal 1/2), anterior and posterior intermuscular septa of leg	Tuberosity of 5th metatarsal, tendinous slip to little toe	**Ankle joint:** Plantar flexion **Talotarsal joint:** Pronation

*Plantar flexion is also known as flexion, dorsiflexion is also known as extension.

330 Lower limb

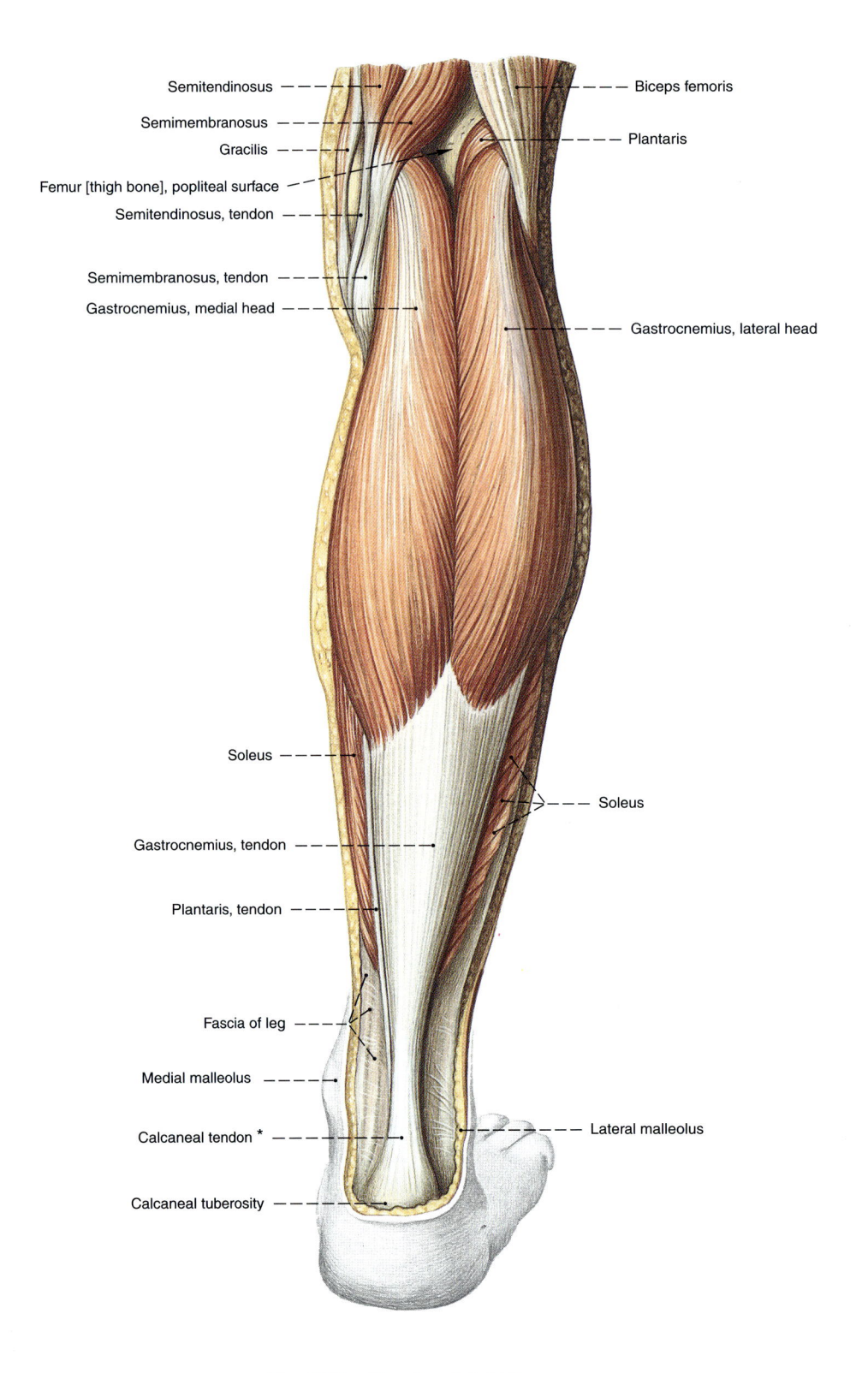

Fig. 1296 Muscles of right leg; fascia of leg removed; posterior aspect.
* Also: ACHILLES tendon.

Muscles of leg 331

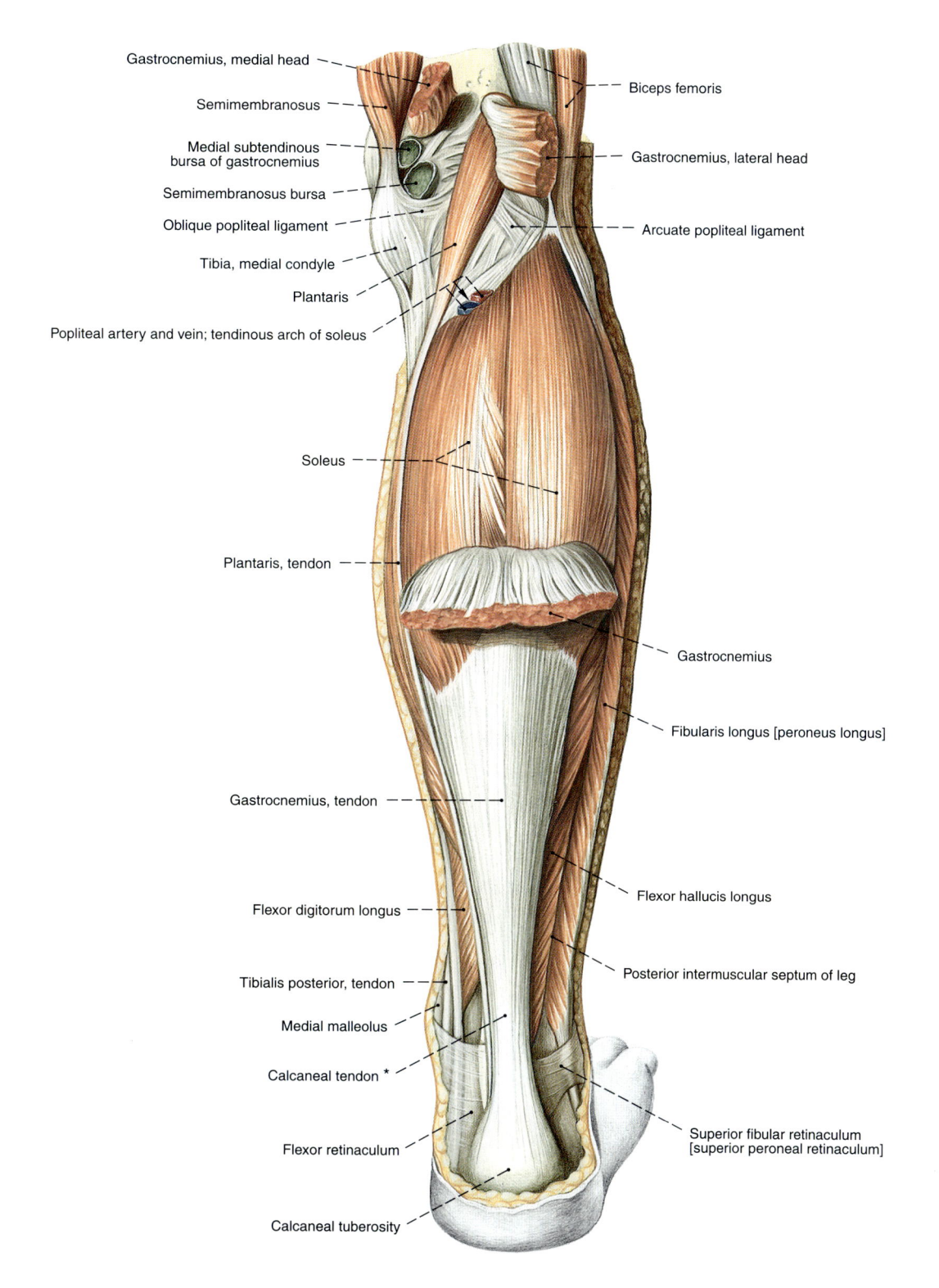

Fig. 1297 Muscles of right leg; gastrocnemius partially removed; posterior aspect.
* Also: ACHILLES tendon.

332   *Lower limb*

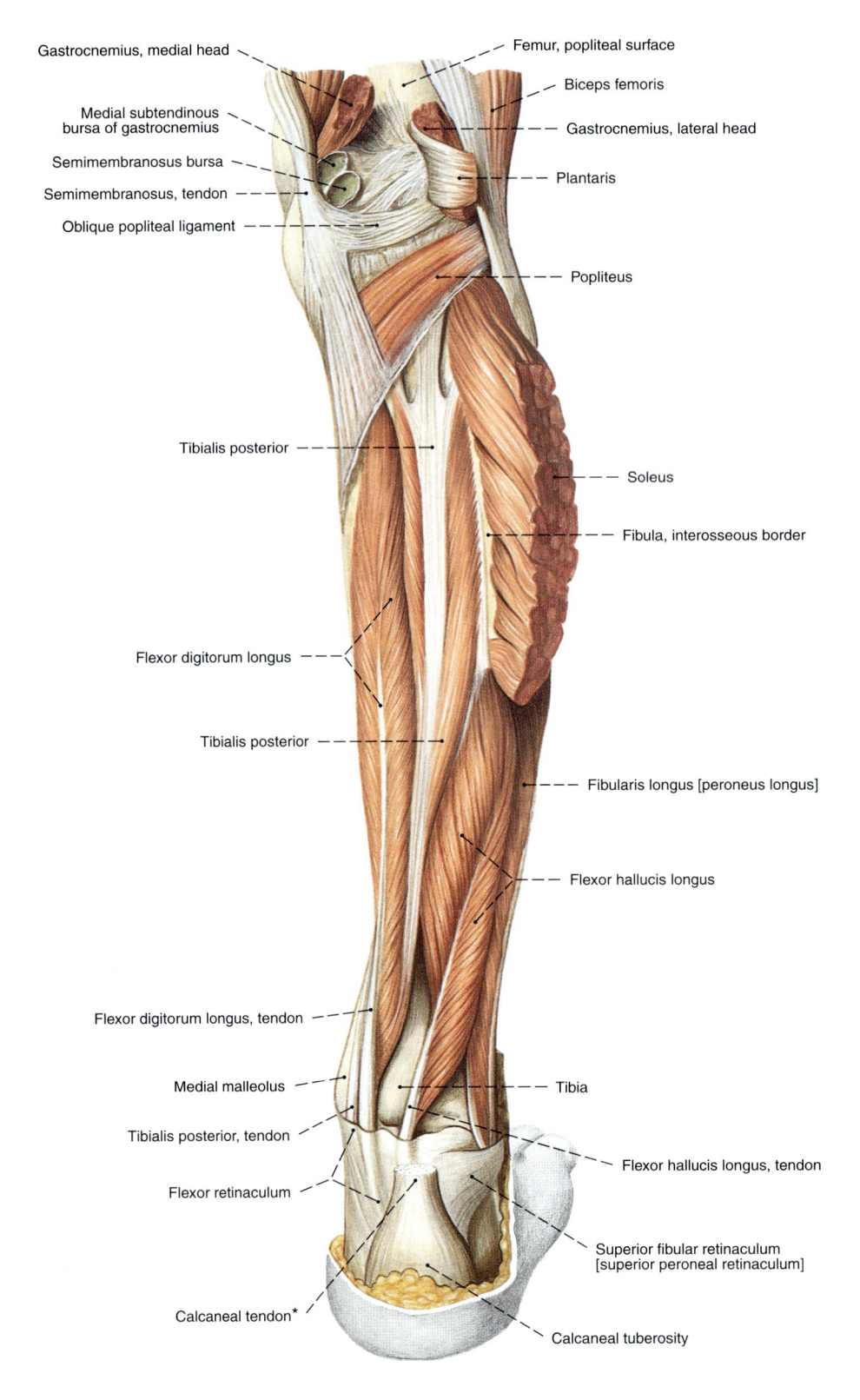

Fig. 1298 Muscles of right leg; superficial muscles extensively removed; posterior aspect.

* Also: ACHILLES tendon.

Muscles of leg

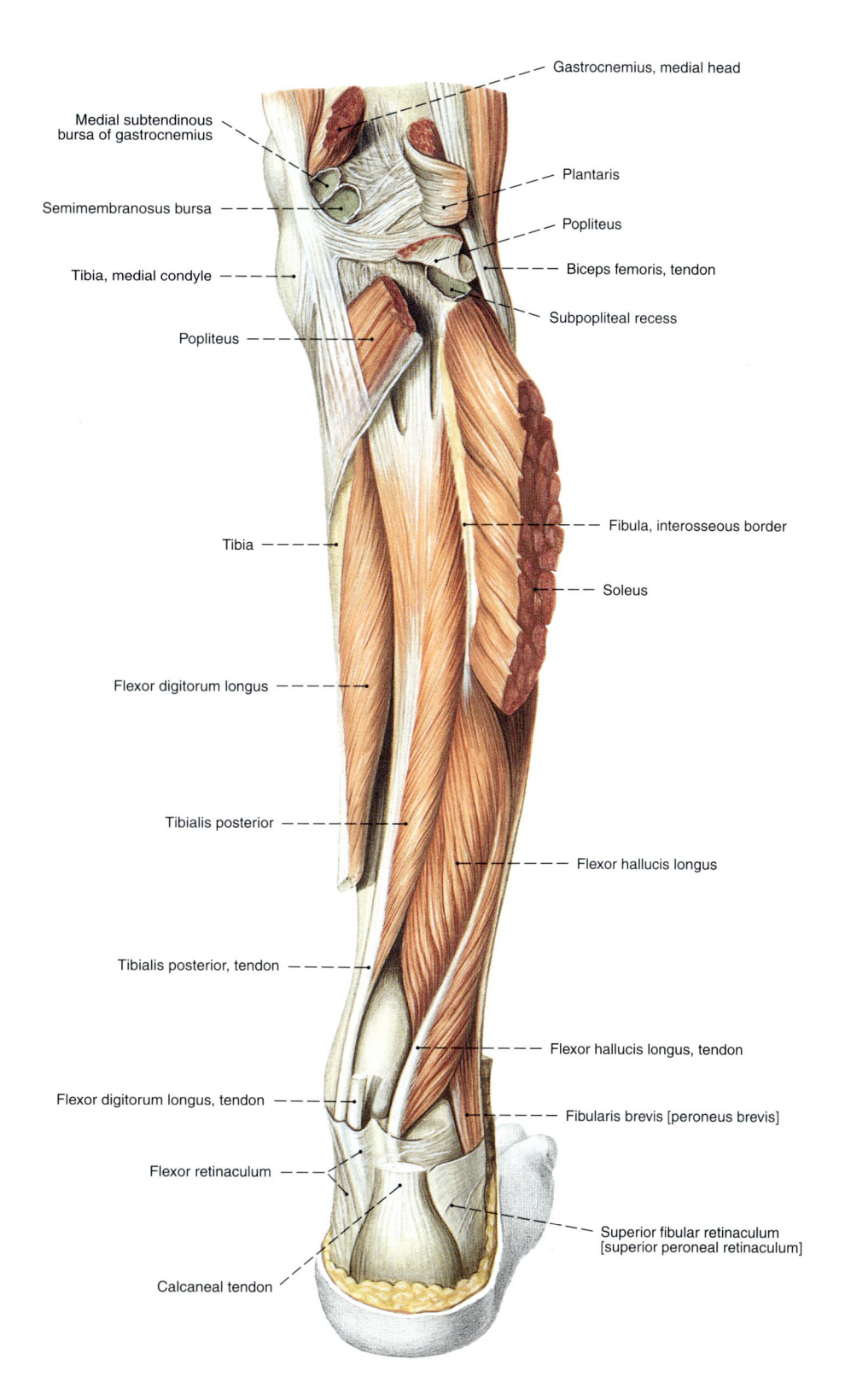

Fig. 1299 Muscles of right leg; superficial muscles extensively removed; popliteus sectioned and tendon of flexor digitorum longus removed at crossing with tendon of tibialis posterior (crural chiasm); posterior aspect.

Superficial dorsal muscles of leg (Figs. 1296, 1297, 1301)

The surface relief of the calf is formed by the two heads of gastrocnemius. It overlies the soleus and together with the soleus forms the triceps surae. The tiny plantaris may be considered a fourth head of this muscle

Muscle *Innervation*	Origin	Insertion	Function
1. **Triceps surae** *Tibial nerve (sciatic nerve)*	**Gastrocnemius, medial head:** popliteal surface of femur (proximal of medial condyle) **Gastrocnemius, lateral head:** popliteal surface of femur (proximal of lateral condyle) **Soleus:** head of fibula, posterior surface and posterior border of fibula (proximal 1/3), posterior surface of tibia (from and beneath soleal line), tendinous arch of soleus **Plantaris:** popliteal surface of femur (proximal of lateral condyle)	Calcaneal tuberosity via calcaneal tenodn [ACHILLES tendon]	**Knee joint** (gastrocnemius and plantaris only): Flexion **Ankle joint:** Plantar flexion **Talotarsal joint:** Supination

* Plantar flexion is also known as flexion; dorsiflexion is also known as extension.

Deep dorsal muscles of leg (Figs. 1298, 1301, 1313, 1314, 1318)

Most proximal the popliteus courses obliquely to the lateral region of the knee joint. Of the muscles in the foot the tibialis posterior is the most superficial. Beneath it are medial the flexor digitorum longus and lateral the flexor hallucis longus.

Muscle *Innervation*	Origin	Insertion	Function
1. **Popliteus** *Tibial nerve (sciatic nerve)*	Lateral epicondyle of femur	Posterior surface of tibia above soleal line	**Knee joint:** Medial rotation, flexion
2. **Tibialis posterior** *Tibial nerve (sciatic nerve)*	Interosseous membrane of leg, posterior surfaces of tibia and fibula (proximal 1/2 adjacent to interosseous membrane)	Tuberosity of navicular, lateral, intermediate [middle], and medial cuneiform (plantar surfaces), bases of 2nd-4th metatarsals	**Ankle joint:** Plantar flexion **Talotarsal joint:** Supination
3. **Flexor digitorum longus** *Tibial nerve (sciatic nerve)*	Posterior surface of tibia (beneath soleal line), tendinous arch between tibia and fibula (above crural chiasm)	Distal phalanges 2nd-5th metatarsals	**Ankle joint:** Plantar flexion **Talotarsal joint:** Supination **Joints of toes:** Flexion
4. **Flexor hallucis longus** *Tibial nerve (sciatic nerve)*	Posterior surface of fibula (distal 2/3), interosseous membrane of leg, posterior intermuscular septum of leg	Distal phalanx of great toe	**Ankle joint:** Plantar flexion **Talotarsal joint:** Supination **Joints of great toe:** Flexion

*Plantar flexion is also known as flexion; dorsiflexion is also known as extension.

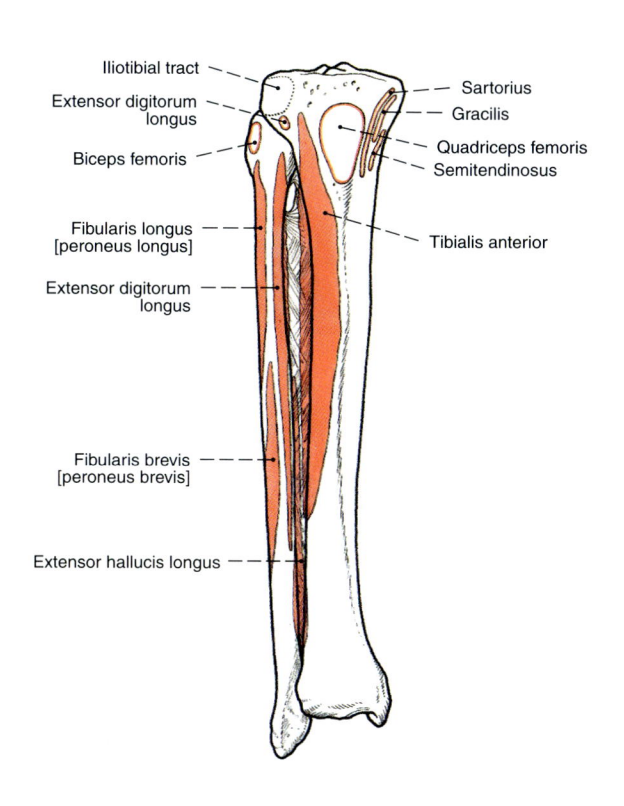

Muscle origins and insertions, mechanics of foot **335**

Fig. 1300 Muscle origins and insertions on the bones of right leg; anterior aspect.

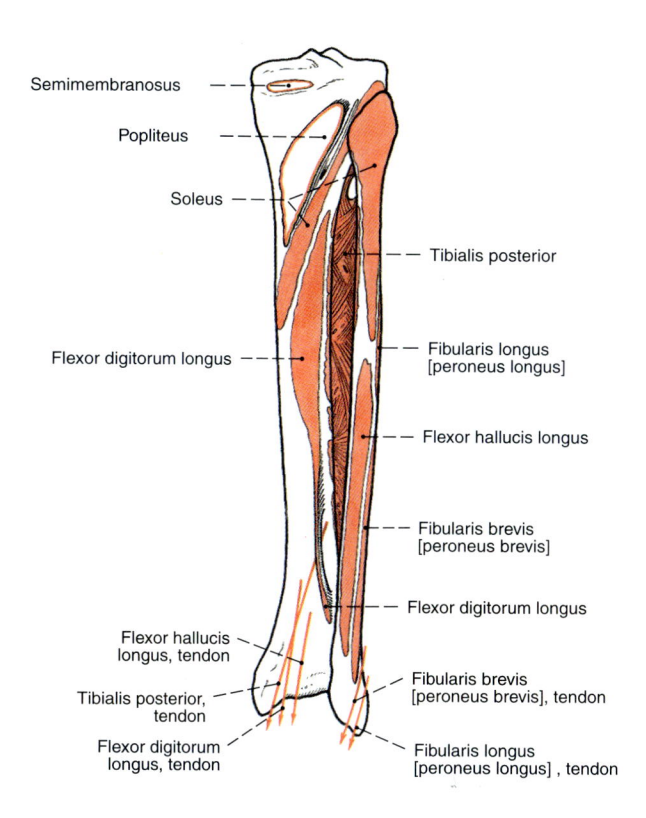

Labels: Iliotibial tract, Extensor digitorum longus, Biceps femoris, Fibularis longus [peroneus longus], Extensor digitorum longus, Fibularis brevis [peroneus brevis], Extensor hallucis longus, Sartorius, Gracilis, Quadriceps femoris, Semitendinosus, Tibialis anterior.

Fig. 1301 Muscle origins and insertions on the bones of right leg; posterior aspect.

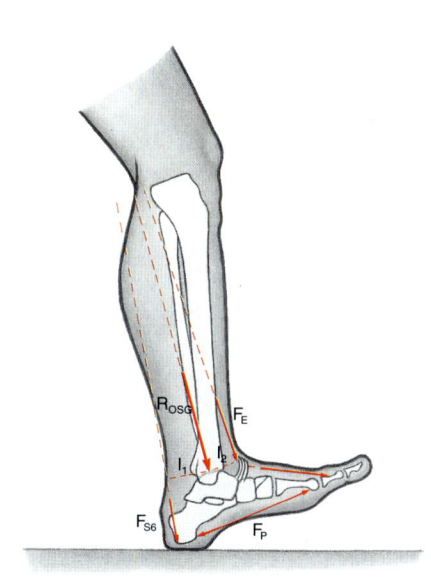

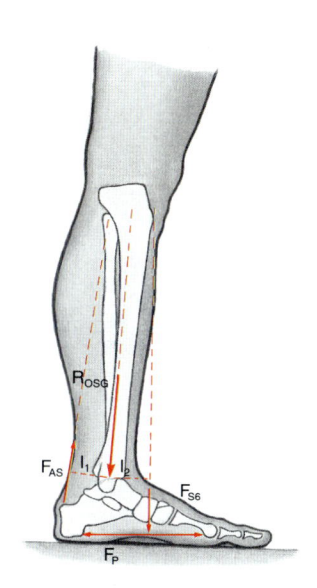

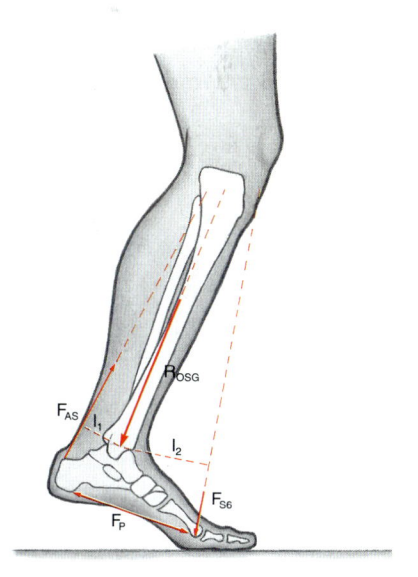

Labels: Semimembranosus, Popliteus, Soleus, Flexor digitorum longus, Flexor hallucis longus, tendon, Tibialis posterior, tendon, Flexor digitorum longus, tendon, Tibialis posterior, Fibularis longus [peroneus longus], Flexor hallucis longus, Fibularis brevis [peroneus brevis], Flexor digitorum longus, Fibularis brevis [peroneus brevis], tendon, Fibularis longus [peroneus longus], tendon.

F_{S6} force of body weight (6/6)
R_{OSG} resulting force in ankle joint
[REMARK: OSG *may* be changed to AJ for ankle joint both in figures and legend]

F_{AS} tractive force of Achilles tendon
[REMARK: AS *may* be changed to AT for Achilles tendon both in figures and legend]
F_E tractive force of extensor muscles

F_P tractive force effective on plantar aponeurosis
I_1 lever arm
I_2 lever arm

Fig. 1302 Forces in the foot during heel-strikeposition (standing on calcaneal tuberosity).

Fig. 1303 Forces in the foot during support phase (static load on sole).

Fig. 1304 Forces in the foot during toe-off position (standing on balls of toes).

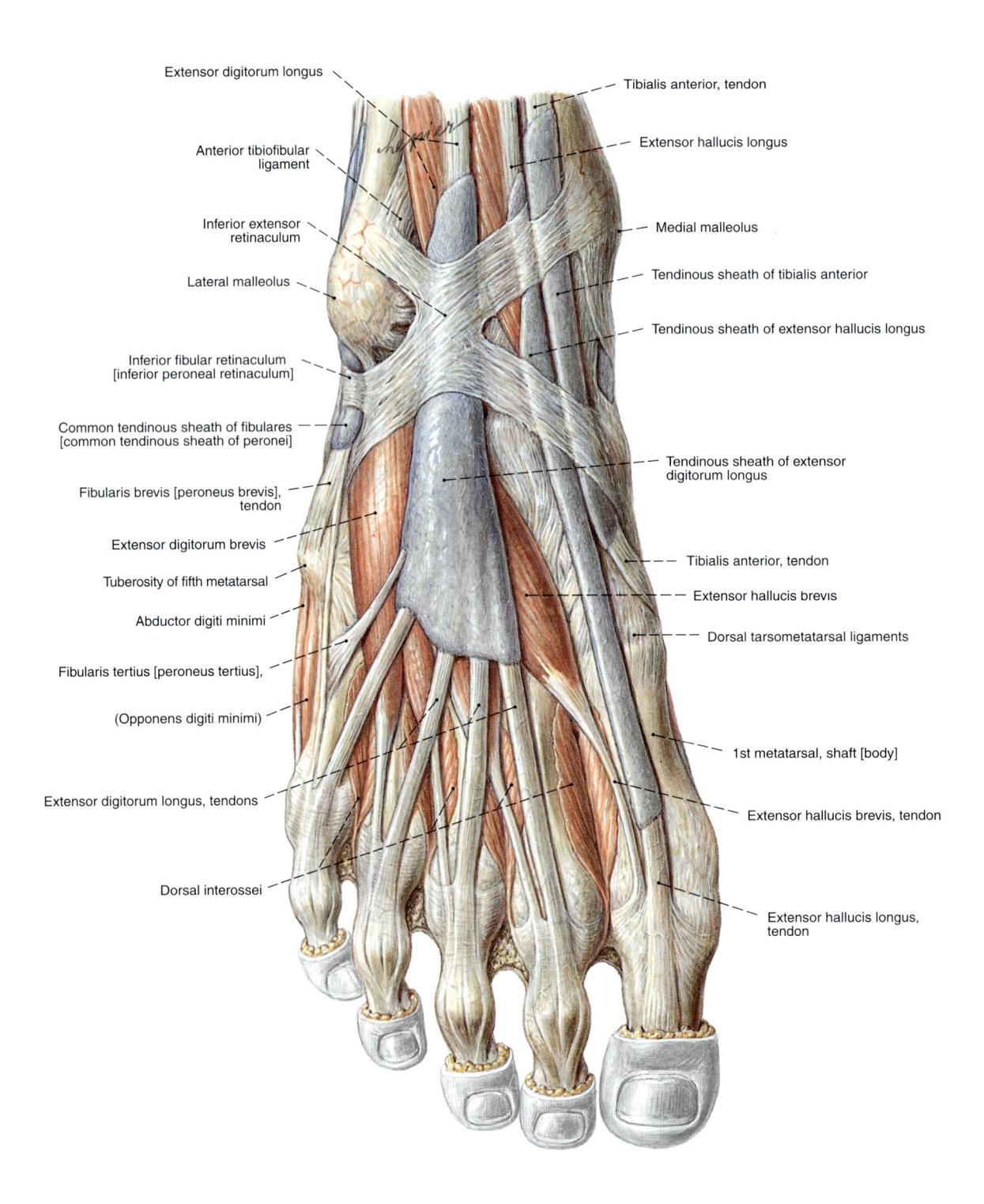

Fig. 1305 Tendinous sheaths of right foot; anterior aspect.

Tendinous sheaths of foot

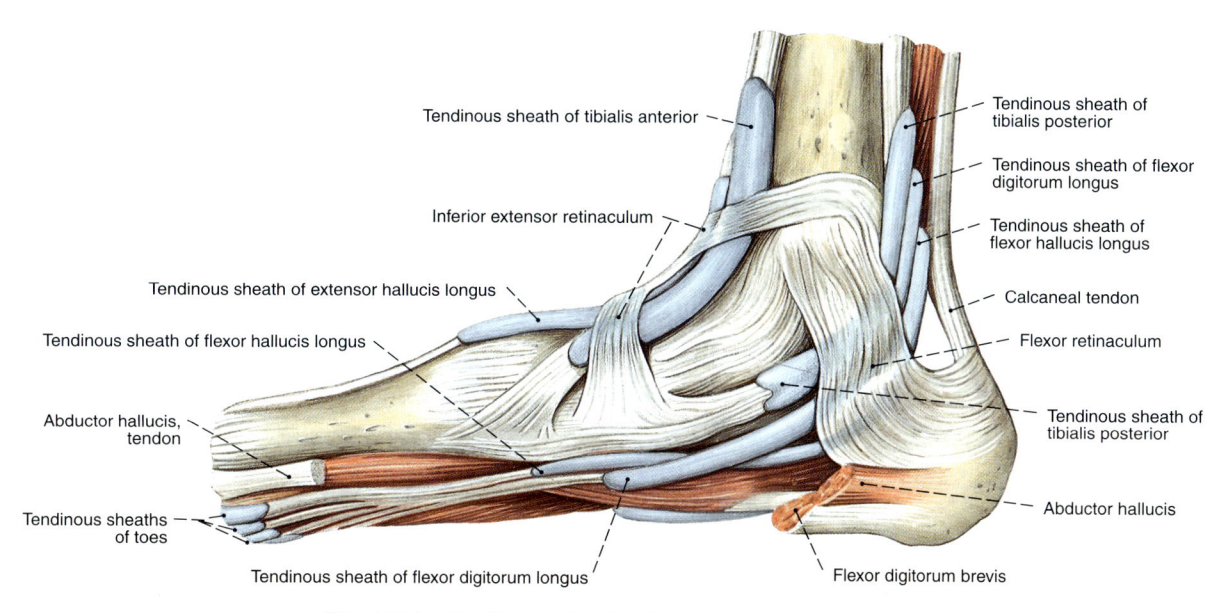

Fig. 1306 Tendinous sheaths of right foot; medial aspect.

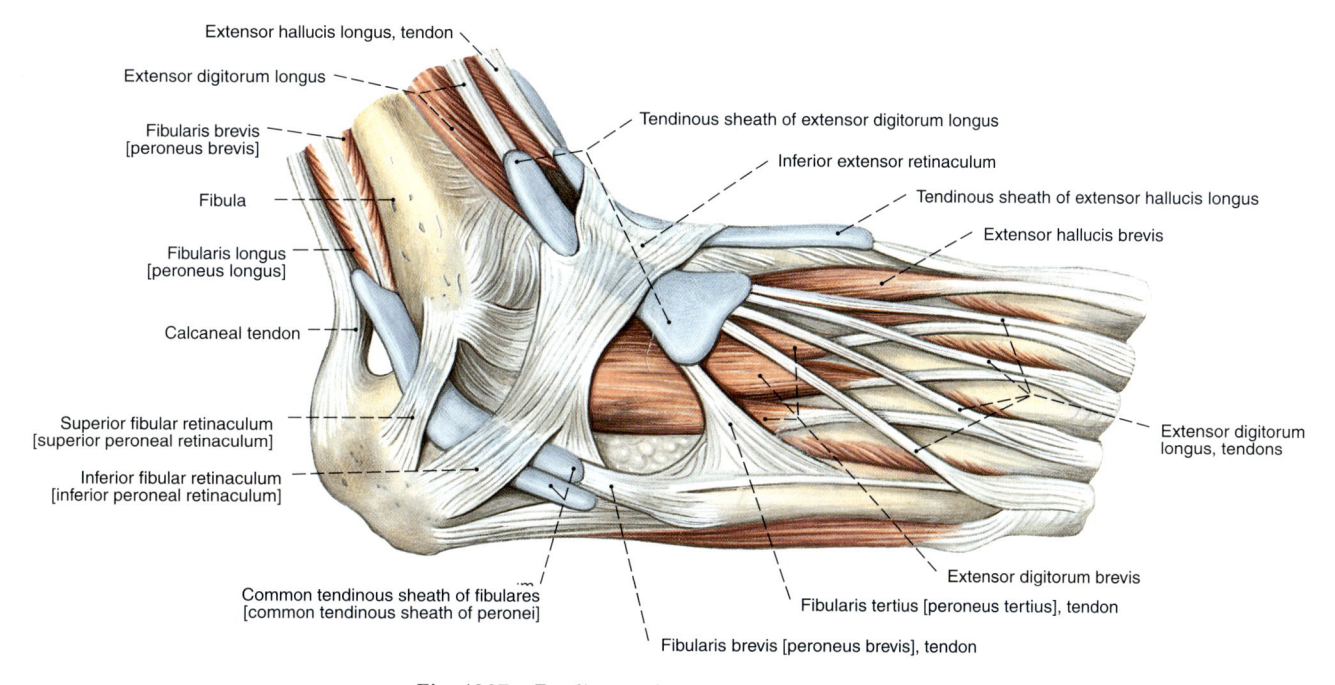

Fig. 1307 Tendinous sheaths of right foot; lateral aspect.

Tendinous sheaths of foot

Anterior tarsal tendinous sheaths: On the dorsum of foot beneath the superior and inferior extensor retinacula for tendons of tibialis anterior, extensor hallucis longus, and extensor digitorum longus.

Tibial tarsal tendinous sheaths: Behind the medial malleolus beneath the flexor retinaculum for tendons of tibialis posterior, flexor digitorum longus, and flexor hallucis longus.

Fibular tarsal tendinous sheaths: Behind the lateral malleolus beneath the superior and inferior fibular [peroneal] retinacula usually a common tendinous sheath for tendons of fibulares [peronei] longus and brevis. The tendinous sheath of fibularis [peroneus] longus extends further distally under the long plantar ligament to the insertion at the plantar surface of the base of the 1st metatarsal and the medial cuneiform.

Tendinous sheaths of toes: On the plantar side of toes for flexor digitorum longus and flexor digitorum brevis.

338　Lower limb

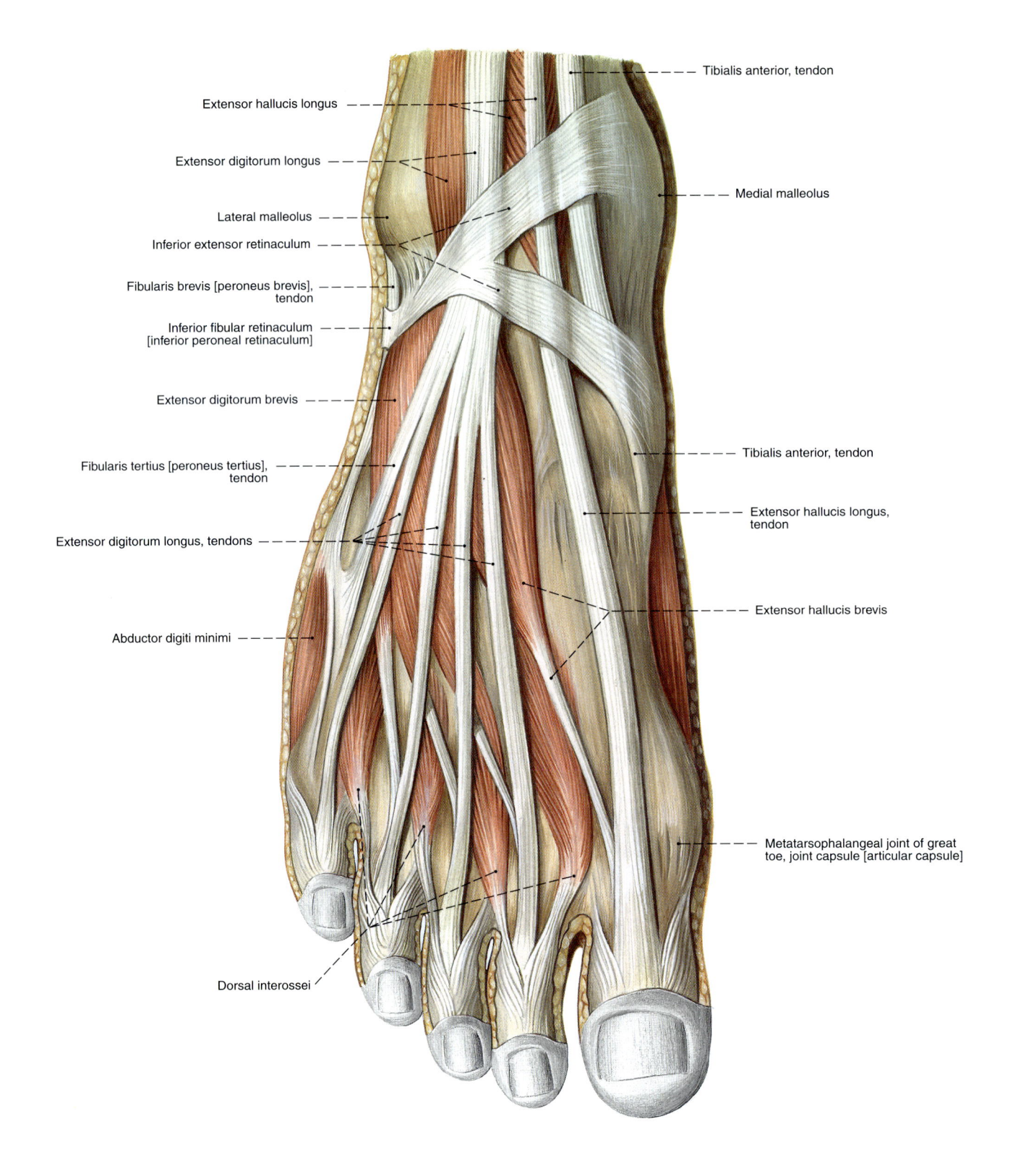

Fig. 1308　Muscles of right foot; tendinous sheath removed; anterior aspect.

Muscles of foot

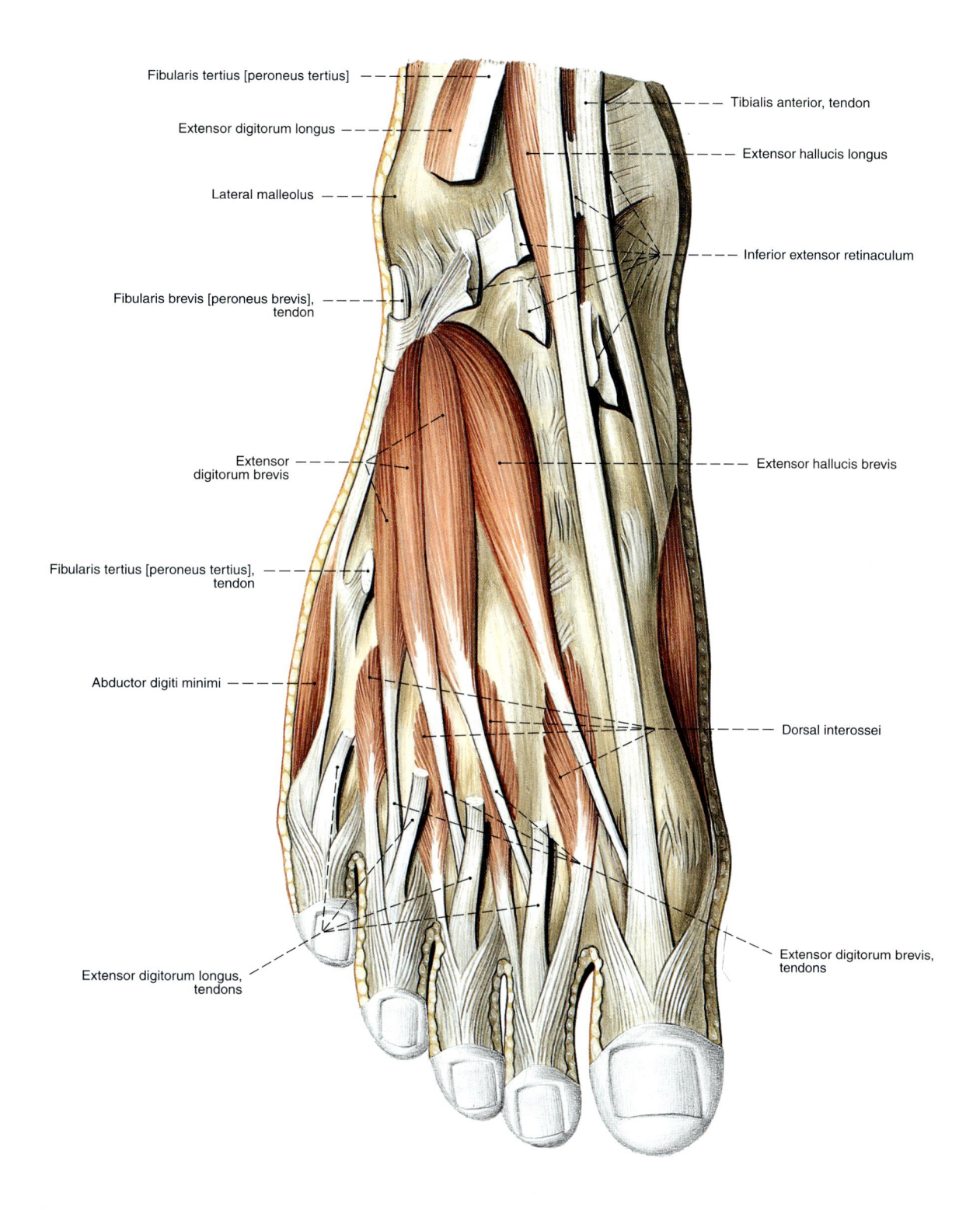

Fig. 1309 Muscles of right foot; inferior extensor retinaculum split and extensor digitorum longus extensively removed; anterior aspect.

Lower limb

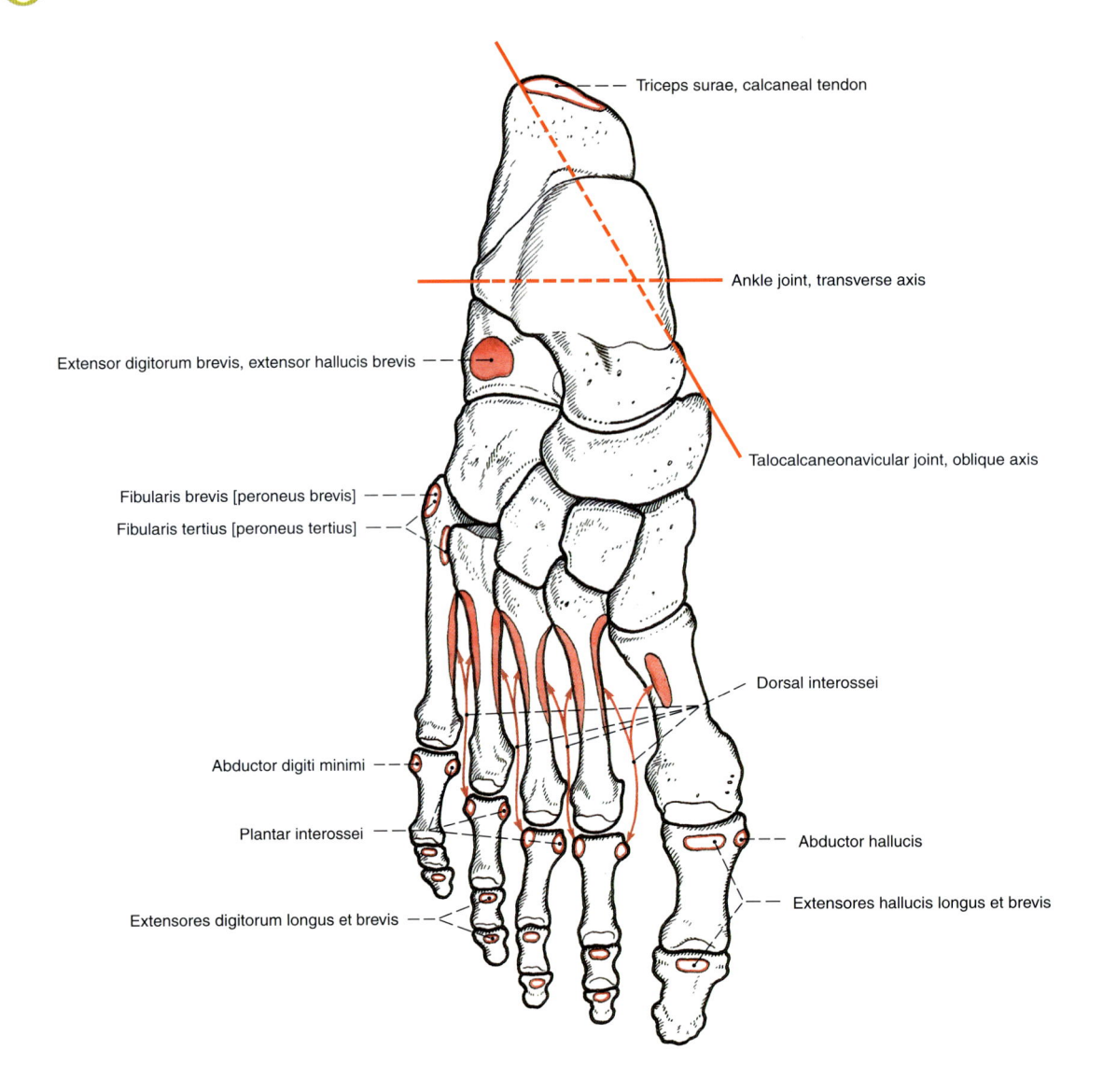

Fig. 1310 Muscle origins and insertions on bones of right foot; dorsal aspect.
The axes of the ankle joint and the talotarsal joints are indicated.

Muscles of dorsum of foot (Fig. 1308)

Both muscles of the dorsum of foot protrude only little through the skin. From a small area of origin the extensor hallucis brevis courses to the great toe and the extensor digitorum brevis to the other toes.

Muscle *Innervation*	Origin	Insertion	Function
1. Extensor digitorum brevis *Deep fibular [peroneal] nerve (Common fibular [peroneal] nerve)*	Calcaneus (dorsal and lateral surface)	Extensor expansion of 2nd–4th toes	**Joints of toes:** Extension
2. Extensor hallucis brevis *Deep fibular [peroneal nerve (Common fibular [peroneal] nerve)*	Calcaneus (dorsal and lateral surface)	Proximal phalanx of great toe	**Joints of great toe:** Extension

* Plantar flexion is also known as flexion, dorsiflexion is also known as extension.

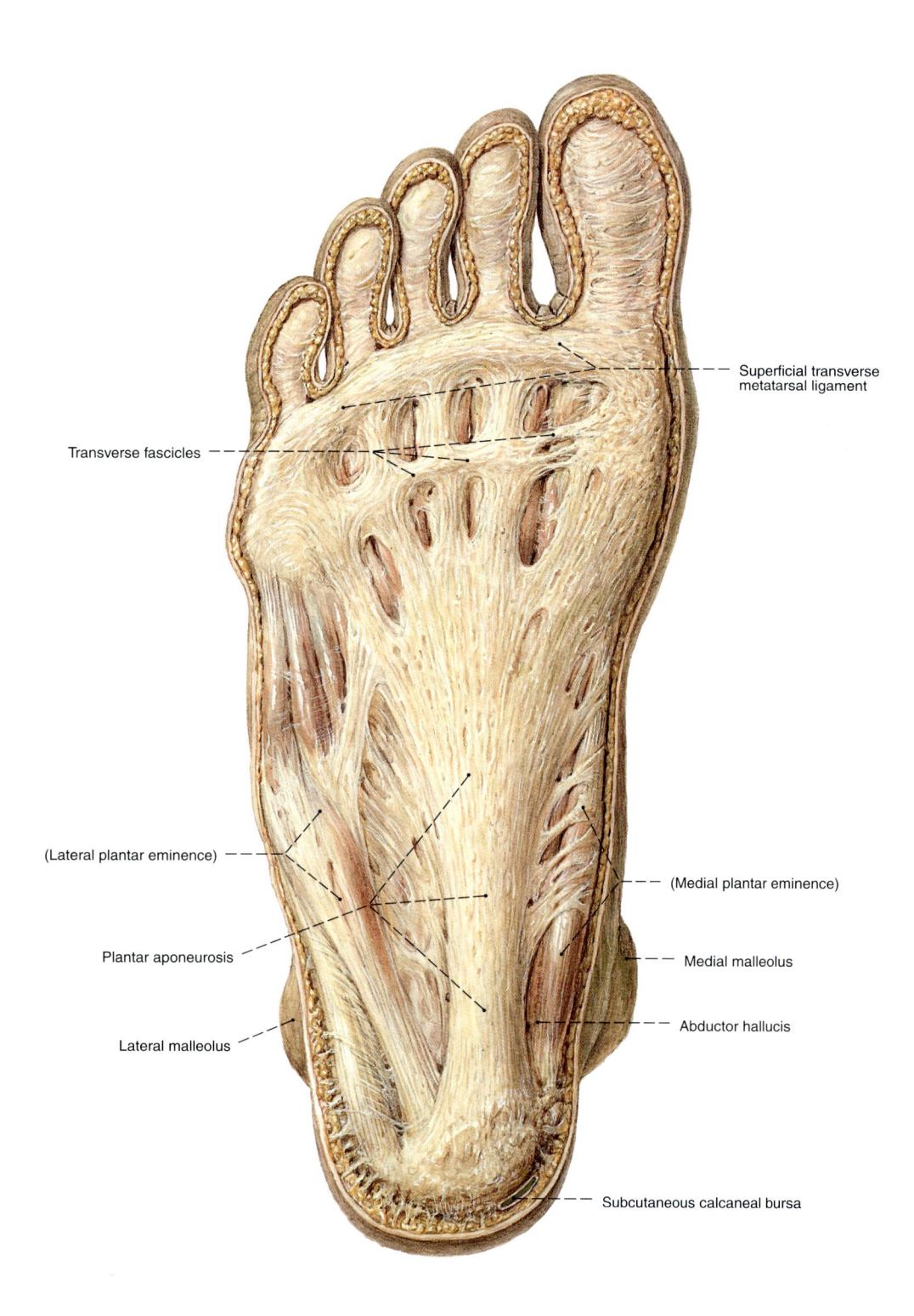

Fig. 1311 Muscles of right foot; demonstration of plantar aponeurosis; plantar aspect.

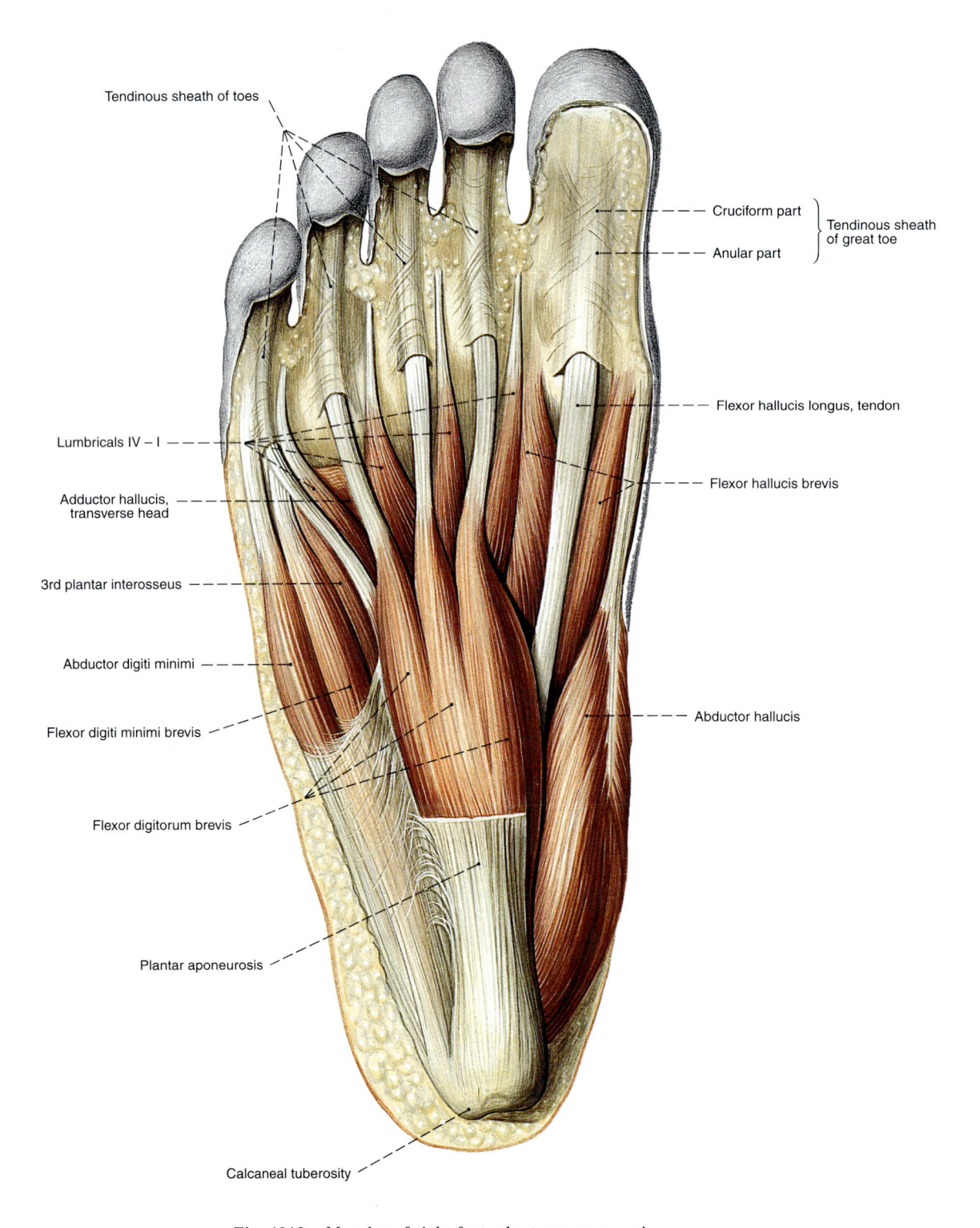

Fig. 1312   Muscles of right foot; plantar aponeurosis extensively removed; plantar aspect.

Muscles of foot 343

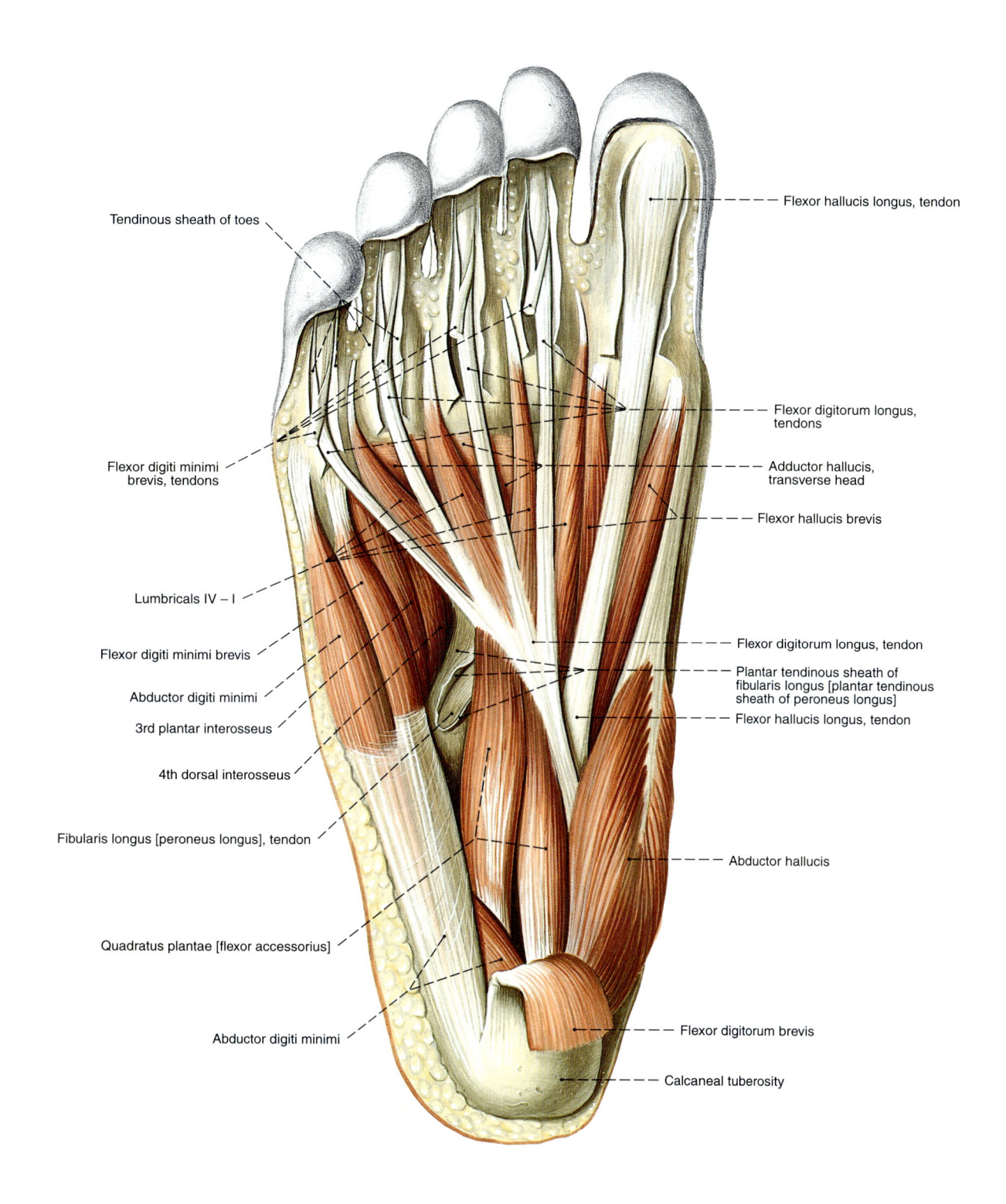

Fig. 1313 Muscles of right foot; middle layer; plantar aponeurosis and adhering flexor digitorum brevis extensively removed; plantar aspect.

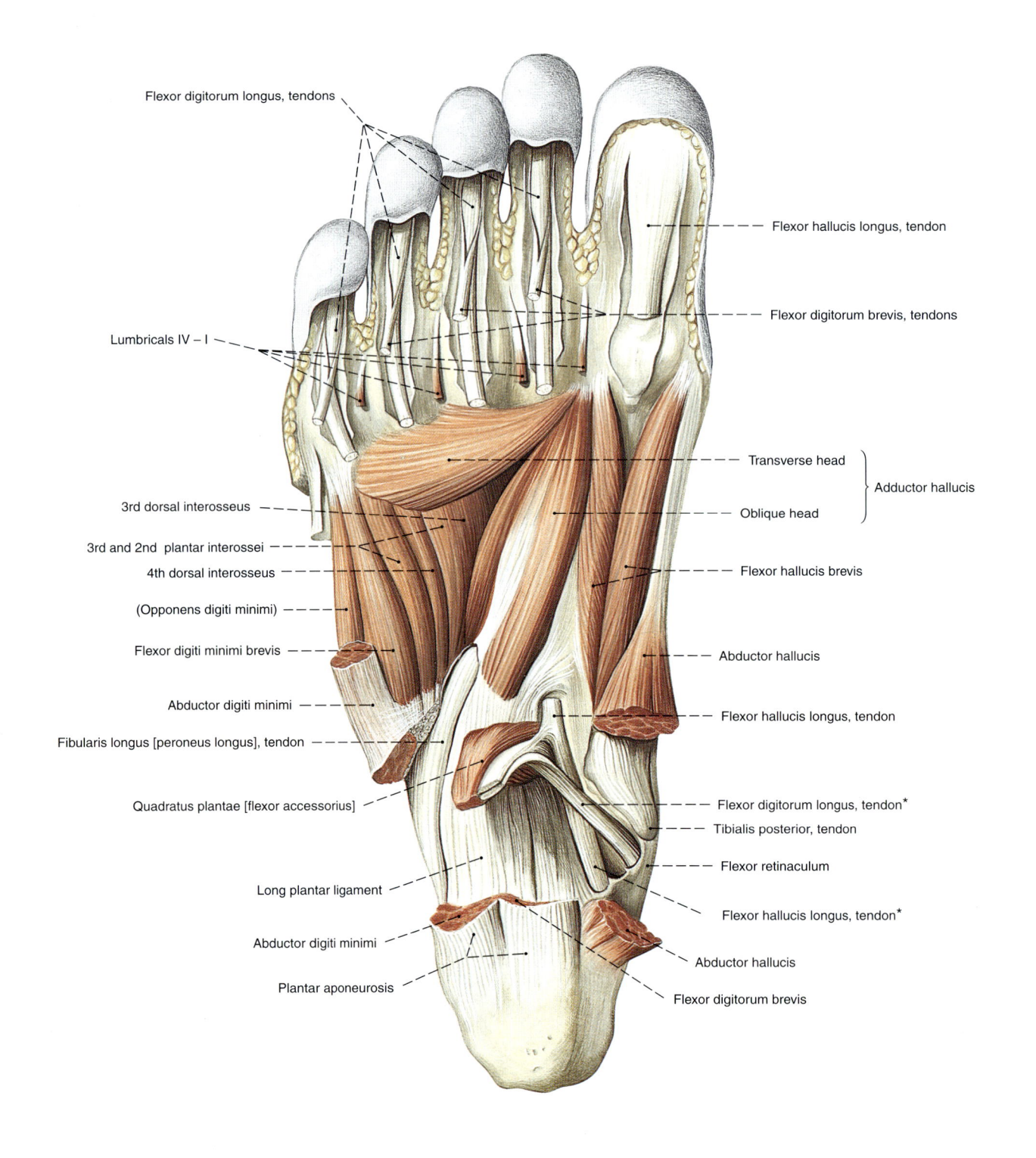

Fig. 1314 Muscles of right foot; deep layer; superficial muscles, flexor digitorum and hallucis longus extensively removed; plantar aspect.

* The crossing over of the tendons of flexor digitorum longus and flexor hallucis longus is also known as plantar chiasm.

Muscles of foot 345

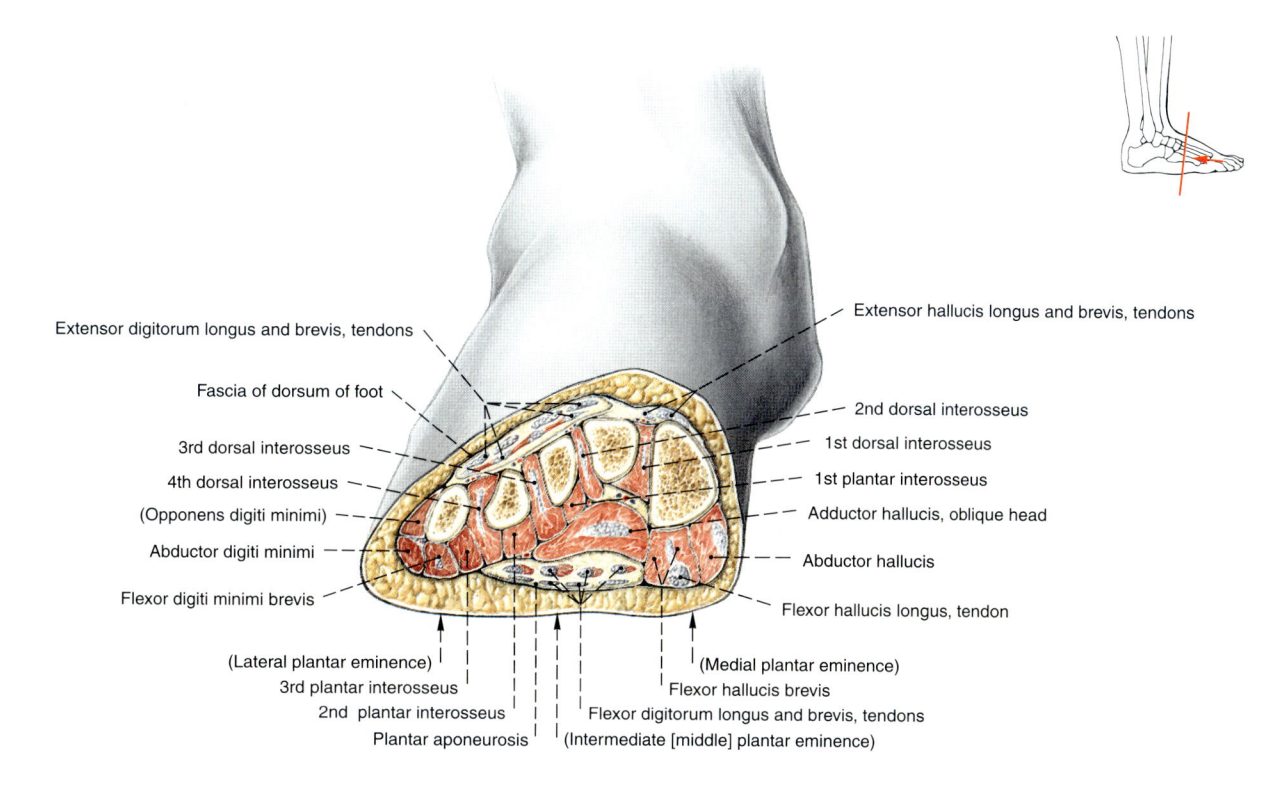

Fig. 1315 Osseofibrous tubes of right foot; frontal section through metatarsus; distal aspect.

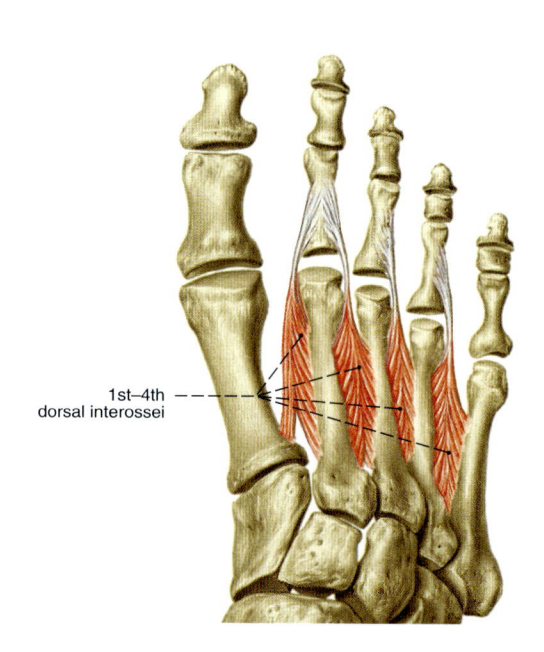

Fig. 1316 Muscles of right foot; dorsal interossei; dorsal aspect.

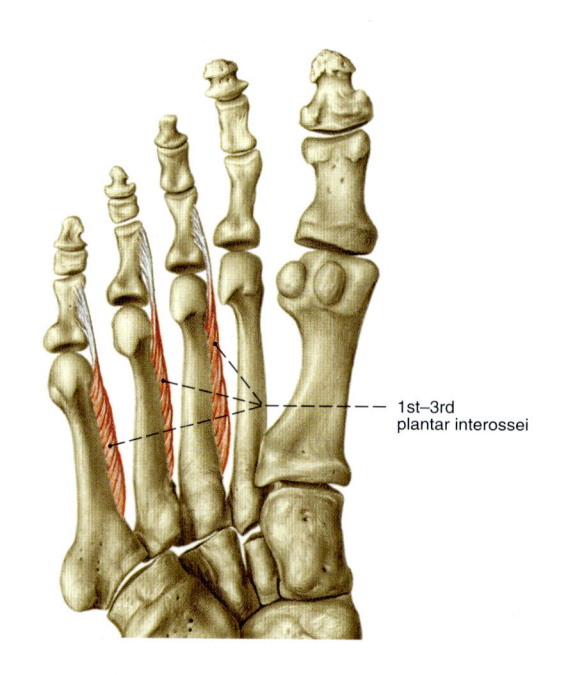

Fig. 1317 Muscles of right foot; plantar interossei; plantar aspect.

Medial plantar muscles (Figs. 1312, 1318)

The medial border of the foot, the medial plantar eminence, is formed mainly by the abductor hallucis. Neighboring are the flexor hallucis brevis and the adductor hallucis laterally.

Muscle Innervation	Origin	Insertion	Function*
1. Abductor hallucis *Medial plantar nerve (tibial nerve)*	Medial process of calcaneal tuberosity, plantar aponeurosis, flexor retinaculum	Medial sesamoid bone of capsule of metatarsophalangeal joint of great toe, base of proximal phalanx of great toe (medial edge)	**Metatarsophalangeal joint of great toe:** Abduction, flexion
2. Flexor hallucis brevis *Medial part: medial plantar nerve (tibial nerve)* *Lateral part: lateral plantar nerve (tibial nerve)*	Cuneiform bones (plantar surface), plantar calcaneocuboid ligament [short plantar ligament], tendon of tibialis posterior	**Medial part:** medial sesamoid bone of capsule of metatarsophalangeal joint of great toe, base of proximal phalanx of great toe **Lateral part:** lateral sesamoid bone of capsule of metatarsophalangeal joint of great toe, base of proximal phalanx of great toe	**Metatarsophalangeal joint of great toe:** Flexion
3. Adductor hallucis *Medial plantar nerve (tibial nerve)*	**Oblique head:** cuboid, lateral cuneiform, long plantar ligament, plantar calcaneocuboid ligament [short plantar ligament] **Transverse head:** joint capsules of metatarsophalangeal joints of 3rd–5th toes; deep transverse metatarsal ligament	Lateral sesamoid bone of capsule of metatarsophalangeal joint of great toe, base of proximal phalanx of great toe	**Metatarsophalangeal joint of great toe:** Adduction toward 2nd toe, flexion

* Explanation see page 347.

Middle plantar muscles (Figs. 1312, 1318)

Small muscles are located in the depth of the longitudinal arch of foot. The flexor digitorum brevis is attached to the plantar aponeurosis proximally. Beneath this muscle the quadratus plantae [flexor accessorius] blends with the main tendon of the flexor digitorum longus. The four lumbricals originate from its four tendons. The three plantar and the four dorsal interossei fill the space between the metatarsals.

Muscle/*Innervation*	Origin	Insertion	Function*
1. Flexor digitorum brevis *Medial plantar nerve (tibial nerve)*	Calcaneal tuberosity (plantar surface), plantar aponeurosis	Middle phalanges of 2nd–4th toes (penetrated by tendons of flexor digitorum longus)	**Metatarsophalangeal joints of toes:** Flexion **Interphalangeal joints of toes:** Flexion
2. Quadratus plantae [flexor accessorius] *Lateral plantar nerve (tibial nerve)*	Calcaneal tuberosity (plantar surface), long plantar ligament	Tendon of flexor digitorum longus (lateral border before its division)	Changes direction of flexor digitorum longus
3. 1st–4th lumbricals *Medial(1st) and lateral (2nd–4th) plantar nerve (tibial nerve)*	**1st lumbrical:** tendon of flexor digitorum longus of 2nd toe (medial side) **2nd–4th lumbricals:** tendons of flexor digitorum longus of 3rd–5th toes (adjacent sides)	Proximal phalanges of 2nd–5th toes (medial side), occasionally into the extensor expansion [extensor hood]	**Metatarsophalangeal joints of toes:** Flexion
4. 1st–3rd plantar interossei *Lateral plantar nerve (tibial nerve)*	3rd–5th metatarsals (plantar surface), long plantar ligament	Bases of proximal phalanges of 3rd–5th toes (medial sides)	**Metatarsophalangeal joints of toes:**
5. 1st–4th plantar interossei *Lateral plantar nerve (tibial nerve)*	Adjacent sides of 1st–5th metatarsal (by two heads), long plantar ligament	**1st dorsal interosseus:** Base of proximal phalanx of 2nd toe (medial side) **2nd–4th dorsal interossei:** Bases of proximal phalanges of 3rd and 4th toes (lateral side), blend with the extensor expansions [extensor hoods]	**Metatarsophalangeal joints of toes:** Flexion, lateral abduction (3rd and 4th toes), medial abduction (2nd toe) **Interphalangeal joints of toes:** Extension

* Explanation see page 347.

Lower limb

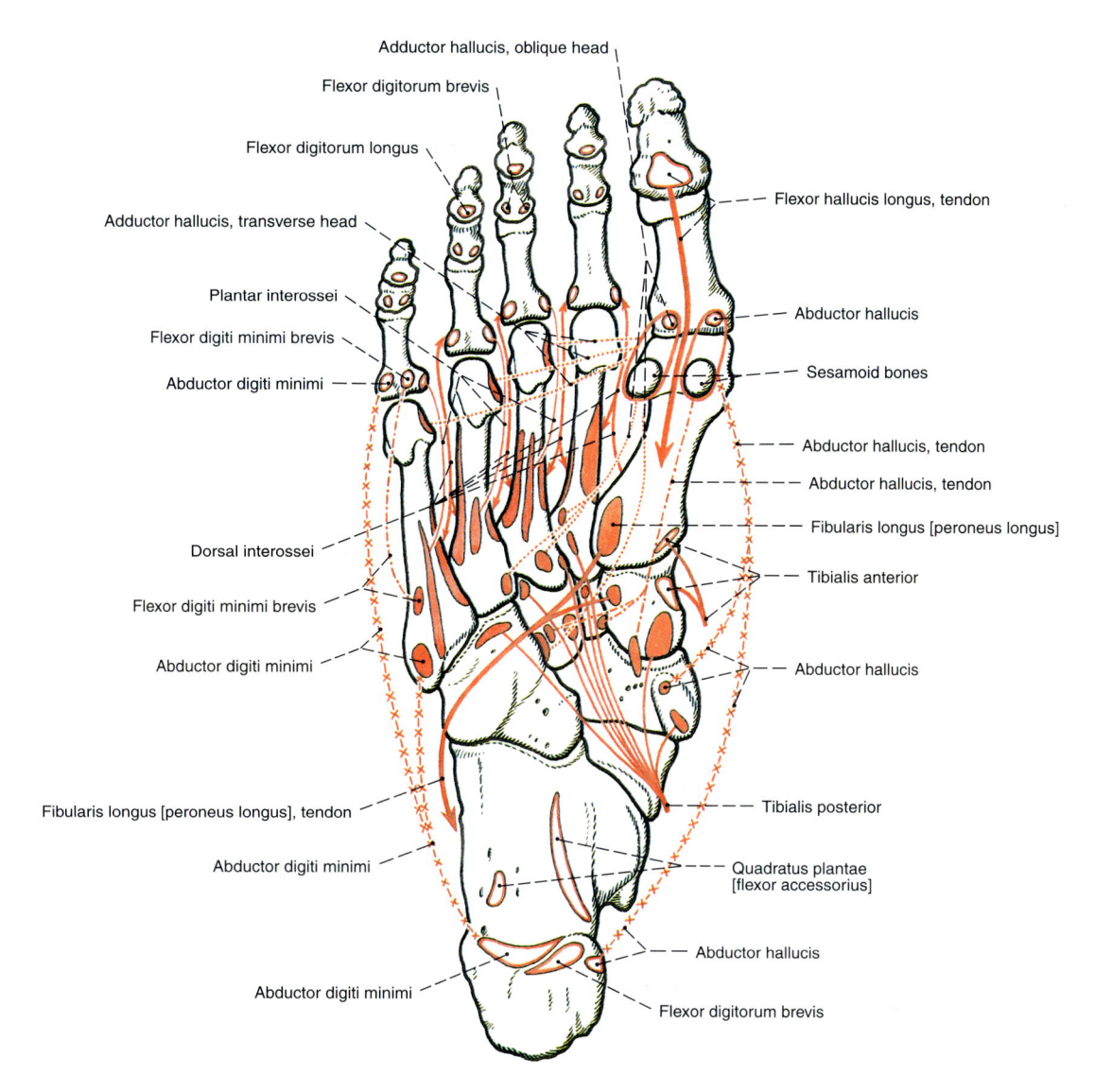

Fig. 1318 Muscle origins and insertions on the bones of right foot; plantar aspect.

Lateral plantar muscles (Fig. 1312)

The lateral border of the foot, the lateral plantar eminence, is formed mainly by the abductor digiti minimi. Beneath are the flexor digiti minimi brevis and opponens digiti minimi.

Muscle/Innervation	Origin	Insertion	Function
1. Abductor digiti minimi *Lateral plantar nerve (tibial nerve)*	Lateral and medial process (deep head) of calcaneal tuberosity, plantar aponeurosis	Base of proximal phalanx of 5th toe, tuberosity of 5th metatarsal	**Metatarsophalangeal joint of 5th toe:** Abduction, flexion, opposition
2. Flexor digiti minimi brevis *Lateral plantar nerve (tibial nerve)*	Base of 5th metatarsal, long plantar ligament, plantar tendinous sheath of fibularis [peroneus] longus	Proximal phalanx of 5th toe	**Metatarsophalangeal joint of 5th toe:** Abduction, flexion, opposition
3. Opponens digiti minimi *Lateral plantar nerve (tibial nerve) (variable)*	Base of 5th metatarsal, long plantar ligament, plantar tendinous sheath of fibularis [peroneus] longus	5th metatarsal (lateral border)	**Metatarsophalangeal joint of 5th toe:** Abduction, flexion, opposition

* Plantar flexion is also known as flexion; dorsiflexion is also known as extension.

348   Lower limb

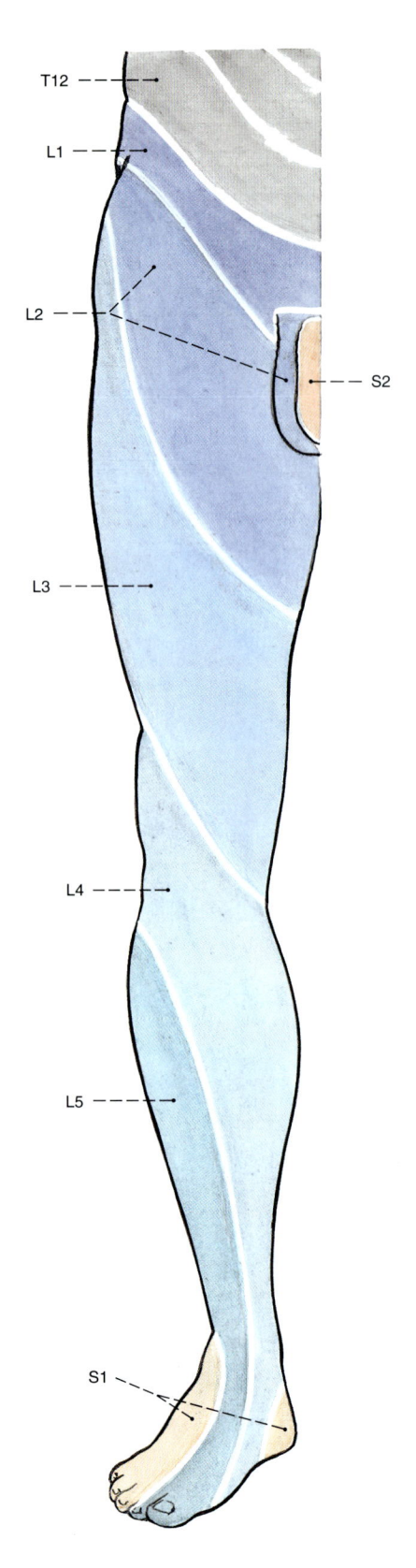

Fig. 1319 Segmental cutaneous innervation (dermatomes) of right lower limb; anterior aspect.

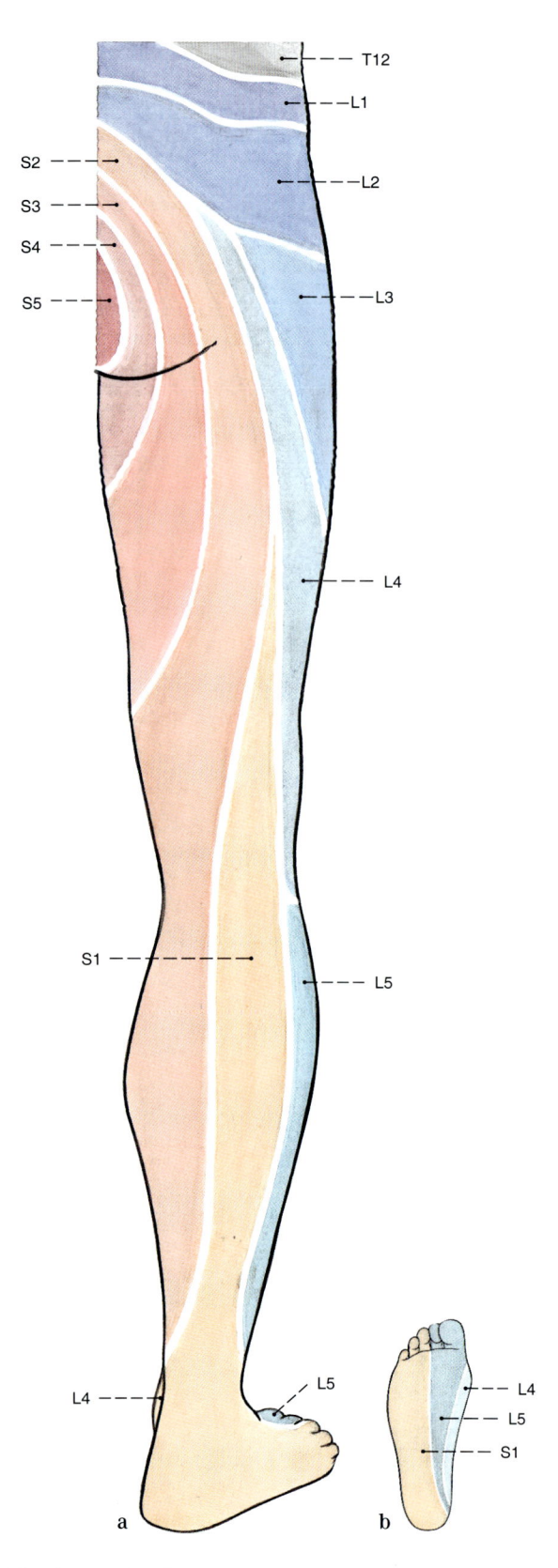

Fig. 1320 a, b Segmental cutaneous innervation (dermatomes) of right lower limb.
a Posterior aspect
b Plantar aspect

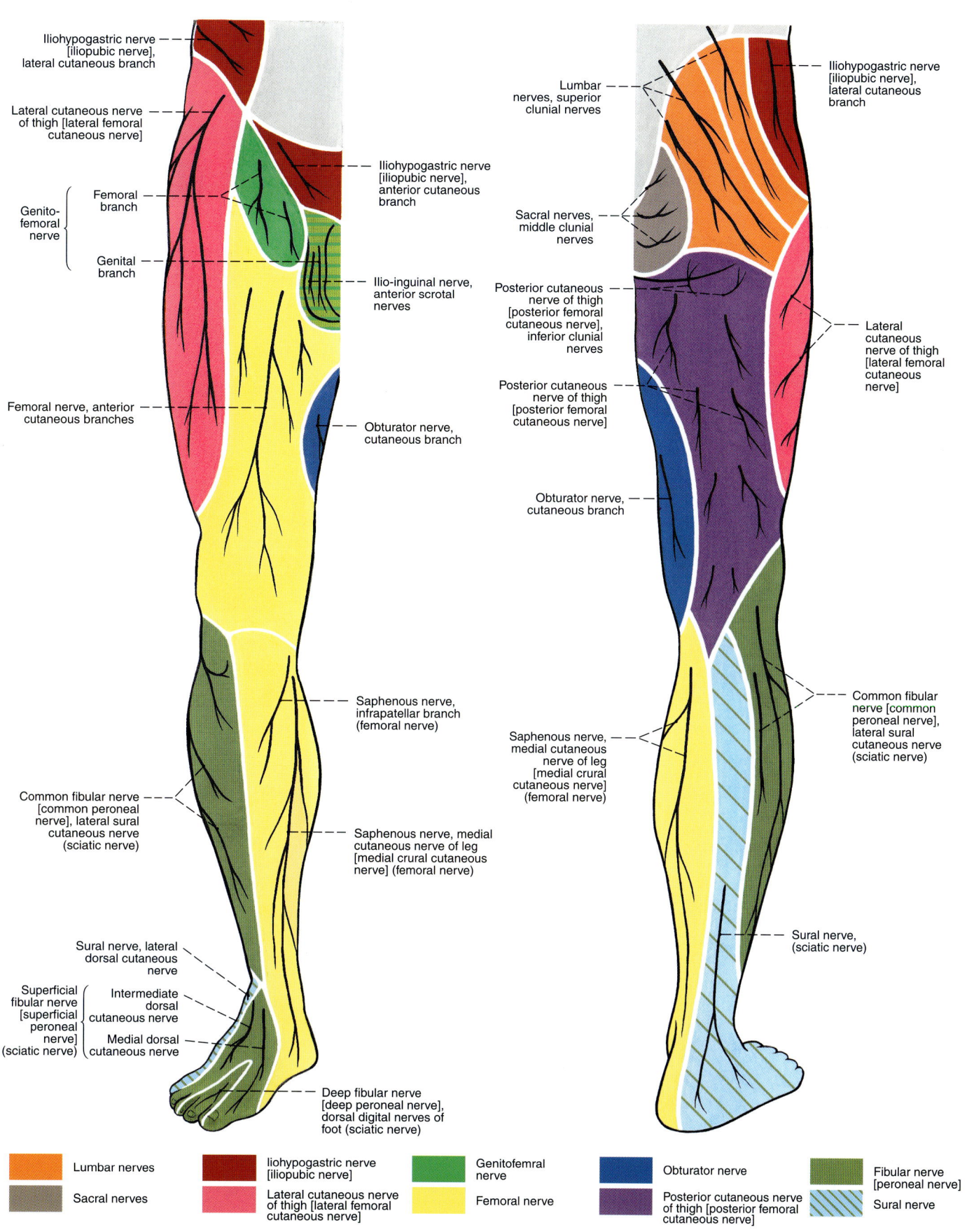

Cutaneous nerves of lower limb 349

Fig. 1321 Cutaneous nerves of right lower limb; anterior aspect.

Fig. 1322 Cutaneous nerves of right lower limb; posterior aspect.

Lower limb

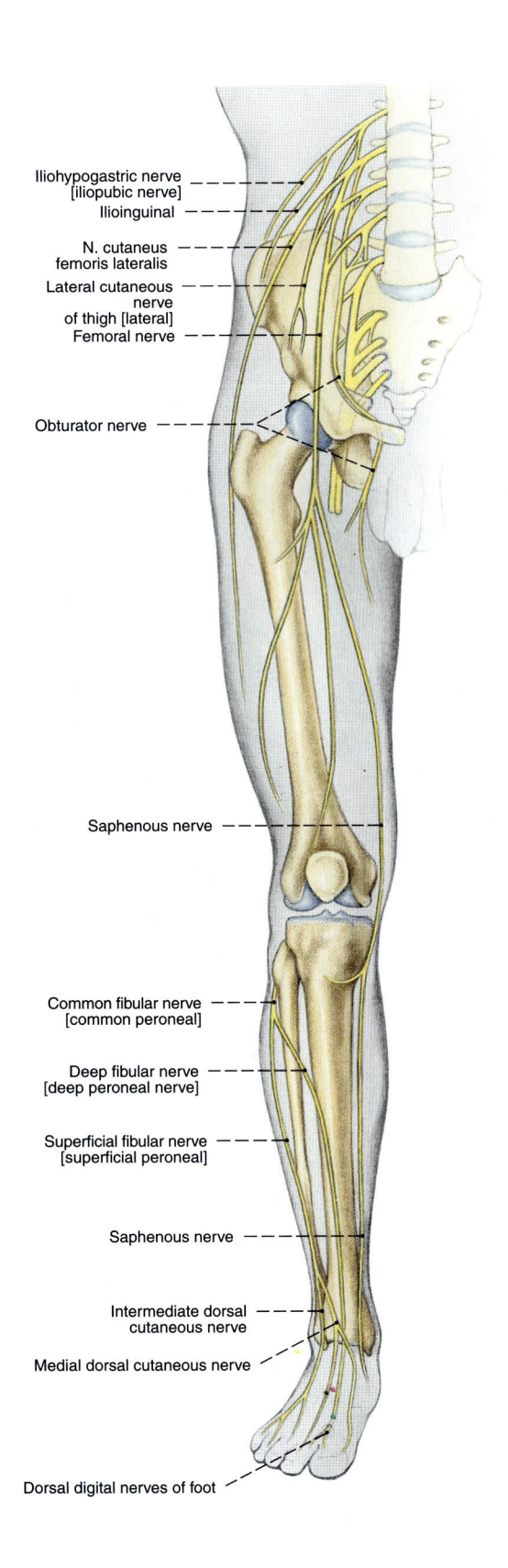

Fig. 1323 Nerves of right lower limb; general survey; anterior aspect.

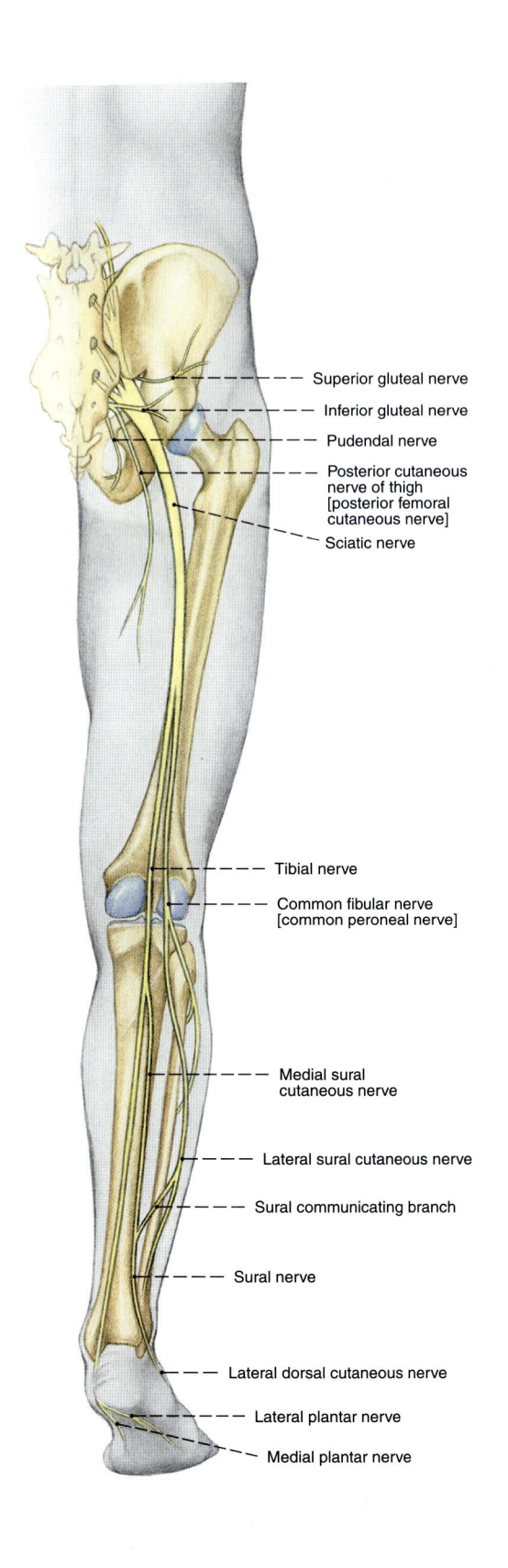

Fig. 1324 Nerves of right lower limb; general survey; posterior aspect.

Arteries of lower limb 351

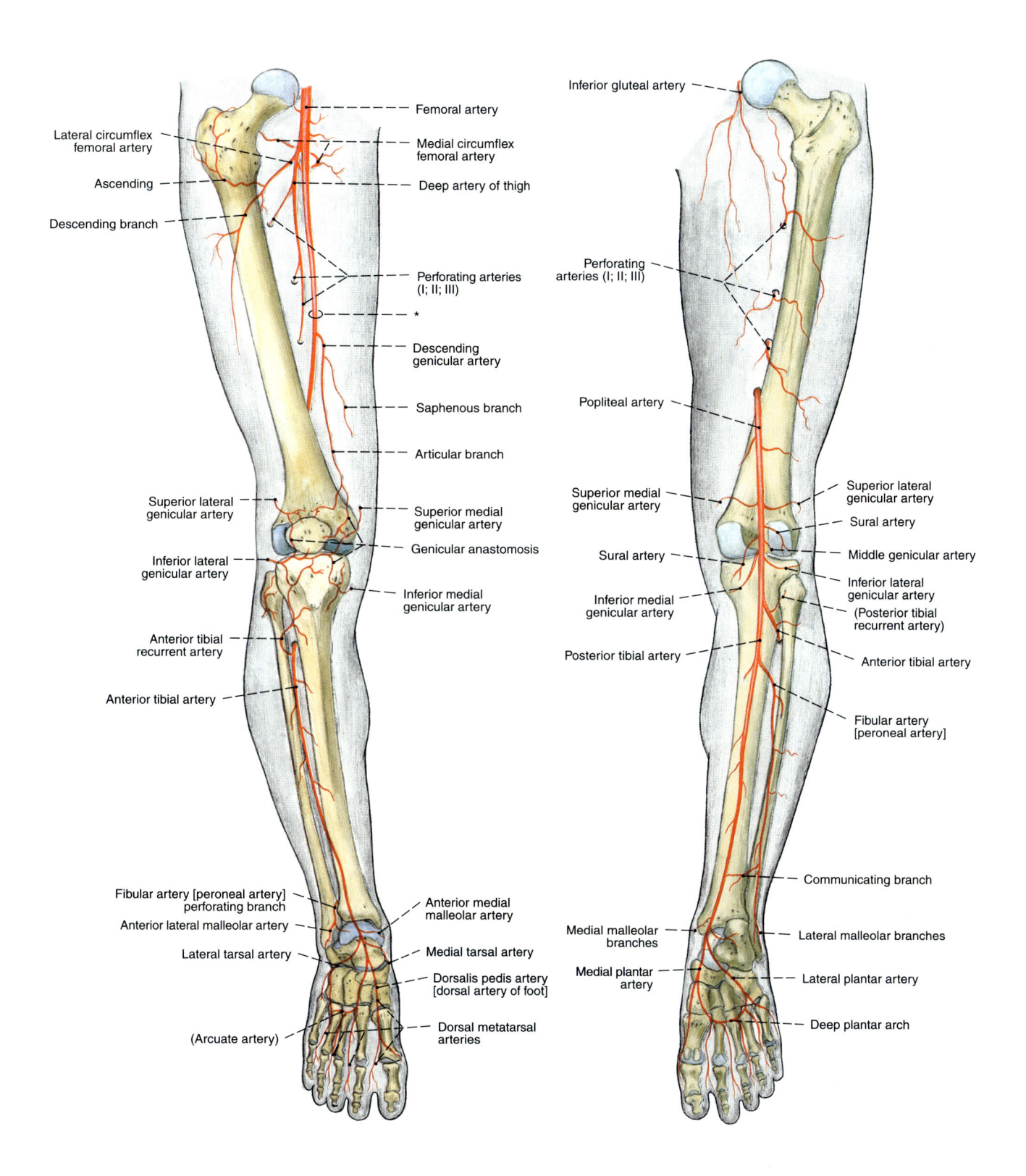

Fig. 1325 Arteries of right lower limb; general survey; anterior aspect.
The segment of the femoral artery between the origin of the deep artery of thigh and its entrance into the adductor canal (*) is clinically also known as superficial femoral artery.

Fig. 1326 Arteries of right lower limb; general survey; posterior aspect.

352 Lower limb

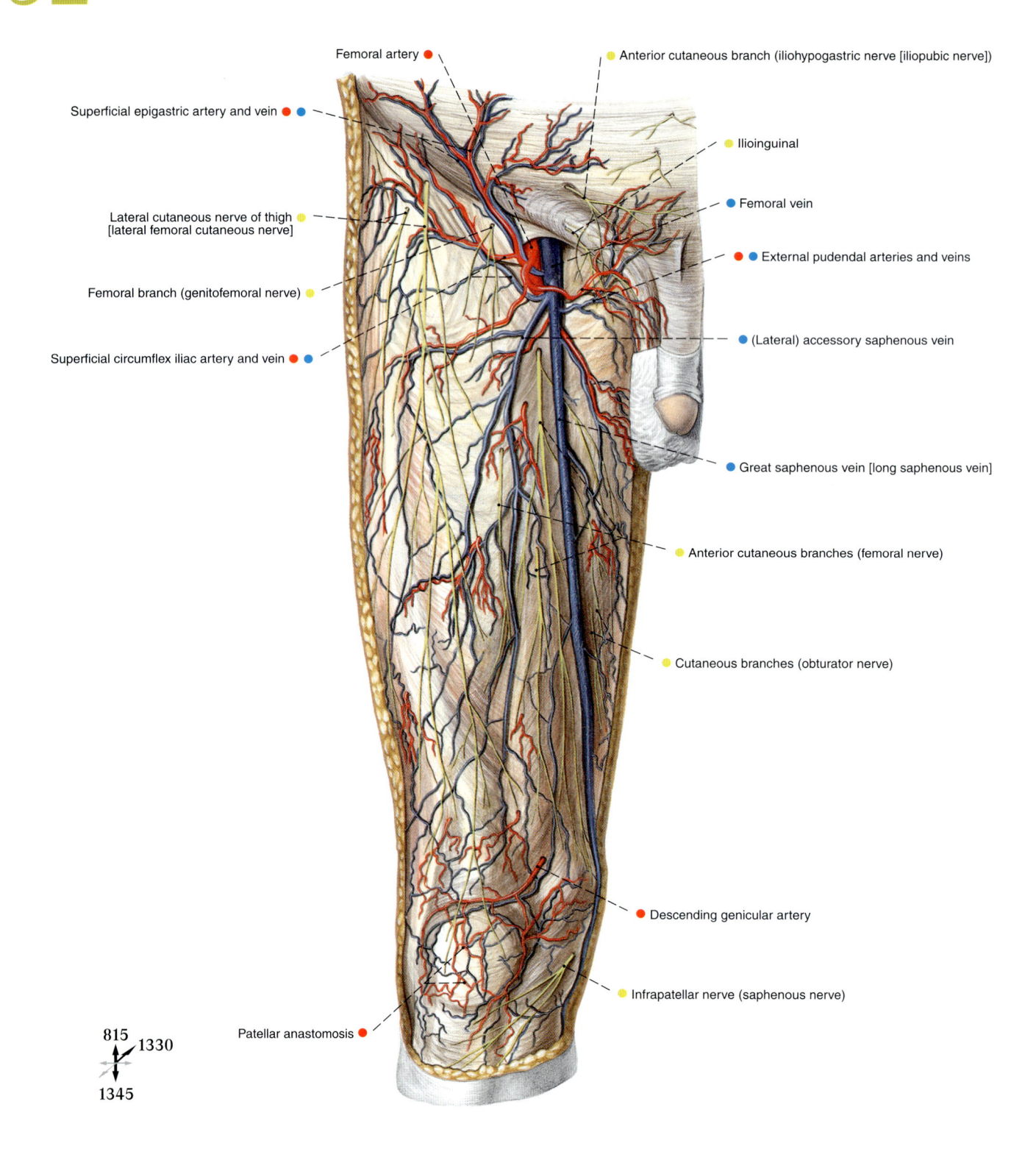

- Femoral artery 🔴
- Superficial epigastric artery and vein 🔴🔵
- Lateral cutaneous nerve of thigh [lateral femoral cutaneous nerve] 🟡
- Femoral branch (genitofemoral nerve) 🟡
- Superficial circumflex iliac artery and vein 🔴🔵
- Anterior cutaneous branch (iliohypogastric nerve [iliopubic nerve]) 🟡
- Ilioinguinal 🟡
- Femoral vein 🔵
- External pudendal arteries and veins 🔴🔵
- (Lateral) accessory saphenous vein 🔵
- Great saphenous vein [long saphenous vein] 🔵
- Anterior cutaneous branches (femoral nerve) 🟡
- Cutaneous branches (obturator nerve) 🟡
- Descending genicular artery 🔴
- Infrapatellar nerve (saphenous nerve) 🟡
- Patellar anastomosis 🔴

815 / 1330 / 1345

Fig. 1327 Epifascial blood vessels and nerves of right groin [inguinal region], anterior regions of thigh and knee; anterior aspect.

Groin [inguinal region]

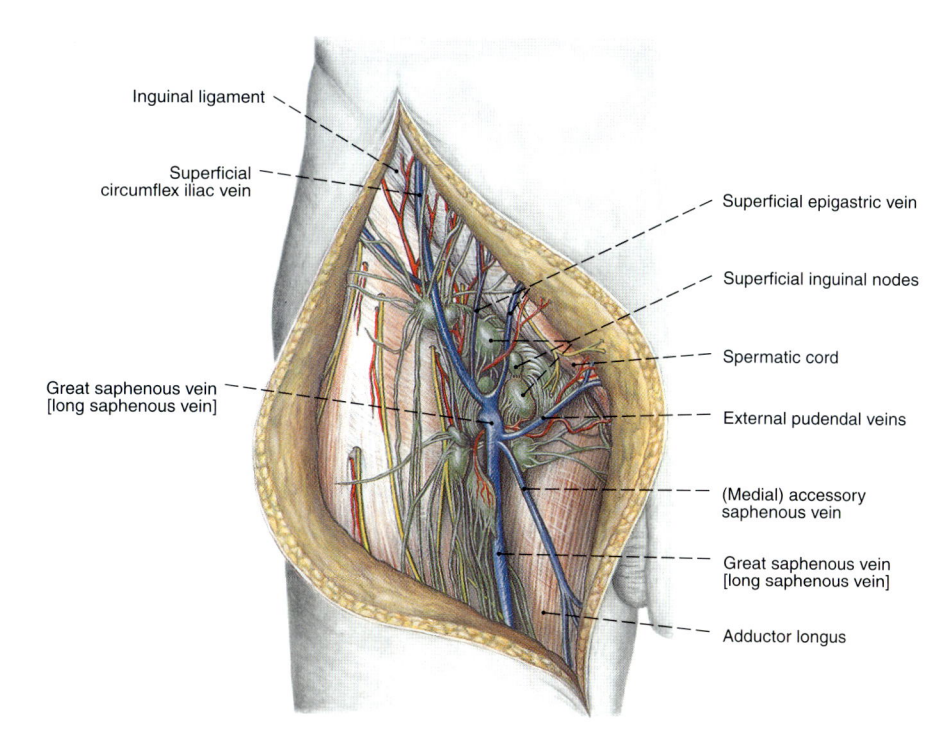

Fig. 1328 Superficial lymphatic vessels and venous trunks of right groin [inguinal region]; anterior aspect.

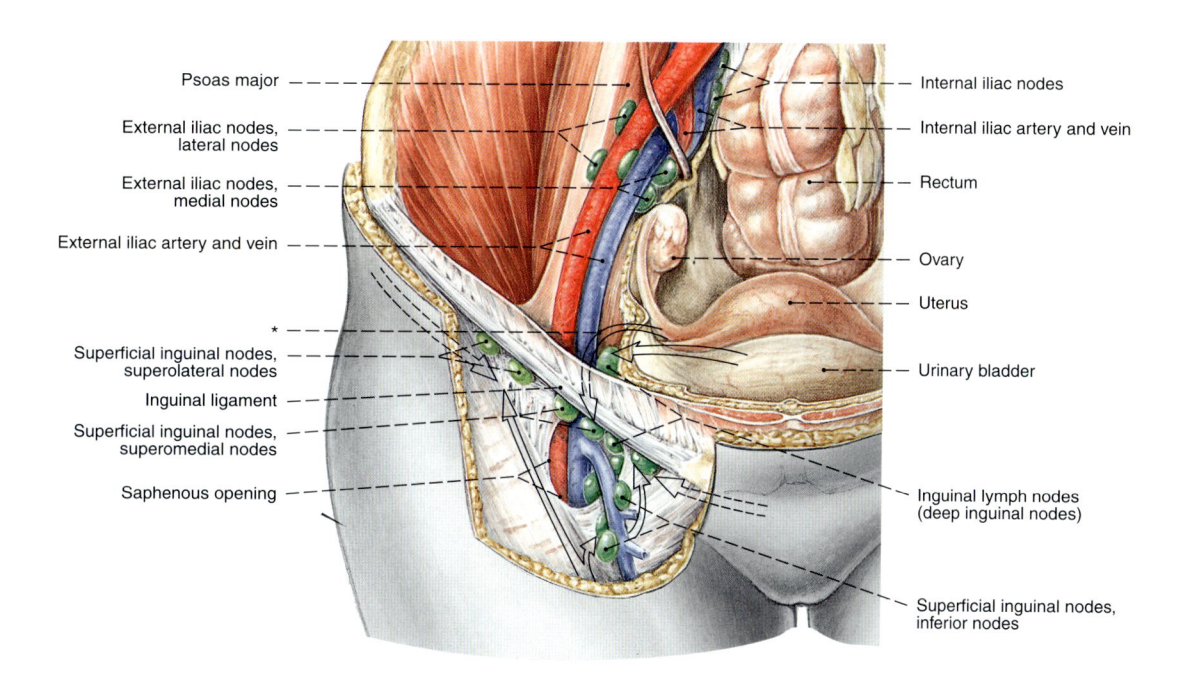

Fig. 1329 Tributaries of right inguinal nodes in the female; general survey; anterior aspect.
Arrows indicate possible directions of lymphatic flow.

* The medial part of the uterine tube and the fundus of uterus lymph also may drain into the superficial inguinal nodes via the round ligament of uterus.

354 Lower limb

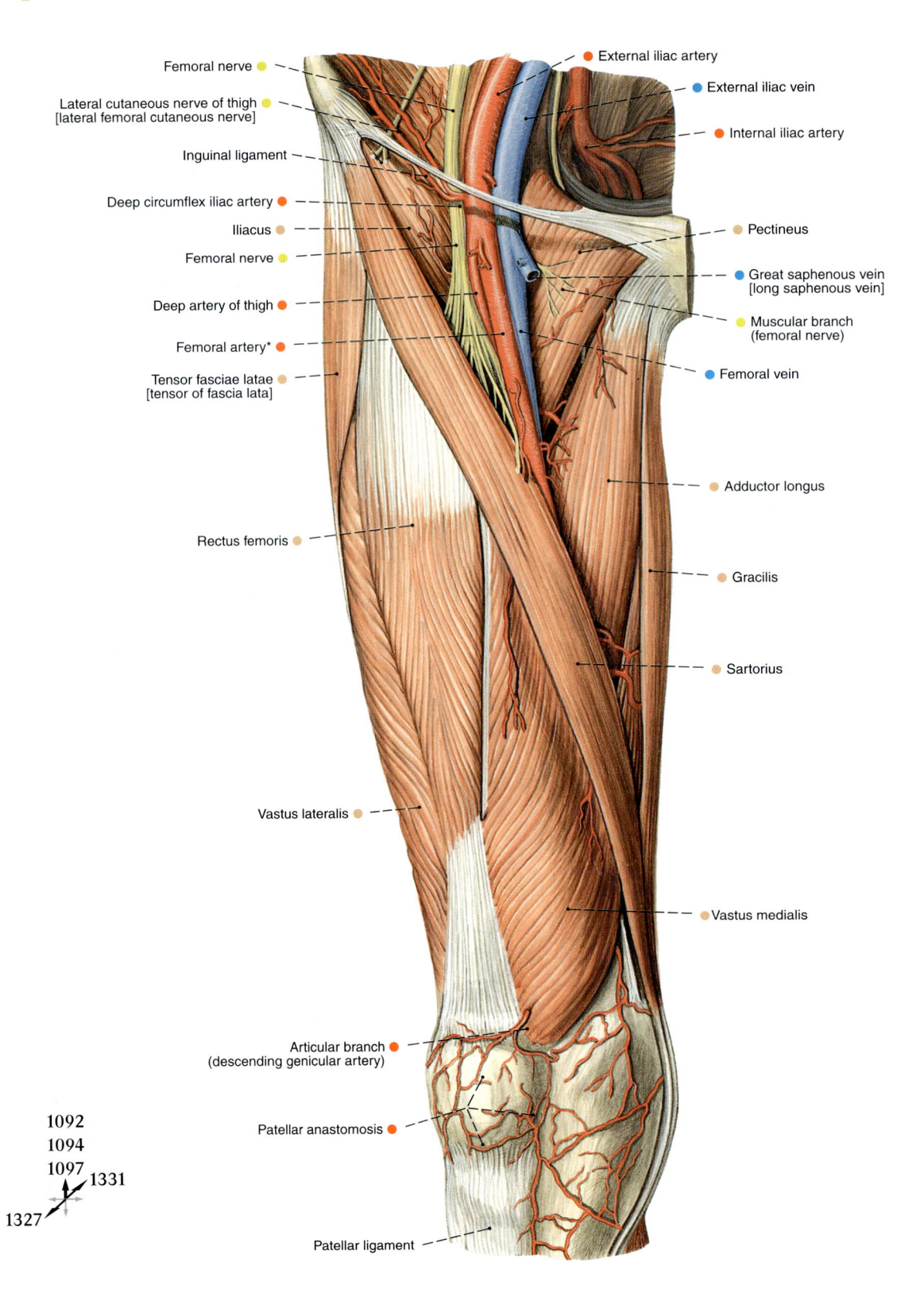

Fig. 1330 Blood vessels and nerves of anterior region of right thigh; fascia lata, except iliotibial tract removed; anterior aspect.

* Clinically, the femoral artery is frequently also known as superficial femoral artery, compared to the deep femoral artery (= deep artery of thigh).

Blood vessels and nerves of thigh 355

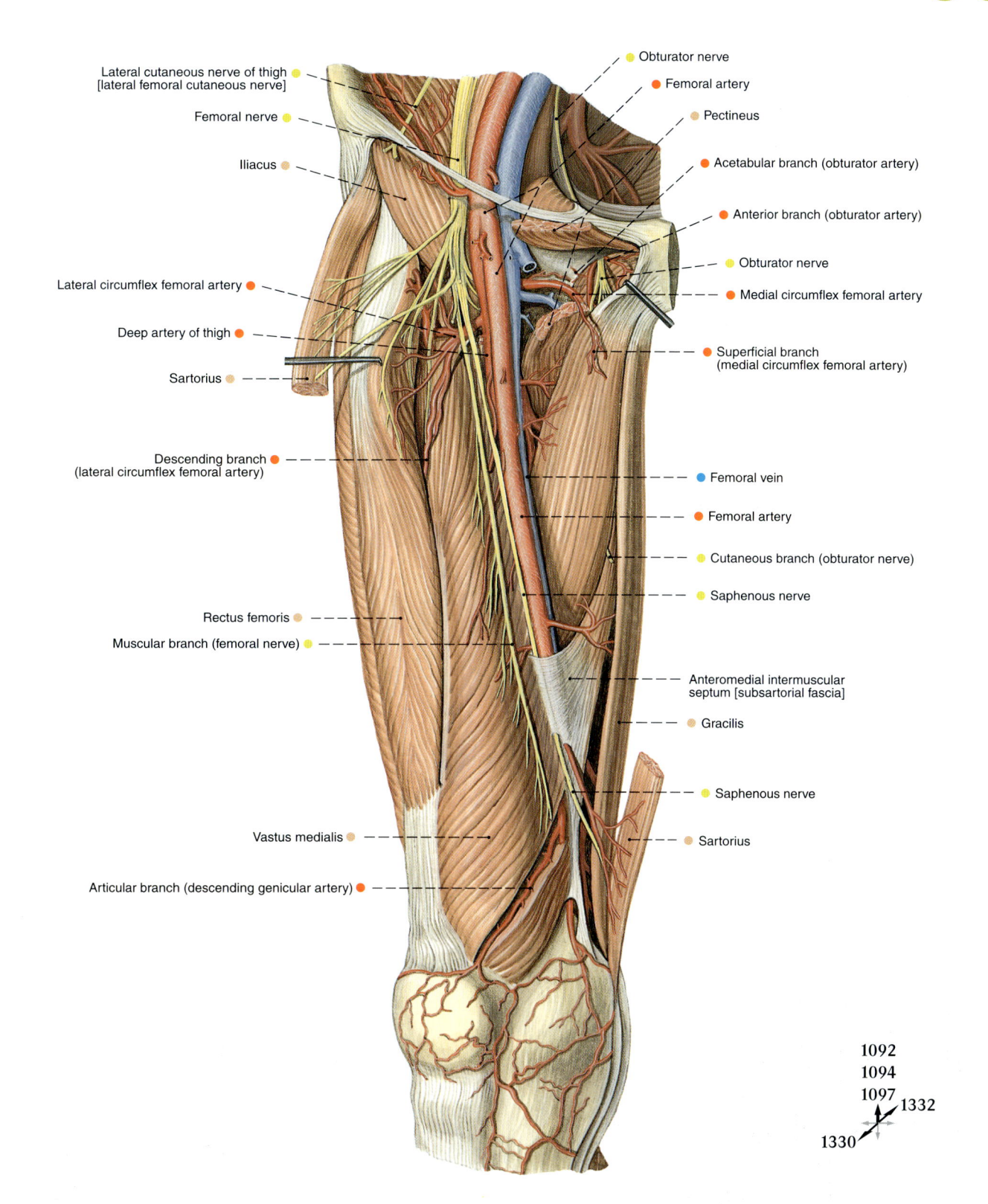

Fig. 1331 Blood vessels and nerves of anterior region of right thigh; sartorius partially removed and pectineus sectioned; anterior aspect.

* The entrance into the adductor canal is formed by the vastus medialis and the adductor longus, as well as by the anteromedial intermuscular septum [subsartorial fascia], which stretches between them.

356   Lower limb

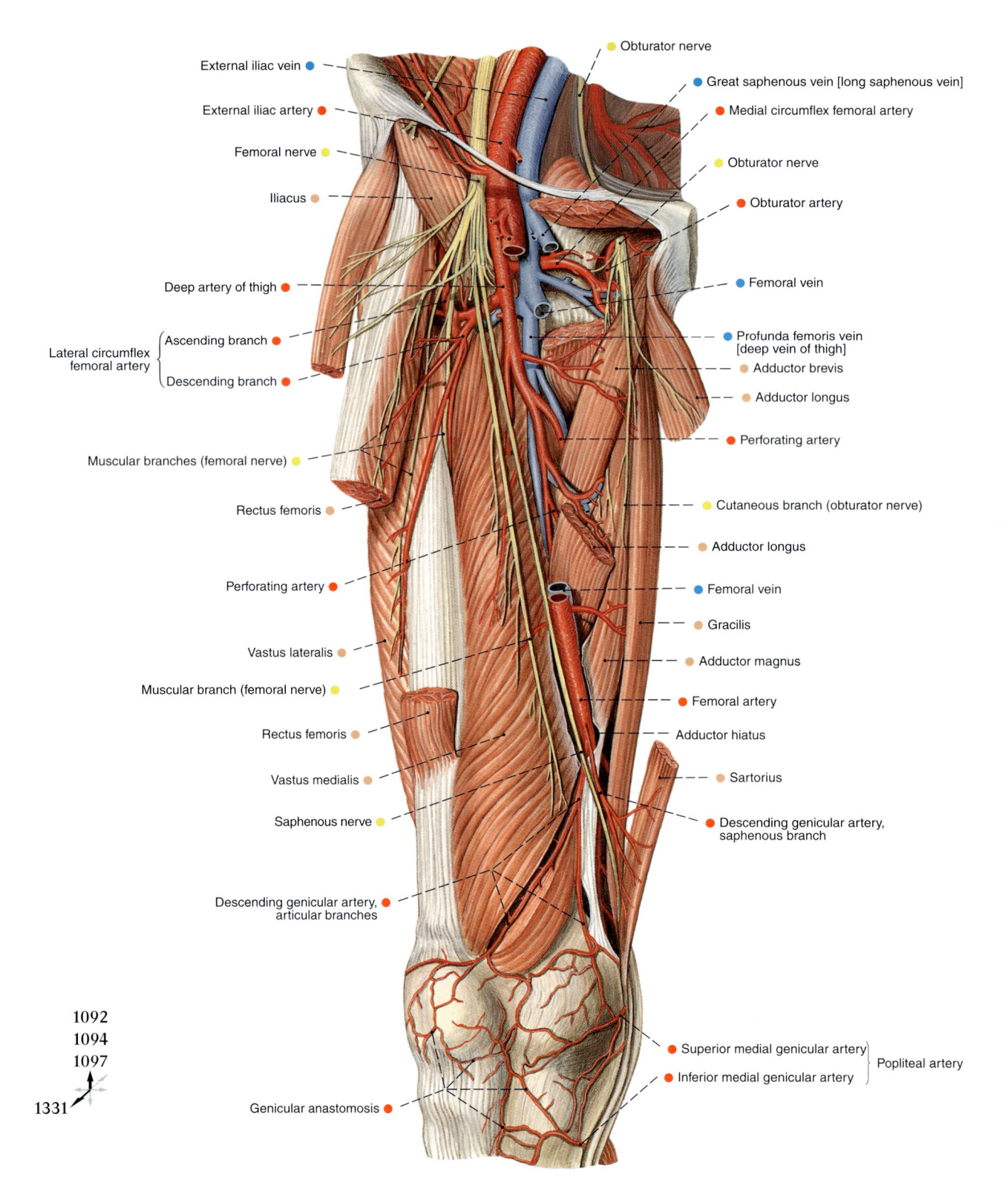

Fig. 1332 Blood vessels and nerves of anterior region of right thigh; deep layer after partial removal of sartorius and rectus femoris as well as sectioning pectineus and adductor longus; anteromedial intermuscular septum [subsartorial fascia] cut longitudinally to expose the adductor canal; anterior aspect.

Arteries of hip and thigh 357

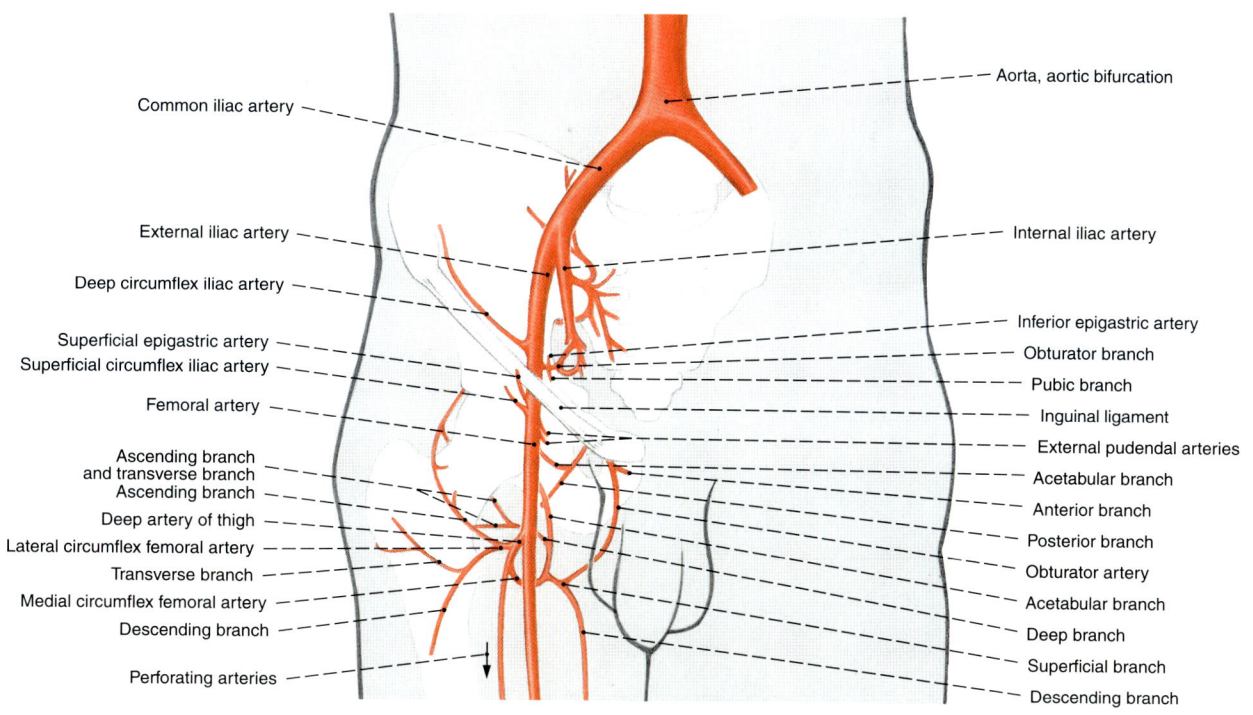

Fig. 1333 Arteries of right hip and thigh; general survey; anterior aspect.
The shown origin and branching pattern of the deep artery of thigh can be observed in approximately 58% of cases.

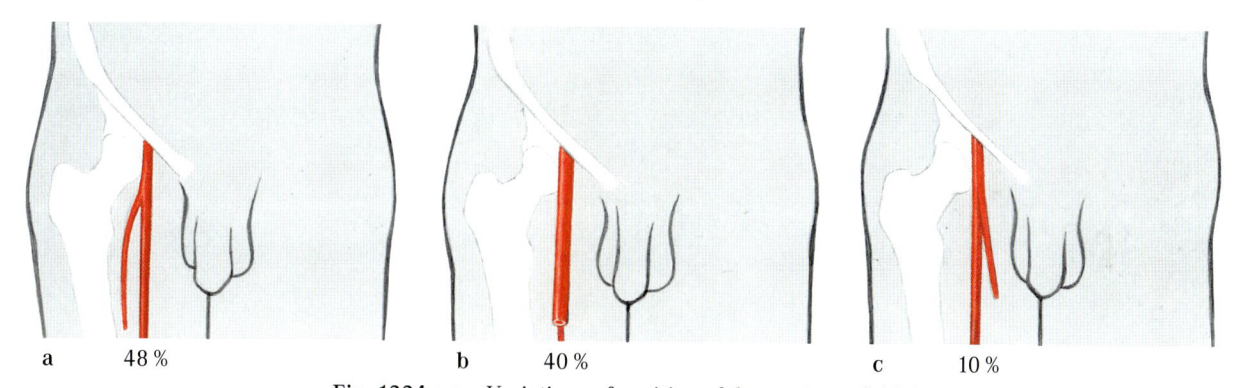

Fig. 1334 a–c Variations of position of deep artery of thigh.
 a Lateral or laterodorsal to femoral artery
 b Dorsal to femoral artery
 c Medial to femoral artery

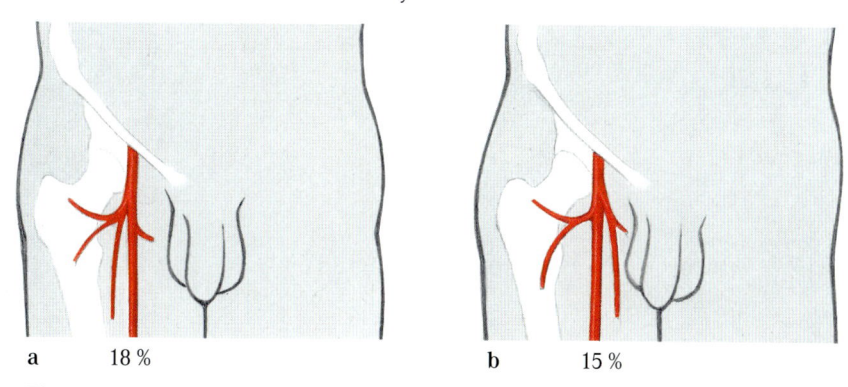

Fig. 1335 a, b Variations of origin of circumflex femoral arteries.
 a Separate origin of medial circumflex femoral artery from femoral artery
 b Separate origin of lateral circumflex femoral artery from femoral artery

358 Lower limb

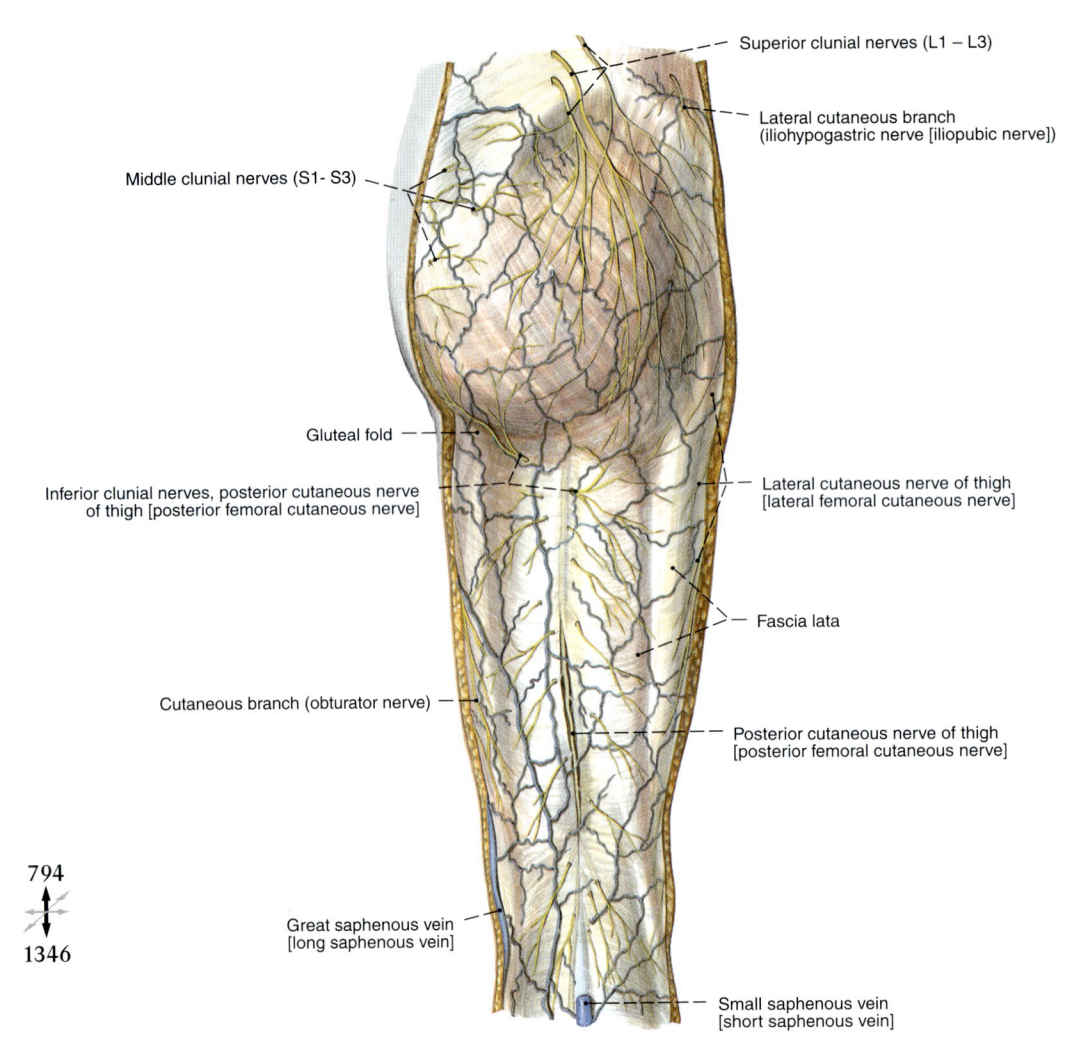

Fig. 1336 Epifascial blood vessels and nerves of posterior regions of right thigh, gluteal region, and popliteal fossa; posterior aspect.

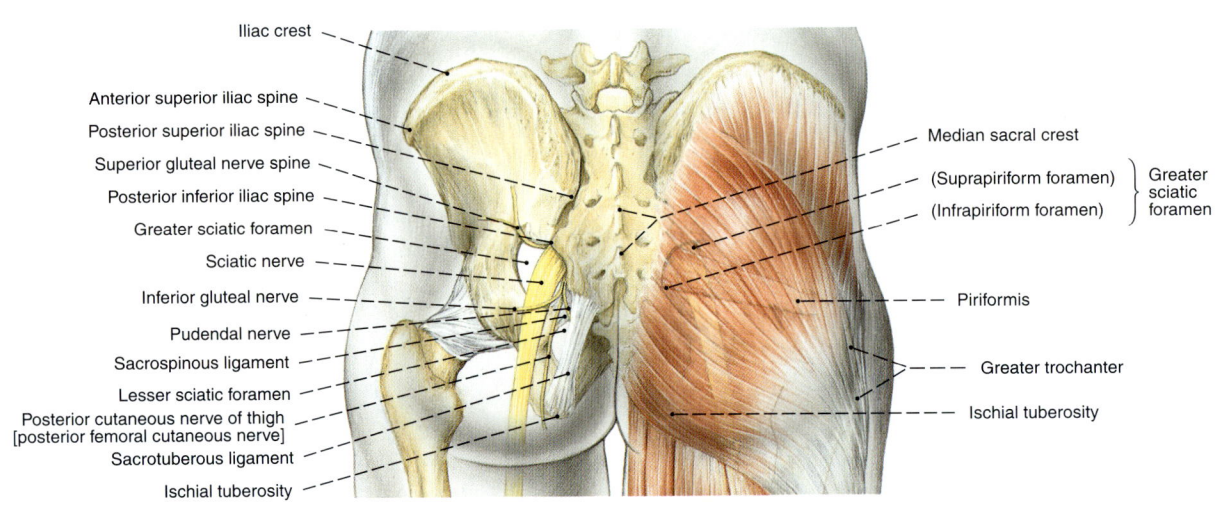

Fig. 1337 Projection of skeleton and sciatic nerve onto the surface of the gluteal region; posterior aspect.

Blood vessels and nerves of gluteal region

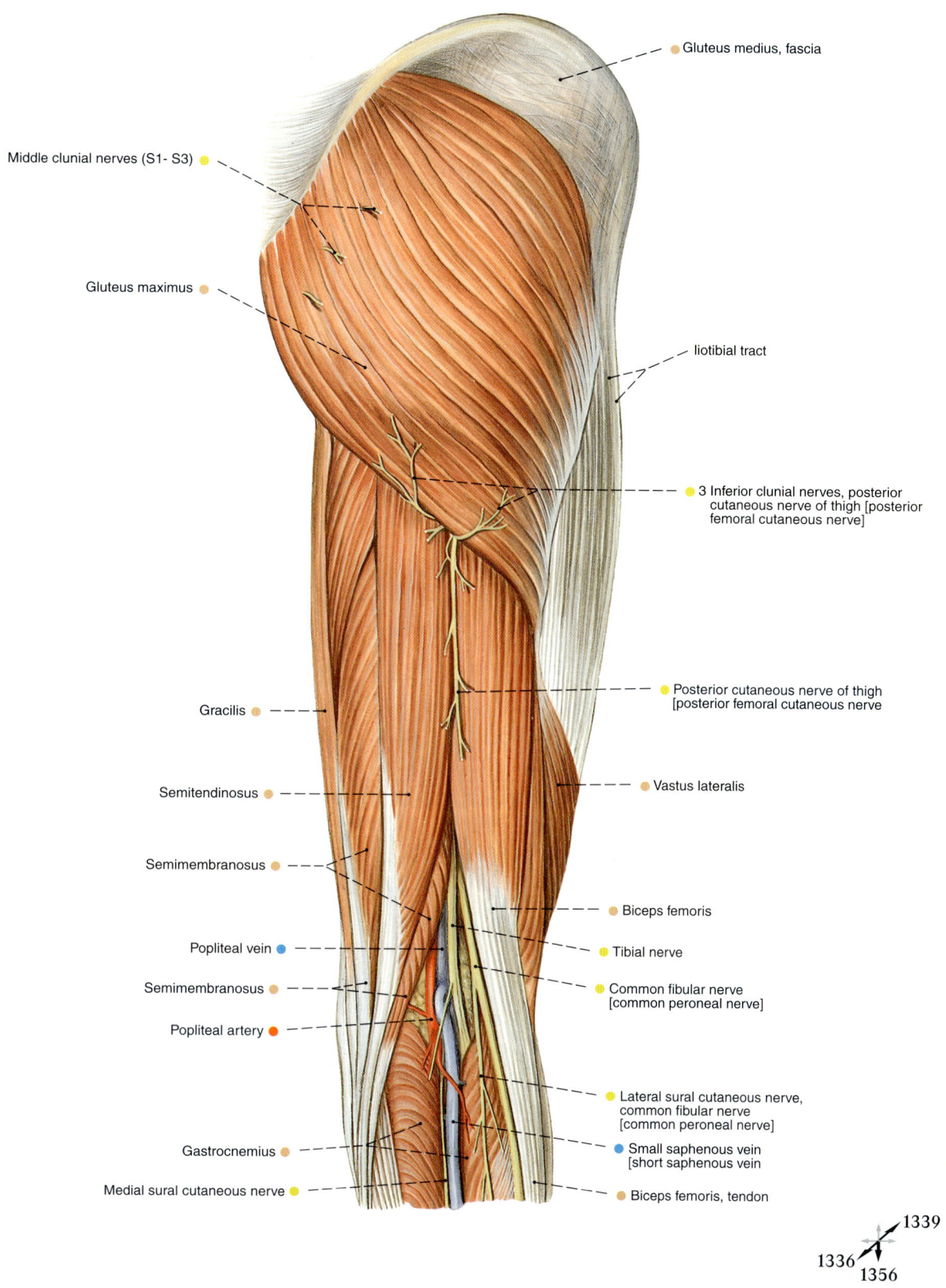

Fig. 1338 Blood vessels and nerves of right gluteal region, posterior region of thigh, and popliteal fossa; fascia lata, except iliotibial tract removed; posterior aspect.

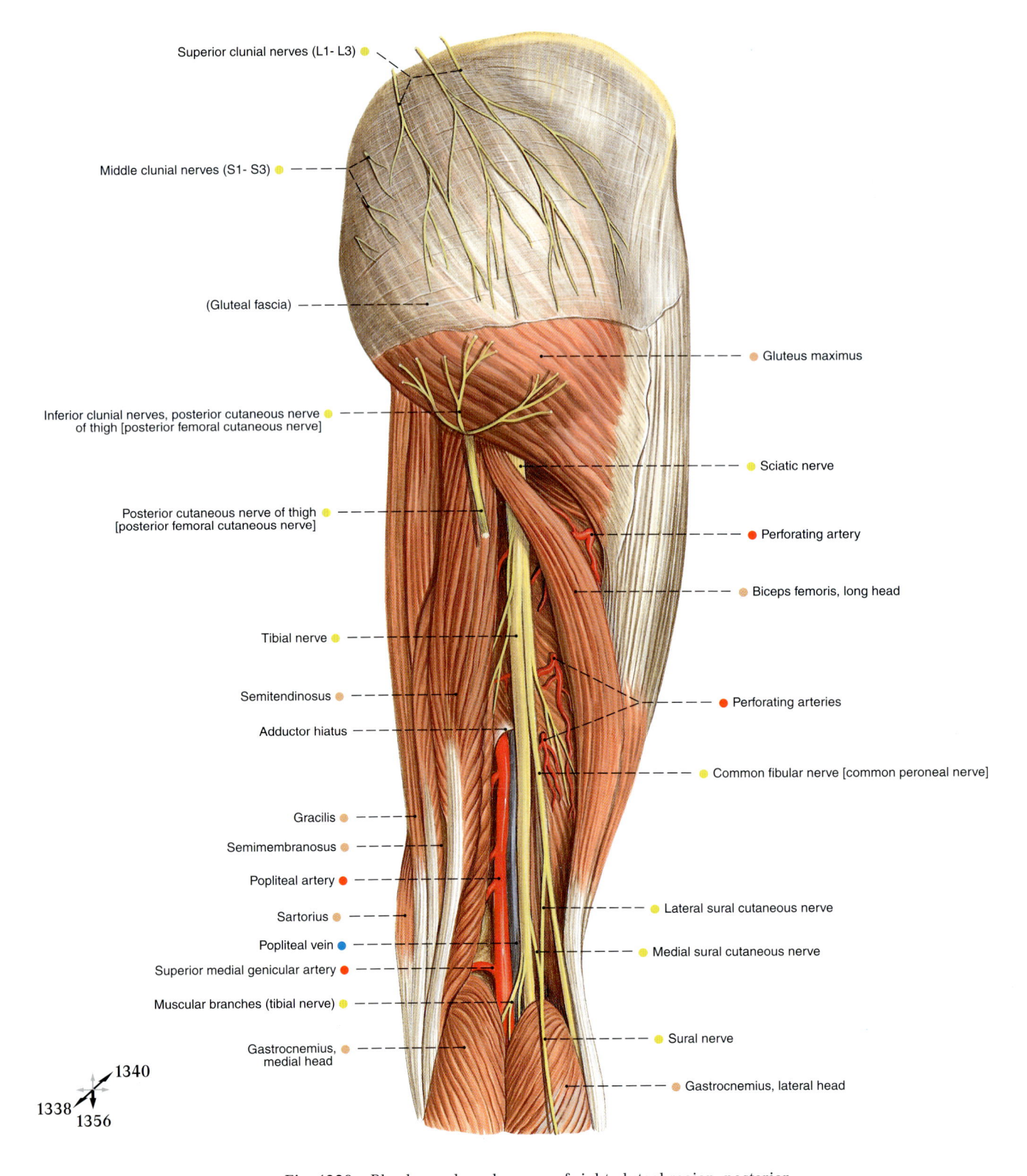

Fig. 1339 Blood vessels and nerves of right gluteal region, posterior region of thigh, and popliteal fossa; fascia lata removed; long head of biceps femoris retracted laterally; posterior aspect.
In this specimen the medial and lateral sural cutaneous nerves branch off somewhat far proximal.

Blood vessels and nerves of gluteal region

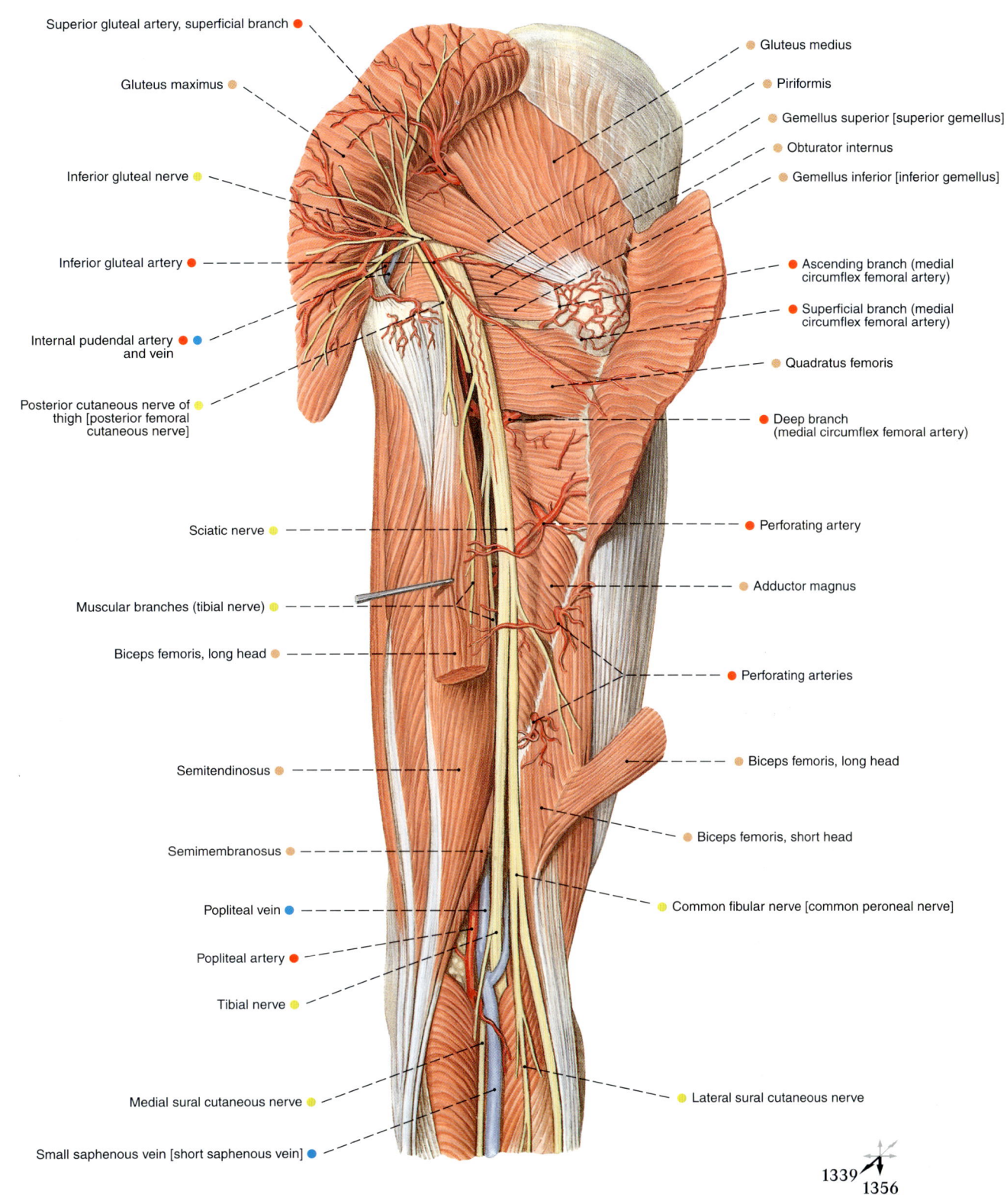

Fig. 1340 Blood vessels and nerves of right gluteal region, posterior region of thigh, and popliteal fossa; gluteus maximus and long head of biceps femoris sectioned; posterior aspect.

362 Lower limb

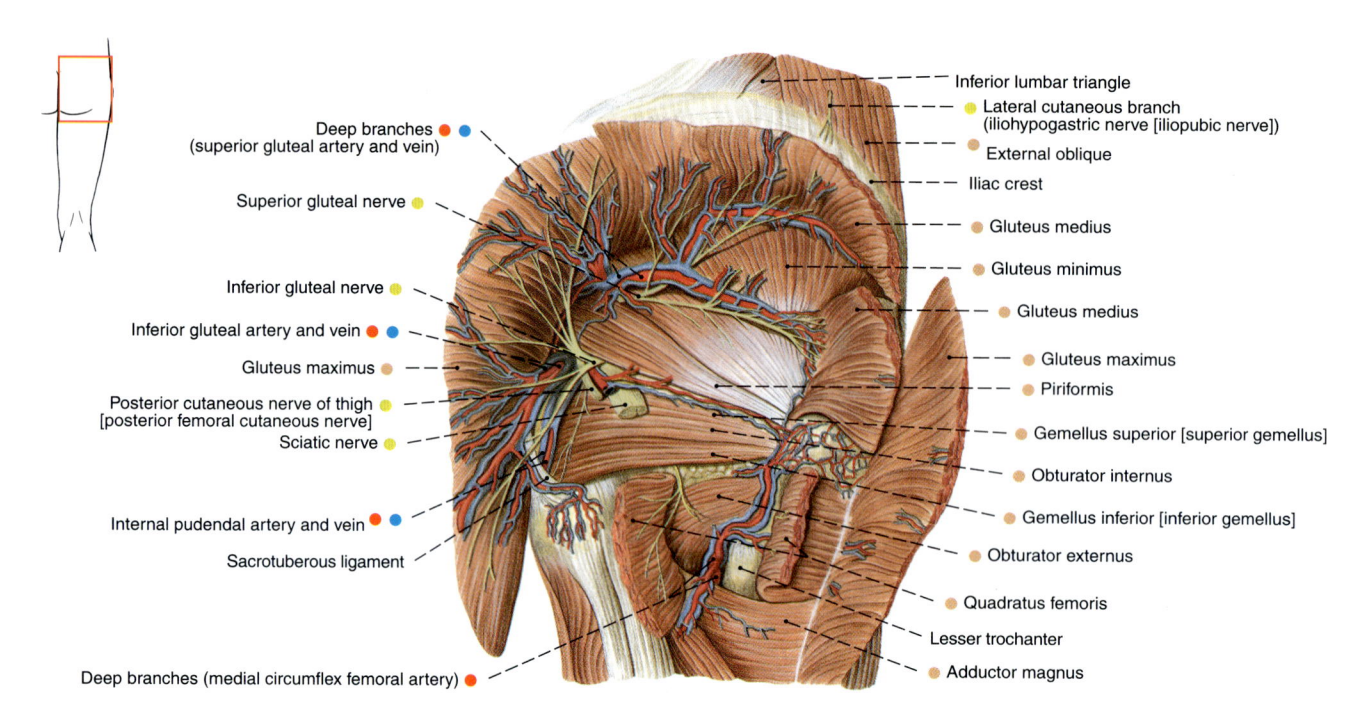

Fig. 1341 Blood vessels and nerves of right gluteal region; gluteus maximus and medius sectioned and partially removed; sciatic nerve after passage through infrapiriform foramen removed; posterior aspect.

The **greater sciatic foramen** is divided into two passages for blood vessels and nerves by the piriformis.
The **suprapiriform foramen** contains the superior gluteal artery, vein, and nerve; the **infrapiriform foramen** contains the sciatic, inferior gluteal, and pudendal nerves, the posterior cutaneous nerve of thigh [posterior femoral cutaneous nerve] as well as the inferior gluteal and internal pudendal arteries and veins. Through the **lesser sciatic foramen** pass the tendon of obturator internus, the pudendal nerve, and the internal pudendal artery and vein.

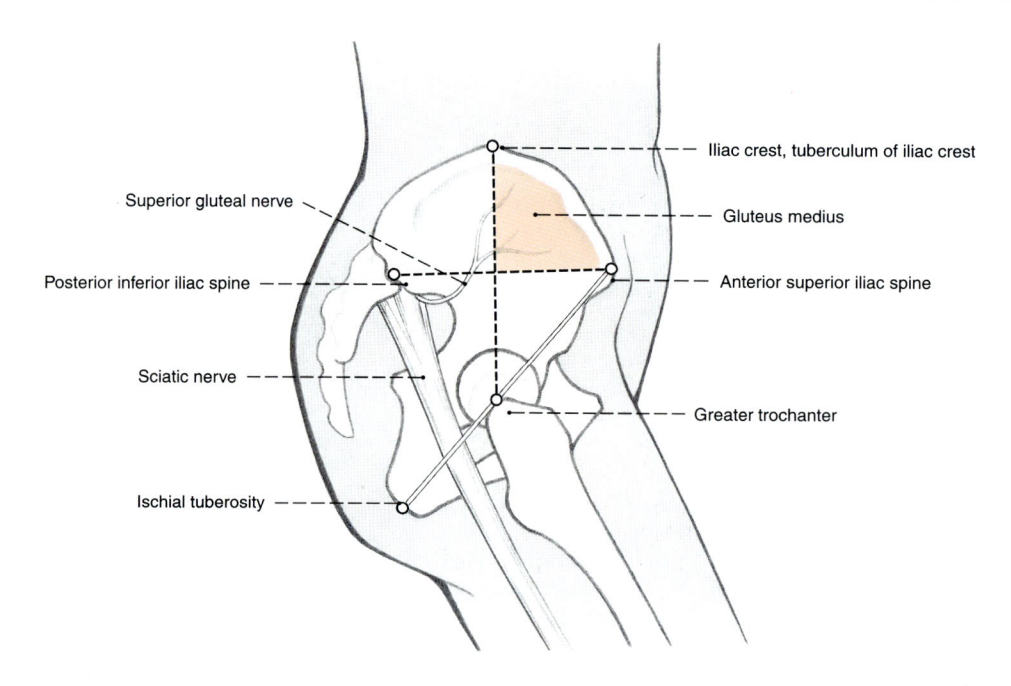

Fig. 1342 Projection of skeletal structures of right hip important for injection into the gluteus medius, lateral aspect.

Intramuscular injections

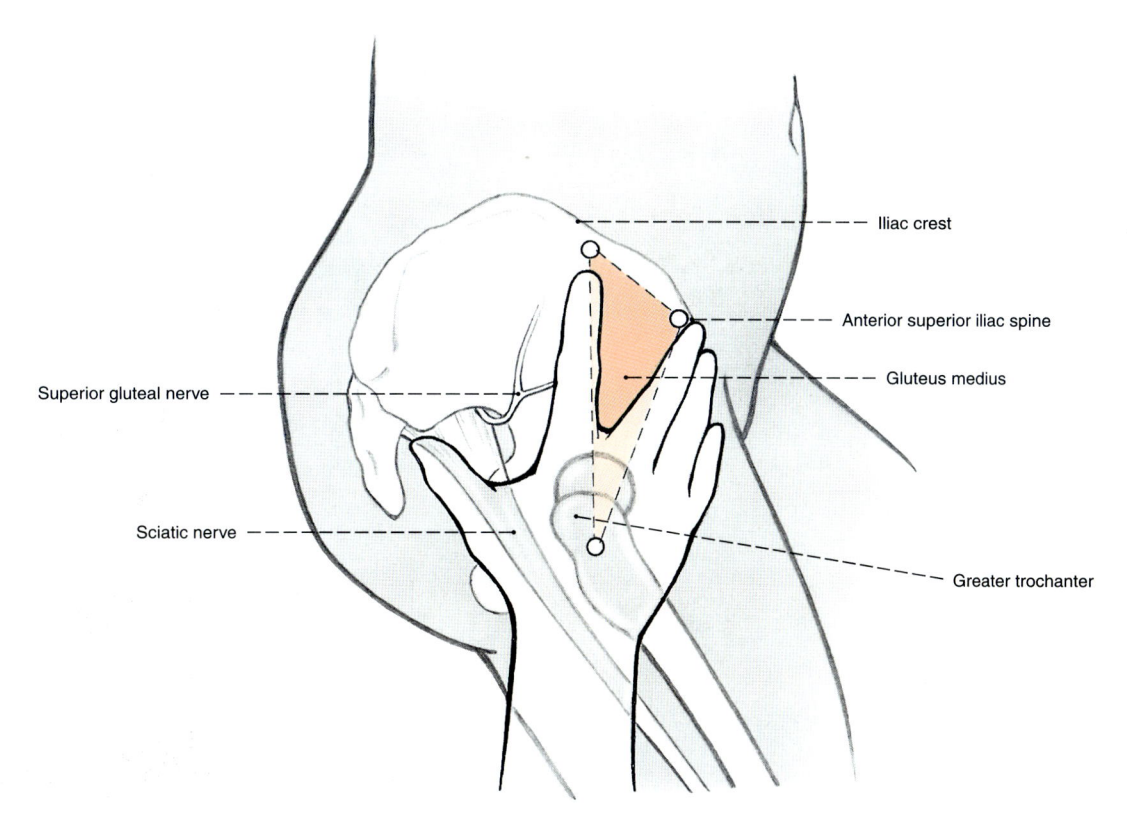

Fig. 1343 Intragluteal injection (according to A. v. HOCHSTETTER). To safely avoid the superior gluteal nerve, and particularly the superior gluteal artery, the injection is made into the triangular area bordered by the two spread fingers and the iliac crest. The middle finger—or when using the left hand the index finger—lies on the anterior superior iliac spine, the palm on the greater trochanter. Because the injected medication should be placed in the belly of the gluteus medius as far as possible from any blood vessels, the direction of the needle must not cross under the fingers. Some risk, however, remains for the branch of the superior gluteal nerve to the tensor fasciae latae [tensor of fascia lata].

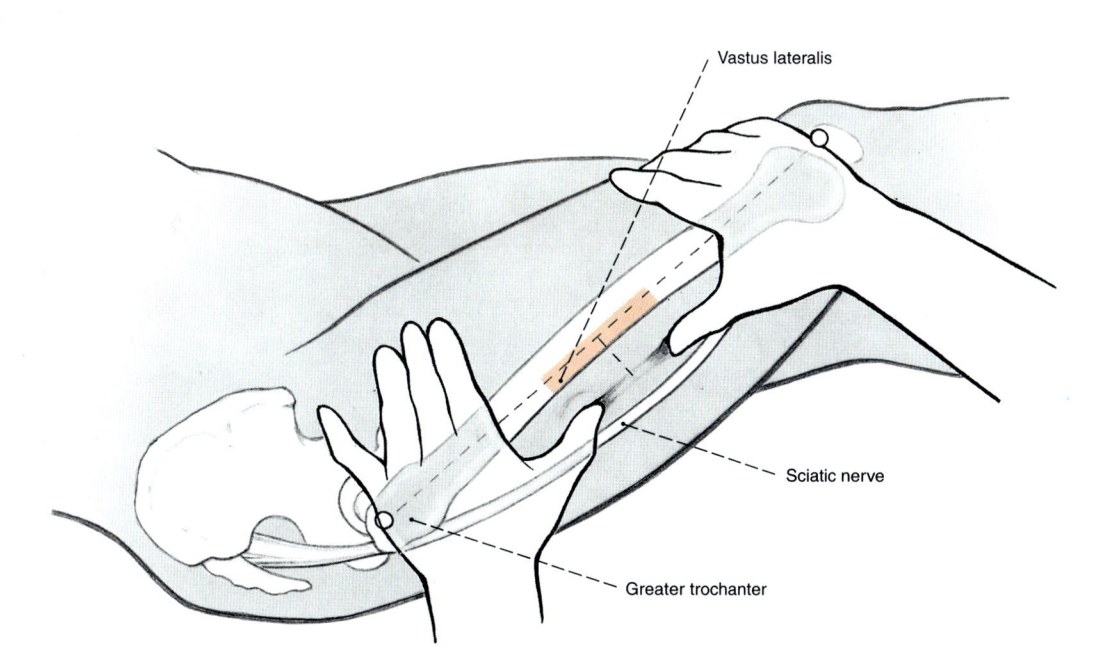

Fig. 1344 Intramuscular injection into the vastus lateralis (according to A. v. HOCHSTETTER). Except for the tiny branches of the lateral cutaneous nerve of thigh [lateral femoral cutaneous nerve] there are no large nerves or blood vessels in the middle of the lateral surface of the thigh. After orientation as to the position of the femur [thigh bone] the needle is inserted transversally directed towards the bone into the belly of the vastus lateralis.

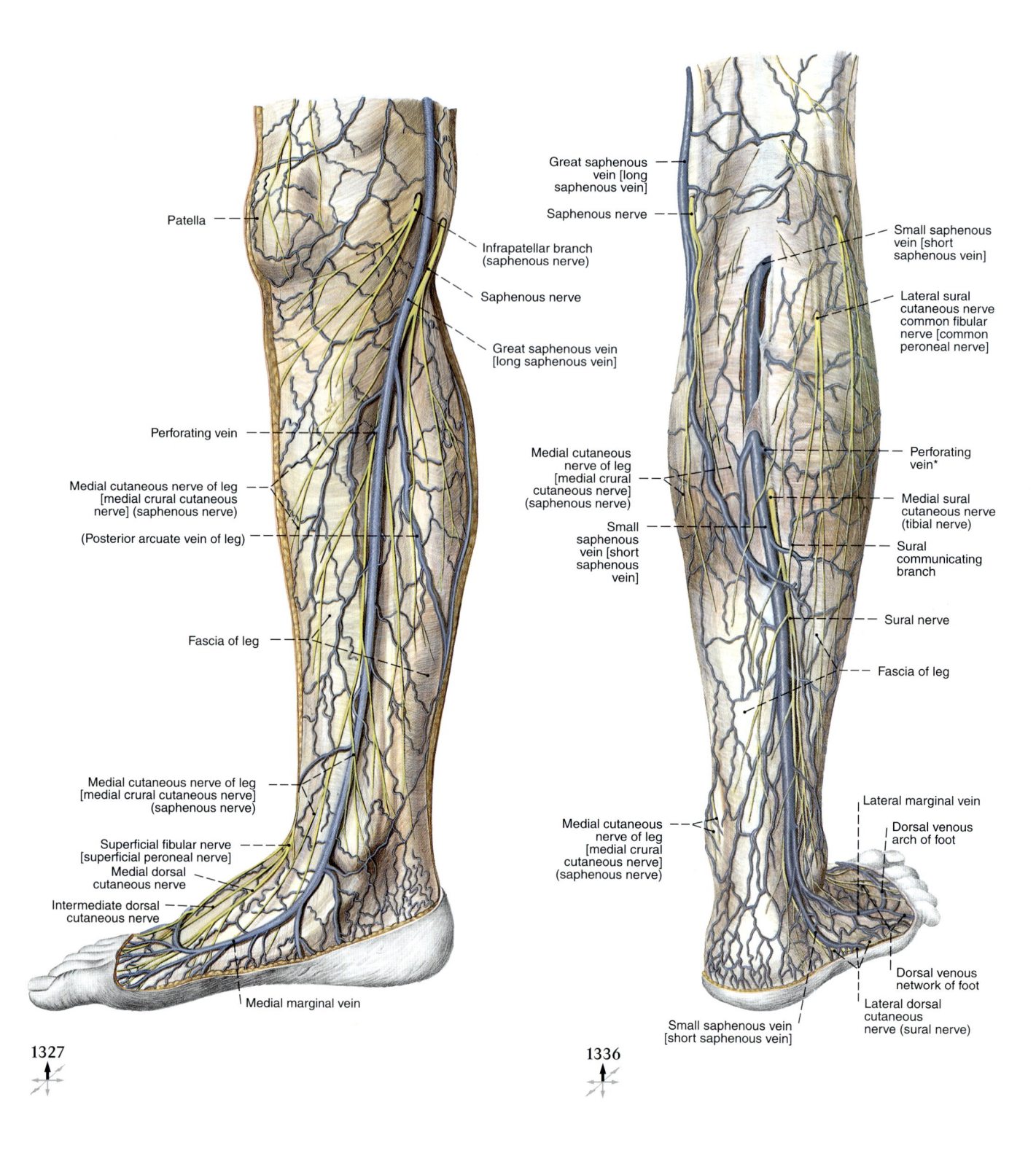

Lower limb

Fig. 1345 Epifascial veins and nerves of right leg and foot; medial aspect.

Fig. 1346 Epifascial veins and nerves of right leg and foot; fascia of leg split proximally; posterior aspect.
* Clinically also: MAY's vein.

Veins of lower limb

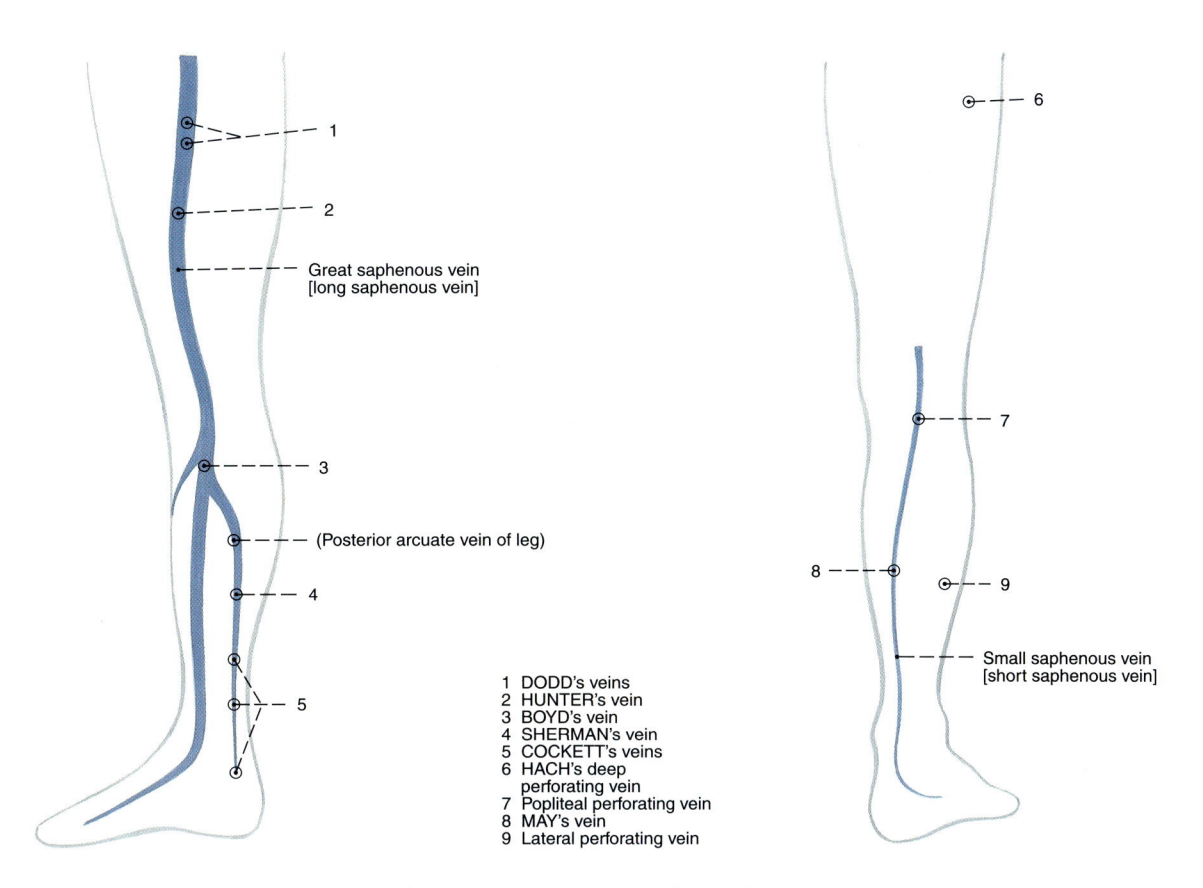

1 DODD's veins
2 HUNTER's vein
3 BOYD's vein
4 SHERMAN's vein
5 COCKETT's veins
6 HACH's deep perforating vein
7 Popliteal perforating vein
8 MAY's vein
9 Lateral perforating vein

Fig. 1347 Connections between epifascial and deep veins in the tributary of the right great saphenous vein [long saphenous vein]; general survey (according to HACH, 1986); medial aspect.

Fig. 1348 Connections between epifascial and deep veins in the tributary of the right small saphenous vein [short saphenous vein]; general survey (according to HACH, 1986); posterior aspect.

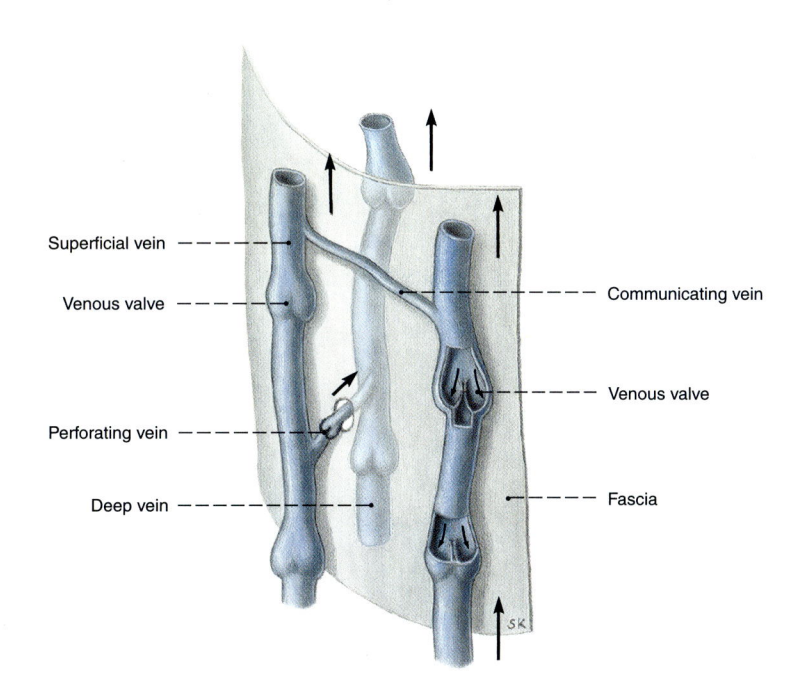

Fig. 1349 Veins of lower limb; principles of arrangement.
Disturbances in drainage from veins of the lower limb, particularly varicosities, are frequent vascular diseases. If one of the venous systems is completely closed, the perforating veins obtain an important role in venous drainage.

366 Lower limb

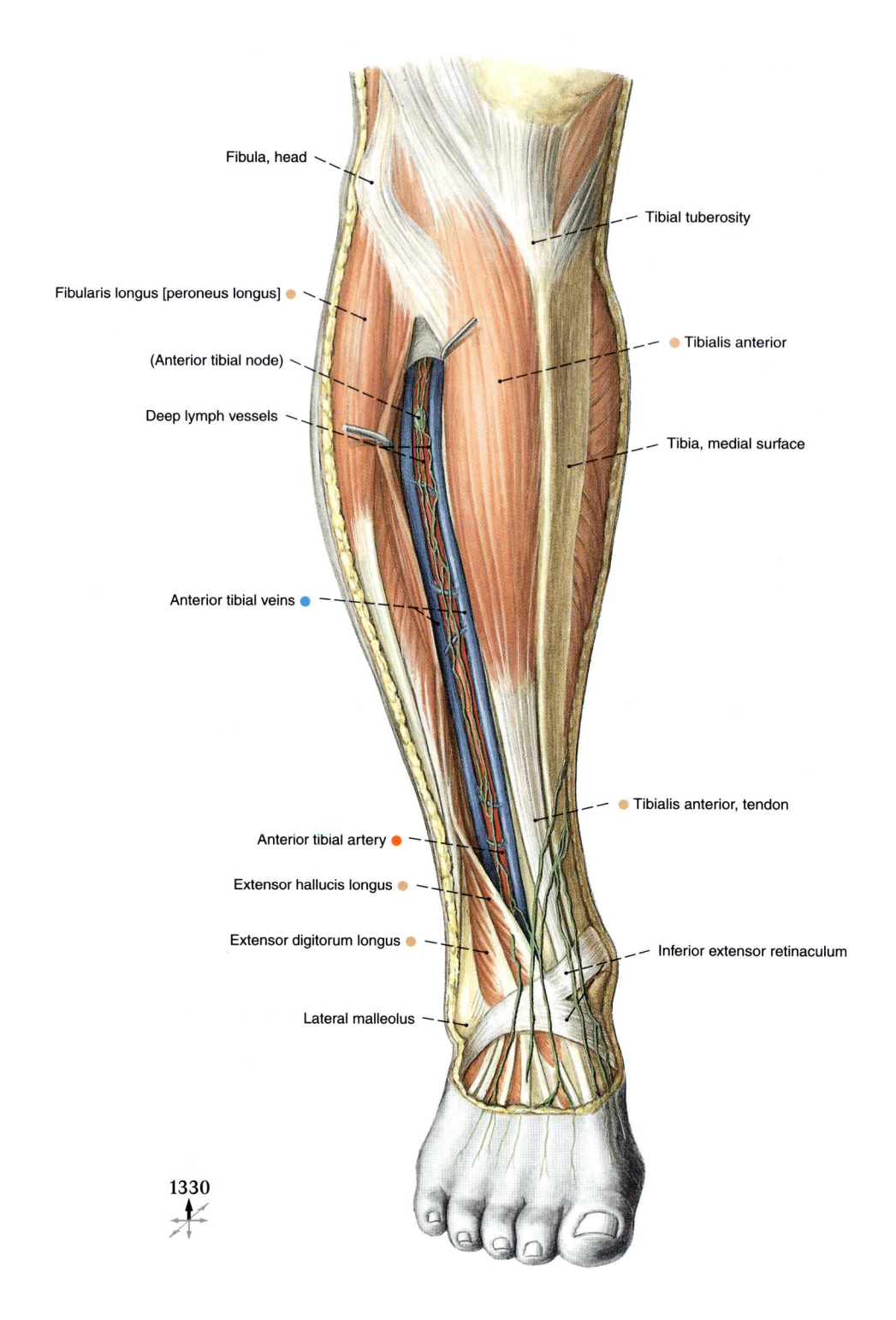

- Fibula, head
- Fibularis longus [peroneus longus]
- (Anterior tibial node)
- Deep lymph vessels
- Anterior tibial veins
- Anterior tibial artery
- Extensor hallucis longus
- Extensor digitorum longus
- Lateral malleolus
- Tibial tuberosity
- Tibialis anterior
- Tibia, medial surface
- Tibialis anterior, tendon
- Inferior extensor retinaculum

1330

Fig. 1350 Blood vessels of anterior region of right leg; fascia of leg removed and extensors spread apart; anterior aspect.
The superficial lymph vessels accompany the epifascial veins. They converge along the great saphenous vein [long saphenous vein] on the medial side of the leg. The deep lymph vessels accompany the deep veins and arteries in their connective tissue sheaths.

Blood vessels and nerves of leg

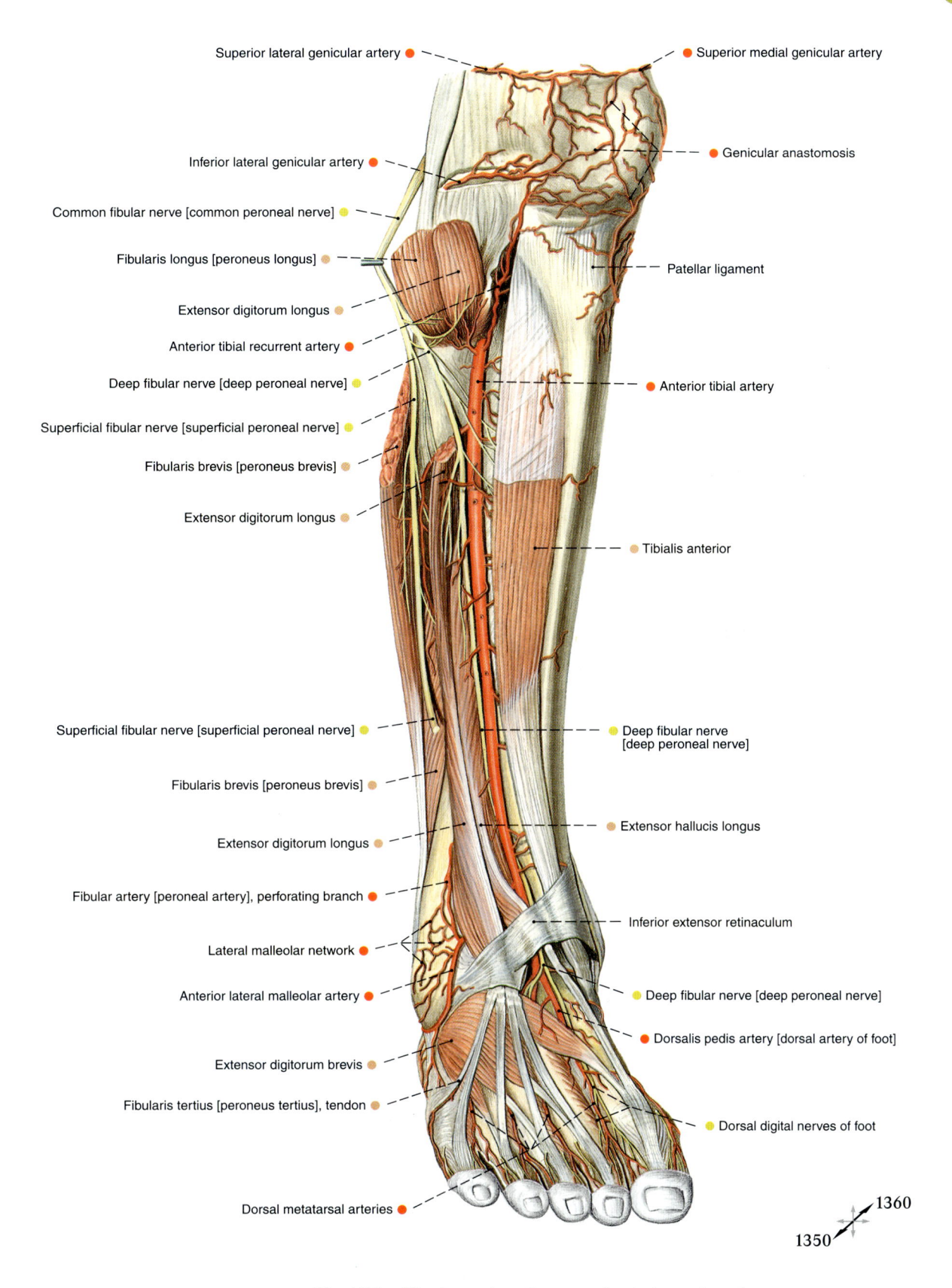

Fig. 1351 Blood vessels and nerves of anterior region of right leg and dorsum of foot; fascia of leg removed and extensor digitorum longus and fibularis longus [peroneus longus] sectioned; anterior aspect.

Lower limb

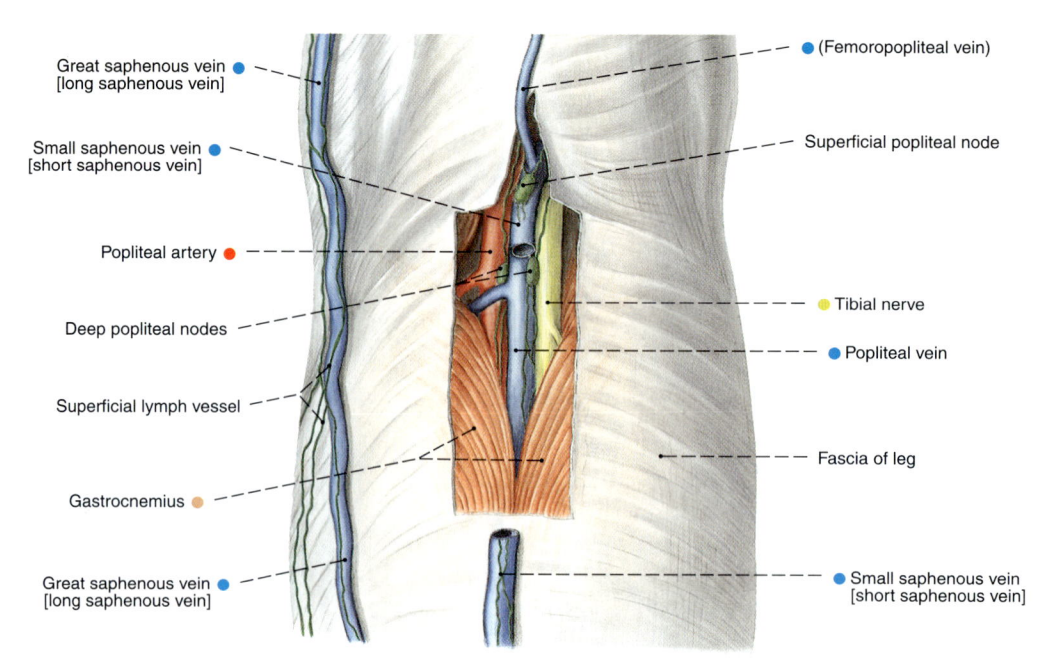

Fig. 1352 Blood vessels and nerves of right popliteal fossa; fascia of leg split and small saphenous vein [short saphenous vein] removed; posterior aspect.

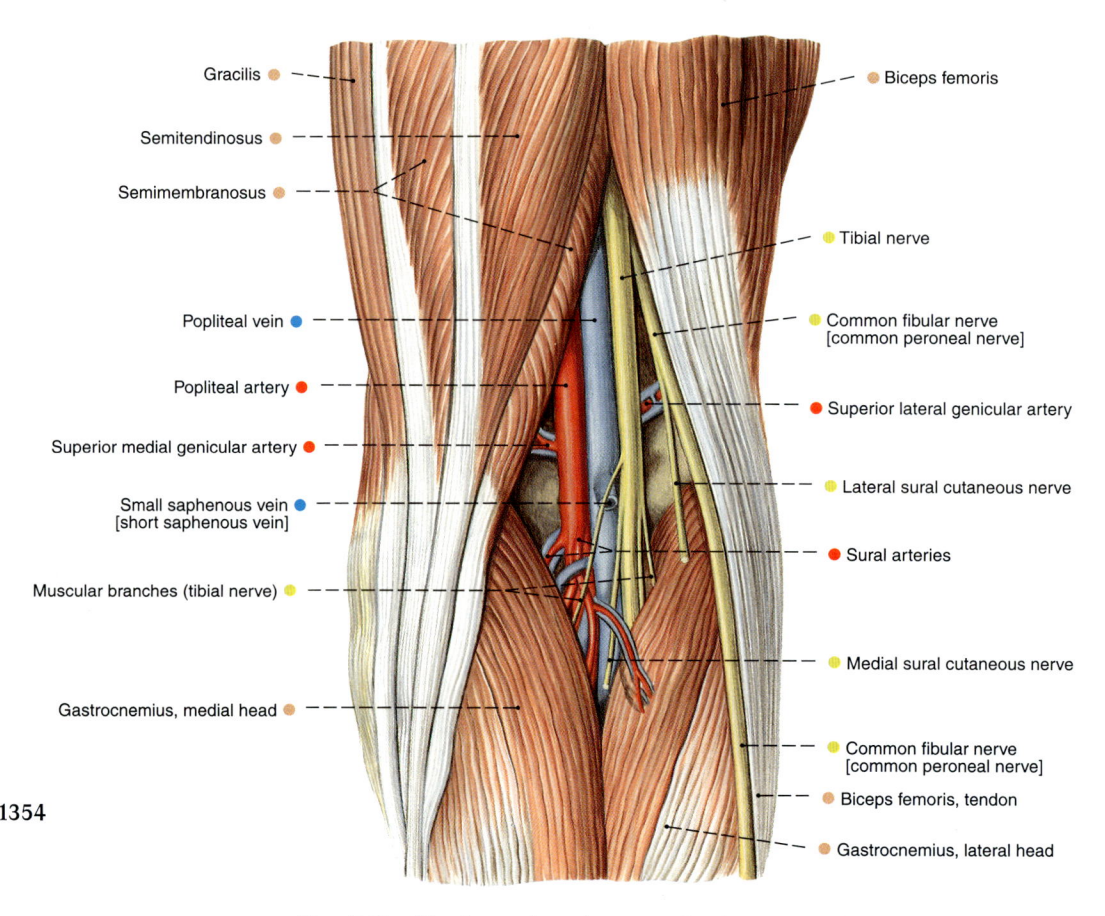

Fig. 1353 Blood vessels and nerves of right popliteal fossa; fascia lata and fascia of leg split removed; posterior aspect.

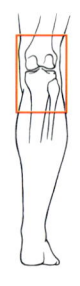

Arteries of popliteal fossa 369

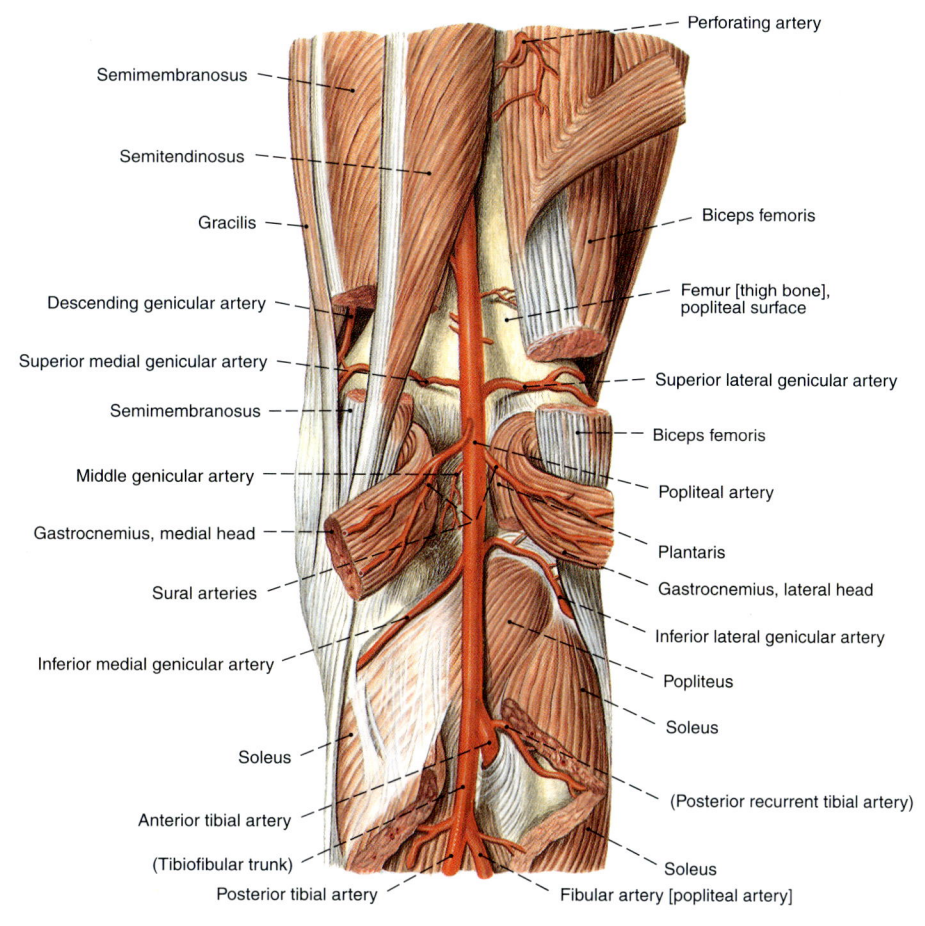

Fig. 1354 Arteries of right popliteal fossa; covering muscles partially removed; posterior aspect.
This branching pattern can be observed in approximately 90% of cases.

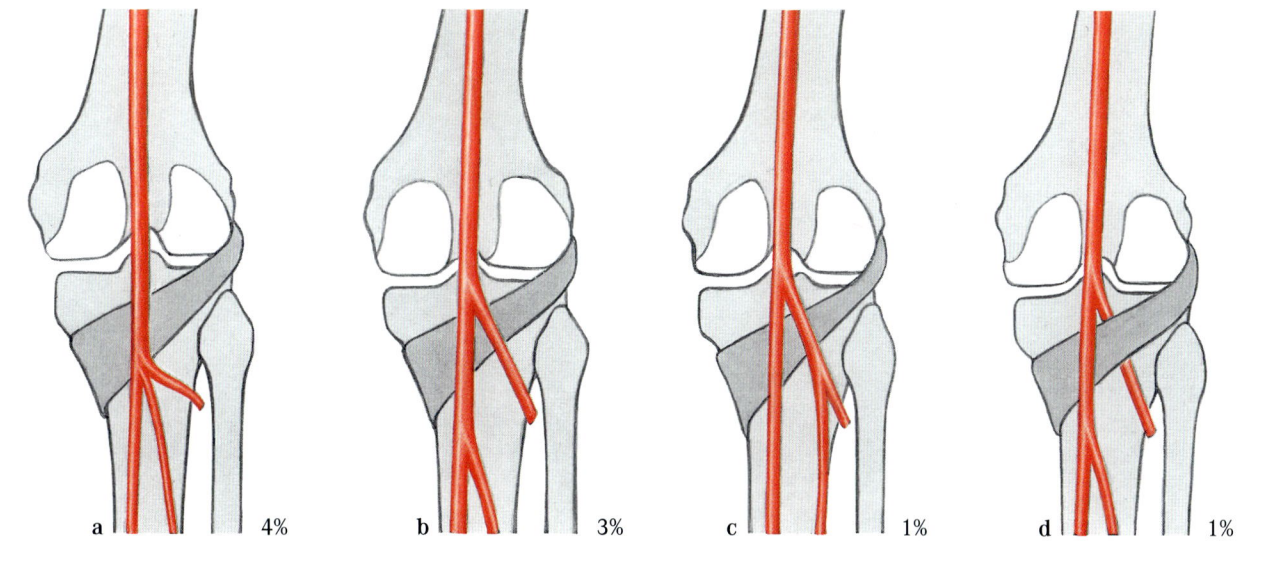

Fig. 1355 a–d Variations in the branching pattern of popliteal artery.
a Common trunk of anterior and posterior tibial arteries and fibular [peroneal] artery
b Division of popliteal artery proximal to upper border of popliteus
c Proximal trunk formation of posterior tibial and fibular [peroneal] arteries
d Course of anterior tibial artery ventral to popliteus

Lower limb

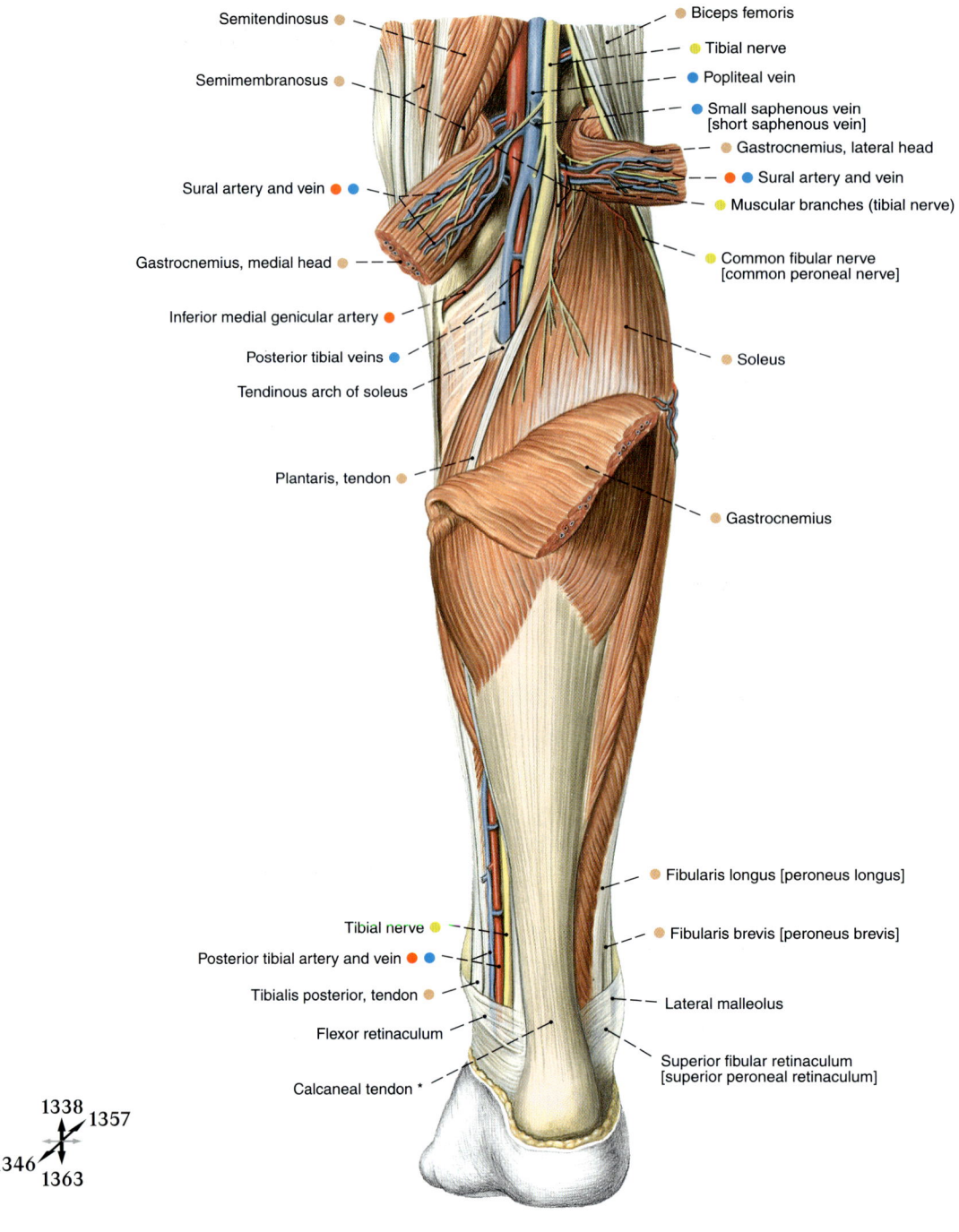

Fig. 1356　Blood vessels and nerves of popliteal fossa and posterior region of right leg; fascia of leg removed and gastrocnemius sectioned; posterior aspect.

* Also: ACHILLES tendon.

The medial retromalleolar space, covered by the flexor retinaculum, connects the calf to the deep layer of the sole. From anterior to posterior it contains the tendons of tibialis posterior, flexor digitorum longus, tibial blood vessels, tendon of flexor hallucis longus, and the tibial nerve. The distal continuation of this space is known as the tarsal tunnel (see Fig. 1364).

The lateral retromalleolar space is covered by the superior and inferior fibular [peroneal] retinacula. From anterior to posterior it contains the tendons of fibularis [peroneus] brevis and longus.

Blood vessels and nerves of popliteal fossa 371

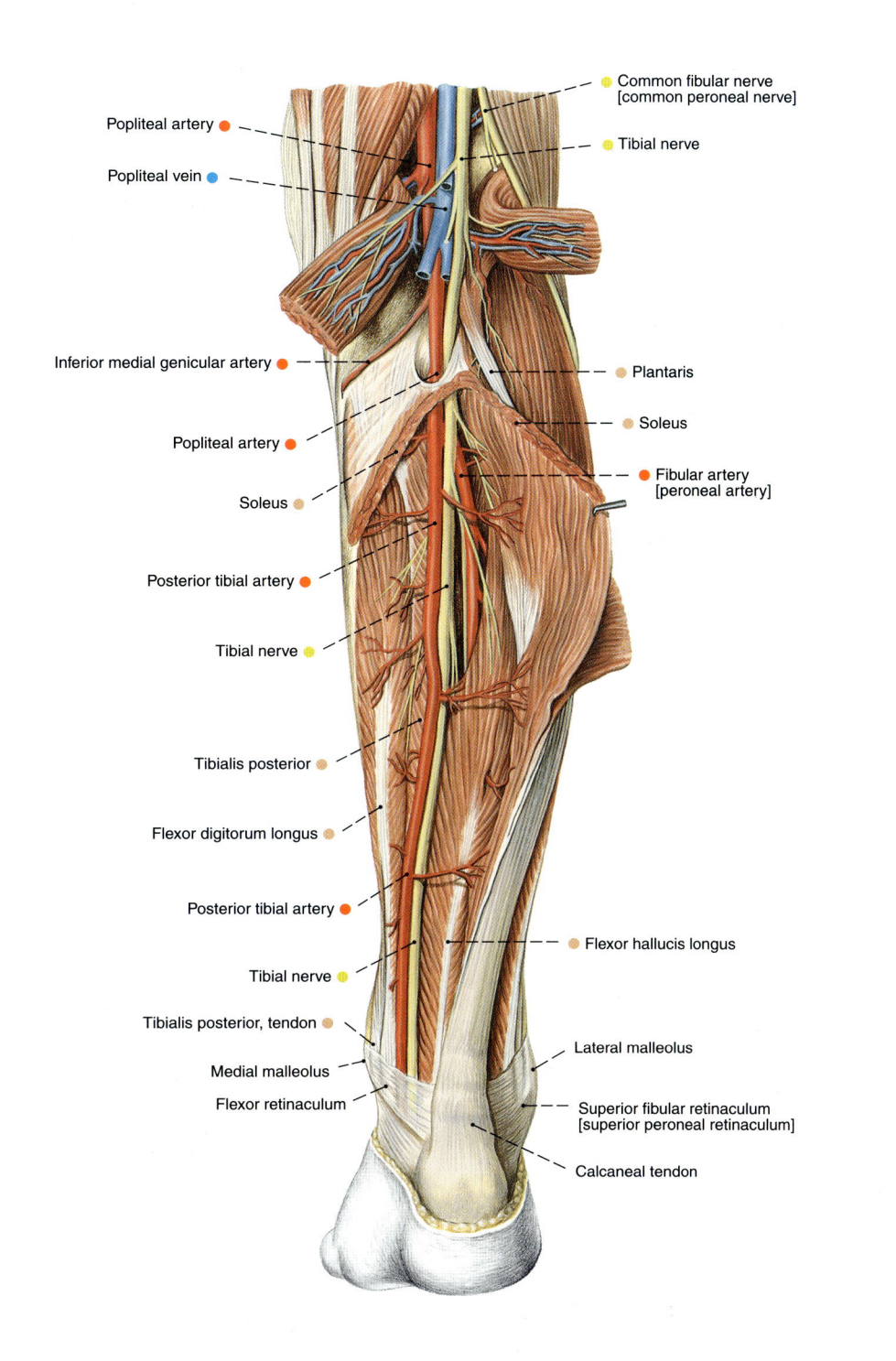

Fig. 1357 Blood vessels and nerves of popliteal fossa and posterior region of right leg; gastrocnemius extensively removed and soleus split to expose the deep layer; posterior aspect.

372 *Lower limb*

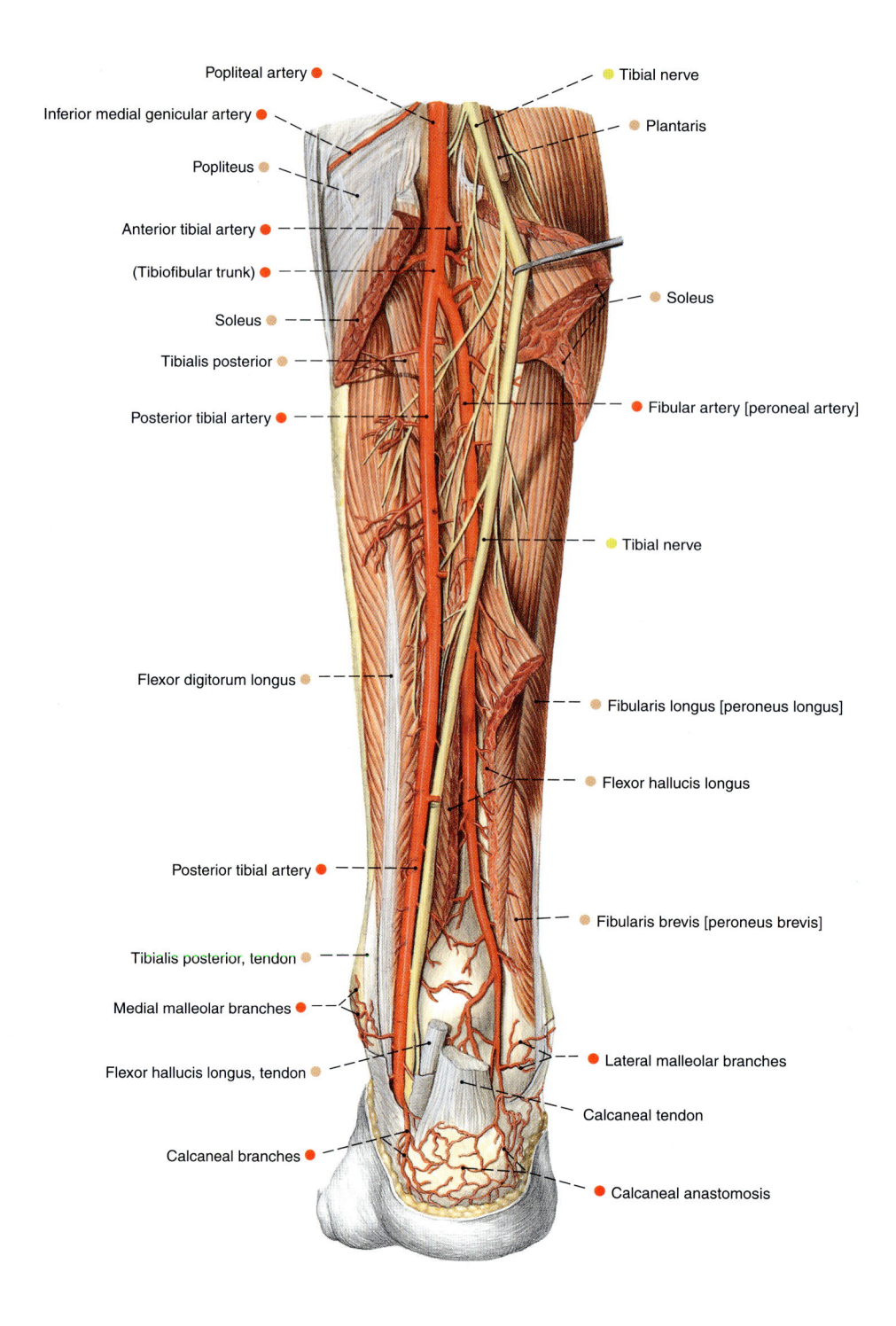

Fig. 1358 Arteries and nerves of popliteal fossa and posterior region of right leg; triceps surae and extensor hallucis longus extensively removed; posterior aspect.

Blood vessels and nerves of foot 373

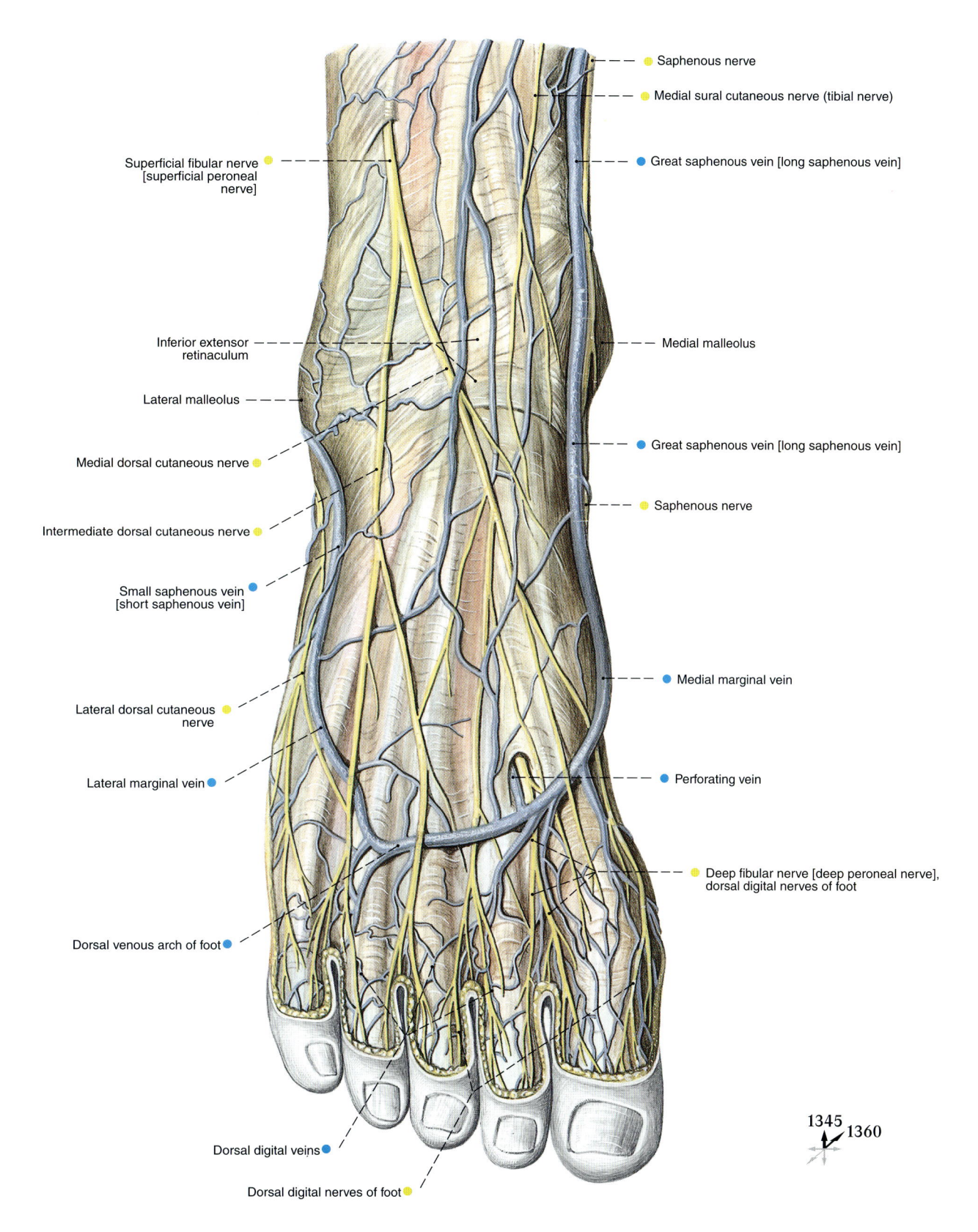

Fig. 1359 Epifascial veins and nerves of right dorsum of foot [dorsal region of foot]; dorsal aspect.

374 Lower limb

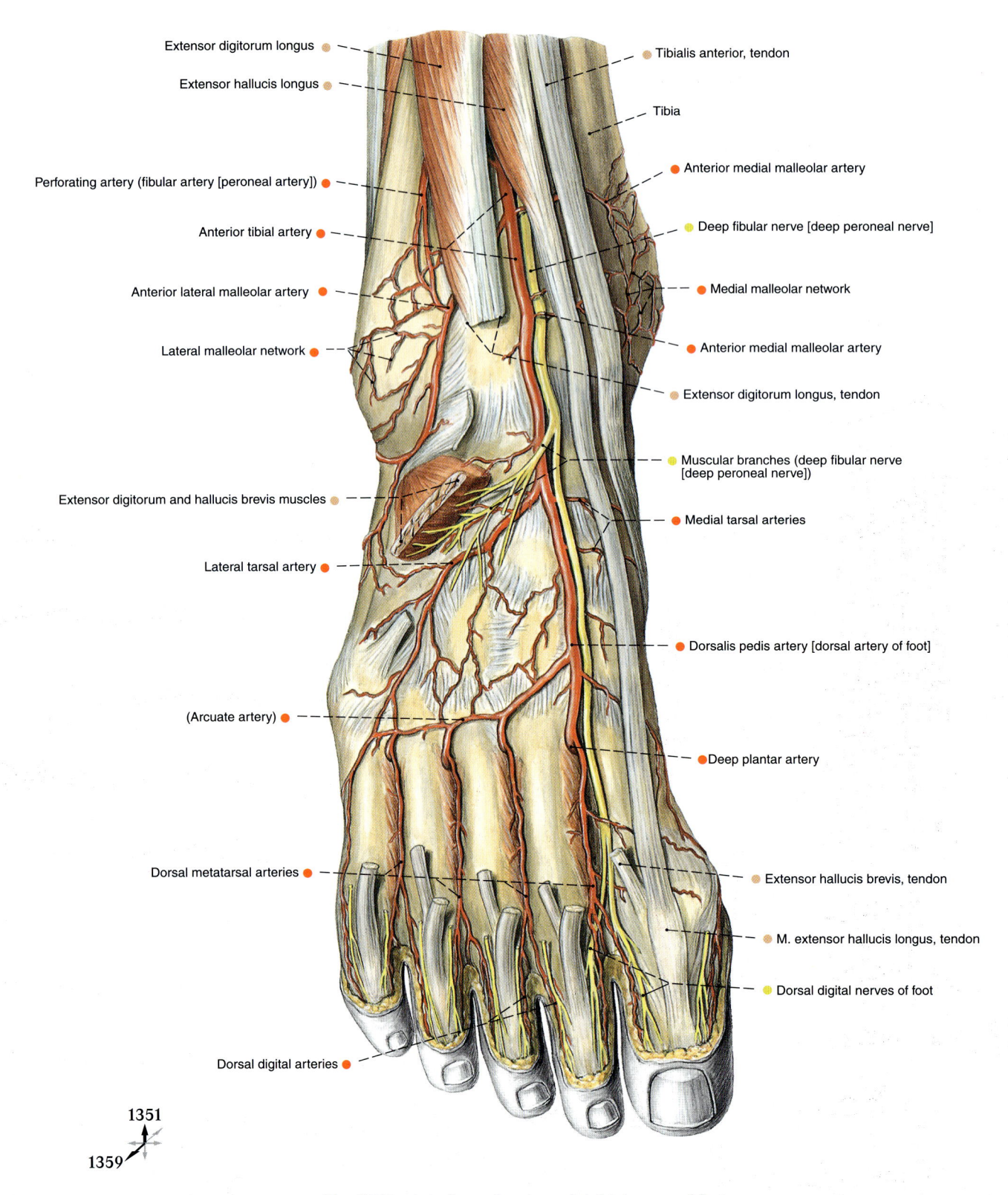

Fig. 1360 Arteries and nerves of right dorsum of foot [dorsal region of foot]; dorsal fascia of foot and extensor digitorum and hallucis muscles partially removed; dorsal aspect.

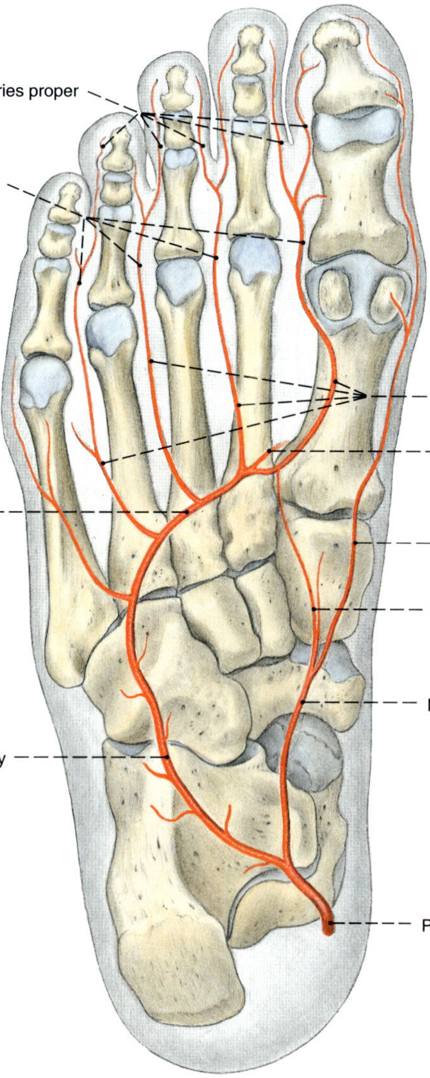
Plantar digital arteries proper
Common plantar digital arteries
Plantar metatarsal arteries
Deep plantar artery (dorsalis pedis artery [dorsal artery of foot])
Deep plantar arch
Superficial branch
Deep branch
Medial plantar artery
Lateral plantar artery
Posterior tibial artery

Fig. 1361 Arteries of right sole; general survey; dorsal aspect.

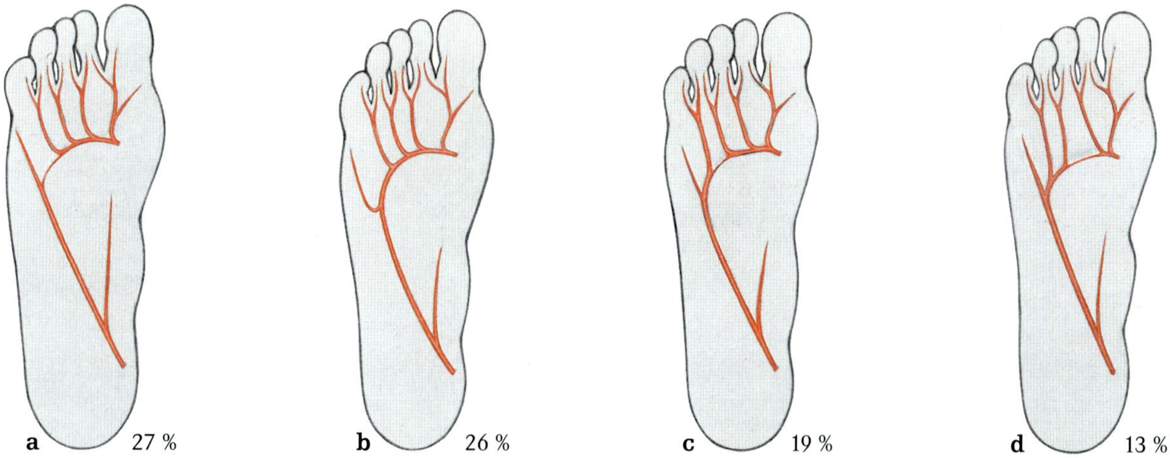
a 27 %
b 26 %
c 19 %
d 13 %

Fig. 1362 a-d Variations of arteries of sole.

- **a** Deep plantar arch supplied mainly by the dorsalis pedis artery [dorsal artery of foot]
- **b** Deep plantar arch supplied mainly by the tibialis posterior artery
- **c** 5th and lateral part of 4th toe supplied by the posterior tibial artery, medial toes supplied by dorsalis pedis artery [dorsal artery of foot]
- **d** 5th, 4th, and lateral part of 3rd toe supplied by the posterior tibial artery, medial toes supplied by dorsalis pedis artery [dorsal artery of foot]

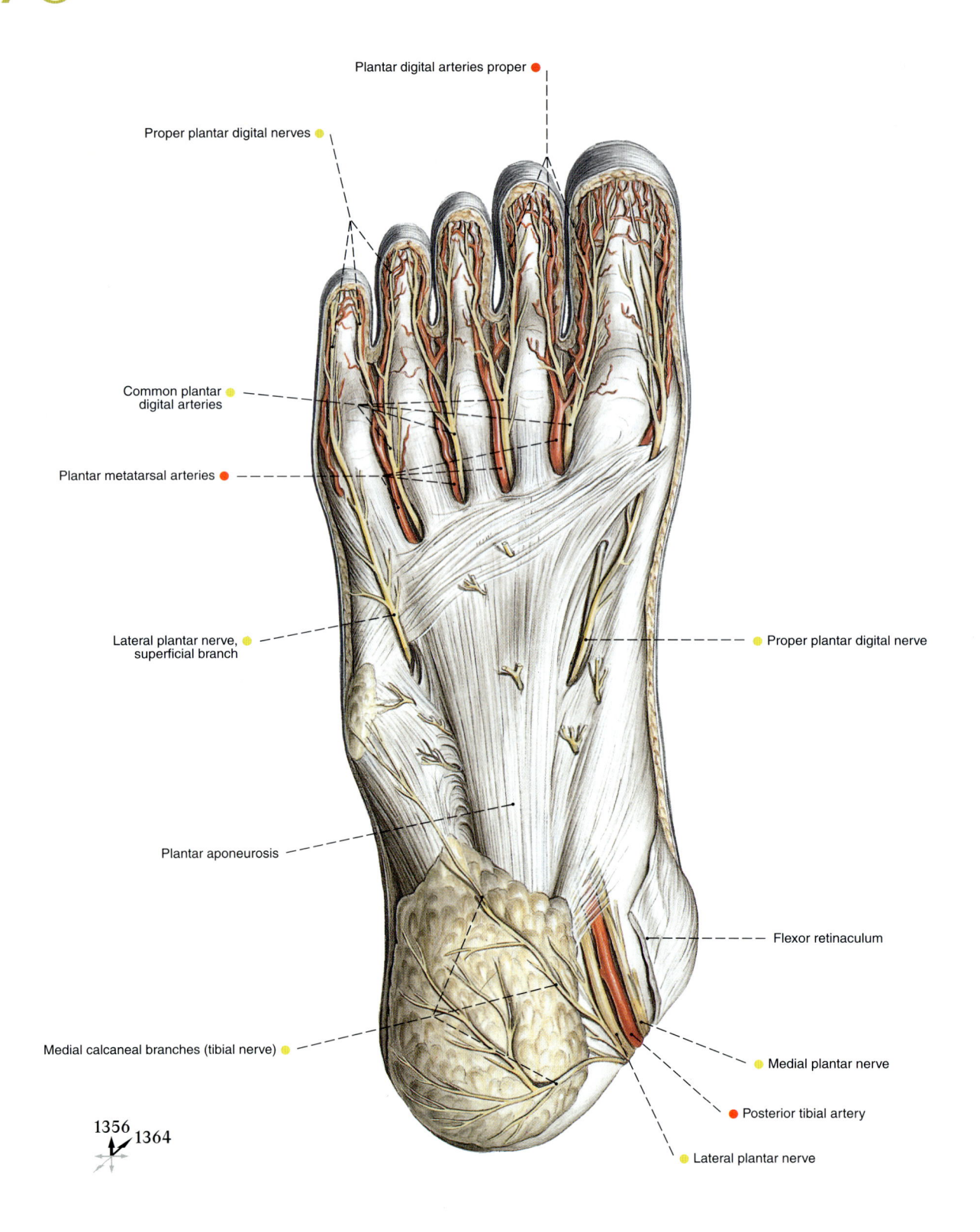

Fig. 1363 Arteries and nerves of right sole; flexor retinaculum split; plantar aspect.

Blood vessels and nerves of foot 377

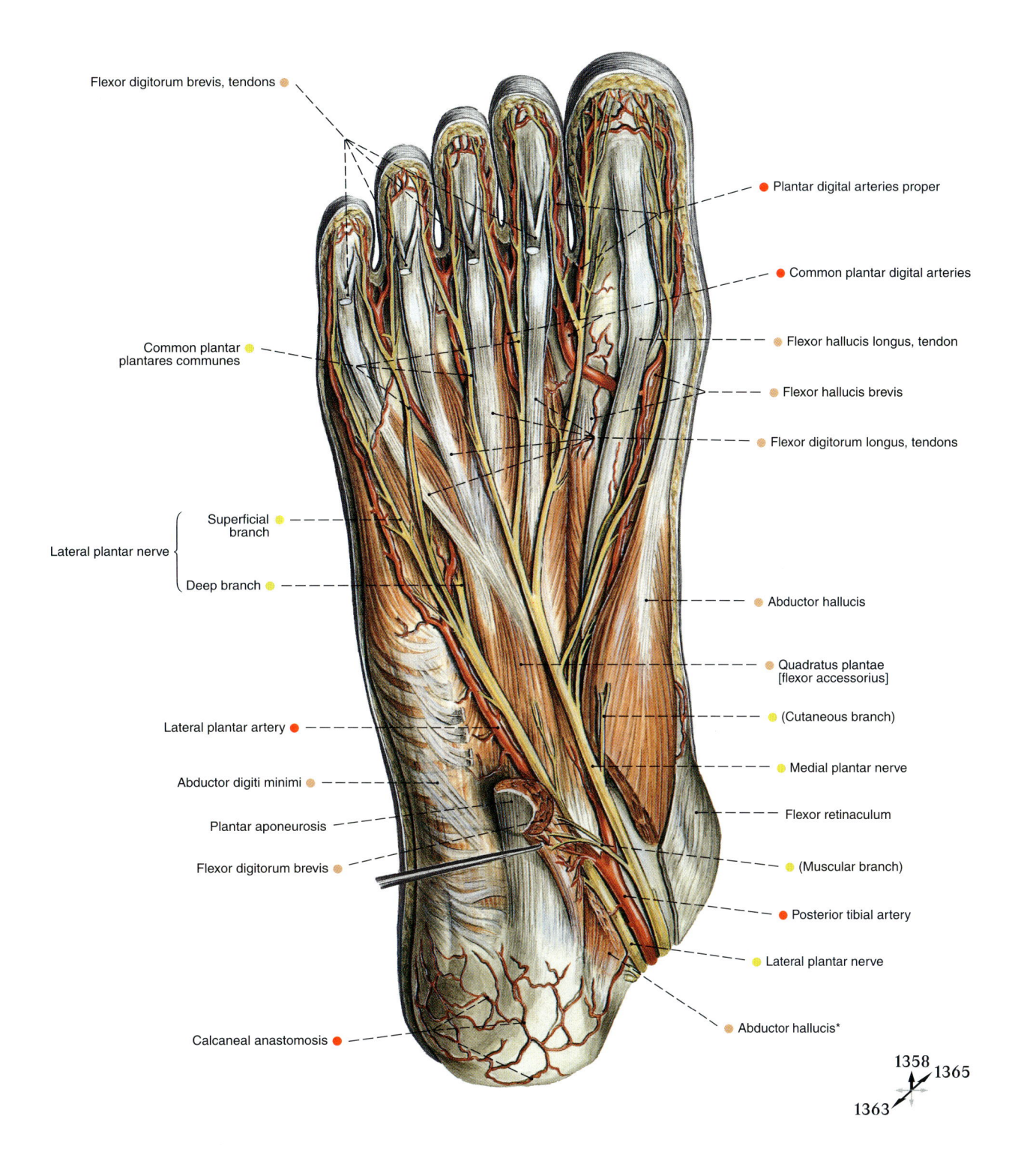

Fig. 1364 Arteries and nerves of right sole; plantar aponeurosis and flexor digitorum brevis extensively removed and abductor hallucis split; plantar aspect.

* The distal continuation of the medial retromalleolar space beneath the abductor hallucis is also known as tarsal tunnel (see also page 370).

378 Lower limb

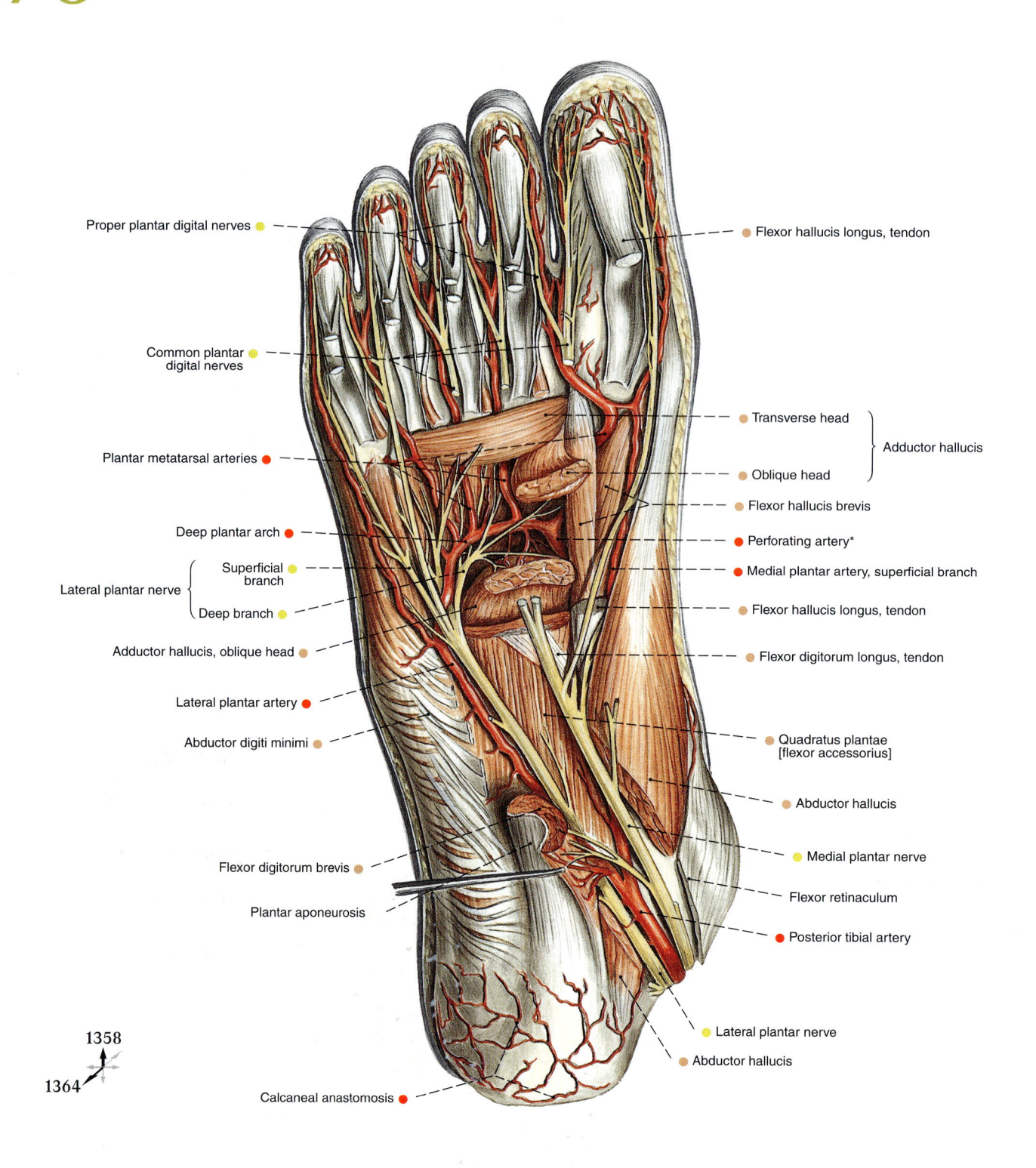

Fig. 1365 Arteries and nerves of right sole; flexor digitorum brevis and longus and flexor hallucis longus extensively removed; abductor hallucis and oblique head of adductor hallucis split; plantar aspect.

* Anastomosis with dorsalis pedis artery [dorsal artery of foot].

Spaces of foot 379

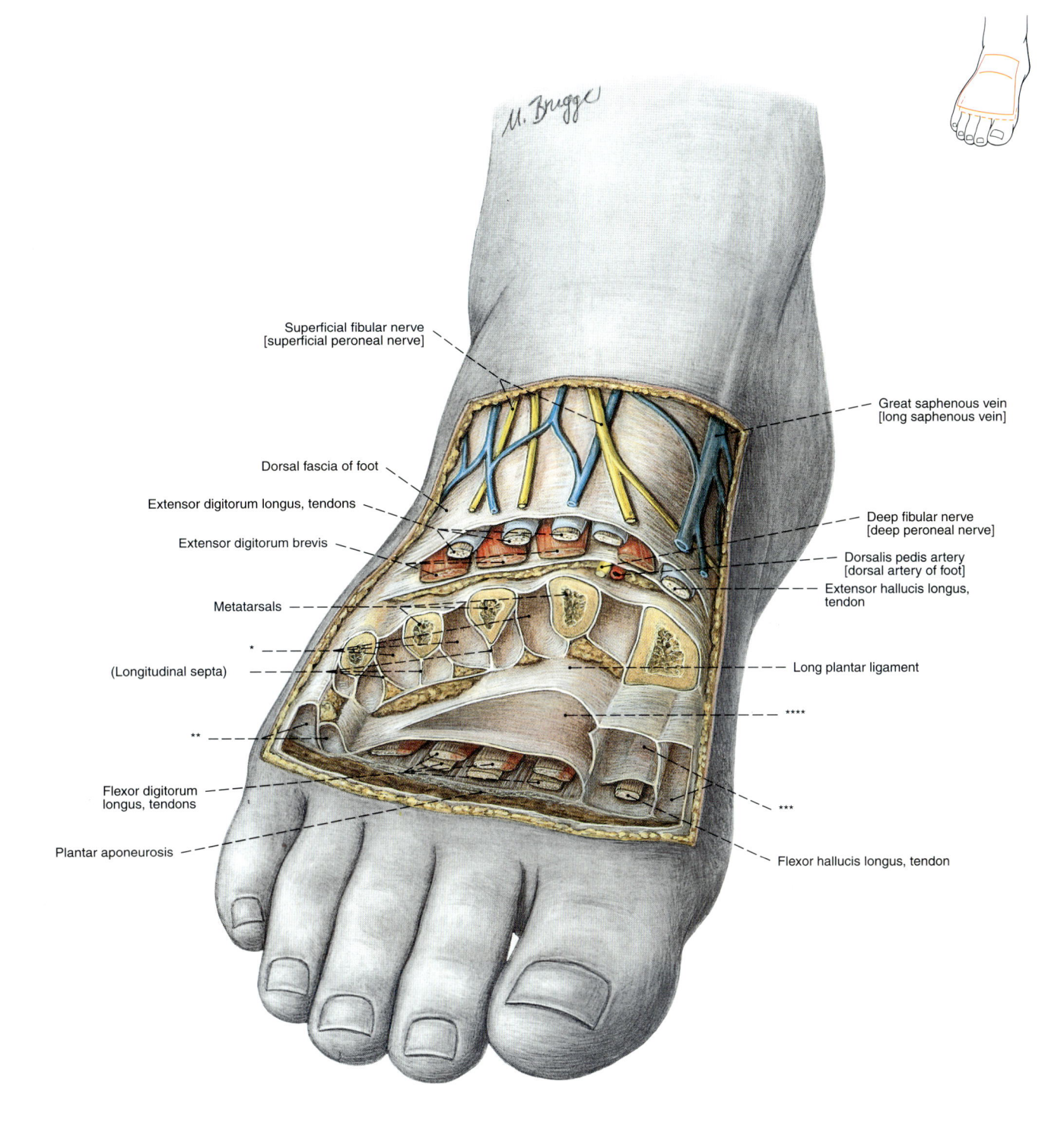

Fig. 1366 Compartments of right foot opened layer by layer; anterior dorsal aspect (30%).

*   Spaces for interossei.
**   Lateral compartment.
***   Medial compartment.
**** Intermediate [middle] compartment.

380 Lower limb

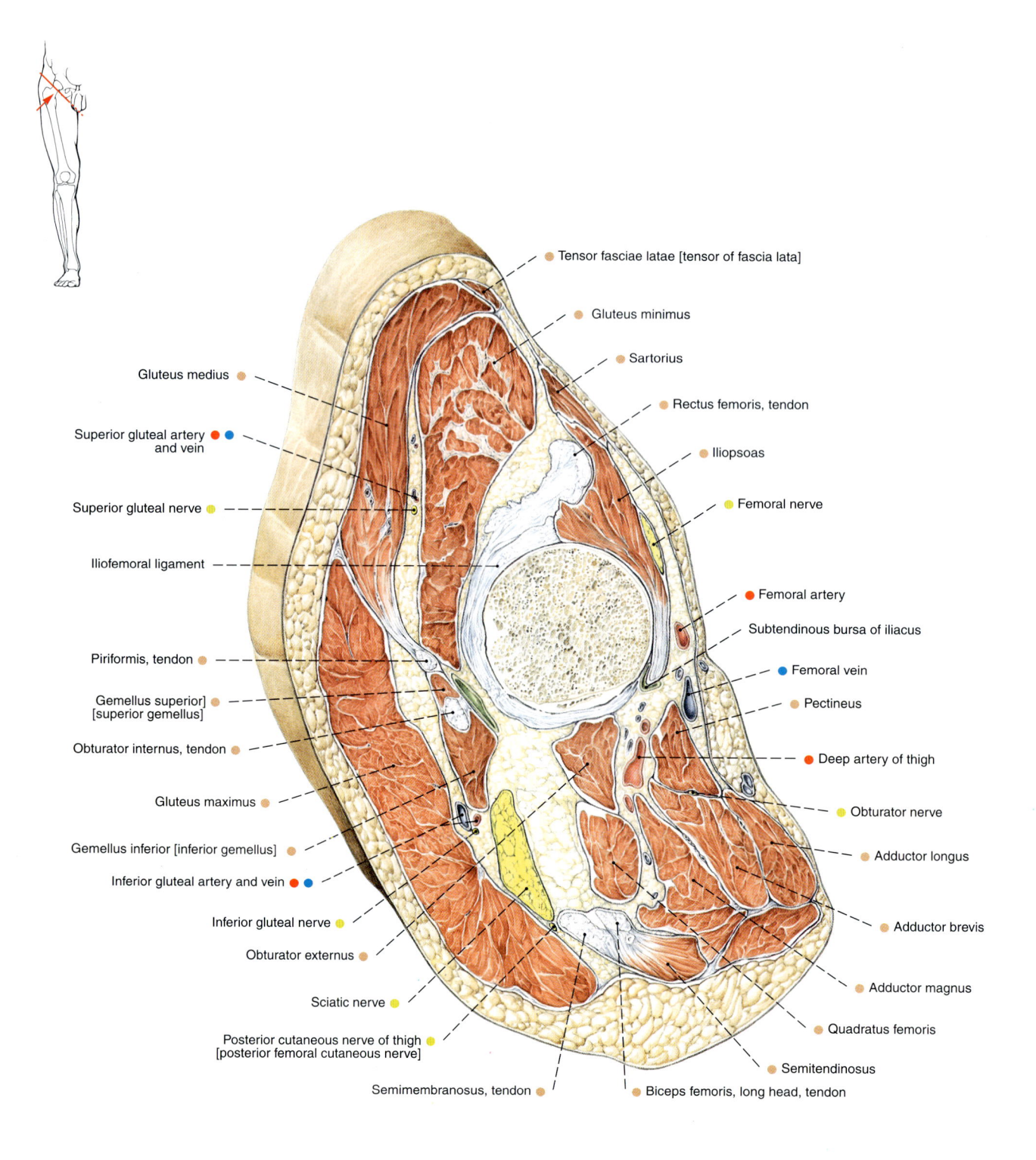

Fig. 1367 Right thigh; oblique section through hip joint; distal aspect.

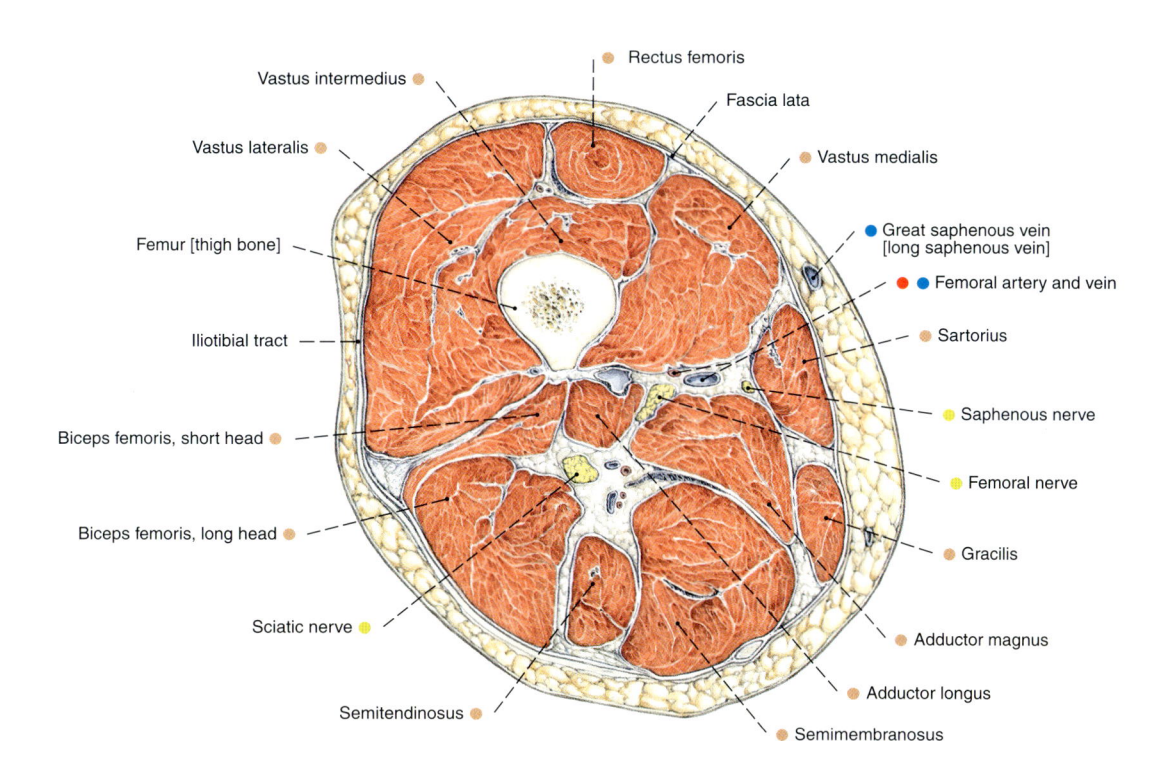

Cross-sections through thigh

Fig. 1368 Right thigh; cross-section through middle of thigh; distal aspect.

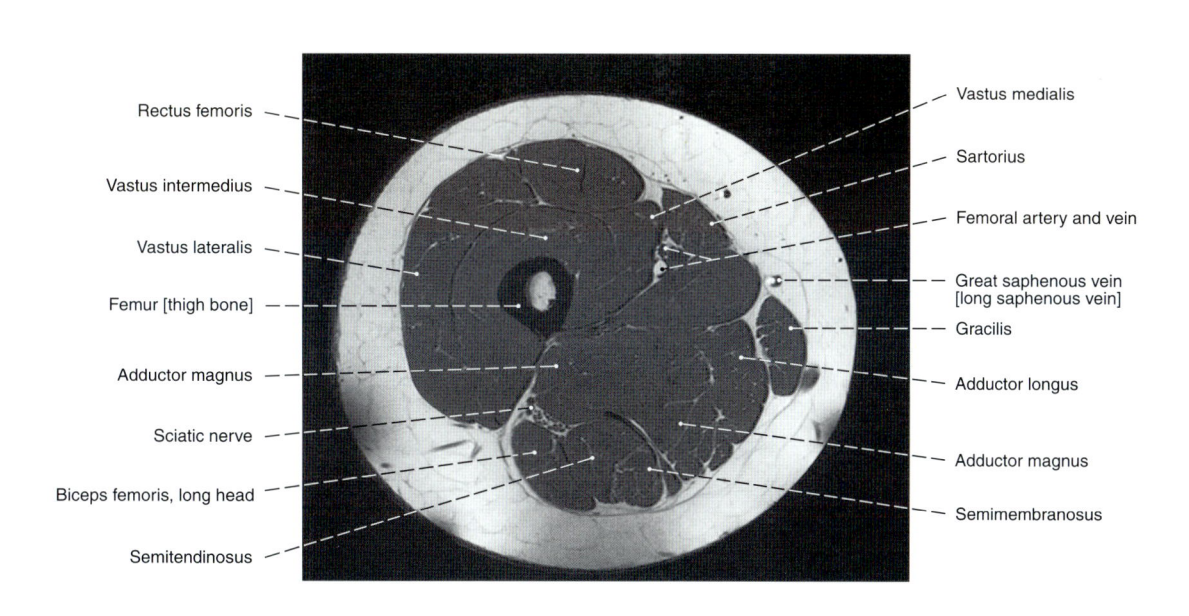

Fig. 1369 Right thigh; magnetic resonance image (MRI); cross-section slightly above middle of thigh; distal aspect.

382 Lower limb

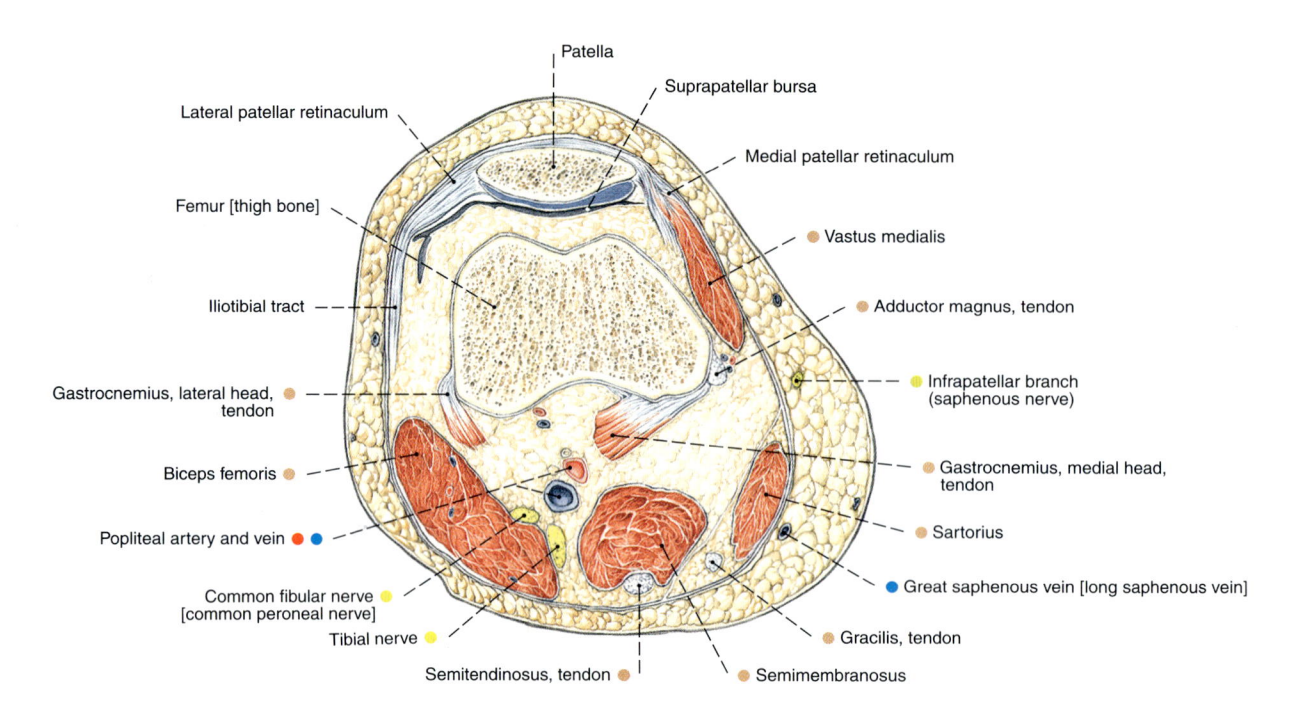

Fig. 1370 Right thigh; cross section through distal extremity of femur [thigh bone] and patella; distal aspect.

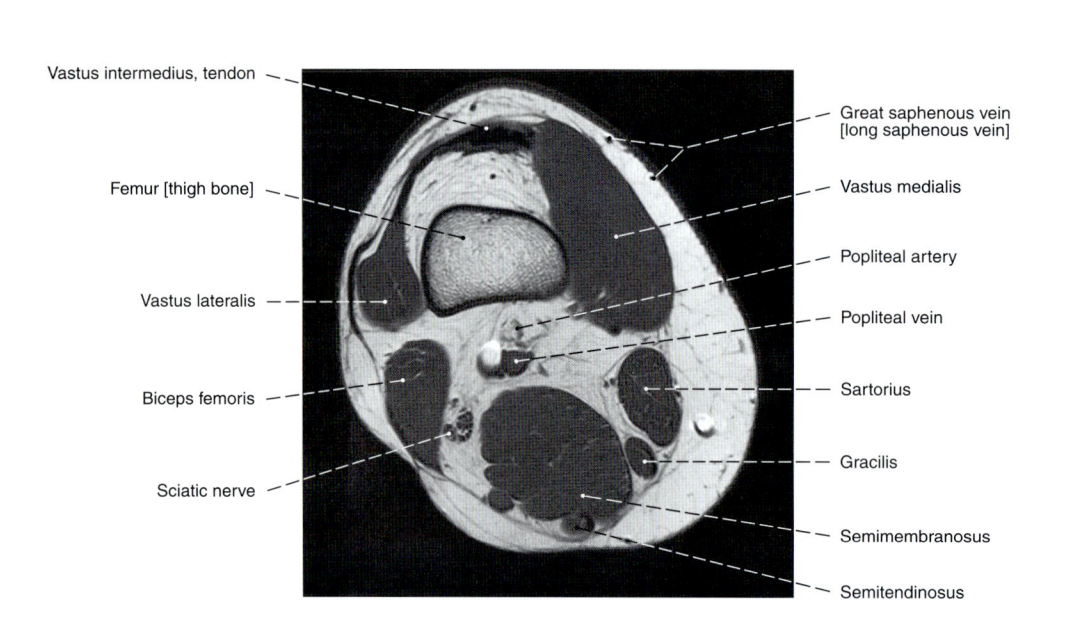

Fig. 1371 Right thigh; magnetic resonance image (MRI); cross-section through lower third of thigh slightly above patella; distal aspect.

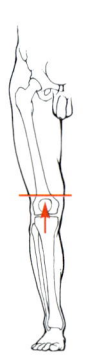

Cross-sections through leg

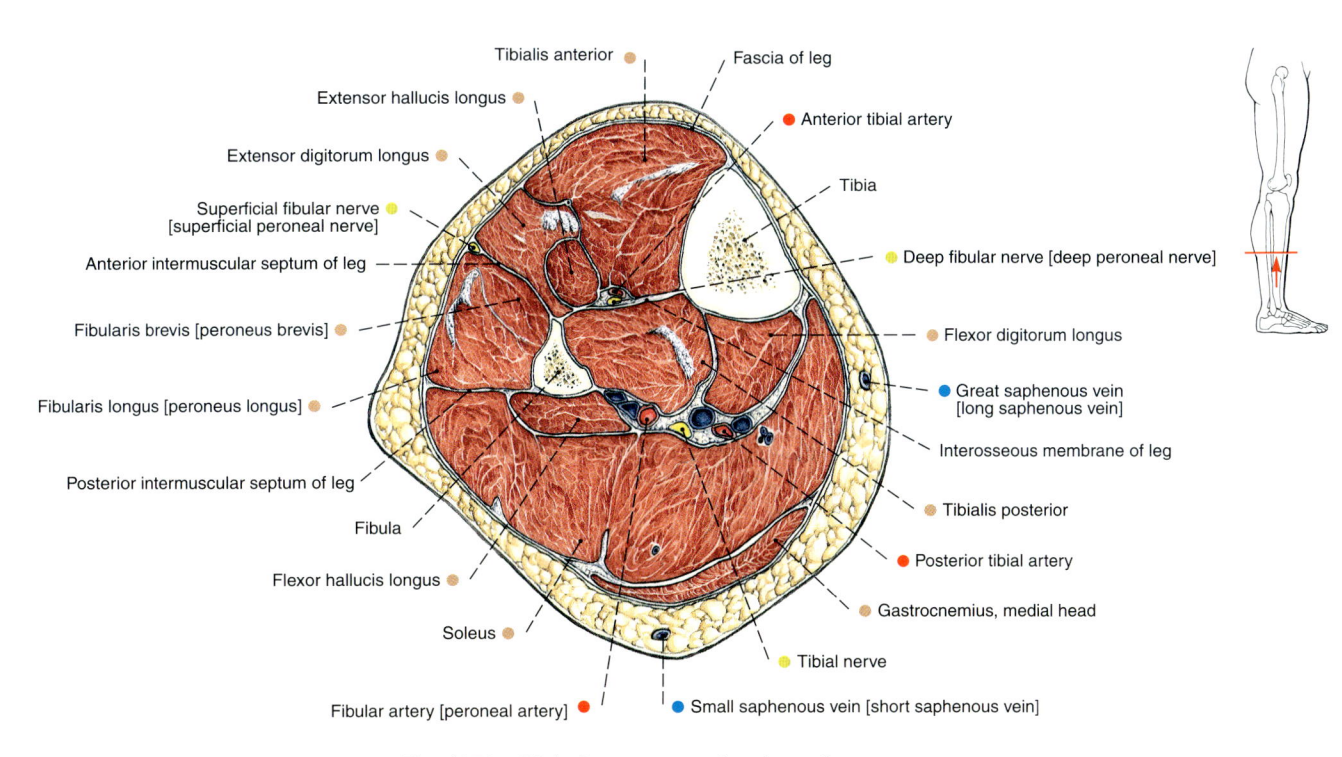

Fig. 1372 Right leg; cross-section through middle of leg; distal aspect.

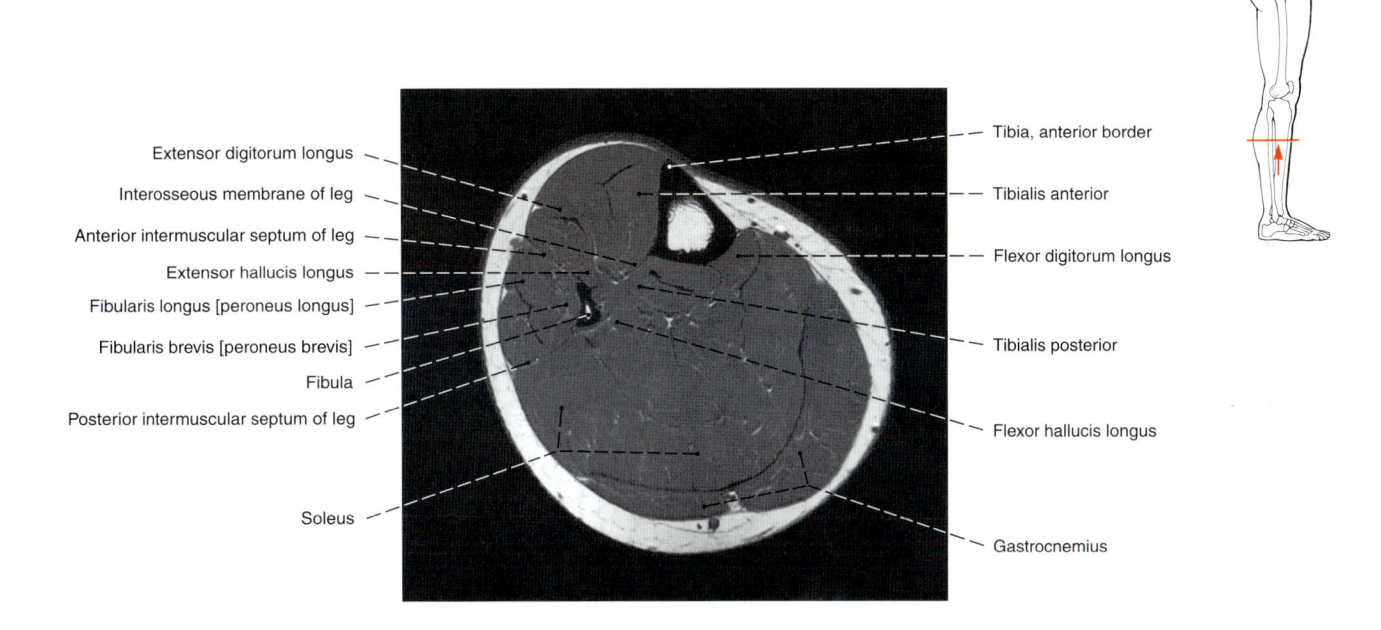

Fig. 1373 Right leg; magnetic resonance image (MRI); cross-section through middle of leg; distal aspect.

Lower limb

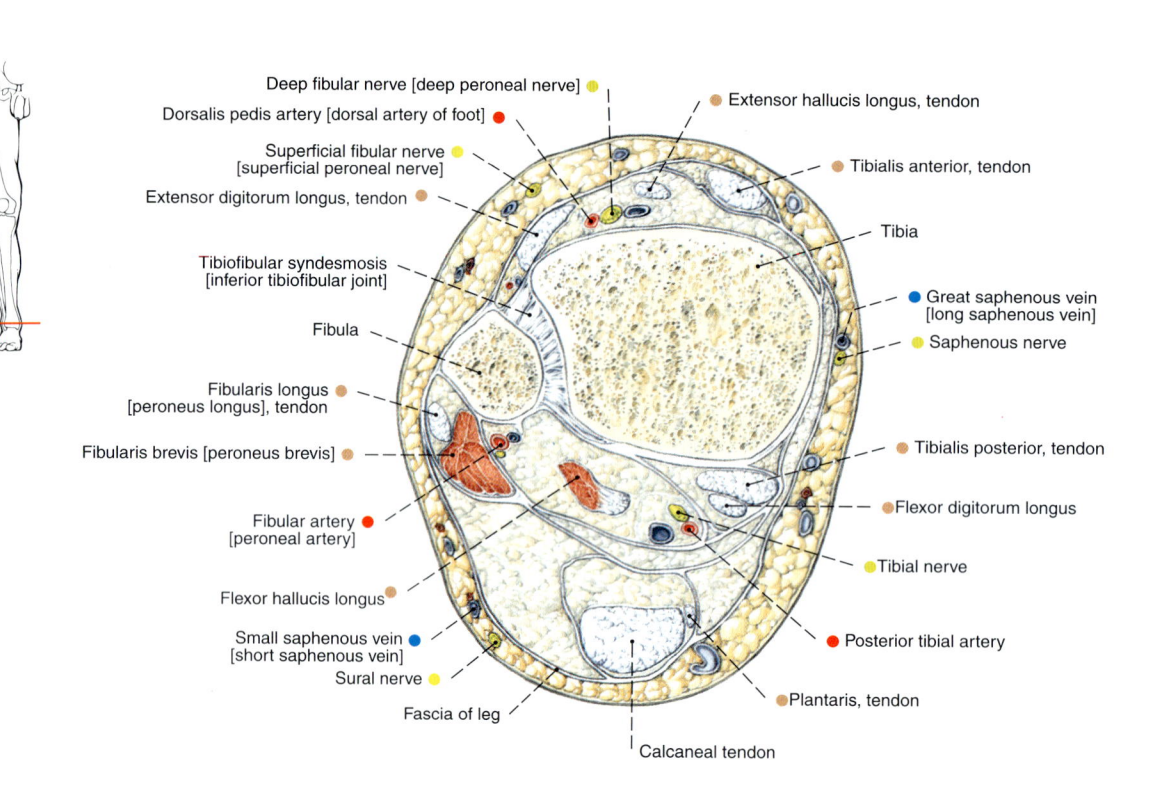

Fig. 1374 Right leg; cross-section slightly above ankle joint; distal aspect.

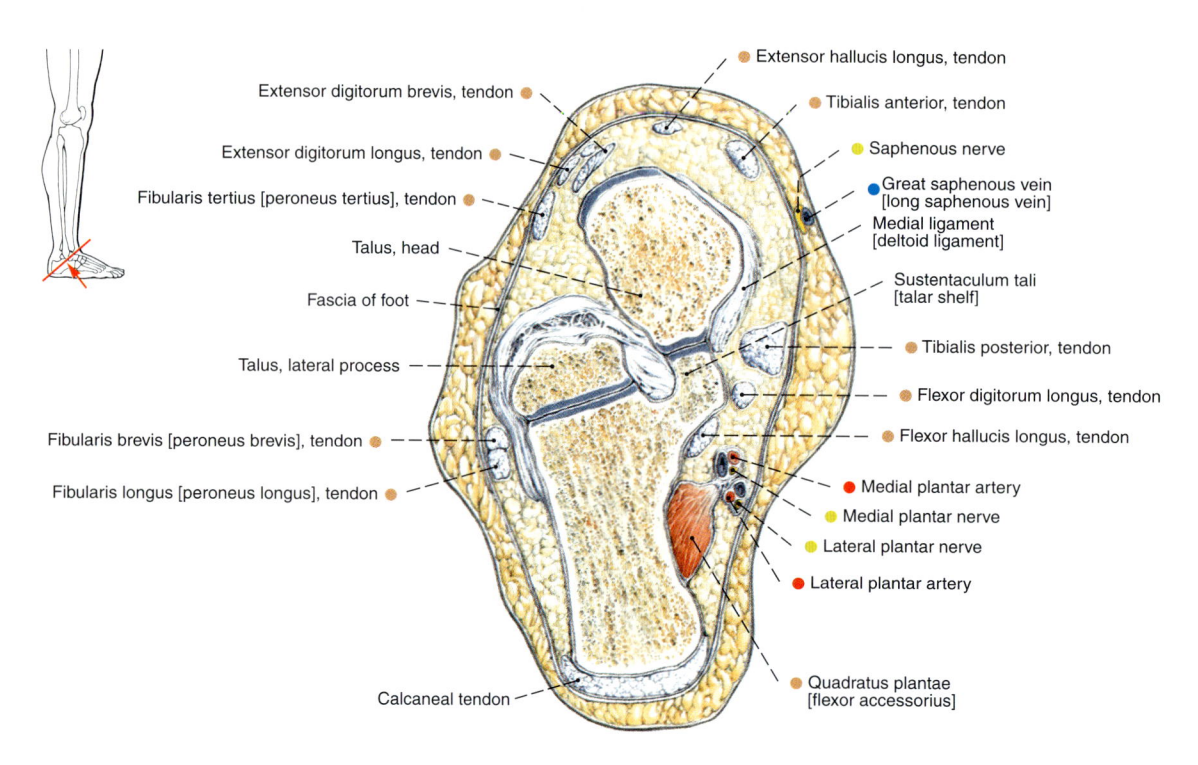

Fig. 1375 Right foot; oblique section through calcaneus and head of talus; distal aspect.

Frontal sections through foot

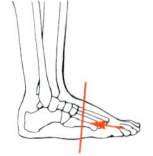

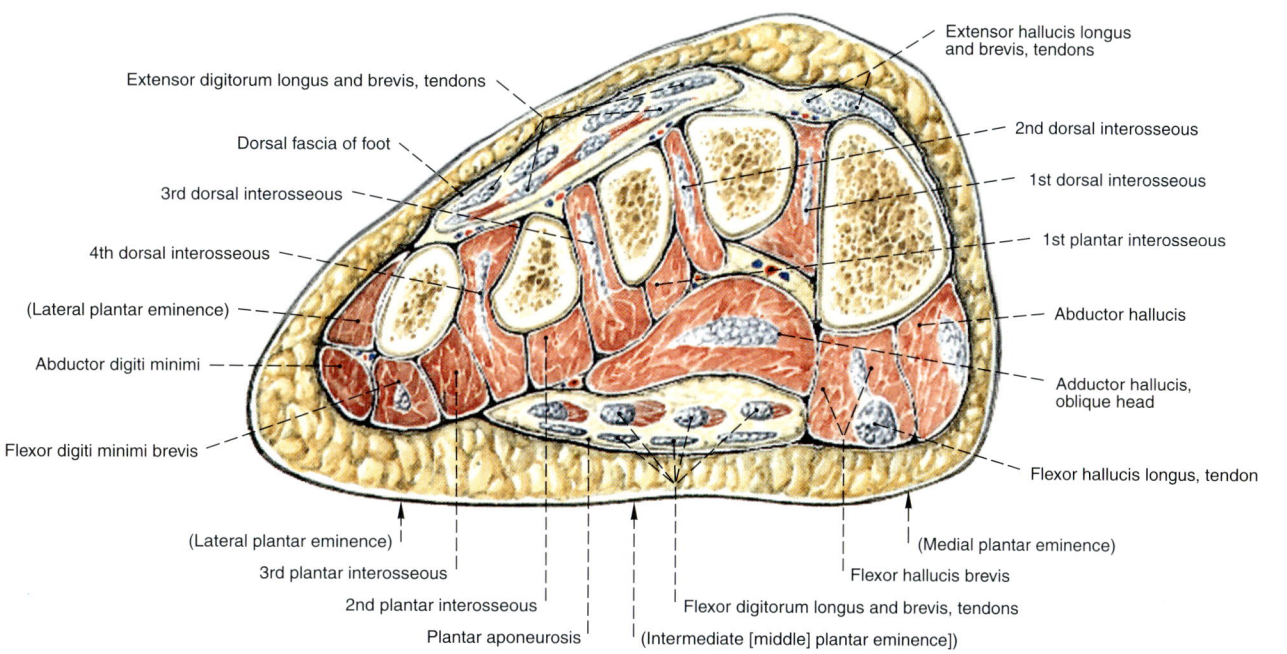

Fig. 1376 Right foot; frontal section through metatarsus; distal aspect.

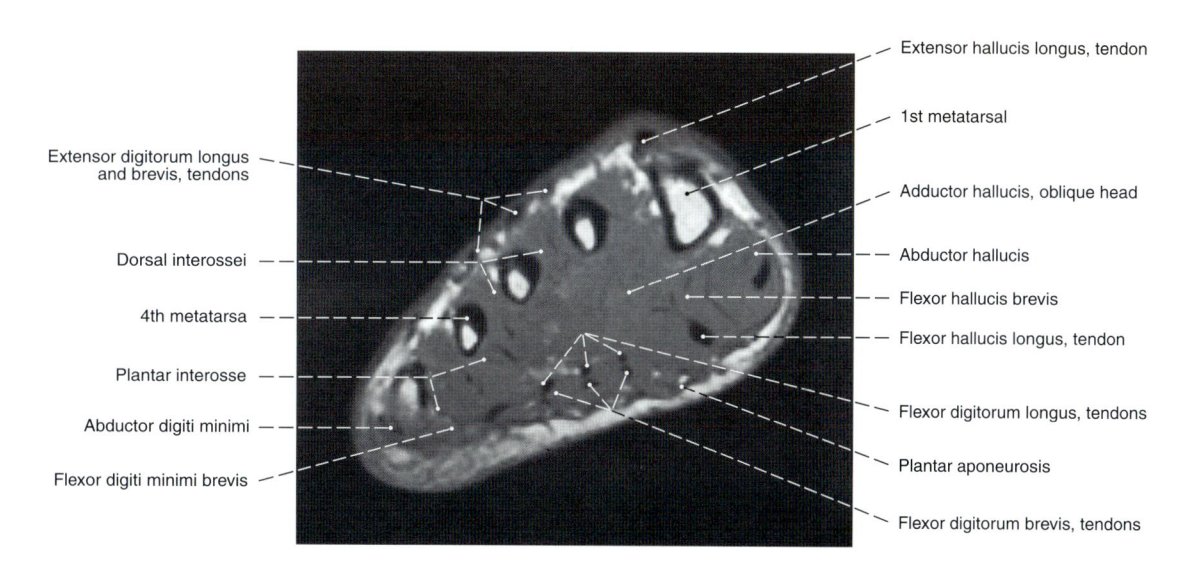

Fig. 1377 Right foot; magnetic resonance image (MRI); frontal section through metatarsus; distal aspect.

Lower limb

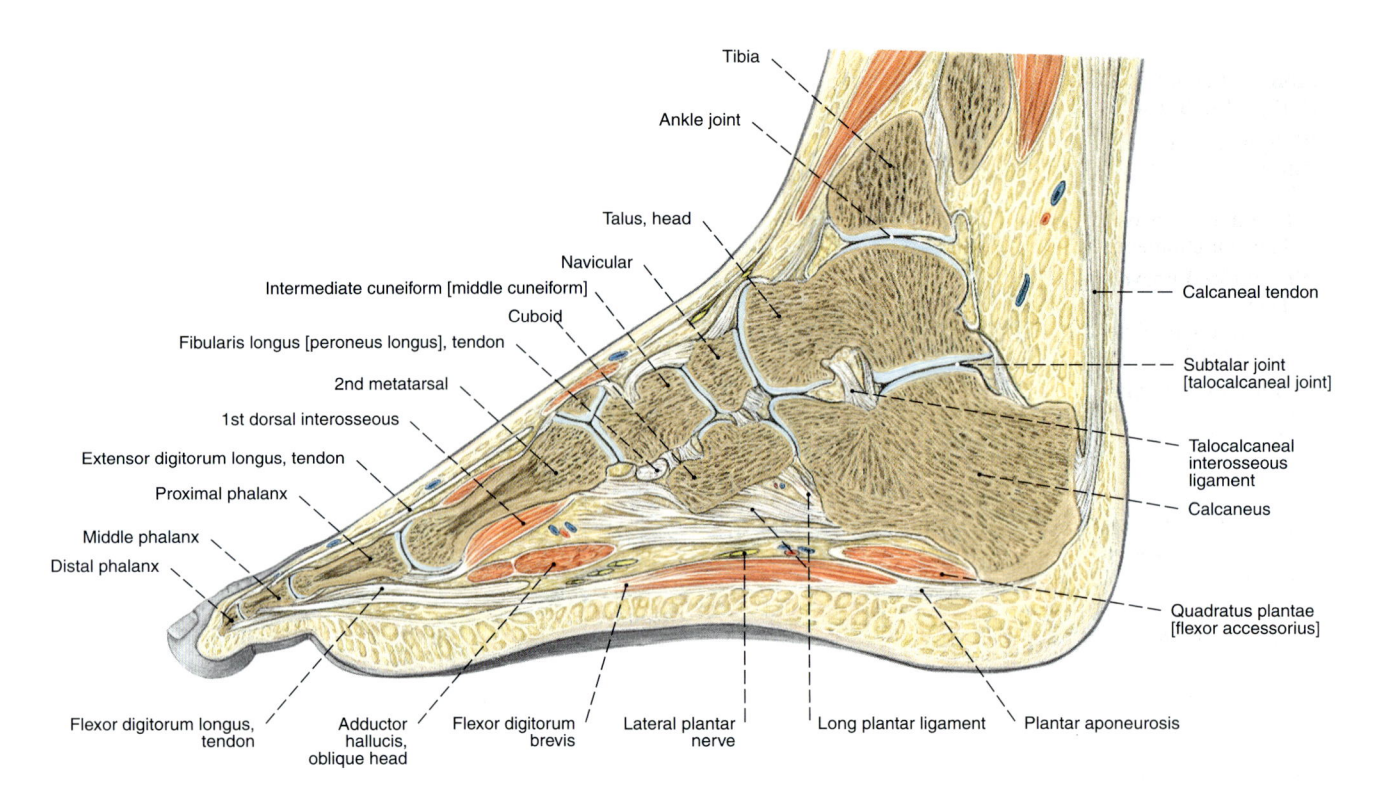

Fig. 1378 Foot; sagittal section through 2nd toe; medial aspect.

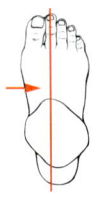

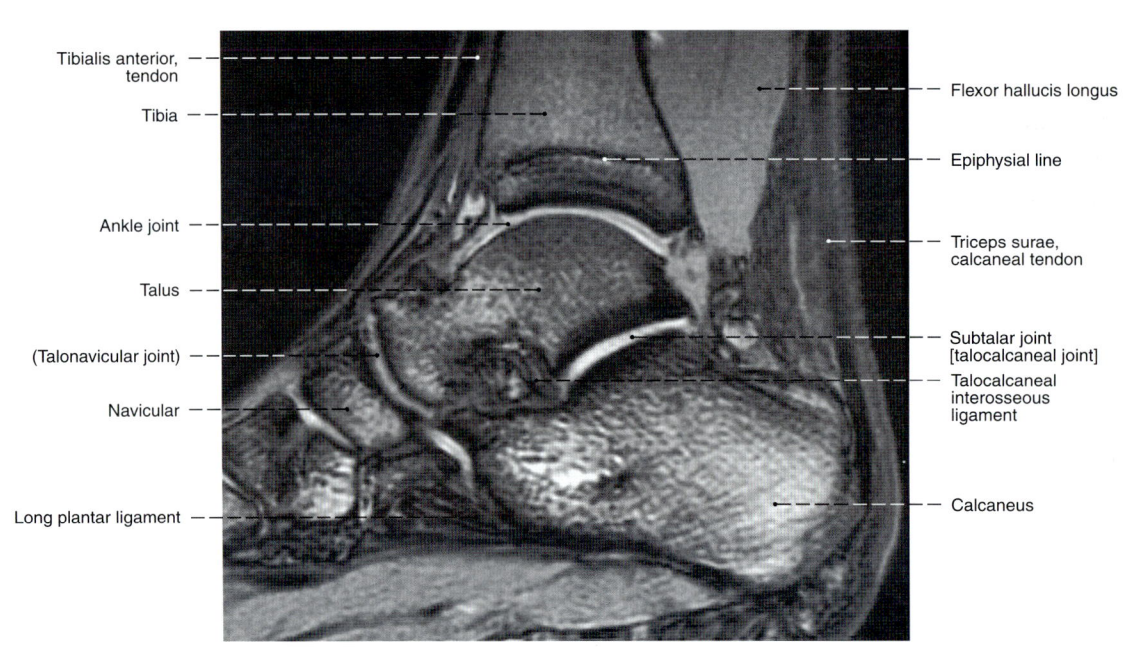

Fig. 1379 Foot; magnetic resonance image (MRI); sagittal slightly medial to longitudinal axis of neck of talus; medial aspect.

Lumbosacral plexus

	Motor	Sensory
Lumbar plexus (T 12) L 1–L 3 (L 4)		
Iliohypogastric nerve [iliopubic nerve] T 12, L 1 Lateral cutaneous branch Anterior cutaneous branch	Rectus abdominis, external oblique, internal oblique, transversus abdominis [transverse abdominal]	Skin of hip Skin of external inguinal ring and mons pubis
Ilio-inguinal nerve (T 12) L 1 (L 2) Anterior scrotal nerves/ anterior labial nerves	Rectus abdominis, external oblique, internal oblique, transversus abdominis [transverse abdominal]	Skin of inguinal region, root of penis, and scrotum Skin of inguinal region and labia majora
Genitofemoral nerve L 1, L 2 Genital branch Femoral branch	Cremaster	Layers of testis (including dartos fascia)
Lateral cutaneous nerve of thigh [lateral femoral cutaneous nerve] L 2, L 3		Skin over saphenous opening Skin of lateral and anterior side of thigh proximal to knee
Obturator nerve L 2–L 4 Anterior branch Cutaneous branch Posterior branch Muscular branches	Obturator externus, pectineus, adductor brevis, adductor longus, gracilis Adductor magnus, (adductor brevis), adductor minimus	Joint capsule of hip joint Skin of medial side of thigh proximal to knee Joint capsule of hip joint, periosteum of posterior surface of femur [thigh bone]
Accessory obturator nerve L 3, L 4	Pectineus	Joint capsule of hip joint
Femoral nerve L 2–L 4 Muscular branches Anterior cutaneous branches Saphenous nerve Infrapatellar branch Medial cutaneous nerve of leg	Iliopsoas, pectineus, sartorius, quadriceps femoris	Joint capsule of hip joint Skin of anterior and medial side of thigh proximal to knee, periosteum of anterior surface of femur [thigh bone] Skin of medial and anterior side of knee and medial side of leg and foot
Sacral plexus (L 4) L 5–S 3 (S 4)		
Nerve to obturator internus L 5–S 2	Obturator internus	
Nerve to piriformis S 1, S 2	Piriformis	
Nerve to quadratus femoris L 5–S 1 (S 2)	Quadratus femoris	
Superior gluteal nerve L 4–S 1	Gluteus medius and minimus, tensor fasciae latae [tensor of fascia lata]	
Inferior gluteal nerve L 5–S 2	Gluteus maximus	
Posterior cutaneous nerve of thigh [posterior femoral cutaneous nerve] S 1–S 3 Inferior clunial nerves Perineal nerves		Skin of posterior side of thigh and proximal leg Skin of gluteal region Perineum, skin of scrotum resp. skin of labia majora
Sciatic nerve L 4–S 3	Flexors of thigh, all muscles of leg and foot	
Common fibular nerve L 4–S 2 Lateral sural cutaneous nerve Sural communicating branch	Biceps femoris, short head	Joint capsule of knee joint Skin of calf up proximal to lateral malleolus Communicating branch with sural nerve
Superficial fibular nerve Muscular branches Medial dorsal cutaneous nerve Intermediate dorsal cutaneous nerve Dorsal digital nerves of foot	Fibularis [peroneus] longus and brevis	Skin of leg and dorsum of foot down to 1st–3rd toe Skin of lateral border of foot Skin of dorsum of toes except 1st interdigital space and lateral border of 5th toe

Continued → 388

Lower Limb

	Motor	Sensory
Deep fibular nerve	Tibialis anterior, extensor digitorum longus, extensor hallucis longus, extensor digitorum brevis, and extensor hallucis brevis	Periosteum of tibia and fibula and joint capsule of ankle joint
Muscular branches		
Dorsal digital nerves of foot		Skin of 1st interdigital space
Tibial nerve L 4 - S 3	Triceps surae, plantaris, popliteus, tibialis posterior, flexor digitorum longus, flexor hallucis longus	Joint capsule of knee joint
Muscular branches		
Interosseous nerve of leg [crural interosseous nerve]		Periosteum of tibia and fibula and joint capsule of ankle joint
Medial sural cutaneous nerve		Merges with lateral sural cutaneous nerve to form the sural nerve
Sural nerve		
Lateral dorsal cutaneous nerve		Skin of lateral border of foot up to lateral border of little toe
Lateral calcaneal branches		Lateral skin of heel
Medial calcaneal branches		Medial skin of heel
Medial plantar nerve	Abductor hallucis, flexor digitorum brevis, flexor hallucis brevis (medial head), 1st and 2nd lumbricals	Medial skin of sole
Common plantar digital nerves		Skin of plantar side of medial 3 1/2 toes and nail area
Proper plantar digital nerves		
Lateral plantar nerve	Abductor digiti minimi, quadratus plantae [flexor accessorius], flexor digiti minimi brevis, opponens digiti minimi, interossei of 4th interdigital space	
Superficial branch		
Common plantar digital nerves		Skin of plantar side of lateral 1 1/2 toes and nail area
Proper plantar digital nerves	2nd - 4th lumbricals, adductor hallucis (transverse head), interossei of 1st - 4th interdigital space	
Deep branch		
Pudendal nerve (S 1) S 2 - S 4		Skin of anal triangle and perineum
Inferior anal [rectal] nerves S 3, S 4		
Perineal nerves	Superficial and deep transverse perineal muscles, bulbospongiosus and ischiocavernosus, external anal sphincter	Dorsal skin of scrotum resp. labia majora and minora, mucosa of urethra, vestibule of vagina
Posterior scrotal nerves/ posterior labial nerves		
Muscular branches		
Dorsal nerve of penis/ dorsal nerve of clitoris	Deep transverse perineal muscle	Skin of penis, glans penis/ clitoris, prepuce
Coccygeal nerve S 4, S 5 (Co 1)	Ischiococcygeus [coccygeus], levator ani	Skin over coccyx and between coccyx and anus
Coccygeal plexus S 4, S 5, (Co 1)		
Anococcygeal nerve		

Muscles used in clinical diagnosis of segmental innervation of lower limb

Spinal segment resp. segmental spinal nerve	Resp. muscle(s) / tendon(s) reflex
L 3	Quadriceps femoris (paralysis and loss of patellar tendon reflex)
L 4	Quadriceps femoris and tibialis anterior (weakening of patellar tendon reflex)
L 5	Extensor hallucis longus, possibly also brevis (paralysis and atrophy)
S 1	Fibular [peroneal] muscles, possibly also triceps surae and glutei (loss of Achilles tenodn reflex)

Index

Bold numbers indicate pages in which terms occur also in legends or tables.

A

Abdomen
- cross-section **246-249**
- CT **246**
- frontal section **242-243**
- median section **240**
- sagittal section **241, 244-245**

Abdominal aorta 41, 68, **106**, 117, **117**, 119, 145, 152, 154-155, 169, 172, 175-176, **176**, 177, 183-184, 206, 208-210, 213, 217, 219, 221, 226, 240, 243, 248-250
- ultrasound image **176**

Abdominal viscera **156, 160, 164, 169**

Abdominal wall **56, 58, 67, 72-73**
- anterior **69**
- innervation, segmental, sensory **57**
- male **250**
- posterior **69, 212-213**
- surface **48**

Abduction (hip joint) 314
Acetabular fossa 279
Acetabular margin 256, 267-268
Acetabulum 256, 261, 267
ACHILLES tendon *see* calcaneal tendon
Achilles tendon reflex **388**
Acromion 1, 26-27, 53, 126
Adduction (hip joint) 314
Adductor canal 313, **355-356**
Adventitia 108
Ala [wing]
- of ilium 74, 255, 263, 266-268, 273, 275
- of sacrum 10

ALCOCK's canal **223, 258**
Ampulla
- of ductus deferens 67, 187, 192-193, 236
- (duodenum) 132, 134-135, 139, 177
- hepatopancreatic 139, 150, 152
- rectal 205, 225, 240, 252-253, 257-258
- of uterine tube 165-166, 195-196, 203-204, 253

Anastomoses, portocaval **108, 179, 207**

Anastomosis
- calcaneal 372, 377-378
- genicular 351, 356, 367
- patellar 352, 354

Angle
- inferior 1, 27, 29
- infrasternal 48
- of mandible 12
- of pubis 267
- of rib 49-50, 103
- sternal 48, 51

Angle
- subpubic **268**, 270-271

Angle of inclination **277**
Angle of neck of femur **277**
Anorectal junction 205
Ansa subclavia 119-120
Anteflexion (uterus) **196**
Anteversion
- (hip joint) 314
- (uterus) **196**

Anthracotic lymph node **97**
Anthracotic pigment **96**
Anular epiphysis 4-5, 7-9, 24-25
Anulus
- fibrosus 24-25, 30
- - left 79, 81, 85
- - right 79, 85

Anus 205, **205**, 206-207, 223, 226-229, 238, 251
- sphincters **205**

Aorta 30, 41, **71**, 78, 90, 119, **119**, 126, 130, 172, 240, 246, 248-249, 357

Apex
- of bladder 187-188, 252
- of cusp (tooth) 6
- of head of fibula 285, 293
- of heart 76-77, 79-82, 85, 88, 90, 100-101, 103
- of lung 96-97, 100-101, 113, 127
- of patella 286, 292-293
- of sacrum 10-11

Aponeurosis
- of latissimus dorsi 32
- plantar 301, 306, 341-342, 344-345, 376-379, 385-386

Appendix(-ces)
- of epididymis 190, 232
- fibrous (of liver) 142-143, 158
- omental 140, 160, 163, 177, 218, 258
- of testis 189-190, 232
- vermiform 140, **140**, 141, 161-164, 167, 173, 204
- - projection 167
- - variations of position **166-167**
- vesicular 194-195, 197, 204

Arachnoid mater
- cranial 46
- spinal 46-47, 252

Arch
- anterior (of atlas) 6, 12, 19
- of aorta 76-77, 83, 85, 88, 91, 100-101, 103, 106-107, 109-110, 116, **116**, 117, 122-124, 126, 128-129
- - branches **116**
- - radiograph (ap) **116**
- - variations **116**
- of azygos vein 118
- costal 3, 48, 62, 69, 201
- of cricoid cartilage 92
- deep plantar 351, 375, 378

Arch
- dorsal venous (of foot) 364, 373
- iliopectineal 271, 309-310, 318
- jugular venous 113
- posterior (of atlas) 6, 12, 18-19, 38, 40, 45-46
- of psoas **70**
- pubic 268, **271**
- of quadratus **70**
- tendinous (of levator ani) 223-224, 318
- - (of soleus) 324, 331, 370
- vertebral 6-8, 15, 17, 20, 22, 30, 37

Arch of psoas **70**
Arch of quadratus **70**

Area(s)
- anterior intercondylar 284, 295
- bare 123, 142-143, 240
- gastric 132
- posterior intercondylar 284

Areola 54, **54**

Artery(-ies)
- anterior lateral malleolar 351, 367, 374
- anterior medial malleolar 351, 374
- anterior superior pancreaticoduodenal 168, 171
- anterior tibial **285, 329**, 351, 366-367, 369, 372, 374, 383
- anterior tibial recurrent 351, 367
- appendicular 172
- arcuate 208, 351, 374
- ascending 174
- axillary 59, 90, 115, 124, 126, 128
- of bulb of penis 230, 237
- - of vestibule 230
- of caudate lobe 142
- circumflex scapular 43, 126
- common carotid 76-77, 91, 100-101, 106-109, 112-113, 115-116, 119-120, 122, 124-128
- common hepatic 134, 151, 168, **168**, 169-171, 176-177, 210, 246
- - radiograph (ap) **168**
- common iliac 165, 177, 203, 206, 209-210, 213, 216-221, 224, 226, 240-241, 250, 254-255, 259, 357
- coronary **85-86**
- cremasteric 190, 217, 231
- cystic 142, 168-169
- deep
- - (of thigh) 256-257, 261, 351, 354-357, 380
- - variations **357**
- - (of penis) 218-219, 232-234, 242
- deep cervical 45, 117
- deep circumflex iliac 177, 213,

Artery(-ies)
219, 224, 354, 357
- deep plantar 374-375
- descending genicular 351-352, 354, 356, 369
- dorsal (of clitoris) 230
- - (of foot) 351, 367, 374-375, 379, 384
- - (of penis) 219, 230-232, 234, 237, 242
- dorsal digital (foot) 374
- dorsal metatarsal 351, 367, 374
- dorsal pancreatic 168
- external iliac 67, 72, 177, 193, 206, 213, 216-217, 219-221, 224, 236, 250, 253, 318, 353-354, 356-357
- external pudendal 56, 231, 352, 357
- femoral 68, 75, 210, 242, 256-257, 309, **309**, 311, 318, 351-352, 354-357, 380-381
- fibular **329**, 351, 367, 369, 371-372, 383-384
- gastroduodenal 151, 168-171, 240, 242
- helicine 233
- hepatic proper 134, 142, 148, 151, 165, 168, **168**, 169-170, 177, 241-242, 246
- hepatic, variations **168**
- ileal 151, 172-173, 249
- ileocolic 172, **172**, 173
- iliolumbar 209, 213, 216-217, 221
- inferior epigastric 56, 72, 74, 156-157, 171, 173, 177, 193, 203, 209, 213, 217, 219, 221, 224, 236, 250, 253, 255, 357
- inferior gluteal 206, 216-217, 256-257, 351, 361-362, **362**, 380
- inferior lateral genicular 291, 351, 367, 369
- - medial genicular 291, 351, 356, 369-372
- inferior lobar 100-101, 130
- inferior mesenteric 151, 165, 172, 174-175, **175**, 177, 206, 209, 213, 217, 219, 226, 248-249
- - radiograph (ap) **174**
- - variations **174**
- inferior pancreatic 168
- inferior pancreaticoduodenal 171, 175
- inferior phrenic 106, 169, 171, 209-210, 213
- inferior rectal 206, 219-220, 237, 239
- inferior suprarenal 180, 209
- inferior thyroid 108
- inferior vesical 217, 219-220
- - arteriography **208**

Index

Artery(-ies)
- intercostal 124, 131
- interlobar 182, 208
- internal iliac 206, 209, 216-217, **217**, 219-221, 224, 353-354, 357
- - variations 216
- internal pudendal 206, 216-217, 219-221, 224, 230, 236-237, 239, 256-258, 260-261, 361-362, **362**
- internal thoracic 56, 72, 90, 113-114, 116-117, 122, 124, 128, 130
- jejunal 151, 172-173, 175, 240, 242
- lateral circumflex femoral 61, 351, 355-357
- lateral plantar 306, 351, 375, 377-378, 384
- lateral sacral 216-218
- lateral tarsal 351, 374
- lateral thoracic 56
- left colic 165, 173-175, **175**, 177, 209
- left coronary 76-77, 81-82, 84-86, **86**, 87, **87**, 88, 100, 123-124, 131
- - coronary angiography **87**
- left gastric 108, 134, 151, 158, 168, **168**, 169-170, **170**, 171, 176-177, 210, 242, 245-246
- left gastro-omental 134, 158, 168, **168**, 169-170, 170, 245
- lumbar 177, 209, 213, 243, 250
- marginal 172-174, **175**
- medial circumflex femoral 260-261, 351, 355-357, 361-362
- medial plantar 306, 351, 375, 378, 384
- medial tarsal 351, 374
- median sacral 175, 177, 206, 209, 213, 217, 219-221, 253
- middle colic 151, 161-162, 172-175, **175**
- middle genicular 291, 351, 369
- middle lobar 100
- middle rectal 206, 216-217, 219-221
- middle suprarenal 180, 209
- musculophrenic 72
- obturator 206, 216-217, 219, 221, 224, 236, 250, 256-257, 261, 309, 318, 356-357
- - variations **221**
- occipital 43-45
- ovarian 151, 165, 195, 197, 204, 215, 220-221, 253
- perforating 351, 356-357, 360-361, 369, 381
- pericardiacophrenic 72, 90-91, 114-115, 122, **122**
- perineal 230, 237
- plantar digital 375, 377
- plantar digital proper 375-377
- plantar metatarsal 375-376, 378, 385
- popliteal 286, 291, 319, 331, 351, 356, 359-361, 368-369, 371-372, 382
- - variations **369**

Artery(-ies)
- posterior auricular 44-45
- posterior cecal 172
- posterior circumflex humeral 43, 126
- posterior gastric 170, **170**
- posterior intercostal 34, 36, 59, 73, 75, 77, 106-107, 114-115, 117-118
- posterior superior pancreaticoduodenal 168, 170, 176
- posterior tibial **329**, 351, 369-372, 375-378, 383-384
- posterior tibial recurrent 351, 369
- profunda brachii 43
- pulmonary 114
- - left 76-77, 85, 88, 90-91, 100-101, 107, 109, 115, 128
- - right 76-78, 85, 88, 90-91, 97, 100-101, **102**, 103, 107, 109, 123, 129
- renal 151, 180, 182, 184, **185**, 208-210, 213, 240-241, 243-244, 248, 250
- - accessory 209
- - arteriography 208
- - inferior polar 208
- - superior polar 208
- - variations 208
- right colic 151, 172, **172**, 173
- right coronary 76-77, 80-82, 84-86, **86**, 87, **87**, 88, 100, 123-124, 131
- - coronary angiography **87**
- right gastric 134, 168-170
- right gastro-omental 134, 165, 168, **168**, 169-170, 170, 171
- segmental (renal artery) 208
- - anterior (liver)168
- - anterior (lung) 128
- - anterior basal (lung) 100
- - lateral basal (lung) 101
- - medial basal (lung) 101
- - posterior (liver)168
- - posterior basal (lung) 101
- short gastric 134, 164, 170-171
- sigmoid 165, 174-175, 177, 206, 209, 255, 258
- splenic 151-153, 159, 165, 168-170, **170**, 171, 176-177, 210, 243, 246-247
- subclavian 76-77, 91, 100-101, 106-109, 112, 114-115, 117, 119, 127
- - left 116, 124, 128
- - right 116, 124
- subcostal 117-118, 243
- subscapular 128
- superficial cervical 56
- superficial circumflex iliac 56, 352, 357
- superficial epigastric 56, 352, 357
- superficial femoral 351, **354**
- superior epigastric 56, **71**, 72-74
- superior gluteal 206, 216-217, 255, 361, **362**, 380
- superior lateral genicular 351, 367-369
- - medial genicular 351, 356, 360, 367-369

Artery(-ies)
- superior lobar 100, 103, 129
- superior mesenteric 70, 117, 151-152, 165, 168, **168**, 171-172, **172**, 173-177, 184, 209-210, 213, 240-242, 248-249
- - radiograph (ap) **172**
- - variations **172**
- superior rectal 165, 174-175, 177, 206, 209, 219-221, 255
- superior suprarenal 180
- superior thyroid 113
- superior vesical 73, 216, 219, 221, 250, 260
- suprascapular 124
- supreme intercostal 117
- sural 351, 368-370
- testicular 67, 73, 151, 177, 190-191, 209, 213-214, 231-232, 235, 241, 249-250, 255-256
- - variations **209**
- thoraco-acromial 124
- thoracodorsal 128
- to ductus deferens 190, 219, 235
- transverse cervical 44-45
- umbilical 67, 73, 157, 183, 193, 200, 216-217, 219-221, 236
- urethral 234
- uterine 197, 216, 220-221
- - variations **197**
- vaginal 197, 220-221
- vertebral 24, 40, 43, 45-46, **46**, 108, 116, 124
Arthroscopy, knee joint **294**
Ascending aorta 77, 80, 82, 84-85, 109, 116-117, 119, 123-125, 129-130
ASCHOFF TAWARA-node 84
Atlas 2, 5, 6, 7, 12, 17-19, 34, 38, 40, 45-46
Atrioventricular node **84**
Atrium
- left 77-78, 81, **81**, 82, 85, 88, 91, 101, 103, 116, 123, 130-131
- right 76-78, 80, **80**, 83-84, **84**, 85, 88, 91, 101, 103, 116, 123-125, 131, 241-242
Auricle
- left 76-78, 81, 85, 88, 100, 116, 130
- right 76, 80-82, 85, 100
Axilla **126**
Axis 2, **6**, 7, 12, 17-19, 38
- longitudinal (hip joint) 314
- - (knee joint) 322
- oblique (talocalcaneonavicular joint) 327, 340
- pelvis 269
- sagittal (hip joint) 314
- transverse (hip joint) 314
- - (ankle joint) 327, 340
- - (knee joint) 322

B

Back 1, **1**, 43
- cutaneous innervation, segmental 42

Back
- dermatomes **42**
- planes and axes 1
- surface 1, **1**
BARTHOLIN's gland **194**, 229, **238**
Base
- of lung 97
- of metatarsals 297, 300, 304
- - of great toe 298
- of patella 286, 292-293, 325
- of phalanges (foot) 297
- of prostate 192
- of pyramid 181
- of sacrum 10-11, 275
BAUHIN's valve **140**
Belly
- occipital 44-45
- posterior 34, 38, 40
- superior 113
Bifurcation
- aortic 175, 177, 357
- of pulmonary trunk 77-78, 88, 91
- tracheal 92-93, 101, 104, 106-107, 109, 123, 129
BOCHDALEK's triangle **69-70**
Body(-ies)
- anococcygeal 200, 218, 223-224, 228-229, 237-239, 252, 257
- of bladder 187
- of breast 62
- of clitoris 224, 253
- of epididymis 191
- of gallbladder 146
- of ilium 259, 266, 268
- of ischium 266-268
- of pancreas 149-152, 159, 164, 171
- of penis 235
- of pubis 223, 241, 266
- of rib 49, 103
- of sternum 3, 51, 61, 104, 123, 128-130, 240
- of stomach 125, 132, 134-136, 156, 158-159, 243
- of talus 298-299, 306
- of uterus 195, 197, 251
- vertebral 4-9, 12-17, 19-25, 30, 74, 129, 246
Bone(s)
- coccyx 2-3, 11, **11**, 200, 223, 225, 228-229, 240, 256-257, 273, 275
- cuboid 297-298, 300, **300**, 301, 305, 386
- of foot **297-298**, **301**
- - arrangement **301**
- hip 47, 264, **267-268**
- - development **266**
- hyoid 12, 106
- ilium 3, 15, 47, 67, 75, 203, 223, 242, 258, 263, 266, 274, 279, 282
- intermediate cuneiform 297-298, 300-301, 306, 386
- ischium 236, 256, 263, 266, 279
- lateral cuneiform 297, 300-301
- medial cuneiform 297-298, 300-301, 304

Bones
- metatarsal 264, 297–298, 300, **300**, 305–306, 379, 385–386
- navicular 297–298, 300–301, 305–307, 386
- occipital **6**, 12, 17–19
- phalanges (foot) 264, 297, **297**, 298, **298**
- pubis 69, 193, 218, 225, 230, 240, 242, 256–257, 259, 263, 266, 279–280
- ribs 4
- sacrum 2–3, **4**, 5, **10–11**, 15, 23, 27, 47, 218, 223, 225, 240–241, 251, 255, 262–263, **263**, 273–275, 318
- sesamoid (foot) 297–298, 301, 304, 347
- sex differences 11
- tarsal 264, **297**, 298, **298**, **300**
- temporal 46

Border
- acetabuli s. Limbus acetabuli
- - anterior (fibula) 285
- - - (lung) 96–97, 112–113
- - - (testis) 190
- - - (tibia) 262, 284–285, 325, 383
- - free (ovary) 195
- - inferior (liver) 142–143, 161
- - - (lung) 96–97, 113
- - - (spleen) 153
- - interosseus (fibula) 285, 332–333
- - - (tibia) 284–285
- - lateral (kidney) 180, 208
- - medial (suprarenal gland) 180, 187
- - - (kidney) 180, 208
- - - (scapula) 26
- - - (tibia) 284–285
- - mesovarian 195, 204
- - posterior (fibula) 285
- - - (testis) 190
- - superior (suprarenal gland) 180, 187
- - - (spleen) 153, 159, 164–165
BOYD's vein 365
Branch(es)
- acetabular (medial circumflex femoral artery) 357
- - (obturator artery) 355, 357
- anterior abdominal cutaneous 56
- anterior cutaneous (femoral nerve) 71, 349, 352, 387
- - (iliohypogastric nerve) 56, 349, 352, **387**
- anterior gastric (anterior vagal trunk) 119
- - (right gastro-omental vein) 158
- anterior intercostal 72, 245
- anterior interventricular 76, 81–82, 85–87, 100, 131
- anterior (middle genicular artery) 291
- - (cervical nerve) 120
- - (hepatic portal vein) 244
- - (lumbar nerve) 47, 218
- - (obturator artery) 355, 357

Branch(es) anterior
- - (obturator nerve) 71, **387**
- - (renal artery) 180
- - (sacral nerve) 218
- anterior pectoral cutaneous 56
- anterior scrotal 231
- - (ilio-inguinal nerve) 349
- articular (descending genicular artery) 351, 354–356
- ascending (lateral circumflex femoral artery) 351, 356–357
- - (medial circumflex femoral artery) 361
- atrial (right coronary artery) 85–86
- - (left coronary artery) 86
- atrioventricular 86–87
- atrioventricular nodal 86
- bronchial (aorta) 107–108, 114, 117, 121
- - (vagus nerve) 119–121
- calcaneal (posterior tibial artery) 372
- - lateral (tibial nerve) **388**
- - medial (tibial nerve) 376, **388**
- cardiac
- - inferior cervical 120, 122
- - thoracic (vagus nerve) 114–115, 122
- circumflex (left coronary artery) 76–77, 85–88
- communicating (fibular artery) 351
- - sural 364, **387**
- conus 85, **85**, 86–87
- deep **388**
- - (lateral plantar nerve) 377–378
- - (medial circumflex femoral artery) 357, 361–362
- - (medial plantar artery) 375
- - (superior gluteal artery) 362
- - (superior gluteal vein) 362
- - (transverse cervical artery) 44–45
- descending (lateral circumflex femoral artery) 351, 355–357
- - (medial circumflex femoral artery) 357
- dorsal (lumbar artery) 47
- - (lumbar vein) 47
- esophageal (left gastric artery) 108, 134
- - (aorta) 108
- - (inferior thyroid artery) 108
- - (recurrent laryngeal nerve) 117, 121
- - (thoracic ganglion)
- femoral 56, 71, 209, 213, 250, 309, **309**, 318, 349, 352, **387**
- to fundus of uterus (uterine artery) 197
- (gastro-omental veins) 134, 158
- genital 71, 209, 213, 217, 231, 235, 250, 256, 349, **387**
- helicine 197
- iliac 209, 213
- infrapatellar 349, 352, 364, 382, **387**
- interganglionic 121
- internal (superior laryngeal nerve) 106

Branch(es)
- of ischium 230, 261, 266–268, 275, 317–318
- lateral (left coronary artery) 86
- lateral cutaneous (iliohypogastric nerve) 42, 349, 358, 362, **387**
- - (spinal nerve) 42
- lateral malleolar 351, 372
- left (hepatic artery proper) 148
- - (hepatic portal vein) 148, 152
- left marginal 82, 85–87
- mastoid (occipital artery) 44–45
- medial crural cutaneous 349, 364, 387
- medial cutaneous (spinal nerve) 42
- - (medial plantar nerve) 377
- - (obturator nerve) 349, 352, 355–356, 358, **387**
- medial malleolar 351, 372
- muscular (femoral nerve) 354–356, 387
- - (deep fibular nerve) 374, **388**
- - (medial plantar nerve) 377
- - (obturator nerve) **387**
- - (perineal nerves) **388**
- - (superficial fibular nerve) **387**
- - (tibial nerve) 360–361, 368, 370, **388**
- obturator (inferior epigastric artery) 217, 357
- occipital (posterior auricular artery) 44
- - (occipital artery) 44–45
- omental (gastro-omental arteries) 134, 169
- ovarian 197
- pectoral lateral cutaneous (thoracic nerve) 44, 56
- perforating (fibular artery) 351, 367, 374
- - (deep plantar arch) 378
- - (internal thoracic artery) 72
- pericardial (phrenic nerve) 122
- perineal 237, 239, **387**
- phrenicoabdominal 71, 122
- posterior (middle genicular artery) 291
- - (cervical nerve) 43–46
- - (greater auricular nerve) 42
- - (hepatic portal vein) 247
- - left ventricular 86
- - (obturator artery) 357
- - (obturator nerve) **387**
- - (renal artery) 180
- - (sacral nerve) 43
- - (spinal nerve) **33**, **35**, 42–43, 47
- - (thoracic nerve) 43–44
- posterior cutaneous (cervical nerves) 44
- - (thoracic nerves) 44
- posterior interventricular 77, 82, 85–87, 124
- posterior labial 239
- posterior scrotal 219, 237
- pubic (inferior epigastric artery) 217, 357
- - (obturator artery) 217
- right (hepatic artery proper) 148, 168, 246

Branch(es)
- - (hepatic portal vein) 148, 242, 244, 246–247
- right marginal 82, 85–87
- right posterolateral 86–87
- saphenous (descending genicular artery) 351, 356
- septal interventricular (right coronary artery) 86
- - (left coronary artery) 86–87
- sinu-atrial nodal 86
- spinal (lateral sacral artery) 218
- splenic 171
- superficial (medial circumflex femoral artery) 355, 357, 361
- - (lateral plantar nerve) 376–378, **388**
- - (medial plantar artery) 375, 378
- - (superior gluteal artery) 361
- - (transverse cervical artery) 45
- tracheal (recurrent laryngeal nerve) 120
- transverse 357
- tubal (uterine artery) 197, 220
- ureteric (renal artery) 250
- vaginal (uterine artery) 197
Breast **54–55**
- lymphatic drainage **55**
- radiograph **55**
Bronchogram 95
Bronchoscopy **104**
Bronchus(-i) **92–94**
- inferior lingular (B V) 92, 95
- intrasegmental 124, 128
- left main 92–93, 95, 101, 104, 106–107, 115, 117, 119, 123, 129
- - projection **104**
- lobar **94**, 109
- - inferior 130
- - - left 92–93, 95, 100, 104
- - - middle 92–93, 97, 104, 121, 130
- - - right 92–93, 97, 104, 120–121
- - superior
- - - left 92–93, 95, 100–101, 104
- - - right 92–93, 97, 101, 104, 106, 129
- right main 90, 92–93, 97, 101, 103–104, 106–107, 109, 114, 117, 119–120, 123, 129
- segmental **92–94**, 101
- - anterior [B III] 92, 95, 126, 128–129
- - anterior basal [B VIII] 92, 95
- - apical [B I] 92
- - apicoposterior [B I + II] 92, 95
- - cardiac [B VII] see medial basal segmental bronchus [B VII]
- - lateral [B IV] 92
- - lateral basal [B IX] 92, 95, 131]
- - medial [B V] 92
- - medial basal [B VII] 92
- - posterior [B II] 92, 129
- - posterior basal [B X] 92, 95, 130
- - superior [B VI] 92, 95
- - superior lingular (B IV) 92, 95

Index

BRUNNER's glands **138**
Bulb
- aortic 81
- of duodenum 132, **132**
- of penis 193, 233, 236, 251–252
- of vestibule 194, 220, 238–239, 261

Bundle
- atrioventricular 84
- right (atrioventricular bundle) 84

Bursa
- anserine 313
- deep infrapatellar 287, 290–291
- of gluteus maximus 280, 317, 319–320
- of gluteus medius 256, 280, 320, 324
- iliopectineal 309, 324
- omental 154–155, **159**, 64–165, 245–247
- sciatic (of obturator internus) 320, 324
- semimembranosus 331–333
- subcutaneous calcaneal 341
- - coccygeal 43
- - infrapatellar 308, 310, 325
- - prepatellar 286, 308, 325
- - sacral 43
- - of superior posterior iliac spine 43
- - trochanteric 324
- subfascial prepatellar 290
- subtendinous
- - (of iliacus) 256, 312–313, 380
- - medial (of gastrocnemius) 324, 331–333
- - of obturator internus 256–257
- - prepatellar 310
- - of sartorius 313
- suprapatellar 287, **287**, 290, 292, 294, 382
- trochanteric

Buttocks
- female **227**
- male **227**

C

Calcaneal tendon 302–303, 306, 325–326, 330–333, 337, 340, **370**, 371–372, 384, 386
Calcaneus 297–298, **299**, 300–303, 305–306, 385–386
Calf 262
Calices
- major 181, 183, 243
- minor 181–183, 208, 244, 248
Canal
- adductor 311, **351**
- anal 225
- cervical (uterus) 195–196, 253
- femoral 309
- hypoglossal 18
- inguinal 232
- obturator 206–207, 223, 270, 280–281, 309, 313, 318, **318**
- pudendal 223
- pyloric 132, 139, 150
- sacral **4**, 10–11, 24, 219, 273, 318
- vertebral 3, 24, 318

Cardia 132, 158, 245
Cardiac veins 85, 88–89
Carina of trachea 104, 123
Cartilage(s)
- articular 286
- arytenoid 93
- bronchial 92, 106
- corniculate 93
- costal 52, **52**, 61, 64–65, 70, 73, 117, 129, 131
- cricoid 12, 123
- thyroid 41, 65, 92–93, 106, 113, 120, 123
- tracheal 92–93, 104, 106–107, 123
Carunculae hymenales 229, 238
Cauda equina 24, 30, 203, 240, 248–250, 255
Cavernous spaces of corpora cavernosa 233
Cavity
- articular (hip joint) 273, 275, 280
- glenoid 53, 126
- infraglottic 123
- medullary 278, 283
- nasal 12
- pericardial 123, 129
- peritoneal 154–155, **155**, 165, 240–242, 245–249
- - development 154
- pleural 114–115, **119**, 122, 125, 130, 246–247
- serous (of scrotum) 191
- symphysial 274
- thoracic **122–123**, 129
- - CT **129**
- - frontal section **124**, **126**
- - median section **123**
- - MRI **124–125**
- - transverse section **127–129**, 130
- uterine 195–196, 253
Cecum 140, **140**, 141, 156, 160–164, 166–167, 173, 203–204, 254
- mobile 166
- projection 167
Celiac arteriography 170
Central tendon 61, 68–70, **71**, 75, 106–108, 114–115, 240, 244
Cervical muscles **39**
Cervical pleura 105, 126
Cervical vertebral column
- CT **41**
- radiograph (ap) **13**
- - (lateral) **12**
Cervix of uterus 196–198, 251
Chiasm
- crural 333
- plantar 344
CHOPART's joint 265, **298**
Chorda(e)
- tendineae 81–83
- of umbilical artery 56, **56**, 74, 156, 193, 221, 236, 250, 253
Cistern
- cerebellomedullary 46
- chyli 118, 210
Clavicle 3, 26, 48, 52–53, 62, 103–104, 110, 113–115, 122, 124, 126–127, 157

Cleft, uncovertebral **24**
Clitoris 200, 215, **215**, 224
Clivus 18
CLOQUET's septum **309**, 328
Coccygeal body 253
COCKETT's veins 365
Colon **140**, **161–163**
- ascending 140, **140–141**, 156, 159–160, 163–164, 166–167, 178, 186, 242, 249, 255
- descending 141, 157, 163–164, 166, 175, 178, 186, 242–243, 246, 248–249, 254–255
- - projection **141**
- - radiograph (ap) **141**
- sigmoid 141, 154–156, 160, 162–166, 173, 175, 177, 200, 203, 206–207, 209–210, 218, 225, 240, 242, 249–255, 258
- transverse **140**, 141, 148, 154–156, 158–160, 162–164, 166, 173, 240–242, 244–246, 248
- - layers **140**
- - variations of position **141**
Colonoscopy **141**
Column(s)
- anal 205, 240, 252, 258
- anterior vaginal 238
- renal 181, 244
- vertebral **2–3**
Commissure
- anterior (labium majus) 238
- posterior (labium majus) 227, 238
Compact bone 278
Compartment
- anterior 329, **329**
- lateral **329**
- posterior **329**
- superficial posterior **329**
Compartment syndrome **329**
Computer-tomography (CT)
- abdomen 246
- cervical vertebral column **41**
- female 257
- lumbar vertebral column **41**
- male 256
- muscles of abdomen **75**
- muscles of back **30**
- pelvis 254
- thoracic cage **129**
Conducting system of heart **84**
Condyle
- lateral (femur) 276, 278, 283–284, 287–289, 292–295
- medial (femur) 276, 278, 283–284, 287–289, 292–293, 295, 310–311
- - (tibia) 284, 292–293, 295, 326, 331, 333
- occipital 6
- (tibia) 284, 289, 292–295
Conjoint tendon 69
Conjugate
- anatomical 269
- diagonal 269
- true 268–269
Conus arteriosus 76, 85, 100
Cord(s)
- lateral 126

Cords
- posterior 126
- tendinous 81–83
- of urachus 74, 236
Cornu
- coccygeal 11
- sacral 10–11
Corona of glans 193, 233–234, 252
Coronary angiography **87**
Corpus(-ora)
- albicans 195, 204
- cavernosum of clitoris 200, 238, 253
- - penis 189, 193, 214, 219, 232, 234, **234**, 235, 240–241, 252
- luteum 195
- spongiosum penis 189, 193, **193**, 214, 228, 232–235, 240, 251–252, 260
Cortex
- renal 181–182, 185, 244–245, 248
- (of suprarenal gland) 187
Costal margin 3, 48, 62, 69, 201
Cotyledons 202
COWPERS's gland **218**, **228**, 230
Coxa
- valga **277**
- vara **277**
Craniocervical joints **17–19**
- Radiograph (ap) **19**
Crest
- external occipital 6
- of head of rib 49
- iliac 1, 15, 27, 29, 43, 68, 75, 105, 174, 186, 208, 212, 223, 254–255, 259, 263, 266–268, 271, 275, 308, 316–319, 358, 362–363
- intermediate sacral **4**, 10–11, 15, 272, 358
- intertrochanteric 275–277
- lateral sacral **4**, 10
- medial 285
- medial sacral 10
- of neck of rib 49
- obturator 268
- urethral 188, 233
Cribriform plate 71
Crus
- of clitoris 194, 238, 261
- lateral (superficial inguinal ring) 63, 65, 67, 232
- left (diaphragm) 69–70, **70–71**, 106, 108, 118, 247
- medial (superficial inguinal ring) 58, 63, 65, 67, 232
- of penis 193, 218, 233, 236, 260
- - cross-section **383–384**
- - MRI **383**
- right (diaphragm) 68–69, **70**, 71, **71**, 106, 108, 118, 246
Curvature
- greater 132–135, 156–159
- lesser 132–135, 139, 158
Cusp
- anterior semilunar 79, 85
- - left semilunar (aortic valve) 79, 81–82, 84–85, 123, 130

Cusp
- - posterior semilunar (aortic valve) 79, 81-82, 84-85, 123, 130
- - (pulmonary valve) 79, 84-85
- - right semilunar (aortic valve) 79, 81, 84-85, 123, 130
- anterior (tricuspid valve) 79-80, 83-84
- - (mitral valve) 79, 81-82, 84, 130
- left commissural 79
- posterior (tricuspid valve) 79-80, 82-83
- - (mitral valve) 79, 81-83, 130
- right commissural 79
- septal (tricuspid valve) 79-80, 82

Cutaneous innervation
- back 42
- segmental, lower limb 348

Cutaneous nerves, lower limb 349
Cystoscopy 188

D

Dartos fascia 73, 190-191, 218, 228, 232, 235, 240, 252
Declination [angle of antetorsion] 278
Defecography 225
Dens of axis 6-7, 12, 18-19
Dermatomes
- back 42
- lower limb 348

Descending aorta 77, 116, 129-131, 247
Diameter
- conjugate 269
- - 1st oblique 268
- - 2nd oblique 268
- - sagittal 269
- - transverse 268-269
- - tuberal 269

Diaphragm 57, 59, 61, 68, **68**, 69, **69-71**, 72, 75, 87, 103, 106-110, 112-114, 117-119, 121-125, 142, 145, 148, 151, 155, 157-158
- pelvic 185, **222**, 240-241, 243-248
- - female **223-224**, 229
- - male **228**, **236**
- urogenital **222**, 239, 241, 261
- - female **230**, **238**
- - male **230**

Diaphysis (femur) 279
Digit(s) of foot 264
Disc
- articular 273
- - (sternoclavicular joint) **52**
- interpubic 200, 270, 273-274, **274**
- intervertebral 12, 17, 19, 21-24, **24**, 25, 30, 41, 176, 270

Distance
- anterior interspinous 269
- intercristal 269
- posterior interspinous 269
- pubococcygeal 269

Diverticulum(-a)
- of ampulla 187
- ileal 137

Division
- left lateral **144**
- left medial **144**
- right lateral **144**
- right medial **144**

DODD's veins **308**, **365**
Dome of pleura 105, 126
Dorsum
- of foot 262, **367**, **373-374**
- of penis 235

DOUGLAS, pouch of **155**, **165**, 198, **200**, **221**, **253**
Duct(s)
- bile 142, 146-148, 150-152, 168-169, 177, 241, 246
- - radiograph (ap) 147, **152**
- - variations 146, **150**
- of bulbo-urethral gland 189, 233
- common hepatic 134, 146, **146**, 147, 151-152, 165, 168, 177
- cystic 134, 147, 151-152, 165, 168, 177, 246
- ejaculatory 188-189, 192, **192**, 193, **193**, 233
- excretory 193
- lactiferous 54
- left hepatic 146-148
- longitudinal 194-195
- mesonephric 189, 194
- omphalo-enteric 137
- pancreatic 146, 150-152, 240-241
- - accessory 150
- - radiograph (ap) **152**
- - variations 150
- paramesonephric 189, **189**, 194
- paraurethral 238
- prostatic 188, 233
- right hepatic 146-148
- thoracic **71**, 115, 117-118, **118**, 121, 128-131, 243, 246-247, 250

Ductule(s)
- efferent 191, 252
- inferior aberrant 189, 191
- transverse 194-195

Ductus
- arteriosus [BOTALLO's duct] **76-77**, **90**
- deferens 73, 164, 177, **187**, 188-191, **191**, 192, **192**, 193, **193**, 213-214, **214**, 218-219, 231-232, 235-236, 241, 250, 252, 256, 258
- - radiograph (ap) **192**
- venosus [of ARANTIUS] **143**

Duodenum 119, 132, **132**, 133-134, **134**, 139, **139**, 146-147, 149-150, **150**, 151, **151**, 152, 154-155, 158-159, 161, 163-166, 168, 177-178, 241-242
- endoscopy **139**
- layers **138**
- projection **149**
- radiograph (ap) **135**, **139**

Dura mater
- cranial 19
- spinal 19, 46-47, 123

E

Eminence
- iliopubic 223, 263, 266-267, 275
- intercondylar 284, 292-293
- intermediate plantar 345
- lateral plantar 341, 345
- medial plantar 341, 345

End
- acromial 26, 126
- sternal 3, 110

Endocardium 82
Epicardium 76, **76**, 80-82, 124
Epicondyle
- lateral (femur) 276, 283, 286, 292-293
- medial (femur) 276, 278, 283, 286, 289, 292-293, 312

Epididymis 183, 189, **189-191**, 214, 232, 240-241
Epiglottis 12
Episiotomy 229
Epithelium 108, 132, 137, 140
Epo-ophoron 194, **194**
Eporchium **191**
ERCP (endoscopic retrograde cholangio-pancreaticography) **152**
Erection **214**
Esophageal constrictions **110**
Esophageal varicosis **108**
Esophagoscopy **110**
Esophagus 57, 68, 70, **71**, 106, **106**, 107, **107**, 108-110, 114-115, 117-119, **119**, 120, **120**, 121, 123-125, 127-135, 155, 178, 212, 240, 243
- radiograph **110**
- venous drainage **108**

Extension
- (ankle joint) 327
- (hip joint) 314
- (knee joint) 322

External occipital protuberance 27, 45
External os of uterus 195-196, 198, 200, 253
Extremity
- anterior (spleen) 153, 157
- posterior (spleen) 153
- tubal 195
- uterine 195

F

Facet
- anterior (axis) 6, 19
- anterior (for calcaneus) 299
- articular
- for dens 6, 19
- of head of rib 49
- - of fibula 285
- inferior (lumbar vertebra) 9
- inferior costal 4, 8, 20
- lateral malleolar 298-300
- of lateral malleolus 285, 296, 303
- medial malleolar 298-300
- of medial malleolus 284, 296, 303

Facet
- middle (for calcaneus) 299
- posterior (axis) 6, 19
- posterior calcaneal 299
- superior costal **4**, 8-9, 20-21
- transverse costal 4, 8-9, 21
- of tubercle of rib 49

Fascia
- axillary 58
- brachial 58
- cervical 113, 123
- clavipectoral 58
- cremasteric 191, 232, 235, 252
- cribriform 210, 308
- deep (penis) 231, 234-235
- deltoid 27, 29, 31, 44
- dorsal (foot) 325, 345, 379, 385
- external spermatic 73, 190, 232, 235
- of foot 384
- gluteal 62, 308, 360
- iliac 177
- inferior (pelvic diaphragm) 223, 238
- infraspinous 27, 29, 31, 44
- internal spermatic 3, 190-191, 232, 235
- lata 308, **308**, 309-311, **311**, 312, 317, 358, 381
- of leg 308, 325, **325**, 329, **329**, 330, 364, 368, 383
- nuchal 45
- obturator 223, 228-229, 318
- parietal pelvic 253
- perineal 223, 228-230, 260
- rectal 198
- rectoprostatic 252
- rectovaginal 200, 253
- renal 244-245
- superficial (penis) 234
- thoracolumbar 24-25, 27, 29-30, **30**, 31, **31**, 32, **32**, 34, 36-37, 41, 62, 74, 317
- transversalis 34, 65, 68, 72, 74-75
- vesical 198
- vesicovaginal **200**
- visceral pelvic 252

Fascicle(s)
- transverse (plantar aponeurosis) 341

Fatty layer 58, 74, 205
Female external genitalia 215, **229**, **238-239**
Female internal genitalia **195**, **197**, **203-204**
Female pelvis, dimension, **269**
Female urogenital organs, development **189**, **194**
Femoral hernia **309**
Femur 3, 225, 256-257, 264, 275-276, **276-278**, 279, 282, **283**, 286, **286**, 287-289, 292-295, 310-313, 328, 330, 332, **354**, 369, 381-382
- angle of depression **277**
- anteversion **278**
- arteries **357**
- cross-section **380-382**
- - MRI **382**
- fascias **308**

Index

Femur
- inclination **277**
- MRI **381**
- muscle origins and insertions **324**
- muscles **310-313**, **316-320**
  - - dorsal **322**
  - - medial **315**
  - - ventral **314-315**
- ossification center **279**
- radiograph (ap) **279**
- structure of spongy bone **277**

Fetus
- radiograph (ap) **201**
- ultrasound image **199**

Fibers
- intercrural 58, 63, 67
- oblique 133

Fibrous capsule (kidney) 180, 182, 244-245
Fibrous capsule (spleen) 153
Fibula 264, **284-285**, 287-289, **296**, 302-303, 306-307, 329, 332-333, 337, 383-384
Filum terminale 240, 252

Fimbria(-ae)
- ovarian 195
- of uterine tube 5, 203-204, 253

Fissure
- horizontal (of left lung) 96-97, 124
- for ligamentum teres 142
- oblique 96-97, 101, 125, 128-131
- right portal 144
- umbilical 144

Flatfoot [talipes] 305
Flatfoot 305

Flexion
- (ankle joint) 327
- (hip joint) 314
- (knee joint) 322
- (uterus) **196**

Flexure
- anorectal 205, 218
- duodenojejunal 139, 149-150, 164-165, 175, 242
- inferior duodenal 134, 151, 173
- left colic [splenic] 124-125, 135, 141, 160, 162-164, 173
- perineal s. anorectal flexure
- right colic [hepatic] 141, 152, 158-160, 163-164, 173
- sacral 205, 218
- superior duodenal 151

Fold(s)
- alar 287
- circular 132, 135, 138-139, 146, 150
- fatty 91
- gastric 132, 136
- gastropancreatic 159, 164-165
- ileocecal 160-161, 165
- inferior duodenal 163, 165
- lateral umbilical 67, 74, 156-157, 203, 219, 236, 250
- longitudinal (of duodenum) 146, 150
- medial umbilical **56**, 67, 74, 156-157, 193, 204, 209, 219, 236, 250, 253

Fold(s)
- median umbilical 67, 74, 156-157, 193, 203-204, 209, 236, 250, 252-253
- mucosal 146, 188, 233
- palmate 195, 253
- recto-uterine 195, 220-221, 253
- semilunar (of colon) 140-141, 161
- spiral 146-147
- synovial 303
  - - infrapatellar 287
  - - mediopatellar 286
- transverse (of rectum) 200, 240, 251-253
  - - vesical 67, 236
- of uterine tube 195

Foot 264
- arches **301**
- compartments **379**
- cross-section **384-385**
- forces 335
- frontal section **345**, **385**
- joints **302-305**
- ligaments **304**
- longitudinal section, MRI **386**
- MRI **385**
- muscle origins and insertions **340**, **347**
- muscles **326**, **338-339**, **341-345**
  - - dorsal **340**
  - - plantar **346**
- osseofibrous tubes **345**
- sagittal section **386**
- tendon sheaths **336-337**
  - - digital **337**
  - - dorsal tarsal **337**
  - - lateral tarsal **337**
  - - medial tarsal **337**
  - - plantar **337**

Foramen(-ina)
- anterior sacral 10, 16, 275, 318
- for basivertebral vein 9, 23, 25
- costotransverse 4, 21
- epiploic see omental foramen
- greater sciatic 223, 269, 271-273, 317, **318**, 358, **362**
- infrapiriform 317-318, **318**, 319-320, 358, **362**
- intervertebral 2, 12, 14-15, **21**, 22, 25, 30, 41, 273
- lesser sciatic 269, 271-273, 317-318, **318**, 320, 358, **362**
- magnum 6
- nutrient 284-285, 324
- obturator 221, 267-268, **268**, 269, 271, 273, 275, 282
- omental 158, **164**, 165
- ovale (heart) 80, **80**
- posterior sacral 10-11
- suprapiriform 317-318, **318**, 319, 358, **362**
- transversarium 4, 6-7, 41
- vertebral 4, **4**, 6-9, 20, 41, 129
- of WINSLOW 158

Fornix
- of stomach 132, 134, 136, 240, 245
- vagina 196, 198, 200, 253

Fossa
- acetabular 223, 260, 267-268, 275, 280, 282
- condylar 6
- iliac 263, 267
- infraspinous 26
- intercondylar 278, 283, 293, 295
- ischio-anal 228, **228**, 229, **229**, 236, **239**, 257-258
- lateral inguinal 67, 236, 250
- malleolar 285
- medial inguinal 67, 236, 250
- navicular 233-234, 252
- ovalis 80
- paravesical 250, 260-261
- popliteal 262, 308, 320, 325, **358-361**, **368-372**
- supravesical 67, 236, 250
- trochanteric 277-278, 280
- vestibular 238

Fovea for ligament of head 275-278, 280, 282
FRANKENHAEUSER's ganglion **215**

Frenulum
- of clitoris 238, 253
- of ileal orifice 140
- of labia majora 238
- of prepuce 234

Fundus 164
- of bladder 165, 192-193, 233
- of gallbladder 146, 148, 156, 161, 164
- of stomach 124, 132-135, 158
- of uterus 165, 195-197, 200, 203-204, 253

G

G1MBERNAT's ligament **309**
Gallbladder 57, 142, 144, 146, **146**, 147-148, **148**, 149, 152, 158-159, 166, 168-169, 178, 248
- radiograph (ap) 147, **152**

Ganglion(-a)
- cardiac 120
- celiac 226, 246
- cervicothoracic 119-120
- impar 71
- inferior mesenteric 226
- middle cervical 119-120
- pelvic 214, **214**, 215, 226
- sacral 217
- satellite see cervicothoracic ganglion
- spinal 24, 46-47
- of sympathetic trunk 214-215, 226
- thoracic 114-115, 119-121

Gastric pits 132
Gastroscopy **136**

Genitalia
- female 215
  - - development **194**
  - - external **229**, **238-239**
  - - innervation **215**
  - - internal **195**, **197**, 203-204
- male 214, 232

Genitalia male
  - - development **189**
  - - external **231**, **235**, **237**
  - - innervation **214**

Gland(s)
- areolar 54
- bulbo-urethral 189, 193, 214, **214**, 218, 228, **228**, 230, 233, 236
- duodenal 138
- esophageal 108
- gastric 132
- greater vestibular 194, 229, 238
- intestinal 137, 140
  - - mammary 129-131
- seminal 187, **187**, 189, 192, **192**, 193, **193**, 214, **214**, 218-219, 236, 240-241, 256, 258
  - - radiograph (ap) **192**
- suprarenal 151, 159, 165, 177, 180, **180**, 183, **183**, 187, 209, 243, 246
- thyroid 106-107, 109, 112-113, 122-123
- tracheal 93

Glandular abdomen **158**

Glans
- of clitoris 194, 200, 229, 238
- penis 189, 193, 214, 233-234, **234**, 235, **235**, 240-241, 252

Gluteal fold 262, 308, 317, 358
GRAAF's follicle **195**
Great toe 262, **297**, 301

Groove(s)
- costal 49
- malleolar 284-285
- obturator 267
- for popliteus 283, 293, 295
- for sigmoid sinus 18
- for spinal nerve **4**, 7
- for splenic artery 151
- for subclavian artery 49
- for subclavian vein 49
- supra-acetabular 267-268
- for tendon of fibularis longus 297, 299-300, 302, 304
- for tendon of flexor hallucis longus (calcaneus) 298-300, 304
  - - (talus) 299-300
- for vertebral artery 6, 17

Gubernaculum testis 73, 189

H

HACH's deep perforating vein 365
HALLER's arches **70**
Haustra of colon 140-141, 161

Head
- of epididymis 189-191, 232, 252
- of femur 225, 256, 259-261, 273, 275-278, 280, 282
- of fibula 262, 284-285, 287-289, 293, 295-296, 308, 310, 316, 325, 366
- of fifth metatarsal 298
- of humerus 126-127
- lateral (gastrocnemius) 286, 288-289, 316, 319-320, 328, 330-332, **334**, 360, 368-370, 382

Index

Head lateral
- - (triceps brachii) 62
- long (M. biceps brachii) 126
- - (biceps femoris) 316-320, **322**, 328, 361, 380-381
- - (triceps brachii) 43, 62
- medial (gastrocnemius) 286, 288-290, 319-320, 328, 330-333, **334**, 360, 368-370, 382-383
- of metatarsals 297, 300
- oblique (adductor hallucis) 306, **341**, 344-345, **346**, 347, 378, 385-386
- of pancreas 149-151, 165-166, 171, 177, 241-242
- of phalanx (foot) 297
- reflected 280-281, 312, **314**
- of rib 4, 14, 22, 49
- short (biceps brachii) 59
- - (biceps femoris) 316, 319-320, **322**, 328, 361, 381, **387**
- straight 280-281, 312, **314**
- of talus 297-300, 307, 384, 386
- transverse (adductor hallucis) 342-344, **346**, 347, 378, **388**
HEAD's zones 57
Heart 57, **76-77**, **100**, 116, **116**, 240
- arterial blood supply 86
- axis 82
- balanced distribution 86
- contour 103
- - aortic knob 103
- - left atrial contour 103
- - left ventricular contour 103
- - pulmonary contour 103
- - right atrial contour 103
- coronary arteries 85-86, 87
- - coronary angiography 87
- dominant left distribution 86
- dominant right distribution 86
- left atrium 81
- left ventricle **81-84**
- position 90
- - during expiration/inspiration **104**
- projection 103
- right atrium 80, 84
- right ventricle 80, **82-84**
- ultrasound image 130
- valves 85
- - projection 90
Heel 262
HEISTER's valve **146**
Hemorrhoidal zone **205**
Hiatus
- adductor 312-313, 328, 356, 360
- aortic 68-70, **71**, 106, 151, 177
- esophageal 68-69, **71**, 106, **106**, 107, 109, 177, 209, 213
- sacral 10-11
- urogenital and anal **223**
Hilar nodes 90, **101**
Hilum
- of kidney 180, **180-181**
- splenic 153, 159, 246
- (suprarenal gland) 180
Hip
- arteries 357

Hip
- muscles 310-313, 316-320
- - dorsal 321
- - ventral **314**
HIS, bundle of **84**
Horn
- anterior (lateral ventricle) 292
- inferior (falciform margin) 308-309
- posterior (lateral ventricle) 292
- superior (falciform margin) 308-309
Horseshoe kidney **182**
Humerus 3, 128
HUNTER's vein **365**
Hydatid, stalked **195**
Hymen 238
Hysterosalpingography **196**

I

Ileocecal valve **140**
Ileum 137-138, **138**, 140, 154-156, 160-161, 164, 166-167, 173, 203, 225, 240-242, 249, 254-255
Iliotibial tract 280, 308, 310, **310**, 316, **316**, 317, 326, 335, 359, 381
Impotentia
- coeundi 214
- generandi 214
Impression
- cardiac 97
- colic 142, 153
- duodenal 142
- esophageal 142
- gastric 142
- - (spleen) 153, 164-165
- renal 142
- suprarenal 142
Infrapatellar fat pad 287, 292, 295, 328
Infundibulum
- of paramesonephric duct 189
- of uterine tube 194-195, 197, 204, 220, 253
Inguinal canal **67**, **73**
Inguinal falx 69
Injection, intragluteal **362-363**
Interacetabular line 269
Interarticular portion 8, **15**
Intergluteal cleft 262
Intermediate zone 263, 267-268
Interspinous line 269
Interureteric crest 188, 233, 260
Intervertebral joints
- cervical **25**
- lumbar **25**
Intestinal abdomen **156**
Intestinal villi 137
Intestine
- large 57, **161**, 162, **162-163**
- layers 137
- small 57, **137**, 138, **138**, 157, **161**, 162, **162**, 252
Isthmus 8, **15**
- of thyroid gland 106
- of uterine tube 195, 203-204, 221, 253
- of uterus 195-196, 253

J

Jejunum 135, 138, **138**, 139, 151-152, 154-155, 160-161, 163, 173, 177, 240, 242, 245-246, 248
Joint capsule
- (atlanto-occipital joint) 18
- (costovertebral joint) 21-22
- (hip joint) 270, 272-273
- (knee joint) 287, 292, 328
- (lateral atlanto-axial joint) 17-18
- (metatarsophalangeal joint of great toe) 338
- (sternoclavicular joint) 52
- (zygapophysial joint) 23, 25, 40
Joint(s)
- acromioclavicular 126
- ankle 264, **265**, **303**, 306-307, 340, 385-386
- - axis 327
- - frontal section 306
- - (lateral) 307
- - radiograph (ap) 307
- - sagittal section 306
- atlanto-occipital 17-19
- axes 322
- arthroscopy **294**
- cross-section 286
- forces **323**
- frontal section 292
- (lateral) 293
- MRI **295**
- radiograph (ap) 293
- sagittal section 292
- calcaneocuboid 264, **265**
- costotransverse 4, 14, 20
- costovertebral 20-22
- cuneocuboid 264, **265**
- cuneonavicular 264, **265**
- femoropatellar 264, 286, **291**
- of foot **265**, **302-305**
- of free lower limb **265**
- of head of rib 4, 14, 20, 22
- hip 257, 264, **265**, 270-273, **275**, **280-281**
- - axes 314
- - forces **323**
- - LAUENSTEIN-projection **282**
- - radiograph (ap) **282**
- intercuneiform 264, **265**
- intermetatarsal **265**
- interphalangeal (of foot) 264, **265**
- knee 264, **265**, 286, **287-291**, **294**, 328
- lateral atlanto-axial 17-19
- lumbosacral 270, **270-272**, 273, **273**
- meniscofemoral 264, **291**
- meniscotibial 264, **291**
- metatarsophalangeal 264, **265**, 304, 306
- - of great toe 306, 338
- sacrococcygeal 218, 252, 263
- sacroiliac 1, 16, 174, 223, 254, 263, **263**, 264, 268, 270-271, 273-274, **274**, 275, 282, 318
- sternoclavicular 48, 52, **52**, 123
- sternocostal 52

Joint(s)
- subtalar 264, **265**, 306-307, 385-386
- talocalcaneonavicular 264, **265**, **305**, 307, 340
- - axis 327
- - frontal section **306**
- - (lateral) **307**
- - radiograph (ap) **307**
- - sagittal section **306**
- talonavicular 386
- talotarsal 264
- tarsometatarsal 264, **265**, 298, 306
- tibiofibular 264, **265**, 284, 292-293, 295-296
- transverse tarsal **265**, 298
- zygapophysial 12, 15-16, 23, **23**, 25, 30, 40-41, 274
Joints of pelvic girdle **263**, 270, **270-273**

K

KEITH-FLACK, node of **84**
Kidney 30, 41, 57, 151-152, 158, 162, 164-165, 175, 177, 180, **180-182**, 183, **183**, 185-186, **186**, 189, 194, 208-209, 243-246, 248, 250
- development 183
- projection 186
- radiograph (ap) **186**, 208
- ultrasound image **185**
Knee 264
- fascias 325
- muscles 328
KOEHLER's teardrop **282**
KOHLRAUSCH's fold **205**, 252
KRISTELLER, mucous plug of **200**

L

Labium
- majus 200, 224, 227, 238, 253, 259, 261
- minus 200, 215, 224, 229, 238-239, 253, 261
Labrum
- acetabular 280
Lamina
- of cricoid cartilage 12, 93, 123
- propria (mucosa) 108, 132, 137, 140
- right (thyroid cartilage) 92-93, 106
- of vertebral arch 4, 7-9, 21-23, 25, 30, 41, 47
LANNELONGUE's crypts **89**
v. LANZ's point **167**
Laparoscopy **148**
LARREY's cleft **71**
Larynx 41, **92-93**
Lateral mass 6, 17, 19
LAUENSTEIN-projection **282**
Layer
- anterior (rectus sheath) 58, 62-65, 73-74, 309
- - (thoracolumbar fascia) 30

Index

Layer
- circular 108, 132-133, 137-138, 140
- investing [superficial] (cervical fascia) 123
- longitudinal 108, 132-134, 137-138, 140, 205, 220
- parietal (serous pericardium) 76, **76**, 77, 85, 91, 123-124, 240
- - (tunica vaginalis) 73, 190-191, 232
- posterior (rectus sheath) 65, 69, 72-73
- - (thoracolumbar fascia) 30, 37
- visceral (serous pericardium) 76, **76**, 77, 80-82, 123, 240
- - (tunica vaginalis) 191, 232, 240

Leg 264
- compartments **329**
- deep dorsal **334**
- - muscle origins and insertions **335**
- - osseofibrous tubes **329**
- - ventral **327**
- fascia(s) **325**
- lateral **329**
- - superficial dorsal **334**
- muscles **326**, **330-333**

Ligament(s)
- alar 18, **18**
- anococcygeal *see* anococcygeal body
- anterior cruciate 288-289, 291-292, **295**
- anterior (of fibular head) 288, 296
- anterior longitudinal 17, 20-22, 24-25, 30, 61, 74, 118, 128, 270-271, 273
- anterior sacrococcygeal 223-224, 271
- anterior sacro-iliac 223, **263**, 270-271, 273-274, 318
- anterior sternoclavicular 52
- anterior talofibular 302
- anterior tibiofibular 296, 302-303, 336
- anular 92-93
- apical (of dens) 18-19
- arcuate popliteal 288, 290, 292, 331
- arteriosum 76-77, 85, 90, 101, 106-107, 115
- bifurcate 302, 305
- broad (of uterus) 195, **204**
- calcaneocuboid 302, 305
- calcaneofibular 302-304, 306
- calcaneonavicular 302, 305
- cardinal **195**, 198, **198**
- collateral (interphalangeal joints of foot) 304
- coronary 142-143, 158, 165
- costoclavicular 52
- costotransverse 20-21, 37
- - lateral 20-22, 34, 36
- - superior 21-22, 34
- costoxiphoid 58, 63
- cruciate (of atlas) 18-19
- deep posterior sacrococcygeal 272

Ligament(s)
- deep transverse metatarsal 302, 304
- deltoid 302, 304, 306, 384
- denticulate 46
- dorsal cuboideonavicular 302
- dorsal cuneocuboid 305
- dorsal cuneonavicular 302, 305
- dorsal intercuneiform 5
- dorsal metatarsal 302
- dorsal tarsometatarsal 302, 305, 336
- falciform 67, 74, 142-143, 146, 156-158, 164-165, 241, 246-247
- fibular collateral 287-291, 295, 324
- flavum 20-23, 25, 30, 37, 41, 47, 255
- fundiform (of penis) 58, 67, 231, 240-242, 252
- gastrocolic 155-156, 158-159, 164, 171, 241, 245
- gastrophrenic 165
- gastrosplenic 153, 158-159, 164-165, 243, 245
- of head of femur 236, 256, 260, 272-273, 280
- hepatoduodenal 134, 146, 158-159, 164-165, 246
- hepatogastric 134, 154-155, 158-159, 164, 245-246
- iliofemoral 270-271, 280-281, 312, 380
- iliolumbar 34, 47, 209, 270-272, 274
- inferior (of epididymis) 190
- inferior pubic 230, **263**, 270, 272-274
- infundibulopelvic **204**
- inguinal 64, 67-69, 193, 230, 235, 238, 250, 262, 270 272, 308, **308**, 309, **309**, 310, 318, 353-354, 357
- interclavicular 52
- interfoveolar 69, 250
- interosseous sacro-iliac 223, 255, **263**, 272-274
- interspinous 24-25, 34, 41, 123
- intertransverse 21-22, 34, 36-37, 47
- intra-articular (of head of rib) 22
- intra-articular sternocostal 52
- ischiofemoral 280-281
- lacunar 68, 309, **309**, 318
- lateral arcuate 68-71
- lateral atlanto-occipital 17
- lateral collateral **290**
- lateral sacrococcygeal 271
- lateral talocalcaneal 302-303
- lateral thyrohyoid 106
- left triangular 142, 144, 164-165, 242-243
- of left vena cava 142, **142**, 143
- long plantar 301-302, 304, **304**, 306, 344, 379, 385-386
- lumbocostal 70
- medial arcuate 68-70
- medial collateral (knee joint) **290**
- medial talocalcaneal 303

Ligament(s)
- medial umbilical 56
- median arcuate 69
- median cricothyroid 92
- median thyrohyoid 106
- median umbilical 74, 156, 187, 193, 200, 221, 236, 252
- nuchae 25, 31-32, 39
- oblique popliteal 288-290, 331-332
- of ovary 194-195, 197, 203-204
- patellar 287, 289-292, 295, 310-312, 316, 324-326, 328, 354, 367
- pectineal 271, 309, **309**, 310
- phrenicocolic 158, 164
- phrenicosplenic 245
- plantar 301-302, 304-305
- plantar cuboideonavicular 304
- plantar cuneonavicular 304
- plantar metatarsal 304
- plantar tarsal 304
- plantar tarsometatarsal 302, 304
- posterior (of fibular head) 289, 292
- posterior cruciate 288-292, **295**
- posterior longitudinal 20, 23-25
- posterior meniscofemoral 289-290
- posterior sacro-iliac **263**, 272-273
- posterior talocalcaneal 303
- posterior talofibular 303, 306
- posterior tibiofibular 302-303
- pubofemoral 280-281
- puboprostatic 218, 252
- pulmonary 97, 114, **114**
- radiate (of head of rib) 20-21
- radiate sternocostal 52
- reflected 58, 63, 67
- right triangular 142
- round (of liver) 67, 74, 142, 144, 152, 156, 158, 164, 168-169, 246, 248
- - (of uterus) 165, 194-195, 197, 203-204, 220-221, 253
- round **165**, **195**, **197**, **221**
- sacrospinous 216-217, 221, 237, **263**, 269, 271-273, 281, 311, 324, 358
- sacrotuberous 34, 216, 223, 228-229, 237, **263**, 269, 271-273, 281, 317-320, 358, 362
- sacro-uterine **195**, 198, **253**
- splenorenal 153, 243
- superficial posterior sacrococcygeal 252, 272
- superficial transverse metatarsal 341
- superior (of epididymis) 190
- superior pubic 230, 256-257, **263**, 270-271, 274, 309, 311
- supraspinous 22, 25, 34, 38, 272
- suspensory (of clitoris) 238
- - (of ovary) 165, 195, 197, 203-204, 253
- - (of penis) 58, 231-232
- talocalcaneal interosseous 302, 305-306, 385-386

Ligament(s)
- tarsometatarsal 302
- tibial collateral 286-292, 295
- transverse
- - acetabular 223
- - of atlas 18-19
- - of knee 288, 291
- - perineal 223, 230
- venosum 142
- vocal 123

Limb
- lower **264**
- - arteries **351**
- - cutaneous innervation, segmental **348**
- - cutaneous nerves **349**
- - dermatomes **348**
- - joints **265**
- - muscle origins and insertions **324**, **335**
- - nerves **350**
- - skeleton **264**
- - surface projections **262**
- - surface relief **262**
- - veins **365**

Limbus fossae ovalis 80

Line
- alba 48, 58, 63, 67, 69, 74-75, 200, 203, 240-241, 246-247, 249, 252-253, 255
- anocutaneous 205
- anterior gluteal 268
- arcuate 273, 275
- - (ilium) 263, 267
- - (rectus sheath) 65, 67, 69, 73, 156, 250
- aspera 276-278, 328
- epiphysial 283, 293, 295, 306-307, 386
- inferior gluteal 269
- intercondylar 276
- intertrochanteric 276
- lateral supracondylar 276
- medial supracondylar 276
- paravertebral 1
- pectineal 276-277
- posterior axillary 1
- posterior gluteal 268
- posterior median 1
- scapular 1
- semilunar 65
- soleal 284-285
- terminalis 165, 223, 236, 263, 268-269, **269**, 271, 273, 282

Lingula of left lung 96, 113

Lip
- anterior 196, 198
- inner 263, 267-268
- lateral 276, 278
- medial 276-278
- outer 263, 267-268, 316
- posterior 196, 198

LISFRANC's joint **265**, **298**

Liver 57, 59, 123-125, **134**, **142-143**, 146, 148, **148**, 149, 152, 154-155, 159, **159**, 178, 185, 240-242, 244-248
- arteries, variations **168**
- porta hepatis **142**
- projection **149**
- segments **144**

Index

Liver
- veins, projection **148**
- - ultrasound image **145**

Lobar bronchi **94**

Lobe(s)
- caudate 142-144, **144**, 152, 159, 164, 169, 242, 246
- inferior 96-98, 100-101, 105, 113, 122, 125, 128-129, 145, 157, 241, 243-245
- left (of liver) 124, 134, 142-143, 146, 149, 152, 156-159, 164, 168-169, 240-241, 243, 245-248
- left (of prostate) 192
- of mammary gland 62
- middle (prostate) 192
- pyramidal 113
- quadrate 142, 158-159, 169, 246
- right (of liver) 134, 142-143, 148-149, 156-159, 161, 164, 166, 169, 242-244, 246, 248
- of right lung 96-98, 100, 105, 113, 122, 130-131, 157, 243
- right (of prostate) 192
- superior 96-98, **98**, 100-101, 105, 112-113, 122, 128-131, 157, 243

Lobule(s)
- of mammary gland 54
- of testis 190-191, 252
- of thymus 111

Longitudinal bands (cruciate ligament of atlas) 18-19

Lower abdomen, blood vessels **173**, **175**

Lumbar vertebral column
- CT **41**
- intervertebral joints **23**
- ligaments **23**
- load in upright position **40**
- MRI **24**
- radiograph (ap) **16**
- - (lateral) **15**

Lung **94**, 96-102, 113
- arteries 102
- left 91, **97**, 98, 100-101, 112-113, 122, 124-125, **126**, 128, 130-131, 157, 243, 245
- right 91, **97**, 98, **98**, 100, 112-113, 120-122, 124-125, 127, 129-131, 145, 157, 241, 243-244
- veins **102**

Lunules of semilunar cusps 81

Lymph nodes, anthracotic **97**

Lymphatic vessel(s) **211**, 235
- afferent 211
- central 137
- deep 366
- efferent 211
- radiograph (ap) **211**
- superficial 368

Lymphatic vessels, radiograph (ap) **211**

Lymphography **211**

M

Male external genitalia **231**, 235, **237**

Male internal genitalia **214**, **232**

Malleolus
- lateral 262, 296, 302-303, 306-307, 326, 330, 336, 338-339, 341, 366, 370-371, 373
- medial 262, 284, 296, 303, 306-307, 325-326, 330-332, 336, 338, 341, 371, 373
- third **307**

Mammography **55**

Manubriosternal joint 51-52

Manubrium of sternum 3, 51-52, 61, 72, 110, 123, 128

Margin
- falciform 308-309

MAY's vein **364-365**

MC BURNEY'S point **167**

MECKELS's diverticulum **137**

Mediastinum **114-115**, **117-118**, **122-123**, **129**
- posterior 125
- superior 129, **129**
- of testis 190-191, 252

Medulla
- renal 181-182, 185, 244-245, 248
- (suprarenal gland) 187

Membrane
- anterior atlanto-occipital 17, 19
- internal intercostal 34, 36, 61
- interosseous (of leg) **285**, 288, 296, **296**, 303, 328, 329, **329**, 383
- obturator 236, 260-261, 270, 280-281, 309
- perineal 252
- posterior atlanto-occipital 17, 19, 40
- tectorial 18-19
- thyrohyoid 106

Meniscus
- lateral 288-292, 294-295
- medial 288-292, 295

Mesentery 137, 162-163, **163**, 164, 252
- of diverticulum 137

Meso-appendix 161-165

Mesocolon
- sigmoid 162, 164-165, 177, 209-210, 218
- transverse 140, 155, 158-159, 161, 163-165, 171, 173, 175

Mesosalpinx 195, 204

Metaphysis 306

Metatarsus 264, **300**

Moderator band 80, **80**

Mons pubis 238

Mucous membrane 108, 125, 132, 137, 140, 146, 188, 195-196

MUELLERian duct **189**, **194**

Muscle origins and insertions
- foot **340**, **347**
- leg **335**
- pelvis **324**
- thigh **324**

Muscle(s)
- of abdomen 58, 62-66, 68, 74-75
- - CT **75**
- abductor digiti minimi 306, 336, 338-340, 342-345, 347, **347**, 377-378, 385, **388**

Muscle(s)
- - hallucis 306, 337, 340-345, **346**, 347, 377-378, 385, **388**
- adductor 241, 259
- - brevis 242, 261, 312-313, **315**, 324, 356, 380, **387**
- - hallucis 306, 342-345, **346**, 347, 378, 385-386, **388**
- - longus 242, 261, 310-313, 315, 318, 324, 353-354, **355**, 356, 380-381, **387**
- - magnus 260, 288-290, 292, 310, 312-313, **315**, 317-320, 324, 328, 356, 361-362, 380-382, **387**
- - minimus 260, 313, **315**, 319-320, **387**
- anterior papillary 80-84
- articularis genus 287, **314-315**, 324
- of back 27, 29-32, **34**, 36-39, 41
- - CT **30**
- - lateral tract **39**
- - medial tract **35**
- biceps brachii 59, 62, 126, 288, 380
- - femoris 258, 286, 290, 316-320, **322**, 324-326, 328, 330-333, 335, 359-361, 368-370, 380-382, **387**
- brachialis 62
- broncho-esophageus 101
- bulbospongiosus **214-215**, 218, **222**, 228-229, 237-240, 260-261, **388**
- cervicis 39
- coccygeus *see* ischiococcygeus
- coracobrachialis 59, 126
- cremaster 58, 63-64, 67, 73, 190-191, 218, 232, 235, **235**, 240-241, 252, **387**
- cricothyroid 106, 113, 120
- dartos 73, 218, 228, 232, 252
- deep transverse perineal 200, 218, **222**, 223, 228-230, 236, 238, 240, 252, 260, 324, **388**
- deltoid 1, 43, 48, 58-59, 62, 126-127
- digastric 34, 38, 40
- epicranius 44-45
- erector spinae 1, 29-32, **33**, 36-37, 75, 126, 129, 203, 241, 244-249, 254, 317
- extensor digitorum brevis 326, 336-340, **340**, 345, 367, 374, 379, 383-385, **388**
- - - longus 324-326, **327**, **329**, 335-339, 345, 366-367, 374, 379, 383-386, **388**
- - hallucis brevis 325-326, 336-340, **340**, 345, 374, 385, **388**
- - - longus 306, 325-326, **329**, 335-340, 345, 367, 374, 379, 383-385, **388**
- external oblique 27, 29, 31-32, 34, 43, 48, 56, 58-59, 62-65, 66, 67, 69-71, 73-75, 113, 156, 203, 209, 224, 231-232, 247, 249, 254-255, 309, 316, 324, 362, **387**

Muscle(s)
- fibularis brevis 302, 304-306, 326, **329**, 333, 335-340, 367, 370, **370**, 372, 383-384, **387**
- - longus 304, 306, 324, 326, **329**, 331-332, 335, 337, 343-344, 347, 366-367, 370, **370**, 372, 383-384, 386, **387**
- - tertius 326, **327**, **329**, 336-340, 367, 384
- flexor accessorius *see* quadratus plantae
- - digiti minimi brevis (foot) 342-345, 347, **347**, 385, **388**
- - digitorum brevis 306, 337, 342-345, **346**, 347, 377-378, 385-386, **388**
- - - longus 306, 324, **329**, 331-333, **334**, 335, 343-345, 347, **370**, 371-372, 377-378, 383-386, **388**
- flexor hallucis brevis 342-345, **346**, 347, 377-378, 385, 388
- - longus **329**, 331-333, **334**, 335, 342-345, 347, **370**, 371-372, 377-379, 383, 385-386, **388**
- flexores digitorum 379
- gastrocnemius 262, 286, 288-290, 295, 316, 319-320, 324-326, 328, 330-333, **334**, 359-360, 368-370, 382-383
- gemellus inferior 317, 319-320, **321**, 324, 361-362, 380
- - superior 317, 319-320, **321**, 324, 361-362, 380
- gluteus maximus 1, 32, 34, 43, 62, 218, 225, 228-229, 237, 239, 241, 254-257, 259, 262, 280, 316-320, **321**, 324, 359-362, 380, **387**
- - medius 74, 203, 254-256, 259, 280, 311-313, 317, 319-320, **321**, 324, 359, 361-363, 380, **387**
- - - injection **362-363**
- - minimus 280, 319-320, **321**, 324, 362, 380, **387**
- gracilis 228-229, 261, 286, 310-313, **315**, 317-320, 324, 328, 330, 335, 354-356, 359-360, 368-369, 381-382, **387**
- iliacus 67-68, 70, 74, 203, 209, 212, 224, 242, 250, 254-255, 257, 259, 309-311, **314**, 318, 324, 354-356
- iliococcygeus **222**, 223, 241
- iliocostalis cervicis 31-32, **33**, 38-40
- - lumborum 31-32, **33**, 74
- - thoracis 31-32, 33, 36, 43, 246
- iliopsoas 75, 256, 259-261, 280, 309, **309**, 310-313, 320, 324, 380, **387**
- inferior constrictor 106, 120
- infraspinous 27, 29, 31, 43-44, 62, 127-129

Index

Muscle(s)
- intercostal **61**, 74, 129, 209, 247
- - external 32, 34, 36, 59, **60**, 61, 64–65, 108, 117, 128, 130–131, 246
- - innermost 36
- - internal 34, 36, 59, **60**, 61, 63–65, 69, 108, 117–118, 124, 126, 246
- internal oblique 29–32, 34, 36, 63–65, **66**, 67, 69, 71, 73–75, 156, 203, 209, 224, 232, 249, 254–255, 324, **387**
- interossei **346**, **388**
- - dorsal (foot) 306, 336, 338–340, 343–345, **345**, 347, 385–386
- - - compartments **379**
- - plantar 340, 342–345, **345**, 347, 385, **388**
- interspinales cervicis 34, **35**, 38, 46
- - lumborum 34, **35**
- - thoracis **35**, 123
- intertransversarii
- - anterior cervical **33**
- - lateral lumbar **33**, 34, 36–37, 47
- - medial lumbar **33**, 34, 36–37, 47
- - posterior cervical **33**, 34, 40
- - thoracic **33**, 34
- ischiocavernosus **214–215**, 218, **222**, 228–229, 237–240, 260–261, **388**
- ischiococcygeus 217, 219, 222, 223–224, 256, 318, **324**, 388
- ischiocrural [hamstring] 260
- latissimus dorsi 11 27, **28**, 29–32, 43–44, 58–59, 62, 64–65, 70, 74, 130–131, 246–249, 317
- levator ani 205–207, 218–221, **222**, 223–224, 226, 228–229, 236–237, 239–241, 252, 256–258, 260–261, 324, 388
- prostatae **222**
- - scapulae **28**, 29, 31–32, 39, 43–44
- levatores costarum 32, **33**
- - breves **33**, 34, 36
- - longi **33**, 34, 36
- longissimus capitis 31–32, **33**, 34, 38–40, 43–45
- - cervicis 31–32, **33**, 38–40
- - thoracis 31–32, **33**, 36, 43, 74, 246
- longus *see* fibularis longus
- longus colli 61
- lumbricals (foot) 342, **342**, 343–344, **345**, 385, **388**
- multifidi 34, **35**, 36–38, 40, 43, 45, 246
- obliquus capitis inferior 34, 38, **39**, 40, 45–46
- - superior 34, 38, **39**, 40, 45–46
- obturator externus 236, 257, 260–261, 280, 313, **315**, 320, 324, 362, 380, **387**
- - internus 206–207, 217, 223–224, 236, 256–261, 280, 317–320, **321**, 324, 361–362, **362**, 380, **387**

Muscle(s)
- occipitofrontalis 44–45
- omohyoid 113, 127
- opponens digiti minimi 336, 344–345, **347**, 385, **388**
- pectinati 80
- pectineus 242, 256–257, 309–313, **315**, 324, 354–355, 380, **387**
- pectoralis major 48, 54, 58–59, **60**, 62–65, 113, 122–123, 127, 129–131
- - minor 59, **60**, 122, 124, 128
- perineal 223
- peroneus brevis *see* fibularis brevis
- piriformis 216, 218–219, 224, 241, 311–313, 317–320, **321**, 324, 358, 361–362, **362**, 380, **387**
- plantar 288, 324, 328, **329**, 330–333, **334**, 369–372, 384, **388**
- popliteus 288–292, 295, 324, 332–333, **334**, 335, 369, 372, **388**
- posterior papillary 81–83
- psoas major 30, 41, 47, 68–70, 74, 151, 183, 185–186, 203, 209, 213, 236, 243–245, 249–250, 254–255, 257, 259, 309–311, **314**, 318, 324, 353
- - minor 68, 70–71, 74, 177, 203, 209, 250, 309–310, **314**, 318
- pubococcygeus **222**, 223, 240–241
- puborectalis **222**, 223, 256, 258
- pubovaginalis **222**, 224
- pyramidalis 56, 63, **63**, 64–65, **66**, 73–74, 240
- quadratus femoris 260, 317, 319–320, **321**, 324, 361–362, 380, **387**
- - lumborum 30, 34, **66**, 68–70, 74–75, 121, 151, 209, 212–213, 244–245, 249–250, 324
- - plantae 306, 343–344, **346**, 347, 377–378, 384, 386, **388**
- quadriceps femoris 262, 287, 289–290, 292, 311, **314**, 324–326, 335, **387**
- rectococcygeus 223–224
- recto-uterinus 195
- rectus abdominis 48, 56, 63, **63**, 64–65, **66**, 67–68, 70, 72–75, 113, 123, 156, 203, 209, 218, 240–241, 244–251, 254–256, **387**
- - capitis lateralis **39**, 40
- - - posterior major 34, 38, **39**, 40, 45–46
- - - - minor 34, 38, **39**, 40, 46
- - femoris 242, 256–257, 271, 280–281, 310–313, **314**, 316, 318, 324, 354–356, 380–381
- rhomboid major 27, **28**, 29, 31, 43–45
- - minor **28**, 29, 44–45
- rotatores **35**, 36
- - cervicis **35**
- - lumborum **35**
- - thoracis 34, **35**, 37

Muscle(s)
- sacrococcygeus 223–224, 241
- sartorius 62, 242, 256–257, 262, 286, 310–313, **315**, 316, 318, 324, 328, 335, 354–356, 360, 380–382, **387**
- scalenus anterior 61, 113–114, 119, 122, 127
- - medius 39–40, 46, 61, 124, 126
- - posterior 31–32, 34, 39, 61
- semimembranosus 258, 286, 288–290, 316, 318–320, **322**, 324, 328, 330–332, 335, 359–361, 368–370, 380–382
- semispinalis 32
- - capitis 31–32, 34, **35**, 38–40, 44–46
- - cervicis 31–32, 34, **35**, 38, 45
- - thoracis 32, 34, **35**, 36, 38–39
- semitendinosus 258, 286, 313, 317–320, **322**, 324, 328, 330, 335, 359–361, 368–370, 380–382
- septal papillary 80
- serratus anterior **28**, 29, 31, 48, 54, 58–59, 62–65, 70, 73, 124, 126–131
- - posterior inferior **28**, 29, 31–32, 36, 43, 246
- - superior **28**, 29, 31–32, 43
- soleus 292, 324, 326, 330–333, **334**, 335, 369–372, 383
- sphincter of ampulla 150
- - external anal 200, 205–207, 218, **222**, 223–224, 226, 228–229, 237–240, 252, 258, **388**
- - internal anal 200, 205, 224, 240, 252, 258
- - pyloric 139, 150
- - urethral 200, 218, **222**, 224, 230
- - vesical **214**
- spinalis 33
- - capitis 32, 34, **35**
- - cervicis 32, **35**
- - thoracis 31–32, **33**, 36
- splenius capitis 27, 29, 31–32, **33**, 34, 38–40, 44–45, 126
- - cervicis 29, 31–32, **33**, 38–40
- sternalis 59, **60**
- sternocleidomastoid 27, 29, 31, 41, 44, 58–59, 113, 123, 127
- sternohyoid 113, 127
- sternothyroid 61, 113, 123, 128
- subclavius 59, **60**, 113–115, 122, 124, 126–127
- subcostales **60**
- suboccipital **34**, 37–38, **40**, **46**
- subscapular **60**, 126, 128
- superficial transverse perineal **222**, 223, 228–230, 237–239, 260, **388**
- supraspinous 126–127
- suspensory (of duodenum) 139, 150–151
- tensor fasciae latae 62, 75, 242, 256–257, 262, 280, 308, 310–311, **315**–316, 319, 324, 354, 380, **387**

Muscle(s)
- teres major 1, 27, 29, 31, 43–44, 62, 126, 128–129
- - minor 43, 62
- - tertius *see* fibularis tertius
- of thorax 59–60, **62**
- thyrohyoid 113
- tibialis anterior 292, 302, 304, 324–326, **327**, **329**, 335–336, 338–339, 347, 366–367, 374, 383–384, 386, **388**
- - posterior 302, 304, 306, 324, **329**, 331–333, **334**, 335, 344, 347, 370, **370**, 371–372, 383–384, **388**
- trachealis 93
- transverse arytenoid 123
- transversospinalis 30
- transversus abdominis 34, 36, 65, **66**, 68–71, 73–75, 156, 203, 209, 213, 224, 246, 249–250, 254–255, 324, **387**
- - thoracis 61, 72, 113, 131
- trapezius 1, **26**, 27, 29, 31, 38–39, 44–45, 62, 126–130
- triceps brachii 43, 62
- - surae 306, **329**, **334**, 340, 386, **388**
- vastus intermedius 312–313, **314–315**, 324, 381–382
- - lateralis 257, 259, 280, 292, 295, 310–313, **314–315**, 316, 319–320, 324, 326, 328, 354, 356, 359, 363, 381–382
- - medialis 292, 310–313, **314**, 324, 328, 354–356, 381–382
- Muscles of abdomen 58, 62–66, **74–75**
- - CT **75**
- Muscles of back
- - proper **3**, **31–34**, **36–37**
- - - lateral tract **30**, **33**, **39**
- - - long parts 32
- - - medial tract **30**, **35**
- - - - superficial layer **31**
- - superficial **27**
- Muscles of neck 34, **37–40**, **46**
- - deep 39
- Muscles of thorax **58–60**, **62**
- Muscular layer 107–108, 123, 132–134, 137–140, 167, 187–188, 195–196, 205, 218, 220, 223, 261
- Muscularis mucosae 108, 132, 137, 140
- Myocardium **78–79**, 80–82, 123

N

Neck
- of femur 275–278, 280–282
- of fibula 285
- frontal section **126**
- of gallbladder 146–147
- of rib 4, 49
- of talus 298–300, 307
- Neck of bladder 192
- Nerve(s)
- accessory [XI] **26**, 44–45
- accessory obturator **387**

Index

Nerves
- anal 226
- anococcygeal 217, 237, 239, **388**
- anterior labial **387**
- anterior scrotal **387**
- axillary 42-43, 126
- cavernous (of clitoris) **215**
- cervical 19, **28**, 33, **33**, **42**, 46, 120
- coccygeal 71, 217, **388**
- common fibular 286, **340**, 349-350, 359-361, 364, 367-368, 370-371, 382, **387**
- common plantar digital 376-378, **388**
- crural interosseous **388**
- deep fibular **327**, 329, **329**, **340**, 349-350, 367, 373-374, 379, 383-384, **388**
- dorsal (of clitoris) **215**, 230, 239, **388**
- - (of penis) **214**, 230-232, 237, **388**
- - scapular **28**, 44-45
- dorsal digital (of foot) 349-350, 367, 373-374, **387-388**
- erigentes *see* pelvic splanchnic nerves
- femoral 56, 71, 75, 177, 203, 209-210, 212-213, 236, 242, 250-251, 256-257, 309, **309**, **314-315**, 318, 349-350, 352, 354-356, 380-381, **387**
- genitofemoral 56, **66**, 71, 177, 209, 212-213, 217, 221, 235-236, 250, 256, 309, **309**, 318, 349-350, 352, **387**
- greater auricular 42-44
- greater occipital 43-46
- greater splanchnic **71**, 114-115, 117-121, 212-213, 243, 246
- hypogastric 214, **214**, 215, **215**, 226, **226**
- iliohypogastric 42-43, 56, **66**, 71, 75, 117, 119, 177, 209, 212-213, 250, 349-350, 352, 362, **387**
- ilio-inguinal 56, **66**, 71, 75, 177, 209-210, 212-213, 231-232, 250, 349-350, 352, **387**
- inferior anal 217, 237, 239, **388**
- inferior clunial 42, 237, 239, 349, 358-360, **387**
- inferior gluteal 257, **321**, 350, 358, 361-362, **362**, 380, **387**
- inferior lateral brachial cutaneous 42-43
- inferior rectal *see* inferior anal nerves
- intercostal 34, 36, 42, 44, 56, 59, **66**, 75, 114, 117, **117**, 118-119, **119**, 120, 128, 131, 212, 245, 247
- intercostobrachial 43
- intermediate dorsal cutaneous 349-350, 364, 373, **387**
- labial 215
- lateral dorsal cutaneous 349-350, 364, 373, **388**

Nerves
- lateral femoral cutaneous 42, 71, 75, 177, 209, 212-213, 250, **309**, 318, 349-350, 352, 354-355, 358, **387**
- lateral pectoral **60**
- lateral plantar 306, **346-347**, 350, 376-378, 384, 386, **388**
- lateral supraclavicular 42-43
- lateral sural cutaneous **329**, 349-350, 359-361, 364, 368, **387**
- lesser occipital 42-44
- lesser splanchnic **71**, 117, 119, 121, 243, 246
- long thoracic 126, 128-130
- lumbar **28**, 33, **66**, 218, 349
- lumbar splanchnic 226
- medial clunial 42, 349, 358-360
- medial dorsal cutaneous 349-350, 364, **387**
- medial pectoral **60**
- medial plantar 306, **346-347**, 350, 376-378, 384, **388**
- medial sural cutaneous 350, 359-361, 364, 368, 373, **388**
- middle cervical cardiac 120
- obturator 71, 212-213, 217, 221, 224, 236, 256-257, 261, 309, **315**, 318, 349-350, 352, 355-356, 380, **387**
- to obturator internus **321**, **387**
- pelvic splanchnic 214, **214**, 215, **215**, 226
- perineal 230, 237, 239, 260-261, **388**
- phrenic **70-71**, 90-91, 112-115, 117, 120-122, **122**, 128-131
- to piriformis **321**, **387**
- posterior brachial cutaneous 42-43
- posterior femoral cutaneous 42, 237, 239, 257, 349-350, 358-362, **362**, 380, **387**
- posterior labial **215**, 239, **388**
- posterior scrotal **214**, 237, **388**
- proper plantar digital 376, 378, **388**
- pudendal **214**, 215, **215**, 217, **222-223**, 226, 230, 236-237, 239, 257, 261, 350, 358, **362**, **388**
- to quadratus femoris **321**, **387**
- radial 42-43
- recurrent laryngeal 90-91, 112, 114-115, 117, 119-120, 122
- sacral 215, 217-218, **222**, 241, 252, 349
- saphenous 329, 349-350, 352, 355-356, 364, 373, 381-382, 384, **387**
- sciatic 256-257, 286, **315**, **321-322**, **327**, **329**, **334**, 350, 358, 360-362, **362**, 363, 380-382, **387**
- - projection 358
- spinal 24, 30, **33**, 35, 41-42, 46-47, 203, 249
- subcostal 71, 75, 117, 119, 209, 212-213
- suboccipital **39**, 43, 45-46, **390**

Nerves
- subscapular 43
- superficial fibular **329**, 349-350, 364, 367, 373, 379, 383-384, **387**
- superior clunial 42-43, 349, 358, 360
- superior gluteal 315, **321**, 350, 358, 362, **362**, 363, 380, **387**
- superior laryngeal 106
- superior lateral brachial cutaneous 42
- supraclavicular 56
- suprascapular 127
- sural 349-350, 360, 364, 373, 384, **388**
- third occipital 43, 46
- thoracic **28**, 33, **33**, 34, 36, **42**, 43, 56, **60**, **66**, 73, 114-115, 117-121, 212, 246
- thoracodorsal **28**, 126
- tibial 286, **329**, **334**, **346**, 350, 359-361, 364, 368, 370, **370**, 371-373, 376, 382-384, **388**
- vaginal 215
- vagus [X] **71**, 90-91, 112, 114-115, 117, 119-120, **120**, 121-122, 124, 127-131, 212
Nervous system, autonomic **119-121**
Network
- dorsal venous (of foot) 364
- lateral malleolar 367, 374
- medial malleolar 374
Nipple 54, 62, 131
Node(s)
- atrioventricular 84
- hemorrhoidal **205**
- lymph
- - anterior cervical 55
- - - deep 55
- - anterior mediastinal 90, 112, 115
- - anterior tibial 366
- - apical 128
- - axillary 55, 126, 128
- - brachial 55
- - bronchopulmonary 129-131
- - common iliac 210, 221, 250
- - - medial 250
- - deep inguinal 210, 353
- - deep popliteal 368
- - deltopectoral 55
- - external iliac 210, 221, 236, 250, 353
- - - lateral 221, 353
- - - medial 221, 353
- - gastric 134, 210
- - gastro-omental 134, 246
- - hepatic 134
- - ileocolic 241
- - infraclavicular 55
- - internal iliac 210, 221, 353
- - juxta-esophageal 109
- - lacunar 309
- - - intermediate **309**
- - - lateral **309**
- - - medial **309**
- - lateral aortic 221, 250
- - lateral cervical 124
- - - inferior deep 124

Node(s) lymph
- - of ligamentum arteriosum 90
- - obturator 221, 250
- - pancreatic 248
- - paramammary 55
- - pararectal 126, 221
- - parasternal 55
- - paratracheal 90, 124, 128
- - parietal 210
- - postcaval 241
- - posterior mediastinal 109, 243
- - pre-aortic 221, 249-250
- - precaval 221
- - promontorial 210
- - pyloric 134
- - retro-aortic 221
- - right lumbar 210
- - splenic 243, 246
- - submammary 55
- - superficial inguinal 210, 353
- - - inferior 210, 353
- - - superolateral 210, 353
- - - superomedial 210, 256, 353
- - superficial popliteal 368
- - superior phrenic 90, 123
- - superior rectal 221
- - supraclavicular 55
- - thoracic **109**, 124
- - tracheobronchial 100-101, 115, 126
- - - inferior 90, 97, 109, 123, 131
- - - superior 90, 109, 123
- sinu-atrial 84
Nodule(s)
- aggregated lymphoid 138
- of semilunar cusps 81
- solitary lymphoid 132, 137, 140, 146, 205
Notch
- acetabular 267-268
- angular 132, 134-135, 139, 158
- of cardiac apex 85, 88, 101
- cardiac (of left lung) 96-97, 105, 113
- cardial 132, 134
- clavicular 51
- costal 51
- fibular 284
- greater sciatic 267-268, 282
- inferior vertebral **4**, 8, 12, 15
- jugular (sternum) 48, 51
- lesser sciatic 267-268, 282
- for ligamentum teres 142
- pancreatic 150
- superior vertebral **4**, 12, 15
Nucleus pulposus 24-25, 30

O

Occipital plane 6
Oesophag- *see* Esophag-
Olisthesis **9**
Omental eminence 142, 159
Omentum
- greater 125, 134, 140, 148, 154-156, **156**, 157-158, **158**, 159-164, 166, 169, 240-241, 243-246, 252, 255
- lesser 134, 158-159, 164, 245-246

Opening
- caval 61, 68-69, **71**, 106, 108
- of coronary sinus 80, 84-85
- of inferior vena cava 84
- of smallest cardiac veins 80
- of superior vena cava 80, 84

Orifice
- cardial 110, 125, 132, 164-165, 242-243, 245
- external urethral (female urethra) 194, 224, 229, 238-239, 261
- - (male urethra) 233-234, 252
- ileal 140
- internal (female urethra) 253
- - (male urethra) 188, 192, 233, 252, 260
- left atrioventricular 81, 130
- pyloric 139
- right atrioventricular 80
- ureteric 188, 192, 233, 252-253, 260
- vaginal 194, 229, 238
- of vermiform appendix 140

Orifice of pancreatic duct 146

Ostium
- abdominal (uterine tube) 195, 197, 204, **204**
- uterine (uterine tube) 195-196

Ovarian stroma 195

Ovary 165-166, 194-195, **195**, 197, 203-204, **204**, 215, **215**, 220, 253, 353

P

Palate, bony 12
Pancreas 125, 134, 149-150, **150**, 151, **151**, 154-155, 159, **159**, 161-162, 169, 175, 240-241, 243, 246, 248
- projection **149**

Papilla(-ae)
- bipartite 150
- ileal 140
- major duodenal 139, 146, 150
- minor duodenal 150
- renal 181-182, 186, 243

Paracolic gutters 160-162, 164
Paracystium 198, **260-261**
Paradidymis 189, **189**
Parametrium 198
Paranephric fat 185
Paraproctium 198
Parasympathetic part **214-215**, **226**
Parathymic fat **111**
Paroöphoron 194, **194**

Pars
- abdominal (pectoralis major) 58-59, **60**, 62-63
- - (esophagus) 68, 70, 106, 108, 110, 119, 132, 134
- - (ureter) 161, 208
- anterior (vaginal fornix) 196, 198
- - (liver) 143
- anterior tibiotalar 302
- anular (fibrous sheaths) 342

Pars
- ascending (duodenum) 139, 149-150, 163, 165-166
- - (trapezius) **26**
- atlantic 40, 46
- basal (right inferior lobar arteries) 100
- - (left inferior lobar arteries) 100-101
- basilar 6, 17-19
- cardiac 70, 125, 132, 134, 136, 177, 209, 240
- cervical (esophagus) 106, 108-110, 123
- cervical (vertebral artery) 46
- clavicular 59, **60**
- costal 124
- - of diaphragm 59, 68-69, **70-71**, 75, 177, 244-248
- - (parietal pleura) 59, 113-115, 124-125, 128-129, 157, 244-248
- cruciform (fibrous sheaths) 342
- deep (posterior compartment of leg) 329
- - (external anal sphincter) **222**
- descending (duodenum) 132, 134-135, 139, 149-152, 165-166, 177
- - (iliofemoral ligament) 281
- - (trapezius) **26**
- diaphragmatic 59, 70, 91, 112-115, 122, 157, 243, 246-248
- free (lower limb) 264
- horizontal (duodenum) 139, 149-151, 161, 163, 165, 177
- inferior (serratus anterior) **28**
- infraclavicular 59, 114-115
- intermediate (male urethra) 192-193, 233, 252
- intramural (male urethra) 233
- intrasegmental 124, 126
- lateral (occipital bone) 17
- - (sacrum) **4**, 10-11, 47, 255, 263, 275
- left (liver) **144**
- lumbar (diaphragm) 68-70, **70-71**, 106, 108, 117-118, 123, 125, 169, 240-241, 243, 246-248
- mediastinal 91, 97, 112, 114-115, 129, 157
- membranous (interventricular septum) 81, **81**, 82
- middle (serratus anterior) **28**
- muscular 80-82
- occluded 193, 221, 236, 250
- patent 217, 219-221
- pelvic (ureter) 67, 164-165, 213
- posterior tibiotalar 302-303
- posterior (vaginal fornix) 196, 198, 200, 253
- - (liver) **144**
- prostatic 188, 192, 233
- pyloric 119, 132, 134-135, **135**, 136, 139, 156, 164, 245
- right (liver) **144**
- sternal (diaphragm) 68-70, **70-71**, 112-113, 123, 241
- sternocostal 58-59, **60**, 62-63
- subcutaneous (external anal

Pars
sphincter) **222**, 238
- superficial (posterior compartment of leg) 329
- - (external anal sphincter) **222**
- superior (duodenum) 132, 134, **138**, 139, 149, 151, 158-159, 164-165, 177, 242
- - (liver) 142
- - (serratus anterior) **28**
- supraclavicular **28**
- thoracic (autonomic division) **119-121**
- - (esophagus) 70, 106-110, 115, 117-119, 123, 125, 129, 243
- - (thoracic duct) 115, 117-118
- tibiocalcaneal 302-304, 306
- tibionavicular 302
- transverse (iliofemoral ligament) 281
- - (trapezius) **26**
- uterine (uterine tube) 195

Patella 262, 264, 286-287, 289, 292-295, 308, 311-312, 316, 326, 328, 364, 382
Patellar ridge 294
Patellar tendon reflex **388**

Pecten
- anal 205, 224, 252
- pubis 68, 224, 263, 267-268, 273, 311-312, 318

Pectoral girdle **3**, **26**, 53
Pedicle 4, 7-9, 12, 14-16, 20-21, 23-25, 30, 41, 275

Pelvic floor
- female **223-224**, 229-230, 238
- male **228**, 230, 236

Pelvic girdle **3**, **263**, 264
Pelvic inlet 263, **263**, **268**, **269**, **269**
Pelvic outlet 263, 269, **269**

Pelvic viscera
- female **201**, 220
- male **218-219**, 250

Pelvis 268, 270
- CT 254
- dimensions of female **269**
- female **269**
- - cross-section **257**
- - CT **257**
- - median section **253**
- - MRI **251**, **259**
- - oblique section **261**
- - greater [false] 263
- joints **270-273**
- lesser [true] 165, **263**
- lumbosacral joint **270-271**, **273**
- male
- - cross-section **255-256**
- - CT **256**
- - frontal section **258**
- - median section **240**, **252**
- - MRI **251**, **259**
- - oblique section **260**
- - sagittal section **241**
- muscle origins and insertions **324**
- radiograph (ap) **275**, **279**
- renal 170, 180-181, 183, **183**, 185, **185**, 186, **186**, 189, 194, 208, 243-244, 248
- - radiograph (ap) **186**

Pelvis
- sex differences **268**, **270-273**
Penis 214, 227, **234**, 235, 242, 260
Perforating vein, lateral 365
Pericardium 70, **76**, 77, 88, **91**, 100-101, **107**, 113, **113**, 122, **122**, 245
- fibrous **76**, 91, 109, 112, 114-115, 121, 157
- serous 76, **76**, 77, 80-82, 85, 91, 123-124, 240
Perineal body 223-224
Perineal lacerations **229**
Perineal region
- female **223**, **227**, **229**, 239
- male **227-228**, 237
Perinephric fat 180, 209, 243-246
Perineum 238
- female **223**, **227**, 229
- male **227-228**
Peri-orchium 191
Peristalsis **135**
Peritoneal cavity, development **154-155**
Peritoneum 143
- parietal 59, 68, 75, 124, 156, 165, 177, 193, 209, 218, 240, 246-250, 253, 258
- urogenital 196, 205, 260-261
- visceral 59, 73, 124, 137, 240, 244, 246-247, 249
PEYER's patches 138
Phalanx
- distal (foot) 264, 297-298, 386
- middle (foot) 264, 297-298, 386
- proximal (foot) 264, 297-298, 301, 306, 386
Pigment, anthracotic **96**
Placenta 200, **202**
Platysma 58
Pleura 129
- parietal 59, 70, 97, 112-115, 122, 124-125, 127-129, 157, 243-248
- pulmonary 126, 128
- visceral 59, 124-125, 127, 129, 244-245
Pleural boundaries, projection **105**
Pleural cupula 105, 126
Plexus
- brachial 28, 59, **60**, 90, 112, 114-115, 120, 124, 126-128
- cardiac 115, 119, 122
- celiac 212, 226
- cervical **42**, **43**, 46, **70**
- coccygeal 217, **388**
- common carotid 113
- deferential 214, 235
- esophageal 114, 119, 121, 212
- hypogastric 226
- - inferior 214, **214**, 215, **215**
- - superior 214, **214**, 215, **215**, 226, 250
- inferior mesenteric 212, **214**
- inferior rectal 226
- lumbar 30, **42**, 66, 71, 213, 255, **314-315**, 387
- lumbosacral **71**, 212, 387
- middle rectal 226
- ovarian 215
- pampiniform 73, 190-191, 231,

Plexus
231, 232, 235, 241
- prostatic 214
- pulmonary 114-115, 120-121
- renal **215**
- sacral 71, 212, 215, 217, **217**, **222**, 226, **315**, 321, **321**, 322, **322**, 387
- superior mesenteric **214-215**
- superior rectal 226
- testicular 214, **214**, 235
- thoracic aortic 91, 115, 119, 121
- uterovaginal 215, **215**
- venous
- - anterior external vertebral 252
- - anterior internal vertebral 47, 240
- - areolar 56
- - internal vertebral 127
- - posterior external vertebral 123, 252
- - posterior internal vertebral 47
- - prostatic 236, **260**
- - rectal 179, 207
- - suboccipital 45
- - vaginal 220
- - vesical 219, 236, 256
Pole
- inferior (kidney) 162, 165, 185-186, 208
- superior (kidney) 158, 164, 185, 208
- lower (testis) 190
- upper (testis) 190
Popliteal perforating vein 365
Porta hepatis **142**
Portal hypertension **108**
Portocaval anastomoses **108**, 179, **207**
Position
- of abdominal viscera **156-157**, **160**, **164**, **169**, **171**, **173**
- of heart **90**
- of retroperitoneal viscera **177**, **209-210**
Position (uterus) **196**
Posterior attachment of linea alba 69
Posterior rootlets 46
Pouch
- recto-uterine 155, 165, 195-196, 198, 200, 221, 253, 257
- recto-vesical 164, 193, 205, 209, 218, 236, 241, 252
- vesico-uterine 155, 165, 196, 200, **204**, 253
Prepuce of clitoris 229, 238
- (penis) 233-234, **234**, 240-241, 252
Process(es)
- accessory 4, **4**, 5, 8-9
- caudate 142
- coracoid 53, 126
- costal **4**, 5, 9, 16, 23, 26, 30, 36-37, 41, 47, 53, 69-70, 208, 271, 274-275
- falciform 272
- inferior articular 4, **4**, 6, 8-9, 12, 15-16, 22-23, 25, 30, 41, 255

Process(es)
- lateral (talus) 297, 299-300, 384
- - (calcaneal tuberosity) 297, 299-300
- mammillary **4**, 8-9, 41
- mastoid 12, 38, 46
- medial (calcaneal tuberosity) 297-300, 304
- papillary 142, 164, 246
- posterior (talus) 298-300, 307
- spinous 1, **4**, 5-9, 12-16, 19-20, 22-25, 27, 30-31, 38-39, 41, 123, 128, 246, 249, 275
- styloid (temporal bone) 38, 40
- superior articular 275
- - (sacrum) 10-11, 47, 223, 255
- - (vertebra) 4, **4**, 5-9, 12, 15-16, 20-21, 23, 25, 30, 41, 47, 247
- transverse 4, **4**, 6-8, 13-14, 18, 20, 22, 34, 36, 40-41, 129
- uncinate (pancreas) 150-151, 171, **171**, 177, 241
- - (vertebra) *see* uncus of body
- xiphoid 51, 61, 69, 73, 90, 123, 131, 136, 201, 240
Promontory (sacrum) 2-3, 10-11, 15, 68, 175, 183, 209, 219, 240, 263, 268, **268**, 273, **273**, 311
Pronation (talocalcaneonavicular joint) 327
Prostate 67, **187**, 188, **188**, 192, **192**, 193, **193**, 214, **214**, 218-219, **233**, 236, **236**, 240-241, 251-252, 259-260
Prostatic utricle 188-189, 233, 252
Pubic hair 227, 235
Pubic symphysis 75, 200, 217, 223, 230, 238, 242, 251-252, 256-257, 263, **263**, 268, 270, 273, **274**, 275, 279, 309, 318
Pudendal cleft 227, 238
Pulmonary angiogram **102**
Pulmonary boundaries, projection **105**
Pyelography, intravenous **208**
Pyloric antrum 132, 134-136, 139, 245
Pylorus 132, **132**, 133-134, 139, 158-159

Q

Quadrangular space **43**

R

Ramus(-i)
- anterior (spinal nerve) **33**, 46
- inferior pubic 193, 225, 230, 260, 266-268, 274-275, 317-318
- of mandible 12
- superior pubic 69, 193, 230, 263, 266-267, 274-275, 318
Raphe
- perineal 228-229, 238

Raphe
- of scrotum 191, 227, 232
Recess(es)
- axillary 126
- costodiaphragmatic 59, 103, 105, 113, 122, 124-125, 158, 244-245, 247-248
- costomediastinal 113, 115, 128, 131
- inferior duodenal 162, 164-165
- inferior ileocecal 161-165
- inferior (omental bursa) 159
- intersigmoid 162, 165
- phrenicomediastinal 125, 241
- piriform 110
- retrocecal 164
- splenic 159, 165, 246
- subpopliteal **290**, 292, 333
- superior (bursa omentalis) 159, 165, 246
- superior duodenal 162, 164-165
- superior ileocecal 161, 163-165
- suprapatellar **294**
- vertebromediastinal 128, 130
Rectal glomerulus **205**
Rectoscopy **205**
Rectum 68, 141, 163-165, 175, 178, 183, 204, **205**, 206-207, 212-213, 218, 220-221, 224, 226, 241, 251, 256-257, 353
- arteries **206**
- innervation **226**
- radiograph (ap) **141**
- - (lateral) **225**
- veins **207**
Rectus sheath **63-65**, **74-75**
Rectus sheath 58, 62-65, 69, 72-74, 246, 309
Red bone marrow 381
Region(s)
- anal 227
- anterior (of knee) 262, **352**
- anterior (of leg) 262, **366-367**
- anterior (of thigh) 262, **352**, **354-356**
- deltoid 1
- female perineal 227, **239**
- foot 364
- gluteal 1, 227, 262, **358-362**
- - female 227
- - male 227
- infrascapular 1
- inguinal 262, **352-353**
- leg 364
- lumbar 1, **47**
- - radiograph (ap) 211
- male perineal 227, **237**
- occipital **44-45**
- posterior cervical 1, **44-46**
- posterior (of knee) 262
- posterior (of leg) 262, **371-372**
- posterior (of thigh) 262, **358-361**
- sacral 1, 227
- urogenital 227
- vertebral 1
Renal pyramids 181-182, 185, 243
Retinaculum
- flexor (foot) 306, 331-333, 337, 344, 370-371, 376-378

Retinaculum
- inferior extensor 325-326, 336-339, **339**, 366-367, 373
- inferior fibular 306, 326, 336-338
- lateral patellar 286-287, 324-325, 382
- medial patellar 286-287, 328, 382
- superior extensor 325
- superior fibular 306, 326, 331-333, 337, 370-371
- superior/inferior peroneal *see* superior/inferior fibular retinaculum
Retromalleolar region
- lateral 370
- medial 370
Retroperitoneal organs **151**
Retroperitoneal space **177**
Retroperitoneal viscera **209-210**
RETZIUS, cave of 198, **200**, 252
Rib(s) 3-5, 14, **14**, 15-16, 20-22, 26, 29-30, 34, 37, 39, 49, **49**, 50, **50**, 53, 59, 65, 69-70, 72, 75, 113, 115, 117-118, 122-124, 126, 128-130, 136, 208-209, 212, 243-248
- false [VIII-XII] 53
- floating [XI, XII] 53
- true [I-VIII] 53
Rim of vertebral body **4-5**, **25**
Rima glottidis 116
Ring
- deep inguinal 67, 69, 217, 250
- femoral 221, **309**
- superficial inguinal 63-65, 67, 67, 73, 231-232
- umbilical 48, 56, 58, 62-63, 69, 73-75, 157, 167, 179, 235, 240
Roof of acetabulum 279, 282
Root
- anterior (spinal nerve) 47, 226
- of mesentery 161, 164-166, 175
- parasympathetic 214, **214**, 215, **215**, 226
- posterior (spinal nerve) 47
ROSENMUELLER's node **309**
Rotation
- lateral (hip joint) 314
- - (knee joint) 322
- medial (hip joint) 314
- - (knee joint) 322

S

Sacral width **269**
SANTORINI's duct **150**
Saphenous opening 308, **309**, 353
Scapula 1, 3, 26-27, 29, 53, 103, 110, 126-129
Scrotum **191**, 235, 252
Segment(s)
- anterior [S III] (lung) 98
- anterior basal [S VIII] (lung) 98
- anterior inferior (kidney) 184
- anterior lateral [III] (liver) 144, **144**
- anterior medial [V] (liver) 144, **144**

Index

Segment(s)
- apical [S I] 98
- apicoposterior [S I-II] (lung) 98
- bronchopulmonary **98-99**
- inferior 184
- inferior lingular [S V] (lung)98
- lateral [S IV] (lung) 98
- lateral basal [S IX] (lung) 98
- left medial [IV] (liver) 144, **144**
- left posterior lateral [II] (liver) 144, **144**
- [I] (liver) 144
- medial [S V] (lung) 98
- medial basal [S VII] (lung) 98
- posterior (kidney) 184
- posterior [S II] (lung) 98
- posterior basal [S X] (lung) 98
- posterior lateral [VII] (liver) 144, **144**
- posterior medial [VIII] (liver) 144, **144**
- renal **184**
- right lateral [VI] (liver) 144, **144**
- superior (kidney) 184
- superior (kidney) 184
- superior [S VI] (lung) 98
- superior lingular [S IV] (lung) 98

Segmental bronchi **92-94**
Seminal colliculus 188, 233
Septa testis 190-191, 252
Septum(-a)
- anterior intermuscular (of leg) 326, 329, **329**, 383
- anteromedial intermuscular 311, 355, **356**
- atrioventricular 84
- femoral (CLOQUET) 309, **309**, 328
- of glans 234
- interatrial 80-81, 123
- interventricular 80-82, 130
- longitudinal 379
- penis 234, **234**, 241
- posterior intermuscular (of leg) **328**, 329, **329**, 331, 383
- rectovaginal 200, 253
- of scrotum 191, 232, 240

Serosa 132, 137-138, 143, 146, 153, 195-196, 218

Shaft
- of clavicle 48
- of femur 276, 278, 293
- of fibula 285, 293
- of metatarsals 297, 300, 336
- of phalanx (foot) 297
- of tibia 284-285, 293

SHERMAN's vein 365
Shoulder girdle **3**, **26**, **53**
Silhouette of heart **103**
Sinu-atrial node **84**
Sinus(es)
- anal 205, 252
- aortic 81-82, 84
- coronary 77-78, 85, 88, **88**, 89, 101
- of epididymis 190-191
- lactiferous 54
- maxillary 12
- oblique pericardial 77, 91
- pericardial 77, 85, 91, 123, 130

Sinus(es)
- prostatic 188
- of pulmonary trunk 78, 84, 100
- renal 181, **181**, 182, 248
- superior sagittal 46
- tarsal 298, 307
- transverse pericardial 46
- of venae cavae 77, 88

Skin 73
Sole 262, **346-347**, **375-377**, 378
- arteries 375
- intermediate muscles 346
- lateral muscles 347
- medial muscles 346
- variations 375

Space(s)
- epidural 24, 47, 247, 252
- intercostal 50
- muscular 71, 271, **309**
- pararectal 198
- paravesical 198
- prevesical 198
- retropubic 73, 198, 200, 252, 257
- retrorectal **198**
- subarachnoid 47, 123, 127, 252
- subdural 47
- vascular 68, 71, 271, **309**

Spermatic cord 58, 63-65, 67, **67**, 71, 190, **190**, 210, 218-219, 231, **235**, 256, 308-309, 353
Spinal cord 46, 123, 127, 214-215, 246-247
Spinal pia mater 47
Spine
- anterior inferior iliac 223, 263, 267-269, 273, 275
- - superior iliac 3, 48, 58, 62-64, 67, 136, 167, 201, 223, 235, 262-263, 267-271, 273, 275, 308-309, 312, 316, 318, 358, 362-363
- ischial 3, 206-207, 223, 263, 267-268, 275, 282, 317
- posterior inferior iliac 267-268, 275, 358, 362
- - superior iliac 34, 62, 186, 223, 255, 263, 267-268, 271-272, 275, 358
- of scapula 1, 26-27, 62, 105, 127

Spinocostal muscles 28
Splayfoot 305
Spleen **153**, 157-159, **159**, 164-166, 168-169, 178, 243, 245-247
- hilum 153
- radiograph (ap) **170**
Splenic pulp 153
Spondylolisthesis 9
Spondylolysis 9
Spongy bone 278, 283
Spongy urethra 233-234, 252
Squamous part of occipital bone 19
Sternum 5, 51, **51**, 52, **52**, 53, 112, 123, 129, 131, 136, 201, 240
Stomach 57, 70, 106, 108, 110, 119, **119**, 125, **132-134**, 136, 139, 154-155, **158-159**, 164, 166, 168-169, 177, 209, 240-242, 244-248

Stomach
- arteries, variations **170**
- layers **132**
- projection **136**
- radiograph (ap) **135**, **170**
- shape 136

Subcutaneous tissue 58, 74, 205, 381
Submucosa 108, 132, 137-138, 140
Subserosa 132, 137, 140
SUDECK's point **174**, **206**
Sulcus
- anterior interventricular 78-79, 82
- calcaneal 300
- coronary 77-78, 88
- posterior interventricular 78-79, 82-83, 88
- tali 299
- terminalis cordis 77, 88

Superficial pes anserinus **310**, **328**
Supination (talocalcaneonavicular joint) 327
Supravaginal part 195-196
Surface
- anterior (suprarenal gland) 187
- - (kidney) 185
- - (patella) 286-287, 292-293
- anteroinferior 162
- anterosuperior 159
- articular
- - anterior talar 299-300, 305
- - for cuboid 299-300
- - fibular 284
- - inferior (atlas) 6
- - middle talar 299-300, 305
- - navicular 299-300
- - (patella) 286-287, 292, 294
- - posterior talar 299-300, 305
- - superior (atlas) 6, 19
- - (tibia) 284, 295, 296, 303
- - auricular 10-11, 267
- - contact (of liver) 209
- - costal (lung) 96-97
- - diaphragmatic (liver) 142-143, 158-159
- - (lung) 97
- - (spleen) 153
- dorsal (sacrum) 27
- gluteal 268
- intervertebral 4, 7-9, 12, 14-16, 25
- intestinal 195-196, 203-204, 221, 253
- lateral (fibula) 285
- - (testis) 190
- - (tibia) 284-285
- lunate 223, 267-268, 280
- medial (fibula) 285
- - (ovary) 195, 204
- - (tibia) 284-285, 325-326, 366
- patellar 276, 283, 286-288, 292, 294
- pelvic 11
- popliteal 276, 278, 293, 328, 330, 332, 369
- posterior (fibula) 285
- - (kidney) 185
- - (prostate) 187

Surface posterior
- - (tibia) 284-285
- renal (spleen) 152-153
- sacropelvic 267
- superior (talus) 299
- symphysial 3, 267, 273, 280
- vesical 196, 203-204, 253
- visceral (liver) 143, 158
- - (spleen) 153
Sustentaculum tali 297-300, 302, 304, 307, 384
Sympathetic division 214-215, **226**
Synchondrosis of rib 52

T

Tail
- of epididymis 189-191, 252
- of pancreas 149-152, 159, 164-165, 177, 242, 246
Talus 297-298, **299**, 300-301, 303, 386
Tarsal tunnel **370**, **377**
Tarsus 264
Tendinous intersection 48, 63-65, 69
Tendinous sheath(s)
- common (of fibulares) 306, 336-337
- of extensor digitorum longus 336-337
- of extensor hallucis longus 336-337
- of flexor digitorum longus 306, 337
- of flexor hallucis longus 337, 342
- (of foot) **336-337**
- plantar (of fibularis longus) 343
- of tibialis anterior 336-337
- of tibialis posterior 306, 337
- of toes 337, **337**, 342-343
Tenia
- free 140, 156, 159-163
- mesocolic 140, 159
- omental 140, 156, 158-159, 161, 164
Terminal ileum 138, 161
Testis 57, 183, 189, **190-191**, 214, **214**, 227, 240-241
Thigh bone *see* femur
Thoracic aorta 70, 106, **106**, 107, **107**, 108, 115, 117, **117**, 119, 121, 125, 128-129, 151, 176
Thoracic cage **26**, **53**, **61**
- radiograph (ap) **103**
Thoracic vertebral column
- radiograph (ap) **14**
- - lateral **14**
Thoracic wall **56**, **58**, **72**
- innervation, segmental **57**
- surface **48**
Thorax
- cross-section **129**
- frontal section **122**, **125**
- median section **123**
Thymus 111, 112, **112**, 113, **113**, 114-115, 123, 157

Tibia 264, **284-285**, 287-289, 292-295, **296**, 302-303, 306-307, 325-326, 329, 331-333, 366, 374, 383-384, 386
Tibiofibular syndesmosis 264, **265**, 296, 306, 384
Toe(s) 264
- fifth *see* little toe
- fourth 262, **297**
- great 262, **297**, 301
- little262, **297**
- second 262, **297**
- third 262, **297**
Tongue 12
Trabecula(-ae)
- carneae 81-82
- of corpora cavernosa 233
- septomarginal 80, 82-83
- splenic 153
Trachea 91, **92-93**, 100-101, 103-104, **104**, 106, **106**, 108-109, 112, 116-119, 122-125, 127-128
- bifurcation **104**
- projection **104**
Transverse ridges 10
TREITZ, muscle of **139**, **150**
Triangle
- clavipectoral 58
- lumbar 27, 29, 43, 62, 362
- lumbocostal 70
Triangular space **43**
Trigone
- of bladder 188, 192, 233
- left fibrous 79, 85
- right fibrous 79, 85
Trochanter
- greater 256, 262, 270-272, 275-282, 317, 319-320, 358, 362-363
- lesser 275-282, 313, 320, 362
- third 276
Trochlea
- fibular 298-299
- of talus 297, 299-300, 307
Trunk
- anterior vagal 119
- brachiocephalic 76-77, 91, 100-101, 106-107, 109, 112, 116-117, 120, 122-125, 128
- celiac 68, 106, 108, 117, 151, 168-171, 176, **176**, 177, 184, 209-210, 212-213, 226
- costocervical 117
- gastrosplenic **176**
- hepatomesenteric **176**
- hepatosplenic **176**
- intestinal 210
- lumbar 210-211
- lumbosacral 71, 212-213, 217
- posterior vagal 120-121
- pulmonary 76-78, 81, 84-85, 100, 103, 116, 124-125, 129-130
- sympathetic 71, **71**, 114-115, 117, **117**, 118, **118**, 119, **119**, 120-121, 128-129, 131, 203, 212-214, **214-215**, 217, 243, 247-250
- tibiofibular 369, 372

Trunk-arm muscles **28**
- deep layer **29**
- superficial layer **27**
Trunk-pectoral girdle-muscles **26**, **28**
- deep layer **29**
- superficial layer **27**
Tubercle(s)
- adductor 276, 278
- anterior (cervical vertebrae) **4**, 6-7, 41, 61
- anterior obturator 268
- carotid *see* anterior tubercle
- of iliac crest 263, 268, 362
- intervenous 80
- lateral intercondylar 284, 293
- lateral (talus) 298-300
- medial intercondylar 284, 293
- medial (talus) 298-300
- posterior (cervical vertebrae) **4**, 6-7, 12, 17, 34, 38, 41
- posterior obturator 267-268
- pubic 223, 230, 238, 263, 267-268, 271, 275, 309
- quadrate 276-277
- of rib 4, 20, 22, 49
- scalene 49
Tuberosity
- calcaneal 297-300, 302-307, 330-332, 342-343
- of cuboid 297-298, 300, 304
- of distal phalanx (foot) 297
- of fifth metatarsal bone 297-298, 300, 304-305, 336
- of first metatarsal bone 297, 300
- gluteal 276-277, 281, 317
- for gluteus maximus 268
- iliac 263, 267
- ischial 3, 206-207, 223, 225, 228-230, 238, 257-258, 266-269, 271-272, 275, 282, 317-319, 358, 362
- of navicular 300, 304
- sacral 10-11
- for serratus anterior 49
- tibial 262, 284, 287-289, 293, 296, 326, 366
Tunica
- albuginea 190, 242
- of corpora cavernosa 233-235, 240, 252
- of corpus spongiosum 234
- muscularis
- vaginalis 73, 190-191, 232, 240

U

Umbilical cord 73, **202**
Umbilical cord knot, false **73**
Umbilicus 74
Uncovertebral cleft **24**
Uncus of body 4, 7, 13, 24-25, 41
Upper abdomen
- blood vessels **169**, **171**
- viscera **158**
Urachus 73, 157, 183, 189, 194

Ureter 67, 151, 161-162, 164-165, 170, 177, 180-184, 186, **186**, 187, 189, 193-195, 203-204, 208-210, 213-214, 218-221, 224, 236, 243, 249-250, 253, 255, 258
- radiograph (ap) 186
Urethra 188, 193, **193**, 233, **233**, 252
- female 194, 200, 223, 230, 261
- male 188, 192-193, **193**, 214, 230, 232-233, **233**, 234, 242, 259-260
Urethral lacunae233
Urinary bladder 57, 68, 73, 157, 163-166, 177, 183, **187-188**, 189, 193, **193**, 194, 200, 203-204, 209, 214, 218-221, **233**, 236, **236**, 240-241, 250-251, 256-257, 259-261, 353
Urogenital hiatus **223**
Uterine tube 165, 194-195, **195**, 196, **196**, 197, 203, **204**, 215, **215**, 220, 259
Uterus 166, 194, **195-196**, **198**, **200**, 203-204, **215**, 220-221, 253, 353
- during pregnancy **199-201**
- position **196**
- ultrasound image **199**
Uvula of bladder 188, 233

V

Vagina 194-195, **195**, 196, **196**, 197-198, 200, **215**, 220, 223-224, 230, 251, 257
Vaginal orifice 215
Vaginal part 195, 198, **198**, 200, 253
- Nullipara **198**
Vaginal rugae 195, 198, 229
Valve(s)
- anal 205
- aortic 79, 82, 84-85, 90, 116, 123-124, 130-131
- of coronary sinus 80, 84-85, 89
- EUSTACHIAN 80
- of foramen ovale 81
- of heart **79**, **85**
- of inferior vena cava 80, 84
- left atrioventricular 79, 81-84, 90, 130-131
- mitral *see* left atrioventricular valve
- of navicular fossa 233
- pulmonary 79, 84-85, 90
- right atrioventricular 79-80, 82-84, 90, 123-124, 131
- tricuspid *see* right atrioventricular valve
VATER, tubercle of **139**, **146**, **150**
Vein(s)
- anterior interventricular 76, 82, 85, 89
- anterior jugular 123
- anterior (right superior pulmonary vein) 100, 124, 126

Vein(s)
- anterior (of right ventricle) 85, 89
- anterior tibial **329**, 366
- apical 100
- apicoposterior 100
- appendicular 178-179
- axillary 90, 115, 124, 126, 128
- azygos **71**, 77, 101, 107-109, 114, 117-118, **118**, 121, 128-131, 179, 246
- basivertebral 123, 240
- brachiocephalic 100, 113, 115, 122
- - left 77, 91, 107-108, 112, 118, 122-123
- - right 77, 91, 107, 112, 114, 118
- bronchial 114
- of bulb of penis 230
- - of vestibule 239
- central 187
- cephalic 56, 58, 126
- circumflex scapular 43
- common iliac 165, 177, 203, 207, 209, 213, 217, 219-220, 224, 240-241, 255
- cremasteric 231
- cystic 169, 178-179
- deep cervical 45
- deep circumflex iliac 177, 213, 219, 224
- deep dorsal (of clitoris) 224, 230
- - (of penis) 230-232, 234, 252
- dorsal digital 373
- esophageal 108,**108**, 178-179
- external iliac 67, 177, 179, 193, 207, 213, 218-221, 224, 236, 253-254, 318, 353-354, 356
- external jugular 44
- external pudendal 56, 231, 235, 309, 352-353
- femoral 68, 75, 210, 242, 256-257, 309, **309**, 311, 352, 354-356, 380-381
- femoropopliteal 368
- fibular **329**
- gastroduodenal 151
- great cardiac 76-77, 81, 85, 88-89, 131
- great saphenous 56, 71, 210, 257, 286, 308-309, 329, 352-354, 356, 358, 364-365, **365**, 368, 373, 379, 381-384
- of heart 85, **88-89**
- hemi-azygos **71**, 108, 118, 123, 179, 243, 246
- - accessory 108, 115, 118, 179
- hepatic 70, 91, 124-125, 143, **145**, 165, 177-179, 209-210
- - intermediate 145, 148
- - left 145, 148, 241-242
- - projection **148**
- - right 145, 148, 241, 244, 247
- - ultrasound image **145**
- hepatic portal 142, **145**, 148, 151-152, 165, 168-169, 171, 177-178, **178**, 179, **179**, 241-242, 244, 246-248
- - projection **148**
- - ultrasound image **145**
- ileal 178-179, 249

Index

Vein(s)
- ileocolic 178-179
- iliolumbar 209
- inferior basal 11
- inferior epigastric 56, 72, 74, 156-157, 171, 173, 177, 179, 193, 209, 213, 219, 221, 224, 236, 250, 253
- inferior gluteal 207, 256, 362, **362**, 380
- inferior mesenteric 151, 165, 175, **175**, 177-179, 207, 250
- inferior phrenic 108, 179, 209
- inferior rectal 179, 207, 219-220
- inferior thyroid 90-91, 108, 112-113, 118
- inferior vena cava 41, 70, 71, 77-78, 80, 88, 91, 101, 107-109, 116, 118, 121, 125, 142-145, 148, 151-152, 165, 169, 171, 177-179, **179**, 183-184, 207, 209-210, 213, 241-242, 246-250
- intercostal 73, 130-131
- - anterior 245
- - posterior 34, 36, 59, 75, 108, 114-115, 117-118
- internal iliac 179, 207, 209, 218-220, 224, 254, 258, 353
- internal jugular 91, 107-108, 113, 122, 125-126
- internal pudendal 179, 207, 219-220, 224, 230, 236-237, 239, 256-258, 260-261, 361-362, **362**
- internal thoracic 56, 72, 90-91, 100, 112-113, 128
- jejunal 151, 173, 175, 178-179
- lateral accessory saphenous 352
- lateral circumflex femoral 261
- lateral marginal 364, 373
- lateral plantar 306
- lateral sacral 218
- lateral thoracic 56
- left atrial 77, 89
- left colic 165, 173, 175, 178-179
- left gastric 108, 134, 151, 158, 169, 177-179, 242, 246
- left gastro-omental 108, 134, 158, 169, **169**, 171, 178-179
- left marginal 89
- lumbar 177, 209, 241, 243
- - ascending 117-118, 213, 250
- medial accessory saphenous 353
- medial circumflex femoral 256, 260-261
- medial marginal 364, 373

Vein(s)
- medial plantar 306
- median sacral 177, 209, 213, 221
- middle cardiac 76, 85, 88-89, 101, 123
- middle colic 151, 161-162, 173, 175, 178-179
- middle lobe 100
- middle rectal 207, 219-221
- musculophrenic 72
- oblique (of left atrium) 88-89
- obturator 207, 219, 221, 224, 236, 256-257, 261, 309, 318
- occipital 43-45
- ovarian 151, 165, 179-180, 184, 195, 204, 220-221, 253
- pancreaticoduodenal 178-179
- para-mbilical 56, 74, 179
- perforating **308**, 364, **365**, 373
- pericardiacophrenic 90-91, 112, 114-115, 122
- perineal 230
- popliteal 286, 331, 359-361, 368, 370-371, 382
- posterior arcuate (of leg) 364
- posterior auricular 44-45
- posterior circumflex humeral 43
- posterior (of left ventricle) 77, 88-89
- posterior interventricular 77, 82, 85, 88-89, 101
- posterior (right superior pulmonary vein) 100
- posterior spinal 47
- posterior tibial **329**, 370
- prepyloric 169
- profunda brachii 43
- - femoris 261, 356
- pulmonary 114, 120
- - left 77-78, 88, 90-91, 107, 109, 115, 123, 243
- - - inferior 81, 97, 100, 130-131
- - - superior 81, 97, 100-101, 129
- - right 77-78, 80-81, 88, 91, 97, 100, **102**, 107, 109, 114, 121, 243
- - - inferior 130-131
- - - superior 101, 124, 128, 130
- renal 151-152, 179-180, 182-184, **185**, 209, 213, 240-241, 243-244, 248
- right atrial 89
- right colic 151, 173, 178-179
- right gastric 134, 178-179
- right gastro-omental 134, 165, 169, **169**, 171, 178-179

Vein(s)
- short gastric 134, 164, 178-179
- sigmoid 175, 177-179, 207
- small saphenous 286, **308**, 329, 358-359, 361, 364-365, 368, 370, 373, 383
- splenic 151-153, 159, 165, 171, 175, 177-179, 242-243, 246-248
- subclavian 91, 107-108, 112, 114, 118, 122, 125, 127
- subcostal 117-118
- subcutaneous abdominal 56
- superficial cervical 56
- superficial circumflex iliac 56, 309, 352-353
- superficial dorsal (of penis) 219, 231, 234, 252
- superficial epigastric 56, 179, 309, 352-353
- superior epigastric 56, **71**, 72-74
- superior gluteal 207, 255, **362**, 380
- superior mesenteric 151, 165, 171, 173, **173**, 175, 177-179, 240-242, 249
- superior rectal 175, 178-179, 207, 219-221
- superior thyroid 113
- superior vena cava 76-78, 80, 84-85, 88, 90-91, 100-101, 103, 107-109, 112, 114, 116, 118, 120, 122, 124, 128-130
- suprarenal 180, 184, 209
- sural 370
- testicular 67, 151, 177, 179-180, 184, 190, 209, **209**, 213, 231, 249-250
- thoraco-epigastric 56
- thymic 91
- transverse cervical 44
- umbilical 67, 73, 143, 157, 200
- uterine 220-221
- vertebral 45, 77, 108
- vesical 73, 220
- - inferior 219
- - superior 219
Venous cross 91
Ventricles of heart
- left 76-78, 81, **81**, 82, **82-83**, 84, **84**, 88, 100, 103, 107, 116, 124-125, 130-131
- right 76-78, 80, **80**, 82, **82**, 83, **83**, 84, **84**, 88, 100-101, 116, 124-125, 130-131, 242
Versio (uterus) **196**

Vertebra(-ae)
- anular epiphysis **5**, **24-25**
- cervical 2-3, 4, 5, 7, 12, **12**, 13, 17-19, 26, 41, 46, 53, 123
- - radiograph (ap) **13**
- - - (lateral) **12**
- coccygeal 11
- development 5
- features 4, **4**
- lumbar 1-3, **4**, 5, **8-9**, 15-16, 23-24, 26-27, 31, 36-37, 47, 53, 68-70, 74, 152, 176, 203, 208, 246, 248-249, 251, 255, 270-271, 274-275, 318
- - radiograph (ap) **16**
- - - (lateral) **15**
- ossification centers 5
- prominens 1-3, 7, 27, 39, 105, 123
- thoracic 2-3, **4**, 5, **8-9**, 20, 26-27, 36, 53, 125-130, 246-247
- - radiograph (ap) **14**
- - - (lateral) **14**
Vertebral column **3**
- ligaments **20**
Vesicular ovarian follicles 195, 253
Vestibule
- (of omental bursa) 159, 164
- (of vagina) 238
Viscera
- newborn **157**
- upper abdomen **158-159**
Vortex of heart 79

W

Wall
- anterior (stomach) 136, 158-159
- membranous (trachea) 93, 101, 104, 109, 123
- posterior (stomach) 136
WINSLOW, foramen of **158**
WIRSUNG, duct of **150**
WOLFFian duct **189**, **194**

X

Xiphosternal joint 51

Z

Zona orbicularis 256, 273